SOCIETY'S CHOICES

Social and Ethical Decision Making in Biomedicine

Ruth Ellen Bulger, Elizabeth Meyer Bobby,
and Harvey V. Fineberg, *Editors*

Committee on the Social and Ethical Impacts of
Developments in Biomedicine

Division of Health Sciences Policy

INSTITUTE OF MEDICINE

NATIONAL ACADEMY PRESS
Washington, D.C. 1995

31609904   11/20/96

NATIONAL ACADEMY PRESS • 2101 Constitution Avenue, N.W. • Washington, D.C. 20418

NOTICE: The project that is the subject of this report was approved by the Governing Board of the National Research Council, whose members are drawn from the councils of the National Academy of Sciences, the National Academy of Engineering, and the Institute of Medicine. The members of the committee responsible for the report were chosen for their special competencies and with regard for appropriate balance.

This report has been reviewed by a group other than the authors according to procedures approved by a Report Review Committee consisting of members of the National Academy of Sciences, the National Academy of Engineering, and the Institute of Medicine.

The Institute of Medicine was chartered in 1970 by the National Academy of Sciences to enlist distinguished members of the appropriate professions in the examination of policy matters pertaining to the health of the public. In this, the Institute acts under both the Academy's 1863 congressional charter responsibility to be an adviser to the federal government and its own initiative in identifying issues of medical care, research, and education. Dr. Kenneth I. Shine is president of the Institute of Medicine.

Support of this project was provided by the Howard Hughes Medical Institute and National Research Council, National Academy of Sciences/National Academy of Engineering independent funds, and Institute of Medicine independent funds.

Library of Congress Cataloging-in-Publication Data

Society's choices : social and ethical decision making in biomedicine
  / Ruth Ellen Bulger, Elizabeth Meyer Bobby, and Harvey V. Fineberg,
  editors ; Committee on the Social and Ethical Impacts of
  Developments in Biomedicine, Division of Health Sciences Policy,
  Institute of Medicine.
      p.   cm.
    Includes bibliographical references and index.
    ISBN 0-309-05132-0
    1. Medical ethics. 2. Bioethics. I. Bulger, Ruth Ellen.
  II. Bobby, Elizabeth Meyer. III. Fineberg, Harvey V. IV. Institute
  of Medicine (U.S.). Committee on the Social and Ethical Impacts of
  Developments in Biomedicine.
  R724.S598   1995
  174'.2—dc20   94-39354
                                                             CIP

Printed in the United States of America.

The serpent has been a symbol of long life, healing, and knowledge among almost all cultures and religions since the beginning of recorded history. The image adopted as a logotype by the Institute of Medicine is based on a relief carving from ancient Greece, now held by the Staalichemuseen in Berlin.

COMMITTEE ON THE SOCIAL AND ETHICAL IMPACTS OF DEVELOPMENTS IN BIOMEDICINE

HARVEY V. FINEBERG, M.D., Ph.D.,* *Chair,* Dean, Harvard School of Public Health, Boston

W. FRENCH ANDERSON, M.D., Director, USC Gene Therapy Lab, University of Southern California, School of Medicine, Noris Cancer Center, Los Angeles

JOHN ARRAS, Ph.D., Associate Professor of Bioethics, Albert Einstein College of Medicine, Montefiore Medical Center, Bronx, N.Y.

ALEXANDER CAPRON, LL.B.,* University Professor of Law and Medicine, The Law Center, University of Southern California, Los Angeles

TROY DUSTER, Ph.D., Director, Institute for the Study of Social Change, University of California, Berkeley

ALFRED P. FISHMAN, M.D.,* Chairman, Department of Rehabilitation Medicine, Hospital of the University of Pennsylvania, Philadelphia

THEODORE FRIEDMANN, M.D., Professor of Pediatrics and Bioethics, Department of Pediatrics, Center for Molecular Genetics, University of California, San Diego

WILLIAM D. FULLERTON,* Consultant to "Health Policy Alternatives," Crystal River, Fla.

WALTER HARRELSON, Professor Emeritus, The Divinity School, Vanderbilt University

SHEILA JASANOFF, J.D., Ph.D., Professor and Chair, Department of Science and Technology Studies, Cornell University

ALBERT R. JONSEN, M.D.,* Chairman, Department of Medical History/Ethics, School of Medicine, University of Washington

PATRICIA KING, J.D.,* Professor of Law, Georgetown University Law Center

JOANNE LYNN, M.D., Center for the Evaluative Clinical Sciences, Dartmouth Medical School

JAMES A. MORONE, Ph.D., Associate Professor, Department of Political Science, Brown University

STANLEY REISER, M.D., Ph.D., Director, Program on Humanities and Technology in Health Care, University of Texas Health Sciences Center, Houston

DANIEL WIKLER, Ph.D., Professor, Departments of Medical Ethics and Philosophy, University of Wisconsin, Madison

---

*Member, Institute of Medicine

Staff

RUTH ELLEN BULGER, Ph.D., Study Director and Division Director (until August 1993)
VALERIE P. SETLOW, Ph.D., Division Director (from August 1993)
ELIZABETH MEYER BOBBY, Research Associate
PHILOMINA MAMMEN, Study Assistant and Administrative Assistant
NANCY DIENER, Budget Analyst

Preface

So often, new developments in biomedicine are hailed as panaceas, as answers to problems, as hopes of finally having conquered an adversary. Even when a discovery may lead to a valuable treatment or even a cure for disease, it can also bring with it troublesome social and ethical issues. This report illustrates—through examples like genetic technology, with its power to alter human nature, and health care reform, with its emphasis on cost control—how developments in biomedicine can affect the fabric of society in significant and lasting ways. The report explores mechanisms for confronting these challenges and describes the strengths and weaknesses of various approaches to social and ethical deliberation. Appreciating the subjective nature of their own judgments, members of the committee endeavored to synthesize the available literature, the judgments of its consultants, and the relevant experiences of its members into a thoughtful analysis of mechanisms for bioethics deliberation. The result is a report that differs from many Institute of Medicine reports in that it constitutes an interpretive essay rather than a predominantly data-based analysis.

The development of renal dialysis and transplantation technologies is a salient example. Dialysis and transplantation were (and are today) tremendous advantages for patients with permanent kidney failure, because the procedures gave them many more years of life than they would have had prior to the advent of these technologies, when a diagnosis of end-stage renal disease meant certain death. When more patients needed the technology than could be treated, however, society was faced with a troublesome question: How do we decide who should benefit from these lifesaving technologies, and who should die? This question stimulated philosophers and theologians to study the criteria for fair allocation of a life-saving resource. Is it ethical, they asked, to choose persons on the basis of their social worth or by a lottery? At the same time, a political response to the problem began to build momentum to cover affected patients under Medicare. Congress passed such legislation in 1972 In so doing, it removed the financial barrier to access yet left untouched the remaining social and ethical quandaries. The arguments of the philosophers and theologians were set aside as no longer relevant. Society continues today to struggle with many of the questions related to allocation of scarce life-saving technologies.

Often individuals making biomedical decisions must contend with personal moral dilemmas: a woman who is pregnant with a desired child learns that the fetus she carries is afflicted with a serious genetic or congenital disorder and agonizes over whether she should have an abortion; parents agonize about discontinuing life support for a child who the doctors say has permanently lost all brain function. These are deeply personal dilemmas, and, as a rule, American society has given latitude to such private choices. We have made our own the dictum of the British philosopher, John Stuart Mill, who wrote a century ago,

> The individual is not accountable to society for his actions, insofar as these concern the interests of no person but himself.

> (Mill, *On Liberty*, 1859)

However, the qualifying clause, "insofar as these concern the interests of no person but himself" may loom large. Indeed, even when individual choices may benefit another, we may hesitate to endorse them. Thus, the prospect that some person ill with a neurological or metabolic disorder might be cured by transplantation of tissue from an aborted fetus, or that the organs of a brain-dead child might save the life of another, immediately raises ethical questions that go beyond the personal and private. They become matters of public policy because other parties now enter into the range of those who can be harmed or can benefit. Examples such as these suggest that ethical decisions that are exclusively matters for personal deliberation may be exceptional in modern biomedicine

Despite the difficulty of resolving ethical dilemmas in the public sphere, society has made notable progress in the past two decades in confronting the social and ethical impacts of developments in biomedicine, partly to the credit of a number of "ethics" bodies. The work of many of these bodies, including the National Commission for the Protection of Human Subjects of Biomedical and Behavioral Research (National Commission), the President's Commission for the Study of Ethical Problems in Medicine and Biomedical and Behavioral Research (President's Commission), and the Human Genome Project's Ethical, Legal, and Social Implications (ELSI) Working Group, among others, is described in this report. While the contributions of these groups have been significant, their work is not complete. Technologies and practices in biomedicine continue to evolve, and as they do, novel social and ethical quandaries will undoubtedly take shape. Moreover, many of the social and ethical dilemmas that arose in the past are still in need of resolution. In fact, a principal motivating factor behind this report was indeed the fact that little public bioethics activity took place in the 1980s when the country was sharply divided on several ethical issues. After the closing of the President's Commission, no mechanisms for public discussion and consensus building were being employed effectively.

The charge to this committee had two parts, the first of which was to assess the mechanisms employed by our society to deliberate social and ethical issues stemming from developments in biomedicine. The committee's first step in addressing this charge was to come to an understanding of the circumstances defining such issues. The committee recognized early in its deliberations that not all ethical dilemmas related to biomedical developments have resulted from a new discovery or novel technology. Some scientific developments diffuse into medical practice quickly, and ethical issues related to these developments get overlooked. The development becomes part of accepted practice and, while not novel, ethical quandaries about the application of the development remain and may eventually assert themselves. Techniques of assisted reproduction, such as in vitro fertilization, provide an example.

Social and ethical quandaries can also be raised when numerous small developments accumulate to present a novel situation. An example lies in this country's growing population of elderly persons. Immunization and antibiotics have reduced the risk of death due to infectious disease; surgical advances save more and more people from early death due to cardiovascular disease and cancer. The aggregate effect of these and other medical advances has been the prolongation of life, which in turn raises social and ethical concerns about quality of life and end-of-life care.

Lastly, social and ethical dilemmas can arise from organizational innovation and change. As our society restructures its health care system, for example, ethical issues related to allocation and rationing of health resources will undoubtedly surface.

The second part of the committee's charge was to provide guidance to professionals, institutions, and the general public about utilizing and improving existing mechanisms for deliberation and, where applicable, creating new mechanisms. The value of such mechanisms was clear to this committee from the outset, as was the idea that the more our society can recognize and effectively deal with the social and ethical impacts of developments—through whatever mechanism—the greater the likelihood that these developments will affect society positively.

One of the key steps in the committee's work was to identify and review the groups that have functioned in this capacity in the past. Several groups convened during the past two decades to deliberate ethical issues in biomedicine have been widely recognized as having made important contributions. The impact of these groups is evident in, for example, the enduring nature of their guidance on the protection of human research subjects (National Commission) and the continued citation of their arguments in legal cases pertaining to termination of life-sustaining treatment (President's Commission). In addition to reviewing the work of these well-known groups, the committee explored the efforts of a number of other bioethics institutions whose impact has been less conspicuous. It did so with the recognition that bioethics deliberation takes place at many levels: national, state, community, institutional, and individual. The committee found that there were lessons to be learned at each level about the integration of moral reasoning into decisions in medicine and health.

The committee apprehended that just as there are various forms and styles of bioethics deliberation, so are there various definitions of success. Success may be the fulfillment of a group's intended function, which may take numerous different forms; it may be the citation of a group's work in courts and classrooms; it may be the translation of a group's recommendations into legislation; it may be the mere stimulation of thought among others. Success may also be in the eye of the observer; a group may be perceived as successful by one person or faction and not by another, depending upon what each expected the group to achieve.

The members of the committee brought to their task a wide range of expertise. Several had served as members or staff of ethics bodies of the past, such as the National Commission and the President's Commission. Several were active members of ethics bodies such as the ELSI Working Group and the New York State Task Force on Life and Law. Their fields of expertise covered public health, basic science research, bioethics, law, social science, medicine, theology, medical history, clinical sciences research, political science, and science and technology studies.

The committee also benefitted from the expertise of other professionals not on the committee. Papers were commissioned on a variety of topics, including the implications of labeling an issue an ethical issue, the value of consensus, and the dynamics of moral reasoning in public. The committee discussions stimulated by these papers were unfailingly enlightening and helped shape the orientation of the report. The 12 papers commissioned by the committee are compiled in Part II of this report. In an attempt to understand the current environment in which policy-making in science and health takes place, the committee also invited the contributions of several people from federal health and science agencies who balance scientific and ethical concerns on a daily basis. Their insights into the kinds of guidance needed by the scientific community were especially valuable.

In sum, what is presented in this volume is a historical and social analysis of public moral reasoning in medicine and health, from which this committee has drawn conclusions, principles, and recommendations based on its shared judgments. The report is intended to serve as a source of ideas for those wishing to utilize or redefine mechanisms for considering the social and ethical impacts of developments in biomedicine. It sheds new light on criteria that contribute to the success of such mechanisms at a variety of levels and with a variety of intended functions. It speaks to the critical importance of forethought and communication in turning developments into "advances." It is the committee's sincere hope that policymakers, scientists, health care providers, patients and their families, students, and others concerned with the social and ethical impacts of biomedical developments will find the report valuable.

Harvey V. Fineberg, M.D., Ph.D., *Chair*

Acknowledgments

The committee wishes to express its gratitude to many individuals who helped during the course of this study. They included the authors of the background papers published with this volume, those who wrote drafts of materials used in the text, including Beth Kosiak, Katherine Taylor, and Roger Bulger, and the many individuals who shared their insights with the committee, particularly Michael Yesley, Eric Juengst, Jay Moskowitz, and Sandy Chamblee.

The committee would like to thank Philomina Mammen, study assistant, for her unfailing help in planning and logistics, materials distribution, manuscript and report preparation, and general support to the committee.

The committee members also appreciated the many letters we received from scientists concerning the issue and the processes that are currently being followed in their areas of science. These individuals included Alan R. Fleischman, M.D.; Fred Rosner, M.D., F.A.C.P.; Neil A. Hotzman, M.D., M.P.H.; Beverly Torok-Storb, Ph.D.; David W. Martin, Jr., M.D.; Alvin H. Moss, M.D.; Norman G. Levinsky, M.D.; Arnold S. Relman, M.D.; Nancy Boucot Cummings, M.D.; Robert S. Balaban, Ph.D.; Robert G. Shulman, Ph.D.; Gary Nabel, M.D.; and Ralph Crawshaw, M.D. Thanks also to Enriqueta Bond for her support and advice during the study process, Paul Phelps for his improvements and editing of the report, Mike Edington for his help with the publication of the manuscript, Claudia Carl for coordination of the review process, and Nancy Diener for budget oversight.

The committee expresses its special appreciation to Elizabeth Meyer

Bobby and Ruth Bulger for their excellent and constant support. Their contributions permeate this report, which would have been a different and much diminished product without their participation

Finally I would like to thank the members of the committee for their generous sharing of time and knowledge and their stimulating insights expressed during what were very productive meetings of the group.

Harvey V. Fineberg, M.D., Ph.D., *Chair*

Contents

xiii

SOCIETY'S CHOICES

Social and Ethical Decision Making in Biomedicine

Executive Summary

During the past 30 years, social and ethical issues in biomedicine have vaulted to prominence, prompting public debate and deep reflection by governmental commissions, professional societies, and community organizations. The issues have at times demanded immediate public attention, as in the case of abuse of human research subjects, and, at other times, more gradually raised public concern, as have the possibilities provided by advances in genetic technology. More and more, the ethical implications of such issues as health care delivery and commercialization of biotechnology are being examined in a public fashion. Despite the increasing activity in this area, however, there has been little systematic study of the various social processes through which we subject the ethical and social issues in medicine and biotechnology to debate and analysis.

In an attempt to delineate these processes as they are manifested in this country, the committee considered those characteristics that make an issue an *ethical* issue and the circumstances under which it is determined that an ethical issue should be publicly deliberated. The word "ethical" typically connotes human values and ethical judgments—that is, judgments grounded in values. These issues arise during the deliberation and resolution of nearly every public issue. Some public issues especially prompt reference to the kinds of ethical ideas—dignity, freedom, rights, fairness, respect, equality, solidarity, and integrity—that are evoked in efforts to distinguish right from wrong. These are the sorts of issues that come within the purview of public ethics bodies, including congressionally or presidentially appointed bodies, community-centered bodies, institutional

1

bodies, and the like. This report explores how these bodies approach the task of deliberating ethical issues, and how their approaches reflect the character of our society.

SOURCES OF ETHICAL ISSUES IN BIOMEDICINE

The tasks of ethics bodies convened to address issues in biomedicine have originated from clashes of values, norms, principles, and practices that have occurred in a number of arenas, especially: biomedical research involving human subjects; health care decision making, delivery, and financing; advances in medical diagnostics and therapeutics; and academic-industry relationships in biotechnology. From these arenas have come new technologies, the proper use of which is controversial; crises in resource allocation and perplexing questions of distributive justice; changes in the organization and delivery of health care and related concerns about the appropriate role of physicians; and financing challenges that have spawned new relationships of questionable appropriateness between researchers and their sponsors. It was in the arena of human studies research that the ethical dimensions of biomedicine and the need for public involvement in such ethical matters were first recognized.

Abuses of human research subjects by the Nazis during World War II outraged the public and stimulated formal inquiry into the inherent conflict in biomedical investigation between benefit to the subject and benefit to science and society. The Nuremberg Code of 1948, designed to be used as a standard by which to judge the actions of Nazi scientists, was the first formal enunciation of ethical standards that proscribed scientific zealotry and disregard for human consent and dignity. In the 1960s and 1970s, following revelations in the United States of such incidents as the Tuskegee syphilis study, federal regulations were issued to protect human research subjects. The National Commission for the Protection of Human Subjects of Biomedical and Behavioral Research (National Commission), which operated between 1974 and 1978 and became one of the most well-known public ethics bodies, was influential in developing these regulations and in stimulating the design of localized bodies, known as institutional review boards (IRBs), for the protection of human research subjects.

Changes in health care delivery and financing have also raised ethical concerns that have been subject to public deliberation. Informed consent, the linchpin of regulations for research on human subjects, was at the heart of a movement during the 1960s and 1970s toward greater patient autonomy. At issue were questions of information disclosure, decisional authority, and patient self-determination. At the same time, specialized medical technology began to flourish, health insurance companies grew and began to exert influence on health care decisions, and health care began its transformation into the business-like enterprise it is today. Ethical aspects of the resulting specialization, fragmentation, depersonalization, and variable accessibility of health care became the topics put before such public ethics bodies as the President's Commission for the Study of Ethical Issues in Medicine and Biomedical and Behavioral Research (President's Commission), which operated between 1980 and 1983; institutional ethics bodies known as hospital ethics committees; and community-based groups of health care consumers.

Developments in the area of biotechnology have also raised publicly debated ethical quandaries. Some of these quandaries have reflected genuine societal uncertainty about the use of novel technologies; others have related to the propriety of financial relationships between scientists and biotechnology companies. Developments in genetic research illustrate the promise and hazard of scientific discoveries—at the same time that they offer the potential of an end to suffering from gene-linked disease, they also threaten our identity as humans. One product of this apprehension has been the creation of the Ethical, Legal, and Social Implications (ELSI) Program at the National Center for Human Genome Research. Illustrative of the ethical issues raised by the commercialization of scientific discoveries are the pricing and distribution of products developed with public funds and the degree to which they serve the public interest. Also of concern are the ethical issues raised by the increasing tendency of universities and government laboratories to establish closer ties with industry.

Our society's capacity for dealing humanely and wisely with the impact of technological and scientific innovation, in each of the above areas and in others, is enhanced by the creation of forums in which ethical deliberation can be carried out. The deliberation may draw on many resources: experience in the use of these technologies and in the practice of medicine; the personal values and life experiences of participants; bodies of thought, such as economics and the law, which reflect and systematize value-laden judgments; and the intellectual and scholarly resources of the field of ethics. Its character and form are inevitably influenced by the distinctive history and culture of our society.

THE SOCIETAL CONTEXT OF BIOETHICAL PROBLEM SOLVING

American history is replete with examples of stirring ethical debates that have mobilized huge numbers of citizens. Debates about child labor laws, women's suffrage, prohibition, and the abolition of slavery are illustrative. What stimulated these public deliberations in large part was what characterized this country at its founding: a strong will to reject tyranny, to self-govern, and to preserve individual liberty. The American penchant for celebrating the individual and the private fostered the growth and diversity that has characterized this country. At the same time, these values exist in tension with concerns about responsibility for the community and public well-being. Such tension becomes particularly visible when an ethical issue is at stake.

Our society's capacity for deliberation about social and ethical issues in biomedicine has expanded and matured significantly within the past few decades. In the mid-1960s, ambivalence about authority and tension between public and private life combined to produce a wave of social movements in civil rights, feminism, and consumer activism. In biomedicine as in the whole of society, new voices began to gather volume, particularly those of patients and their families demanding to have a say in medical decision making. As medical technology flourished and new treatment options (e.g., life support) challenged long-held ideas about life and death, religious representatives began to voice their opinions. And as health care costs skyrocketed, additional factions—insurers, employers, and hospitals—organized to represent their interests.

SYSTEMATIC APPROACHES TO BIOETHICS

The events of the 1960s lent impetus to a growing interest in systematic thinking about social and ethical issues in biomedicine. In the 1970s, scholars from several disciplines, principally moral philosophy, theological ethics, medicine, and law, began to study and write about the social and ethical issues of modern medical science and health care. A discipline called bioethics began to emerge, with specialized faculty (usually located in schools of medicine), courses, conferences, and journals. Today, academic bioethics has moved far beyond its beginnings. A number of academic programs prepare students for the field, teaching the foundation of ethical reasoning and a variety of analytic methods. In addition, ethics programs in health professional schools prepare care providers to apply these methods in the practice setting.

Systematic thinking about social and ethical issues in biomedicine also takes place in numerous religious communities. Clergy come into frequent contact with the wrenching moral dilemmas of life and death, and many clergy today have spent time in formal training programs in hospital pastoral counseling. Theological seminaries offer courses on bioethics and their faculty often contribute to the denominational literature on its topics. In addition, several centers of theological and religious reflection on bioethics exist with sponsorship from religious communities. Areas of tension remain with respect to religious participation in bioethical decision making for the entire community. Religious views, precisely because they are religious, are likely to be held with great confidence and tenacity, and inconsistent views may be espoused by leaders of different religious communities. Many thoughtful religious specialists and leaders are willing to participate in public ethics deliberation, and many of them are qualified by temperament, knowledge, and experience to be valuable contributors.

Scientists and other technical experts also make unique contributions to deliberation about the social and ethical impacts of developments in biomedicine. Three arguments have been advanced to justify the importance of their participation in this deliberation. First, science, because of its openness and critical tradition, can be thought to provide a useful way of approaching ethical deliberation in a pluralist society. Second, scientists and physicians, because of their closeness to the practice of medicine and the use of technology, may have special insights into ethical issues arising from their practice that would not as easily be apparent to other users or consumers of technology. Third, science can be counted on to remove certain issues from ethical debate because they are "facts" and hence are no longer open to social negotiation. While there are limitations to each of these arguments, they point to the value of scientific and technical input in decisions made at the frontiers of medicine.

THE SPECTRUM OF SOCIETAL RESPONSES

With the growth in society's interest in and understanding of social and ethical issues in biomedicine has come the creation of a number of mechanisms for deliberation and decision making in this area. Some of these mechanisms entail the formation of a group of persons at a local level, as in grassroots organizations, hospital ethics committees (HECs), and institutional review boards (IRBs), while others relate to the activities of long-established social institutions, such as the legal system. Still others involve federally or state-sponsored groups convened to advise on public policy regarding biomedical developments. Despite their variation in location, sponsorship, and other characteristics, these mechanisms for public deliberation of social and ethical issues can share a variety of functions. Such functions include identification of ethical issues at stake in areas of societal controversy, analysis of an issue, development or documentation of areas of consensus, exposure and documentation of areas of disagreement, generation of public awareness and debate, development of factual bases for public policy, and recommendation of new legislation or improvements in existing public policy.

Political and Legal Mechanisms

Government responsibility to consider the ethical and social consequences of biomedical research arises from its support and encouragement of research as a means of advancing human welfare. Although the timeliness of its initiatives in this area has been criticized, the Congress of the United States has in the past two decades established the National Commission, the President's Commission, and the Biomedical Ethics Advisory Committee (BEAC) to advise public policy on and illuminate issues raised by biomedical research. None of these bodies is currently active, and Congress is presently considering the creation of a new national ethics body that might echo the success of the National and President's Commissions.

Federally sponsored ethics bodies have also been situated within federal agencies that conduct biomedical research. Past examples include the Ethics Advisory Board in the Department of Health Education, and Welfare, and the Human Fetal Tissue Transplantation Research Panel of the National Institutes of Health (NIH). Current examples include the NIH Recombinant DNA Advisory Committee and the Ethical, Legal, and Social Implications (ELSI) Program of the Human Genome Project, both of which are housed within the NIH. Ethics bodies housed within federal agencies generally consider issues that are specific to the work of their sponsoring agency; they may also review protocols for proposed research to be conducted or funded by that agency.

The governments of two states, New York and New Jersey, have established ethics commissions to advise the states' executive and legislative branches on a range of bioethical topics, including surrogate parenting, determination of death, the use of advance directives in medical care, and distribution of organs for transplantation. Both the New Jersey Bioethics Commission (closed in 1991) and the New York State Task Force on Life and Law issue(d) recommendations for changes in state policy related to these areas of medicine.

Courts, regulation, and legislation are mechanisms used by governments and others to contend with social and ethical issues related to developments in biomedicine. In our litigious society, in fact, courts often are the arena where ethical quandaries related to biomedicine first make their appearance and demand resolution. Dramatic cases like *Quinlan* or *Cruzan* illustrate how courts provide a forum in which abstract ethical concerns are made concrete.

While government-sponsored activity in bioethics has languished somewhat in this country since the closing of the President's Commission in 1983, several European countries—notably Denmark, France, and the United Kingdom—have recently taken the initiative. Multinational organizations also have begun to deal with bioethical issues. As the U.S. government considers the possible reestablishment of a national bioethics commission, the experiences of these foreign bioethics groups may hold useful lessons.

Professional and Institutional Mechanisms

Professional medical associations and specialty societies have responded individually and cooperatively to social and ethical questions raised by developments in medical technology and medical care. Several of these groups have formed ethics subcommittees or task forces to deal specifically with these questions and, in several cases, to formulate practice guidelines to assist health care providers in rendering appropriate care to their patients. The guidance provided by professional societies is often the best source of up-to-date scientific, legal, and practical information available to practitioners. Organizations like the American Medical Association, American Academy of Pediatrics, American College of Obstetricians and Gynecologists, American College of Physicians, American Thoracic Society, and National Advisory Board on Ethics in Reproduction, along with others, have taken the initiative to understand and advise on the complex issues that confront practitioners every day.

Institutional review boards and hospital ethics committees are institution-based mechanisms for deliberation on ethical issues in biomedical research and health care. IRBs review protocols for research involving human subjects to ensure that the research does not violate ethical standards. HECs exist to ensure that difficult ethical decisions about medical treatment are made in a careful and impartial fashion. By federal law, IRBs must exist in any institution that conducts or funds human subjects research using federal funds; hospital accreditation standards specify that accredited hospitals must have either a formal HEC or some other mechanism for the consideration of ethical issues in the care of patients. As mechanisms for ethical deliberation and decision making at a local level, IRBs and HECs are uniquely positioned to make decisions that are sensitive to local norms and values and to the particular circumstances of individual patients or research subjects.

The Institute of Medicine (IOM) and the Office of Technology Assessment (OTA) have also from time to time engaged in bioethics deliberation. An arm of the National Academy of Sciences (NAS), IOM is a private, nonprofit organization, associated with the government by virtue of the 1863 NAS congressional charter to advise the federal government on matters pertaining to science. OTA is a branch of the U.S. Congress, established to advise congressional committees on technical issues in all areas of science and technology. Both IOM and OTA have issued reports on a variety of ethical issues over the past 20 years, including health care resource allocation, genetic research, life-sustaining technology, and the responsible conduct of research. Both organizations have been sought to advise on complex ethical issues because of their ability to convene well-informed and impartial study committees.

Deliberation about ethical issues arising from developments in biomedicine also takes place at several research and educational centers throughout the world devoted specifically to the study of ethics. Ethics centers such as the Hastings Center and the Kennedy Institute of Ethics influence policy development in the area of ethics through conferences, publications, and educational programs. In addition, experts in ethics from these centers are frequently called upon to serve on the boards of academic institutions, research centers, professional societies, and nonprofit organizations, as well as journal editorial boards. The Clinton administration's task force on health care reform provides a recent example of a public policy activity in which experts in ethics were called upon to participate in national bioethics deliberation. Together, hundreds of bioethics organizations around the world comprise a remarkable resource for policy-making, analysis, consultation, and education in medicine and the life sciences.

Religious bodies, including interfaith and ecumenical bodies, have also examined the import for religion of developments in biomedicine. In recent years, North American religious groups have produced some carefully researched reports on ethical issues in biomedicine; the Presbyterian Church's report on values and choices in health care is one example. Professorships in religious ethics have been established at several universities and a number of centers have been created for the study of religious ethics. The sheer number of individuals and groups now working on these issues offers some encouragement that useful modes of discourse may be developed, and that a variety of religious perspectives will be a constructive part of public deliberation on the ethical consequences of advances in biomedicine.

Individual and Community Responses

Individuals, groups, and communities are often spurred to action in the wake of changes brought about by developments in biomedicine. Their efforts often begin as loosely structured, grassroots organizations. These organizations frequently come into being as a result of a perceived crisis—over abortion, over concerns about justice in clinical trials—as did the National Abortion Rights Action League, the National Right to Life Committee, and the AIDS Coalition to Unleash Power (ACT-UP). Grassroots organizations often inspire the loyal support of individuals who have little else in common other than their interest in resolving the crisis. The broad-based citizen-sponsored forums on health care that have taken place in recent years in Vermont, Maine, California, and Oregon provide additional examples of community-based bioethics deliberation. The work of grassroots bioethics organizations has had a particularly significant impact on public awareness of social and ethical issues raised by biomedical developments, as well as on public policy.

CRITERIA FOR SUCCESS

The committee developed an approach to evaluating the outcomes of public ethics bodies.[1] These criteria apply particularly to those deliberations that lead to issuance of a document or report. While certain general criteria can be articulated, their importance for evaluating a particular public ethics body is crucially dependent upon context, including the nature of the controversy, the specific tasks of the body, the social setting, the legal environment, and the like. Notwithstanding this caveat, it is still possible to develop a number of important criteria that could be used in establishing, participating in, or judging the overall performance of public ethics bodies. The following discussion divides these criteria into three categories: intellectual integrity, sensitivity to democratic values, and effectiveness. As we shall see, however, there is a considerable amount of overlap and interplay among these categories.

In offering a list and discussion of criteria for judging the success of public ethics bodies, the committee does not mean to suggest that the business of evaluating the performance of these bodies might be reducible to some sort of perfunctory checklist. Often, public ethics bodies must grapple with extremely controversial and contested issues that involve our most fundamental individual and social values. The judgments that people bring to bear on the work of these bodies will naturally reflect their differing views on these fundamental controversies concerning life, death, and justice.

Intellectual Integrity: Logic, Scholarship, and Sound Judgment

Logic

Logic is the first prerequisite of a successful product from a public ethics body. At issue here are the soundness of the reasoning and the overall coherence of the document. Does it describe the topics and issues clearly? Do the conclusions, including the policy recommendations, follow

---

[1] The term "public ethics body" is used in the report to denote a group convened to deliberate about social and ethical issues stemming from developments in biomedicine. Such groups may exist at the level of the institution, professional society, community, state, federal agency, or federal government. Generally, these groups address public policy issues that involve moral ideas such as dignity, freedom, rights, fairness, respect, equality, solidarity, responsibility, justice, and integrity.

logically from clearly stated premises, or are they simply announced on the presumption that the authority or prestige of the body will carry over to its conclusions? Does the document present coherent arguments and recommendations, or is there unresolved contradiction between various parts of the report?

A related function of public ethics bodies is to help clarify, through logical analysis, the terms and nature of the debates covered in their reports. These bodies can often help to fully distinguish the various disciplinary perspectives on an issue, e.g., theological, ethical, economic, political, legal, medical, biological, and epidemiological.

Scholarship

Scholarship is another important dimension of intellectual integrity. The work of public ethics bodies must not only be coherent, it must also be competent—that is, based upon the soundest available scholarship. This means, first, that the body's "findings" must be grounded upon solid, empirical, state-of-the-art information about the relevant area of technological innovation. Although it is reasonable to seek a broad range of cultural, professional, ethnic, and ideological diversity for membership, it is vital that the staff and members of these bodies possess the required expertise in ethics, law, medicine, biology, or related fields. If the membership or staff lacks this technical knowledge, it must consult with appropriate experts and seek out empirical studies bearing on the topic at hand.

Secondly, reports of public ethics bodies should reflect a thorough knowledge of the interdisciplinary field of bioethics. In addition to being factually accurate and well reasoned, such reports should be based upon an equally state-of-the-art understanding of the public and professional "conversation" surrounding a particular issue. The reasoning and conclusions of the report should reflect an awareness of "the best that has been thought" in the bioethical literature, journals of opinion, newspapers, and the like.

Sound Judgment

Sound judgment is also an important element—albeit less tangible and more controversial than logic and scholarship—of the intellectual integrity of public ethics bodies. Because ethical consideration is often complicated by uncertainty, lack of information, and conflicting values and principles, sound judgment in this area resides not so much in being able to apply a single ethical theory or principle to a set of facts, as in the ability to discern the unique particularities of the problem in its social setting, to creatively reframe a question, to reason by analogy, to perceive and acknowledge the interests of affected parties, and to judiciously weigh and balance competing principles and considerations. We call "judicious" those reports that strike an appropriate and fruitful balance between the relevant rights and interests, disciplinary perspectives, and cultural traditions of a given society.

Sensitivity to Democratic Values:
Respect, Representation, and Openness

Respect for Affected Parties

Public ethics bodies should be attentive to all the significant contributors to the public conversation about an issue. Rather than focusing on and advancing their own preferred approach to a problem, members and staff should make an honest attempt to hear all plausible, responsible views. Public ethics bodies should be particularly attentive to minority or disenfranchised voices, not only because these voices can enrich public discourse, but also because they may speak to concerns about religion, culture, and individual rights that ought to be respected, so far as possible, by public policy.

Representation of Diverse Views

Public ethics bodies' consideration of the interests of affected parties should manifest itself not only in the solicitation of input from these parties, but also in the presence of representatives of (or advocates for) these parties in the bodies' membership. Representatives should be willing to deliberate in an open-minded fashion and not merely to champion their group's initial position.

Open versus Closed Meetings

The holding of open meetings by public ethics bodies is intuitively more consonant with democratic values than is the holding of private, closed meetings. Open meetings do not allow for the crafting of secret deals. Rather, they generally foster the effectiveness of public ethics bodies by providing an open forum for exchange of ideas and information among interested parties, all of whom are accountable for their positions.

On the other hand, those who argue that public ethics bodies should operate in private, at least occasionally, note that confidentiality fosters mutual trust and candor among members and staff. When people come together to discuss complex issues, they often require a good deal of intellectual elbow room in which to change their minds once confronted with compelling counterarguments. Proponents of closed meetings argue that it is easier to modify one's position in private than in public, where flexibility and openness to new evidence might be wrongly interpreted as feckless-ness and inconsistency. Many of the issues addressed by public ethics bodies represent problems that have been generated in part by the pres-ence of strongly held, conflicting views within society. If complete consen-sus is not possible on an issue, resolution may require compromise, a pro-cess that some believe can be more successful when undertaken in the absence of publicity. If a public ethics body holds closed meetings, it should make every effort to solicit the views of interested parties during the process of data gathering.

Effectiveness: Communication, Authority

Judgments about the effectiveness of a public ethics body must be based upon a clear understanding of the group's purpose, the public need to which it responds, and the social context in which it deliberates. Not-withstanding the importance of purpose and context, the committee notes two preconditions of effectiveness for any group regardless of its specific charge: communication and authority.

Communication

The reports of public ethics bodies must be clearly written, trenchantly argued, and comprehensible to as wide an audience as possible. Reports should also reflect a clear understanding of the makeup of their audiences; reports that respect the sensibilities of their readers will be more persua-sive, and hence more effective, than those that do not. Even the most clearly written and persuasive reports can fail to be effective, however, if they are not disseminated to as broad an audience as possible. Adequate numbers of reports should be printed and made available at reasonable prices to consumers, professional groups, and public libraries; newer meth-ods of dissemination, such as computer networks and CD ROMs, should also be explored. Members and staff should consider discussing findings and recommendations through a wide variety of media, including newspa-pers, editorial columns, book reviews, radio interviews, professional jour-nals, and public and professional forums. If a public ethics body proposes new legislation, its staff and members should attempt to educate members of the legislature about the issues and about the body's views.

Authority

The effectiveness of a public ethics body is enhanced when it is viewed as an authoritative body—one whose recommendations carry weight with policymakers, professionals, and the general public. Authority can be be-stowed through sponsorship by an authoritative figure like the president.

It can also be earned through, for example, the individual reputations of members and staff or a successful history of accomplishment. Authority can also be a function of democratic representation; the recommendations of a public ethics body may be perceived as authoritative if it is clear that all viewpoints have been heard.

Different Goals, Different Yardsticks of Success: Achieving Consensus, Achieving Results

The primary function of many public ethics bodies is to achieve consensus on issues that require some sort of public response. Thus, whatever may be the specific goals of a particular body, achieving consensus will usually be an explicit policy objective. Consensus can be instrumental in obtaining external acceptance and implementation of a body's recommendations, especially (and, some may argue, only) when members of a public ethics body bring to the deliberations an array of different viewpoints on an issue. On the other hand, consensus can be used to obscure deep philosophical issues. Excessive pressure to reach agreement may lead to underestimation of risks and objections, ignoring of unpopular viewpoints, or failure to consider alternatives or additional information.

Social and political circumstances play a significant role in determining not only the value of consensus, but also the possibility of achieving consensus in any form. A particularly salient factor in public ethics deliberation is the "ripeness" of the issue in question for public resolution. In some cases, a body might merely have to place its imprimatur on a consensus that has been gradually building and is now more or less in place. More frequently, however, public ethics bodies are faced with the harder task of forging a consensus that does not yet exist.

Apart from the objective of forging consensus, public ethics bodies may also seek to achieve more specific goals such as education, influencing of public debate, and stimulation of various government actions, including legislation. Public ethics bodies should successfully discharge the specific mandates that they are given. If a body fails to do what is asked of it, it cannot be judged a success. Depending on the circumstances, some specific objectives may be more difficult to achieve than others. Articulating the contours of an emergent consensus for educational purposes, while a demanding and important task, is not nearly as difficult as drafting legislation on controversial topics for a population divided by ideological and religious differences. Assessments of a body's accomplishments should consider the difficulty as well as the nature of the project assigned to it. Educational projects should be judged in part according to pedagogic standards, while judgment of legislative efforts should reflect the quality of the legal craft presented.

Can Bioethics Be Disadvantageous?

Although there has been no systematic research on the downside of public bioethics deliberation, the committee found it useful to identify two potential risks of public bioethical deliberation, if only as a suggestion for future research, evaluation, and monitoring. One such risk is diversion and capture by advocacy or sectarian groups, or by financially self-interested parties. To the extent that such factions could influence or capture a body charged with the task of bioethical deliberation—a task that aims at impartiality—they could undermine the public interest. While the energy and knowledge of advocacy groups can be an important asset to bodies engaged in bioethical deliberation, the possibility for capture, diversion, and conflict of interest in bioethical deliberation must be carefully monitored. This caution may be particularly important in deliberations regarding health care reform, where ethical and financial considerations are inextricably linked.

Another possible risk associated with public bioethical deliberation is that some might expect bioethics to deliver something—answers, certainty, or the morally correct view—that it is not equipped to produce. It must be clear that "ethical analysis" is not a single, straightforward method, like algebra or geometry. Different ethicists favor different approaches and methodologies and claim different philosophical antecedents. Moreover, even if there existed a single logical formula for ethical argument, such a formula could not account for the substantive elements of ethical argument that arise from individuals' deeply held values and norms, which are colored by culture, religion, heritage, personal history, preferences, and tastes. Ethicists can often do little more than ask for clarification about the meaning of these values and norms in the minds of those who hold them, attempt to discover when the values and norms arise from misunderstanding, and invite those who hold them to find practical ways of living together. The best conclusion of an ethical analysis may be the description of alternative views. Thus, while this committee believes that more good than bad can come from public moral discourse, it also recommends prudent caution whenever an ethical analysis of a major problem is proposed. Broad representation of distinct opinions is probably the best antidote.

CONCLUSIONS AND RECOMMENDATIONS

In formulating its conclusions and recommendations, the committee recognized that not all social and ethical quandaries that have confronted society in the context of biomedicine have resulted from a single radical change or the introduction of a unique new technology. While this is certainly the case in some instances—as in the recently reported cloning of human embryos—social and ethical quandaries may also stem from developments that are rapidly integrated into medical practice before related ethical issues can be resolved. In vitro fertilization (IVF) is an example; many physicians employ the technology, which is no longer regarded as new, despite the fact that IVF continues to challenge widely accepted understandings of parenthood and the legal status of the embryo and fetus.

Social and ethical quandaries may also arise when technological changes or developments (that do not by themselves raise ethical questions) accumulate to present a novel circumstance that alters existing practices and beliefs. For example, the accumulation of several developments in health care, such as immunizations and antibiotics that prevent or cure infectious disease and arterial bypasses that avert death from heart disease, have made it possible for people to live longer than ever before. Longer life spans, however, have increased the incidence of chronic disease, which in turn has provoked reflection on social and ethical issues related to death and dying, the rationing of medical care, and the ends of medicine. Significant organizational changes—like the impending health care reform— can also raise new ethical concerns. For example, it is likely that health care reform will necessitate explicit ordering of priorities regarding health resources as well as new judgments about rationing of expensive medical technologies.

A Multilevel Approach to Bioethics Deliberation

Ethical quandaries arise in the context of everyday interactions with medicine as well as from vanguard research laboratories, and effective mechanisms can be valuable at many levels to recognize and resolve social and ethical quandaries in biomedicine. The committee therefore proposes strengthening the multitiered system of public deliberation at local, institutional, professional, community, state, and national levels and particularly recommends filling a key gap through reestablishing a supra-agency ethics commission at the national level. The recommendation for a multitiered system rests on the conviction that capacities for public ethical deliberation (through academic experts, health professionals, religious communities, secular agencies, and an increasingly informed and interested public) have blossomed in all regions of the country. At the same time, certain contemporary ethical quandaries, including many ramifications of molecular genetic research, may best be considered for the nation as a whole through a supra-agency national commission. The committee presents two supra-agency models: a single national commission with a broad mandate, and a set of national commissions, each with a more focused charge. The recommendations elaborate on the elements proposed for the multitiered system and the features the committee deems desirable for any new national commission. In general, the committee believes that decisions about public policy should occur as closely as possible to the levels at which relevant actions are taken, and should involve those likely to be affected by the policy. The committee is not proposing a new focus of policy-making authority, but a system, separate from existing political structures, for reflecting on and informing public policy decisions at all levels.

Nongovernmental Organizations and Individuals

Based on letters solicited by the committee from scientists and practitioners in a variety of medical areas, the committee noted that those who discover, develop, or apply new technologies in biomedicine are often well positioned to recognize the potential for adverse social and ethical consequences of these technologies. One of the most efficient ways to initiate deliberation of and responses to such consequences may therefore be to call upon researchers, developers of technologies, and medical providers who use new technologies to share their special knowledge of these technologies in ways that could facilitate awareness. Such avenues might include publications and professional presentations; perhaps inquiry about such consequences could even be made part of grant applications. The more that it becomes the norm for consideration of these issues to be part of scientific investigation, the greater would be our society's capacity to catch problems in their early stages and address them more effectively.

> **The committee recommends that the people or organizations that conduct, fund, and commercialize research, as well as those medical providers who apply new technologies, establish a formal capacity whereby they can participate in public moral discourse about the ethical implications of developments in their field. They should attempt to anticipate how these developments may affect society for better or worse and to prepare ways in which adverse effects on social values can be prevented.**

> **The committee recommends that the National Institutes of Health provide funding mechanisms to support (1) the exploration by individual investigators of social and ethical aspects of biomedical technologies as they are developed and (2) the creation of a social and ethical knowledge base for all of biomedical science (e.g., extend the ELSI program to other institutes and other programs within the NIH).**

Professions exist as part of a societal contract that grants learned experts a certain latitude of discretion and self-control in return for the expectation of service to the public. In addition, the resources used to support biomedical innovation and development are generated by the community, largely through governmental support of research. These economic considerations support a role for professional organizations in bioethics deliberations.

The committee recommends that organizations of biomedical professionals establish ethics committees that can be easily mobilized to respond to social and ethical issues as they are identified. Collaboration among professional associations dealing with related issues is to be encouraged.

The committee recommends that professional associations, including those for health care providers and biomedical scientists, recognize their special obligation to investigate the ethical implications of biomedical developments and advocate for the interests of the public and of patients, especially when those adversely affected by change are unable to advocate for themselves.

The committee believes that hospital ethics committees or similar committees operating across health plans could help patients and health care professionals deal with social and ethical quandaries arising from developments in biomedicine. However, little is known about the range and characteristics of effectiveness of HECs. This knowledge needs to be expanded so that it can be applied in the design and evaluation of similar ethics committees that may accompany health care reform.

Preliminary evidence indicates that hospital ethics committees provide many useful support functions for staff, patients, and their families relating to the handling of social and ethical issues that arise from developments in biomedicine. The committee nevertheless recommends that formal studies of the optimum roles, use, and outcomes of HECs be undertaken by such groups as the Office of Technology Assessment, Institute of Medicine, and foundations interested in health care issues.

Like HECs, institutional review boards have played a significant role in the democratization of social and ethical decision making in biomedicine. Given the continuing importance of IRBs, the committee believes that the present structure and role of these bodies should be evaluated and, if necessary, modified.

The committee believes that the NIH, in conjunction with other federal agencies (such as the Food and Drug Administration) to which IRBs relate, need to carefully examine the IRB system and assess whether it is functioning well. Some questions that could be assessed include:

1. **Are IRBs successfully representing the interests of human subjects in research and not merely those of their sponsoring institution?**
2. **Do IRBs generally fulfill their goals?**
3. **What lessons can be learned about effective IRB function from the wide variation in actual IRB practices, and should greater uniformity be encouraged?**
4. **Would communication among different IRBs facilitate effective functioning?**
5. **Are there adequate forums for the appeal of institutional rulings or for resolution of issues that an individual IRB cannot easily address?**
6. **How do freestanding IRBs operate, especially with respect to conflict-of-interest considerations?**

The committee believes that improved integration of social and ethical concepts into health professional education is needed, particularly in the training of students in basic and clinical research. The committee believes that it is important for health care providers and research scientists to be part of the process of examining the social and ethical dimensions of science and technology because: (1) the tradition of openness and internal criticism found in science could fruitfully be extended to the deliberation of ethical issues; (2) biomedical scientists and medical practitioners, due to their understanding of the use of technology as part of the practice of medicine, might have special insight into related ethical issues; and (3) scientists may facilitate the discrimination between factual and value-laden components of scientific belief.

The committee recommends that an evaluation be undertaken of the process of education for graduate students in the health sciences on the social and ethical implications of technology as part of the current educational efforts on scientific responsibility. The committee also urges increased efforts to integrate social and ethical issues in biomedicine into the curriculum of undergraduate and graduate health professional programs.

States

The committee believes that states must play an active role in defining a capacity for ethical deliberation, particularly in a reformed health care system. State governments might facilitate public ethical deliberation through their oversight of professional certification, medical practice, health care financing, and legal liability. Examples of issues that might be addressed at the state level include the use of reproductive technologies; laws and regulations concerning the "definition" of death and forgoing life-sustaining treatments; the practice of assisted suicide and active euthanasia; public health measures involving screening, contact tracing, and quarantining for infectious diseases; screening programs to detect either the presence of genetic disease or susceptibility to diseases such as cancer or heart disease; and the procurement and allocation of organs for transplantation. State mechanisms may be effective at shaping a consensus into the particular legislative form that is appropriate for and acceptable to citizens of a particular state (i.e., one that reflects local conditions, constituencies, historical traditions, and legal requirements).

The committee does not recommend a single specific mechanism for public deliberation of ethical issues at the state level, nor does it recommend a formal institutionalized response in each of the 50 states. Some states may want to establish their own ethics commissions, as has New York. Other states lacking the resources or breadth of representation for such undertakings may wish to cooperate with neighboring states to form regional ethics commissions or information exchange programs.

The committee recommends that states foster or participate in a public deliberative process for responding to social and ethical quandaries stemming from technological and organizational developments in biomedicine and health care.

Advisory Bodies in Federal Agencies

The committee perceives a need for a permanent ethics staff within governmental agencies. Ethics panels located within, and related to, specific agencies have provided valuable advice to these agencies in the past. The committee strongly supports the reestablishment of a body similar to the Ethics Advisory Board because the tasks assigned to it in its originating regulation are not being accomplished at present and constitute a national need and a missed opportunity for leadership in this area.

The committee recommends the establishment of a deliberative capacity within relevant government agencies and departments to provide advice on issues relating to biomedical research and applications of biomedical technology. The committee strongly recommends that as a first step, the Ethics Advisory Board or a similar body within the Department of Health and Human Services be reestablished.

A Supra-agency Commission

For certain issues of broad national interest the committee finds it highly desirable to have a supra-agency national commission to address these issues as they concern the broad public interest and span multiple governmental agencies. At the present time there are several issues that might be incorporated into the mandates of one or more national commissions, including: (1) issues related to scientific advances in genetics, including new possibilities for shaping future generations and the impact of genetic knowledge on peoples' insurability and employability; (2) issues related to confidentiality and privacy of medical information, especially in light of health care reform; (3) the interplay of serious disability and life-sustaining treatment, as well as discrimination on the basis of disability; (4) the integration of cost and social and ethical considerations into clinical and allocation policy decisions; and (5) issues related to reproductive technology and research and medical treatment of embryos and fetuses.

A high-level commission has several institutional advantages over lower-level bodies, including greater visibility, prestige, and independence, as well as greater capacity to address a broad mandate. A national body is also in a better position to formulate and represent distinctively American views on bioethics at a time when issues relating to biomedical research and applications are becoming increasingly internationalized.

The committee recommends that the federal government establish a public deliberative body (or bodies, depending on the breadth of the mandate to be addressed) for a limited term at the supra-agency level to consider social and ethical issues stemming from technological and organizational developments in biomedicine that are of concern simultaneously to several governmental agencies or are nationwide in scope.

In the event that one or more national ethics commissions are established, the committee recommends that each have the following attributes:

Mandate. **The body must have a broad yet clearly defined and coherent mandate, as well as the ability to add additional related topics as they become salient.**

The committee was unable to reach consensus regarding the appropriate breadth of a national commission's mandate. The majority of committee members believe that it is no longer feasible for any single national commission to address all aspects of social and ethical issues in biomedicine, since the expertise and experience that such a broad mandate would require could not be encompassed in a membership of reasonable size. These committee members propose that a national commission's mandate include a set of related social and ethical issues. Commissions with a mandate to address interrelated issues will ordinarily have an easier time studying and resolving subsequent issues after they have reached conclusions in one area. If a national commission were to have a mandate limited to a defined set of related issues, it is possible that more than one national commission would be necessary at any one time.

A second group of committee members believed that a single national commission with a broad mandate was preferable if sufficient time and funding were available to hire staff and commission background papers to encompass all of the appropriate expertise needed. In this case, commission members could be generalists, and background papers and staff research would play a far more critical role than in a commission with a thematic mandate.

Sponsorship. **National commissions could be appointed by the president or Congress. Wherever located, each national commission should operate autonomously.**

Both the perception and reality of independence are important to the credibility of a commission's recommendations. In spite of appointment by the president or Congress, a national commission needs insulation from short-term political interests at the same time as it needs strong ties to affected or vulnerable groups, consumers, and public interest groups.

Membership. **Each national commission should have a diverse membership in order to represent the points of view of all those concerned with or affected by the social and ethical issues to be considered. The composition of the body should enhance the qualities of impartiality.**

Public media coverage can help to educate the public about the deliberations of a national commission. Public meetings can also facilitate broad public involvement.

Public Access. **To the extent possible, a national commission should deliberate in public. The committee recognizes that if such public deliberation is not possible, means need to be found to gain input from all persons and groups with interests in the deliberations. A national commission must reach out to segments of the population whose voices are less regularly heard.**

Commissions at all levels should take specific steps to assure that the results of their deliberations are made accessible to the public. In addition to the use of newspaper and radio, thought needs to be given to how newer methods of information transmission (e.g., electronic means) might be utilized to communicate commission conclusions.

Advisory Role. **A national commission should provide advice not only to its authorizing body but to all concerned parties, including the biomedical community; federal, state, and local governmental bodies; and the public.**

Action-Forcing Powers. **Although a national commission should be advisory, its recommendations should be published, and relevant federal agencies should be required to respond to the recommendations within** a defined "comment period" (e.g., 180 days), either by adopting the recommendations or by explaining why they are not being adopted.

Funding and Staff. A national commission should be given adequate resources and staff to accomplish its task. It should be funded by direct appropriation to ensure its independence. It should have authority over its own budget and the hiring and firing of its staff.

Duration. The commission should have a defined term that is adequate to allow for achievement of assigned tasks.

In determining the duration of a national commission's term, considerations of timeliness, as well as commission members' abilities to maintain energy and concentration of focus come into play. Committee members favored two different possibilities: (1) the term of the commission could be approximately three years, with commissioners serving for the entire term, or (2) the commission could have a longer term, with rotating appointments that replace one-third of the membership every two years. Proponents of shorter-term commissions noted that the existence of a date by which work must be completed can result in a high level of productivity and that shorter-term commissions are less likely to become overly bureaucratic in their work approaches. Those who argued for longer-term commissions pointed to considerations of efficiency of group interaction, consistency, and credibility.

The majority of committee members favored commissions with fixed lifetimes. The majority also believed that a mechanism should be created for initiation of new commissions to consider future issues as they arise. Some committee members favored the idea of a fixed-term national commission with a "sunset clause," which sets an initial date for termination but permits extensions of the commission's term if the issues it is addressing merit further attention.

If a national commission has a fixed term, then the value of continuity and the "learning curve" favor a fixed membership. If a national commission has a sunset clause, then a rotating membership with staggered terms seems advisable, in part as a means to ensure diversity of views and avoid bureaucratic narrowing of the group's collective vision.

If a term-limited national commission is appointed, the committee recommends that responsibility be located within some existing government locus for ongoing monitoring/reporting on social and ethical issues in biomedicine and for recommending the appointment of new commissions as serious issues of national scope emerge. This responsibility could be located in the Office of Science and Technology Policy, the Office of the Secretary of Health and Human Services, or at some other location chosen by the president or Congress.

The committee believes that, during times when no national commission is functioning or when issues arise at an agency level but remain unaddressed, a continuing surveillance mechanism should be in place to identify developing unsolved problems that require more focused attention. A governmental locus for such monitoring could provide several specific functions: it could commission or prepare a biennial report to be published in the *Federal Register* on social and ethical issues emerging from biomedical technology; it could serve as a receptor for the input of communities, individuals, institutions, and states that identify issues that need to be addressed in a broad fashion; it could facilitate networking among the various groups addressing social and ethical issues; and it could advise the executive branch about special social and ethical issues that need immediate attention. Most of the committee members felt that this function could be accomplished in an existing governmental office without increasing the bureaucracy by creating a new office. A few of the committee members favored having an external advisory committee, related to the governmental locus, that is charged with identifying issues to be dealt with at a departmental or across-departmental level, developing mandates, and nominating commissioners.

PART I

1

Introduction

During the past 30 years, the study of ethical issues in the life sciences has become a public concern, debated in the press and, increasingly, guided by governmental commissions, professional societies, and community organizations. The issues have sometimes demanded public attention, as have cases of the abuse of human research subjects, and, at other times, more gradually raised public concern, as have the possibilities provided by advances in genetic technology. More and more, the ethical implications of such issues as health care delivery and commercialization of biotechnology are being pursued in a public fashion. The recent Clinton administration task force on health care reform involved ethicists as consultants; the ethical aspects of academic-industry relationships in the biotechnology industry was the subject of recent congressional hearings. Despite the increasing activity in this area, however, there has been little systematic study of the various collective processes through which we subject these ethical and social issues to debate and analysis. In an attempt to delineate the elements of these processes as they are practiced in this country, the committee found it useful to define more clearly one of the central notions of this discussion—namely, *ethical* issues or dilemmas.

DEFINING "ETHICAL" ISSUES

The word "ethical" is often used interchangeably with the word "moral," although both words also have narrower and more specific meanings (e.g., "ethical" may refer to an issue such as conflict of interest in political settings; "moral" may refer to an issue such as sexual conduct as well as very broad and undefined meanings referring to human values in general). It is difficult, perhaps impossible, to define precisely what these words mean. Often the definitions one finds in the ethics literature define ethics and morality in terms of values, moral principles, virtues, and the like, terms that are in turn defined in terms of ethics and morality. Even if we assume that we share a common, intuitive understanding of these terms, moreover, it is not clear how we come to view a given issue or question as an ethical one. For example, cloning a human being is viewed as an ethical issue whereas international trade agreements typically are not—even though both involve moral choices and affect the vital interests of Americans.

Nearly every public issue requires moral judgments in its resolution. These judgments may be visible or invisible, explicit or implicit, addressed as such or ignored. Thus it is not particularly helpful to decide which public issues are inherently "ethical." However, we can usefully distinguish between issues that are discussed and resolved with reference to the ethical questions they pose and issues debated on other grounds. The former are those discussed in terms of moral ideas, such as dignity, freedom, rights, fairness, respect, equality, solidarity, responsibility, justice, and integrity. Some of these are personal virtues, others are features of social life; some are powers, others ideals. What they have in common is that they are mentioned when one tries to speak of right and wrong, and that they are invoked in discussions that go beyond assertions about facts and descriptions of events to claims about why things *ought* to be done in certain ways or what *ought* to be done.

Perhaps there exist (or once existed) societies in which a single code of morality is so universal and so comprehensive that its members know right from wrong in every situation without need of debate and deliberation. Ours is certainly not such a society. Americans often disagree about standards of justice, conceptions of fairness, and the requirements of integrity; and even when they agree they may still not apply these concepts in the same way to a given subject. Moreover, they may disagree over the facts of the case to which moral standards are to be applied. The discussions and debates that ensue are "ethics" discussions and debates. They form an important subset of the social choices that we routinely confront.

Some "ethical issues" consist in deciding how to react to a moral outrage or scandal. In these cases there is virtual unanimity on the wrongness of what has occurred and no moral argument is needed. Other "ethical issues," however, represent genuine quandaries. With these issues the answers are unclear; they provoke moral disagreement, whether between people or in the form of ambivalence or uncertainty in the mind of individuals. The creation of the Ethical, Legal, and Social Implications (ELSI) Program of the Human Genome Project, for example, was stimulated by genuine uncertainty about the possibilities brought about by new capabilities in genetics. While some perceived new genetic technologies to be encroaching on sacred territory—our identity as humans—many others focused on the potential of these same developments to end suffering from gene-linked diseases and disabilities.

People who disagree over ethical issues can attempt to ignore their differences or to outflank or overpower their opponents. Or they can seek to expand their understanding and perhaps reach agreement or compromise through open discussion and rational moral deliberation, investigation, and argument. This is the potential role of bioethics debates, whether undertaken between neighbors concerned over a personal experience in medicine, or between clinicians perplexed by the moral dimensions of a case, or among presidential appointees to a bioethics commission.

One hallmark of moral deliberation is its ideal of impartiality. Ethical deliberation should be distinct from the pursuit of self-interest; it should also be different from advocacy. Each person, when he or she takes the moral point of view, is supposed to put aside self-interest and the emotions of the moment. Though our cultural, psychological, and religious differences may create some barriers to common agreement, each of us expects the considerations and arguments that lead us to our positions on moral issues to be plausible to other reasonable people who deliberate on these same issues. For example, when we oppose experiments on unconsenting human subjects, we argue that the subjects' right of self-determination is violated, and we expect others to agree that these rights exist. If not, we marshall arguments in support of that proposition, and again appeal to considerations that we expect to be persuasive to those who disagree with us. There is no guarantee that unanimity will be reached, nor even that any consensus that emerges will be well advised and without error. Yet there is widespread agreement on the rules of procedure in ethical argument. Few would be persuaded by a person who backed up a claim about right and wrong by an appeal to personal tastes, feelings, or preferences, for none of these have the essential quality of impartiality.

Our society's capacity for dealing humanely and wisely with the impact of technological and scientific innovation is enhanced by the creation of forums in which this kind of impartial deliberation can be carried out. This deliberation may draw on many resources: actual experience in the use of these technologies and in the practice of medicine; the personal values and life experiences of participants; bodies of formal analysis, such as economics and the law, which reflect and systematize moral judgments; and, not least, the intellectual and scholarly resources of the field of ethics. This report emphasizes the wide variety of settings in which these deliberations are occurring and the diversity of intellectual resources that can be brought to bear on public moral discourse.

SOURCES OF ETHICAL ISSUES IN BIOMEDICINE

The tasks of ethics bodies convened to address issues in biomedicine have originated from clashes of values, norms, principles, and practices that have occurred in a number of arenas, especially: biomedical research involving human subjects; health care decision making, delivery, and financing; advances in medical diagnostics and therapeutics; and academic-industry relationships in biotechnology. From these spheres have come new technologies, the proper use of which is controversial; allocation crises and perplexing questions of distributive justice; changes in the organization and delivery of health care and concerns about the appropriate role of physicians; and financial and policy incentives that have spawned new relationships of questionable appropriateness between researchers and their sponsors. It was in the sphere of human studies research that the ethical dimensions of biomedicine and the need for public involvement in defining these dimensions was first recognized.

Biomedical Research Involving Human Subjects

The use of human beings as research subjects has ancient roots. The Hippocratic tradition recognizes the uncertainty of medical practice. In the famous Hippocratic aphorism, "Life is short, the art long, experience fleeting, experiment perilous, judgment uncertain," there is an awareness that innovative practice carries dangers. Yet no explicit discussion of the ethical dimension of experimental medicine is found in this literature; little more is found in the literature of subsequent centuries.

Specific attention to this issue flowered in the mid-nineteenth century through the work of Claude Bernard, who introduced techniques for comparing different treatment methods. In *An Introduction to the Study of Experimental Medicine* (1865), Bernard declared:

> It is our duty and our right to perform an experiment on man whenever it can save his life, cure him or gain him some personal benefit. The principle of medical and surgical morality, therefore, consists in never performing an experiment which might be harmful to him to any extent, even though the result might be highly advantageous to science, i.e., to the health of others. But performing experiments and operations exclusively from the point of view of the patient's own advantage does not prevent their turning out profitably to science.

This linkage of practice and science became crucial in the early twentieth century as medical innovations made possible the noninvasive monitoring of human functions. Inventions such as the blood pressure cuff, electrocardiograph, X-ray, and blood chemistry using small quantities of blood, allowed scientists to monitor physiological functions without the required invasive techniques that previously dictated the use of animals. Also, mathematical models and statistical techniques made possible discriminating analysis of differences between treatments. In the 1920s and 1930s, it was seen as appropriate for patient care to become a venue of scientific teaming, and for the line between treatment and experimentation to be erased. At that time, Alfred Schwitalla, regent of the medical school at St. Louis University, wrote: "The sick human being, it is true, is not a laboratory animal, but neither is he so isolated in his human glory that he must consider himself outside the possibilities of some, carefully controlled, watchfully supervised experimentation" (Schwitalla, 1929).

The need to assert a clear distinction between practice and research became apparent at the end of World War II. The heinous experiments carried out during the war led to the enunciation of ethical standards that proscribed scientific zealotry and the desire for social benefit at the expense of human consent and dignity. The Nuremberg Code of 1948 is probably the most widely recognized of such declarations. Designed as a standard by which to judge the actions of the perpetrators of the wartime experiments, including the physicians involved, the code filled an important void in the existing medical standards.

Consent of the subject is the linchpin of the Nuremberg Code. The first principle of the code states: "The voluntary consent of the human subject is absolutely essential" (Nuremberg Code, 1949). The code's ten principles establish a wall of protection for the subject and place independent responsibility for avoiding harm to the subject on the shoulders of investigators. The ethical principles enunciated in the Nuremberg Code remain important guides for human experimentation today.

The Nuremberg Code stimulated additional influential statements on the ethical use of human subjects in research. One such statement was issued in 1953 by the Clinical Center at NIH. Titled "Group Considerations for Clinical Research Procedures Deviating from Accepted Medical Practice or Involving Universal Hazards," these were the first federal guidelines for human studies research and the first official statement requiring committee review of human studies protocols.

The Declaration of Helsinki, adopted in 1964 by the 18th World Medical Assembly in Helsinki, Finland, was another such statement. The declaration specified that experimental protocols for clinical research should be sent to a "specially appointed committee for consideration, comment, and guidance," making it the first international research guideline to address the concept of independent review (Levine, 1986). The Declaration of Helsinki included no mechanisms for enforcement of its guidelines, however, except for a recommendation that the results of research not complying with the declaration be rejected for publication. The ultimate duty to serve as protector of human subjects of biomedical research remained the physician's.

Many observers assumed that these proclamations would be sufficient to assure ethical behavior by physician investigators, but revelations in the 1960s of further abuses of human subjects made it clear that this was not true. In 1966 came the news that researchers at the Brooklyn Jewish Chronic Disease Hospital had injected live cancer cells under the skin of elderly patients to test immune competence. The patients had not given, and in some cases could not give, adequate consent to participate in the investigation.

Also in 1966, physician Henry Beecher gave a lecture (and later wrote an article) that presented 22 research studies in which there were serious problems related to the use of vulnerable, disadvantaged, and unaware human subjects. In some of the studies the risks were not adequately explained to the subjects; in others, subjects were not even made aware that they were participating in an experiment. Beecher concluded, "It must be apparent that they would not have been available if they had been truly aware of the uses that would be made of them" (Beecher, 1966).

The controversy stimulated by these and other revelations led to a 1966 surgeon general's ruling that required all medical institutions funded by the Public Health Service to empanel human studies committees made up of scientists, clinicians, and lay members of the community. These committees had two major functions: (1) to evaluate whether the consent form to be signed by subjects was complete and clear; and (2) to decide whether the experiment could be conducted in a manner safer for the subjects, or whether it was safe enough to be conducted at all. Human studies committees declared by their presence that biomedical research was a public enterprise, and that members of the public had important views to offer about its ethical dimensions. The tasks of human study committees later became further refined with the promulgation of federal guidelines. In 1971, the Department of Health, Education, and Welfare (DHEW) issued a publication entitled "Institutional Guide to the DHEW Policy on Protection of Human Subjects," which contained detailed considerations of institutional review and informed consent requirements.

While the creation of research review committees raised public and investigator consciousness about the ethical dimensions of biomedical research, the revelation in 1972 of the Tuskegee Syphilis Study, an observational study of untreated syphilis in black men, begun in 1932, revealed the need for even clearer guidelines and more forceful measures for compliance. A now-infamous litany of ethical abuses characterized the study: no informed consent was obtained from the participants, the men were steered away from treatment even after the discovery in the 1940s that penicillin could effectively treat the disease, and they were deceived into believing that they were receiving treatment when they were not. Congress convened an independent panel that concluded that the Tuskegee Study was highly unethical and should be immediately halted. The panel also declared the protection of human subjects to be a widespread problem and expressed concern that no uniform policy existed for the protection of human subjects of federally funded biomedical research. Among other recommendations, the Tuskegee panel advocated the strengthening of guidelines regarding the review of research protocols by independent committees. These recommendations were reflected in formal policies promulgated in 1971 in the DHEW publication entitled "Institutional Guide to the DHEW Policy on Protection of Human Subjects," mentioned above.

In 1973, the Senate Committee on Labor and Public Welfare held a series of hearings regarding human experimentation that included discussion of such issues as research on human fetuses, sterilization of the mentally retarded, and use of prisoners (Senate Committee on Labor and Public Welfare, 1973). The hearings received extensive television coverage and further increased public awareness of and concern about ethical problems in biomedical research. There was considerable public outrage over reports of fetal research, particularly over a research project that had been conducted in Finland using the perfused heads of aborted fetuses. This study, together with the Tuskegee study, was the stimulus for congressional action on research ethics in the form of the National Research Act of 1974 (P.L. 93-348).

The National Research Act established The National Commission for the Protection of Human Subjects of Biomedical and Behavioral Research (see Chapter 4 for more information on this commission). The National Commission was charged to identify ethical principles that would guide research on human subjects and to develop relevant guidelines for researchers and institutions. The Act also formally established the requirement that research institutions must have an institutional review board (IRB) as a mechanism for the protection of human research subjects (see Chapter 3 for more information on IRBs).

Thus, during the 1970s and 1980s, serious efforts were made to distinguish biomedical research from medical practice. The inherent possibility of conflict between benefit to the patient and benefit to knowledge and society has been acknowledged, and, groups like IRBs and commissions have been entrusted to help investigators, research subjects, and society decide how best to judge the trade-offs.

Recently, President Clinton appointed a 15-member Advisory Committee on Human Radiation Experiments to provide advice and recommendations on the ethical and scientific standards applicable to human radiation experiments carried out or sponsored by the United States government between 1946 and 1974. The group has been charged with reviewing several specific experiments about which questions have been raised concerning whether subjects were treated properly. Composed of experts in medicine, science, ethics, and law, the advisory committee will submit its report in 1995. The rapid establishment of the advisory committee in response to reports of potential past abuses demonstrates the capacity of the federal government to respond to ethical issues.

Changes in Health Care

The seed that was planted in the public consciousness by abuses of human research subjects would later sprout in other areas. The doctrine of informed consent, central to the ethics of clinical research, was at the heart of the movement in the 1960s and 1970s toward greater patient autonomy. At the same time, medical technology began to flourish and health care began its transformation into the business-like enterprise it is today. The resulting specialization, fragmentation, and depersonalization of health care became sources of social and ethical quandaries of great concern to individuals and the public.

Making Decisions About Health Care

Revelations that persons had been subjected to medical experimentation without their knowledge or consent led to great concern that similar situations not occur in the context of medical practice. This concern was directed not only at the potential for the recurrence of blatant abuse, but also at routine questions of disclosure and decisional authority. The newfound interest in greater patient autonomy posed a serious challenge to the historical authority of physicians, who had previously seen patient participation in medical decision making as largely discretionary. Joseph Fletcher's pioneering *Morals and Medicine* (1954) had urged physicians to afford patients freedom of choice and "the fullest possible knowledge" of the medical facts and available alternatives, but the true focus of Fletcher's book was on the dying patient's "right to know the truth" (Faden and Beauchamp, 1986). Physicians continued to consider it their professional responsibility to make treatment decisions for patients, and even to employ what has been called "benevolent deception" when communicating with patients. An excellent account of the history of ethics in medical decision making can be found in David Rothman's *Strangers at the Bedside* (1991).

A cluster of legal cases in 1972 explored the issue of disclosure of information by physicians to their patients and the implications of this disclosure for patient self-determination. While traditional practice standards had permitted professional discretion to dictate what physicians told patients, *Canterbury v. Spence, Cobbs v. Grant,* and *Wilkinson v. Vesey* challenged these standards, claiming that even when a medical procedure is skillfully performed, physicians may nevertheless be liable for adverse consequences about which the patient was not adequately informed. The decisions in these cases combined features of negligence and battery theories into a new approach to informed consent in the medical setting that attempted a fairer balance between patients' rights to self-determination and the demands and complexities of both the physician–patient relationship and the legal setting (Faden and Beauchamp, 1986). Partly as a result of these decisions, the traditional model of medical practice, characterized by paternalism and authoritarianism, eventually gave way to a new model of informed consent, where the competent patient's decision-making authority became primary.

Ironically, the triumph of patient autonomy raised a new set of ethical quandaries. Many clinicians fear that strict observance of patient autonomy may override good medical judgment, encourage moral detachment on the part of the physician, and even work against the patient's best interests (Brock, 1991; Pellegrino, 1993). Patient autonomy also raises questions about increased public costs for expensive but not necessarily beneficial technologies, as well as about prolonging the quantity of life at the expense of quality of life. Empirical research in this area would enhance our understanding of the attendant ethical quandaries.

In addition to the changes in patient care engendered by a new emphasis on patient autonomy, the continuing technological revolution in medical diagnosis and treatment has further altered the delivery of health care and the relationship between patient and provider. Where the physician had once been viewed as omniscient, new medical technologies demythologized the individual physician's role. People began to view physicians less as personal therapeutic forces than as accomplished wielders of technology.

Coincident with the growth of new medical technologies has been an increase in specialization in the health establishment and the proliferation of health care delivery "teams" to administer specialized care. It is not always the physician who leads the team or has the initial or greatest contact with the patient or client. For example, health maintenance organizations (HMOs) might assign a nurse practitioner or physician assistant as a primary care provider or gatekeeper to specialized care, instead of a family physician. A cardiac surgeon may lead both the preoperative and operative teams, while a cardiologist and a cardiac nurse intensivist might lead the postoperative aspects of care. All of these caregivers share in the responsibilities for care of a patient, but each may be distant from total accountability for the patient's welfare.

This arrangement has contributed to a sense of isolation on the part of the patient. Sometimes, it seems that no one is in charge; that no one is there to take overall responsibility; that everyone can, with some justification, feel that almost anything should be taken care of by someone else on the extended team. Advanced technology and the increasingly complex organizational styles it has engendered tend to isolate patients as human beings at just the time when and in the settings where their confrontation with suffering and death may be most intense. The impersonal tone of medical care and the surge in the medical expert industry spurred a growing discontent among patients as health care consumers (Reiser, 1993).

These developments, along with physician paternalism, set the stage for the emergence of a distinct patient rights movement in the early 1970s, a movement that primarily addressed patient rights in hospital care. In 1970, several consumer groups successfully petitioned the Joint Commission on the Accreditation of Hospitals (JCAH) to redraft its standards to address patients' concerns. In 1973, the American Hospital Association published the Patient Bill of Rights, the first explicit statement of the rights of patients and the responsibilities of physicians and medical institutions. Considered by many to be a landmark in the quest for patient autonomy, the bill acknowledged patients' rights to complete and current information in terms that they can understand, to informed consent prior to treatment, to refusal of treatment, and to be advised of and refuse to participate in experimental treatments (American Hospital Association, 1973).

Other developments in the 1970s and 1980s further facilitated a growing acceptance of patient autonomy as the hallmark in both clinical decision making and research. The National Commission's *Belmont Report* (1978) emphasized the need for informed consent and protections for research patients in research trials. The commission's work on informed consent was later continued and applied more to the clinical treatment context by the President's Commission, two of whose reports dealt specifically with the patient's right to informed consent and with the right to refuse life-sustaining treatment (President's Commission, 1982, 1983).

In the last decade, the rights and concerns of patients have held a central place in ethical and health policy discourse. Patient advocates are now employed in many hospitals. State court decisions concerning the right to refuse medical treatment have continued culminating with a Supreme Court decision recognizing a competent refusal of treatment as a constitutionally protected liberty (*Cruzan v. Director, Missouri Department of Health,* 1990). Physician-assisted suicide and euthanasia continue to stir divisive national debate. The recent focus on outcomes research, and calls for increased participation of consumer consultants and advocates in health-care decision making and policy, are just a few examples of a growing trend to involve patient consumers in all levels of health care policy (Reiser, 1993). Finally, the national debate on health care reform has focused significant attention on patient concerns and needs.

The Health Care System: Financing and Structure

Over the past 50 years, the structure and financing of health care has changed in many ways: medical care once rendered by a personal physician is now parcelled out among many specialists and often takes place in vast, impersonal institutions. Its costs, once paid out of pocket by the patient or even provided gratuitously by the physician, are now paid by insurers or by government. In many respects, these changes are beneficial: specialists may provide more skilled care, institutions may supply more sophisticated technology, insurers may pay what the individual could not. At the same time, these changes pose threats to the features of human life that we have designated as ethical, such as individual rights, dignity, liberty, and fairness.

The American hospital began as a charitable institution for the sick poor and evolved into an institution that, relying on community support, made its facilities available to those who could pay and those who could not on a nonprofit basis. This was accomplished by philanthropy and the widely accepted practice of cost-shifting, by which those able to pay subsidized those unable to do so. However, by the 1970s, the need to control rising health care costs and pressure from third-party payers to do so forced hospitals to assume an increasingly business-like mentality. One important third-party payer was the government, which administered Medicare. As hospital costs escalated, payers and providers resisted the financial burden of those who could not afford to pay or had inadequate or no insurance. Determinants of hospital economic viability, like occupancy and proper payer mix (i.e., the proper percentage of patients covered by third-party payers), set the stage for concerns about fair access and about conflicts of interest between hospitals' economic health and patients' physical health.

Financial and organizational systems also vary greatly among institutions: some are wealthier than others, resulting in differential availability of care. Sometimes institutions located in the same city, and staffed by the same specialty teams, operate according to widely variant standards of care. For example, a major county hospital in an urban center might offer dialysis to patients only when symptomatic uremia has progressed to a critical stage, because the hospital cannot afford more dialysis capacity. At a major private teaching hospital in the same city, patients may be dialyzed at lower symptomatic levels (perhaps even before they feel ill from renal failure), since reimbursement and private resources allow it.

Insurance companies have adjusted to the changing environment by segmenting the market, leaving more and more of those outside the work force without insurance and health care. Insurers have also attempted to cut costs by excluding innovative, expensive therapies from coverage on the grounds that they are experimental. This means that those with the means to pay for treatment when an insurance claim is rejected have access to care that is closed to persons who are less affluent. In addition, the practice of denying coverage for treatment of preexisting conditions can severely limit many people's freedom to change employers and can cause enormous out-of-pocket expenses even for those with insurance.

As insurance companies try to manage their risks, so too do physicians. In our increasingly litigious society, malpractice suits against physicians are commonplace, especially as the personal physician is replaced by the more remote specialist. Operating under the threat of malpractice, physicians sometimes perform procedures that are medically unnecessary or marginal in order to protect themselves from the accusation that they did not do everything possible. Inappropriate use of tests and technology carries its own risks to patient health and raises the overall costs of health care, as do the large amounts of money paid by physicians for malpractice premiums.

Thus, these changes in the structure and financing of health care put persons in need of health care into a system that may ignore their dignity as individuals, impose on them or on society as a whole costs that are unfair, and distribute services in an inequitable fashion.

New Diagnostic and Therapeutic Capabilities in Medicine

There are many engines driving technological advance in the biomedical sciences, but it is not entirely clear that maximal stoking of those engines is necessarily the route to equitable distribution of the good that new knowledge can bring. Congressman George Brown, Jr., Chairman of the Committee on Science, Space, and Technology of the U.S. House of Representatives, has argued that the free-market drive to technology, based on the notion of sustained economic growth, may not be the most direct path to improved quality of life for all. He observes, on the contrary, that freewheeling market forces and the drive for high-technology solutions to our society's problems may in fact displace nontechnological, readily distributed preventive solutions in favor of inequitable, expensive, and sometimes even less effective solutions (Brown, 1993). Implied in his argument is the notion that high-technology solutions to biotechnological problems are more likely to produce ethically contorted and difficult situations than are the simpler, low-technology solutions that are driven by concern for the fair and equitable access for all to elemental human needs. Our country's experience with biomedical technology lends some credence to this idea.

During the latter half of the twentieth century, federal investment in research and development has fueled a steady stream of advances in science and technology in general and in biomedicine in particular. The federal government, through NIH, is the principal supporter of biomedical research in U.S. universities and research institutes. But despite the effectiveness of this massive technological effort in fields from physics to material science, as well as the development of biomedical procedures, there have been increasing calls to examine the potential harm that might flow from advances in science and technology.

The biomedical advance that perhaps most effectively illustrates the sometimes troubling consequences of technology was the development of kidney dialysis techniques to save the lives of patients with terminal renal disease. The technology was effective but expensive, and therefore not universally accessible. In the early 1960s, a kidney dialysis team in Seattle, recognizing that it would not be able to treat all medically deserving patients, established a selection committee to choose patients who would receive the treatment (Jonsen, 1993). The committee came to be called the "God Committee," and the well-publicized pain of its dilemma and its choices was relieved only by the passage of legislation that provided funding for treatment of all kidney patients. This experience served to alert both the general public and the medical community to the problems created by limited resources and the desperate need to anticipate such situations and institute equitable solutions.

More recently, advances in molecular genetics have delivered the promise of both technical benefits and ethical problems. Large collaborative efforts have already succeeded in isolating and characterizing some of the genes responsible for a number of our society's most burdensome genetic disorders, including cystic fibrosis, Huntington's disease, fragile X syndrome, and certain forms of common cancers (breast, colon, and prostatic). Population-wide screening tests for these and many more disorders may be within reach. The Human Genome Project, well on the road toward its objective of producing a detailed map of the entire human genome, promises to identify many additional targets for genetic screening tests and gene therapy. Yet, it is likely that social and ethical concerns about employment and insurance discrimination and about the value of knowledge about one's future health will develop in concert.

Academic-Industry Relationships in Biotechnology

Recent dramatic changes in the research and development relationships between industry and academia threaten to upset the time-honored traditions of the biomedical sciences. In the past, academic scientists provided a constant stream of basic biomedical research and a cadre of new investigators as a source of renewed talent. Their activities were generously funded by NIH. Industry would center its attention on the development of their ideas into marketable products. Today, however, the process is undergoing radical change as commercial interests seek to direct scientific discovery.

The ethical issues raised by the tendency of universities and government laboratories to establish closer ties with industry through Cooperative Research and Development Agreements (CRADAs) need to be carefully examined. This need is starkly illustrated by a controversial proposed agreement between Sandoz Pharmaceutical Corporation and Scripps Research Institute, which is being renegotiated under pressure from both the NIH and Congress. The agreement would have given Scripps more than $300 million over 10 years, starting in 1997, in exchange for worldwide license to all Scripps medical or manufacturing inventions (excluding existing research agreements). A joint scientific council (with a Sandoz majority in members) would have been able to influence the direction of research by the Scripps scientists. Under the proposed agreement, Sandoz would have reviewed invention disclosures before they could be filed with the government, and even ongoing Scripps research projects could be transferred to Sandoz facilities for further research and development (Anderson, 1993).

A variety of changes in law and science policy have caused scientists to seek such business-related agreements. Although Congress has steadily increased the funding for NIH-supported biomedical research each year, these increases have been inadequate to meet all increased needs and costs of research. The number of scientists working in biomedical research, the number of individual investigator (R01) grant applications, the proportion of each grant that goes to cover indirect costs, and the average size of each grant have all increased steadily over the years. Such factors underlie the declining success rates of applications for NIH support, from a peak of 45.3 percent in 1975 (Institute of Medicine, 1990) to only 29.3 percent in 1991 (NIH, 1992), and the prospects point to continued decline. The emphasis on obtaining funding and producing publications as measures of success for academic promotion and tenure confounds the problem, causing scientists to seek other sources of research funding. Industry is one obvious source.

Additionally, the insights associated with the genetic revolution have been more readily transferable to industry than previous technologies. As a result, many leading molecular biologists in the academic world have established complex ties with the biotechnology industry. Such relationships have become so prevalent that public agencies such as the U.S. Food and Drug Administration that need unbiased advice from knowledgeable scientists have encountered increasing problems avoiding conflicts of interest when empaneling advisory groups. Finally, both Congress and the executive branch have issued laws, regulations, and executive orders that encourage commercial development of government-funded science (e.g., the Patent and Trademark Amendments of 1980; the Stevenson-Wydler Act of 1980; the Small Business Patent Procedure Act of 1980; and the Federal Technology Transfer Act of 1986).

The types of social and ethical issues that arise from these developments include the availability and cost of new DNA-based products, delay in or reduced numbers of academic research publications due to considerations of commercial profit, "pipelining" of information or inventions to preferred companies, diversion of faculty from other university responsibilities such as teaching, delays of benefit to society, and shifts in the focus of research programs in order to optimize profitability, not scientific advance. The implications for the university of university-industry research relationships in biotechnology have been explored in depth by Blumenthal and his colleagues (1986). These issues demonstrate how social changes can have ethical implications. The issues have attracted public attention, and will do so increasingly, because of concern on the public's part that scientists maintain their honesty and integrity (so that the innovations can be reliably beneficial), their openness and cooperation (so that biomedical science can progress as rapidly as possible), and their commitment to public, not personal, gain (so that all will benefit from publicly supported research).

REFERENCES

American Hospital Association. 1973. Statement on a Patient's Bill of Rights. *Journal of the American Medical Association* 47:41.

Anderson, C. 1993. Scripps backs down on controversial Sandoz deal. *Science* 260:1872–1873.

Beecher, H.K. 1966. Ethics and clinical research. *New England Journal of Medicine* 274:1354–1360.

Bernard, C. 1865. *An Introduction to the Study of Experimental Medicine.* New York: Abelard-Schuman.

Blumenthal, D., Gluck, M., Louis, K.S., Stoto, M.A., and Wise, D. 1986. University-industry research relationships in biotechnology: Implications for the university. *Science* 232:1361–1366.

Brock, D.W. 1991. The idea of shared decision making between physicians and patients. *Kennedy Institute of Ethics Journal* 1(1):28–47.

Brown, G.E., Jr. 1993. The mother of necessity: Technology policy and social equity. Presentation given at the American Association for the Advancement of Science (AAAS) Science and Technology Policy Colloquium. April 16, Washington, D.C.

Cruzan v. Director, Missouri Department of Health, 110 S.Ct. 2841 (1990).

Faden, R.R., and Beauchamp, T.L. 1986. *A History and Theory of Informed Consent.* New York: Oxford University Press.

Fletcher, J. 1954. *Morals and Medicine: The Moral Problems of: The Patient's Right to Know the Truth, Contraception, Artificial Insemination, Sterilization, and Euthanasia.* Princeton, NJ: Princeton University Press.

Institute of Medicine (IOM). 1990. *Funding Health Sciences Research: A Strategy to Restore Balance.* Washington, D.C.: National Academy Press, p. 37.

Jonsen, A.R. 1993. The birth of bioethics. *Hastings Center Report* (special supplement) 23(6):1–15.

Levine, R.J. 1986. *Ethics and the Regulation of Clinical Research.* New Haven, CT: Yale University Press.

National Commission (National Commission for the Protect on of Human Subjects of Bio-medical and Behavioral Research). 1978. *The Belmont Report: Ethical Principles and Guidelines for the Protection of Human Subjects of Research.* Washington, D.C.: U.S. Government Printing Office.

NIH (National Institutes of Health). 1992. *NIH Data Book 1992: Basic Data Relating to the National Institutes of Health.* Bethesda, MD.

Nuremberg Code. 1949. Trials of War Criminals Before the Nuremberg Military Tribunals Under Control Council Law No. 10. Vol. 2. Washington. D.C.: U.S. Government Printing Office, pp. 181–182.

Pellegrino, E.D. 1993. The metamorphosis of medical ethics: A 30-year retrospective. *Journal of the American Medical Association* 269:1158–1162.

President's Commission (President's Commission for the Study of Ethical Problems in Medicine and Biomedical and Behavioral Research). 1982. *Making Health Care Decisions: The Ethical and Legal Implications of Informed Consent in the Patient–Practitioner Relationship.* Washington, D.C.: U.S. Government Printing Office.

President's Commission. 1983. *Deciding to Forego Life-Sustaining Treatment.* Washington, D.C.: U.S. Government Printing Office.

Reiser, S. 1993. The era of the patient: Using the experience of illness in shaping the missions of health care. *Journal of the American Medical Association* 269(8):1012–1017.

Rothman, David J. 1991. *Strangers at the Bedside: A History of How Law and Bioethics Transformed Medical Decisionmaking.* New York: Basic Books.

Schwitalla, A.M. 1929. The Real Meaning of Research and Why It Should Be Encouraged. *Modern Hospital* 33:77–80.

Senate Committee on Labor and Public Welfare. 1973. *Quality of Health Care—Human Experimentation: Hearings Before the Subcommittee on Health,* 93rd Congress, 1st Sess. (February 21–23, March 6–8, April 30, June 28–29, July 10). Washington, D.C.: U.S. Government Printing Office.

2

The Social Context of
Bioethical Problem Solving

THE AMERICAN CHARACTER

The distinctive history and culture of our society shapes the range, character, and form of social and ethical responses to developments in biomedical technology. U.S. history is replete with examples of stirring moral debates that have mobilized the entire country; current debates over developments in biomedicine are shaped by some of the same forces that molded the great controversies of the past.

Our nation was born in rebellion against tyranny to preserve individual liberty; tension between the powers of the state and the rights of the individual has persisted, and it colors the public debate and resolution of major moral issues. In addition, our culture is suffused with an optimistic expectation of progress and change for the better, best exemplified in an unwavering belief in the myth of upward social mobility. Ambivalence about the proper role of government, together with a fervent belief in the power and ultimate triumph of individual efforts, is manifested in a pluralistic approach to political, social, and ethical issues, involving the active participation of numerous and diverse groups and individuals in public discourse. The religious commitments of many of this country's early inhabitants both fostered skepticism about the range of governmental authority and favored governmental sanctions on morality. While moral issues in public policy are often settled at the national level, intense debate may occur at both local and state levels and within scientific, religious, and other communities long before the national debate takes definite shape.

Cases illustrative of this multifaceted approach are found in the history of child labor laws, women's suffrage, prohibition, and the abolition of slavery. For example, in the latter case, citizens engaged in heated debates and formed antislavery societies, newspapers editorialized, churches issued proclamations, and local political bodies took stands, all of which led up to the Civil War and culminated in a national solution. Thus, intense debate at the local and state levels contributed to the formation and acceptance of a central governmental response.

The capacities for public debate of ethical issues in our society have expanded and matured within the past few decades. Discussed in this chapter is the overall social and institutional context in which ethical quandaries arise, get debated, and, sometimes, get resolved. We see, for example, that government performs a dual role: on the one hand it formulates policy responses to nationally debated moral quandaries; on the other, it fuels these quandaries through its funding of the research that produces problematic developments.

Over time, and in many contexts, Americans have managed to maintain a tenuous balance between the celebration of the individual and responsibility for the community, between market striving and civic sharing, between the private sphere and the public good. Populist political mobilizations have offered one mode for restoring the balance; religious movements have proved to be another potent mechanism for doing the same. The structure, function, and dominant ideologies of the political and religious spheres have been central in shaping public discourse on important moral issues—both spheres reflect key aspects of the American character.

The struggle between pluralistic diversity and universal standards has been vivid in both secular and religious American thought. In the political realm, the early colonists demanded to participate in governing their society. The chaos of early participatory politics would echo throughout U.S. history as future generations fought new battles over their place in the political realm. Along with demands for participation came sharp limits to the legitimacy of central authority. A very similar dynamic could be seen in the religious sphere. In contrast to the fixed religious establishments of the old world, Americans witnessed an extraordinary sectarianism, driven by the waves of populist revivalism. Generations of American fundamentalists have, ironically, only added to the multiplicity of sects (Butler, 1990).

Ambivalence About Government

Given that public power has long been viewed as a threat to individual liberty, the state occupies an unusually ambiguous place in U.S. society. As a result, political discourse has been preoccupied with limiting state authority (Morone, 1990). Even as the modern administrative state began to take its contemporary form, somewhere between the two Roosevelt administrations, ambivalence remained. For example, Americans developed their social insurance programs far more reluctantly and obliquely than did their European counterparts (Skocpol, 1992). Throughout the twentieth century, new social welfare proposals were greeted with state bashing, threats of looming socialism, and concerns about the erosion of the work ethic. Hartz (1955), in a classic formulation of this ideology, described the result as "American exceptionalism":

> . . . opposition to the state that weakens every move toward government programs, let alone a class-based politics. New forms of government authority evoke the charge that an overreaching state threatens the people's liberty.

Observers of U.S. health care are familiar with this theme. Ambivalence about government has been offered as an explanation for why Americans refused national health insurance long after the rest of the industrialized world had secured it. While this inconsistent reaction to government runs deep in U.S. politics, however, it is often overstated. Other legacies in U.S. political history have offered now familiar visions of a radically different nature—a strong and active state. American distrust of government matters, but it is only part of the story.

The Political Process

Caution around centralized government is built into U.S. political institutions and celebrated as "checks and balances." Political programs must often pass through the executive branch, both houses of Congress, and other points in the federal bureaucracy; then they must negotiate the various layers of federalism—regions, states, substate bodies, counties, municipalities—each with its own government, each itself fragmented in a number of ways. Legal matters must also be addressed at nearly every stage. To pass through this gauntlet, proposed programs are typically oversold by their supporters, who promise all kinds of benefits to all kinds of constituencies at the same time that they heavily compromise their propositions. The combination, while often succeeding in finding common ground among many competing interests, is also a well-tested recipe for disappointment.

This tangled system of checks and balances is rooted in the Constitution and has been further complicated by succeeding generations of reform. In the vain hope of getting beyond politics, wave after wave of American reformers have organized new agencies designed to be independent, expert, apolitical. Each new "apolitical" reform is quickly bogged down in precisely the politics it was designed to avoid (McConnell, 1966;

Morone, 1992). The result is a political framework that is geared toward narrow incremental changes and best negotiated by individual agencies with narrow jurisdictions and parochial interests. The system is especially resistant to broad policy changes that require coordination from the political center.

In this institutional context, U.S. politics is characterized by broad and persistent participation at every point in the political process. Political scientists once celebrated the resulting play of interest groups as a bulwark for democratic participation. Today, they call it "hyperpluralism" and, generally, lament the resulting stalemate. In sum, an activist interest group culture operates within a sprawling, fragmented state that is always vulnerable to challenges of illegitimacy (Greenstone, 1975; Morone, 1992).

One result is that organized interests can influence policies at multiple points in the political process. The broader consequence is that ideology, institutional design, and the politics of both interests and groups all reinforce the same biases in U.S. politics. Change is difficult to introduce, and the broader the change, the more difficult the task. The overwhelming bias is toward incremental adjustments in the status quo.

How, then, do Americans change their politics and their society? One answer lies in the recurring impulse to organize great democratic movements—a populist urge to remake government, organize direct participation, foster a renewed sense of community. This "democratic wish" has been pursued in a wide variety of contexts across the generations: Anti-Federalists resisting the Constitution, Jacksonians remaking the federal government, abolitionists redefining citizenship, New Left students seeking a more democratic society, and African American activists demanding civil rights.

Broad participatory movements have had a powerful influence throughout U.S. history. It may be difficult to dent the political status quo, but great gusts of democratic sentiment regularly break the impasse. Popular mobilizations create new coalitions, new political rules, new institutions, an entirely new status quo. Precisely when U.S. politics grows most contentious, Americans look beyond their adversary pluralism for direct participation in a shared communal fate.

The Religious Sphere

Religious values permeate U.S. culture. This is the case even for those who are little involved with religious practice, for the substance of religious thought is spread throughout arts, literature, popular culture, and all of the media. Indeed, one can speak of a "civil religion" that throughout the centuries of U.S. history has held the nation together and helped define its character (Bellah, 1985). The question is how this rich fund of human thought and experience can appropriately contribute to public debate and decision making in a democratic society, in which religion is neither to be favored nor curtailed.

The separation of church and state has worked to prevent the dominance of any sectarian theology or religious ideology within U.S. society. As both secularism and religious pluralism have grown with great rapidity during recent decades, some religious groups that had rarely been politically active in former times have developed coalitions that have become a political factor. Some of these groups have mastered the use of the mass media (radio and television, advertising, mass mailings, and political action committees). They have been enlisted by politicians and political parties to further general, national programs, and they have themselves enrolled politicians in their own causes. This public activity by some religious groups has, on the whole, contributed positively to the clarification of issues in the field of biomedicine (Bishop and Coutts, 1994). Religious zeal can, however, lead politically active groups to insist that their religiously derived norms must be accepted by the society at large. Out of such religious zeal, some individuals have resorted to violence against their opponents.

Naturally enough, virtually all religious groups have given major attention to fundamental moral questions raised in the fields of medical science and medical technology. Some of these issues divide the religious communities sharply; issues related to the inception and end of life are particularly divisive. This division is not unique to religious communities, nor is the division merely between the more conservative and the more liberal portions of the religious community, as the issue of abortion makes clear. Persons committed to a traditional or conservative theology may nevertheless be forceful advocates of a more liberal social, economic, and political agenda (see background paper by Swezey in this volume).

At the same time, much religious thought and activity has been directed toward more effective ways of presenting commonly held religious values, such as respect for the views of others, honesty in individual, group, and public life, and the overcoming of racial, ethnic, and sexual biases. Representatives of many religions, including Islam, Buddhism, Hinduism, Judaism, and Christianity often have joined in this effort. Note, for example, the effort by the World Parliament of Religions to articulate a set of common moral commitments and understandings.

Religious organizations are not the only groups that have actively debated and responded to major moral issues, including those brought on by developments in biomedical technology; many other groups are notable for their participation in such debates. Moreover, in addition to the response of diverse social groups, institutions (e.g., the scientific research community and biotechnology industry) also react to and change in accordance with developments in biomedicine. Both specific actors (e.g., minorities, women) and arenas (government, industry, hospitals) shape public ethical discourse on biomedical developments.

ACTORS SHAPING THE SOCIAL
CONTEXT FOR BIOETHICS

Advances in biomedicine do not occur in a vacuum—they are applied within a rich and varied cultural context, with different impacts on diverse social groups. Over the past three decades, the empowerment of certain groups within U.S. society, from minorities to women, from gays and lesbians to health care consumers and patients, has contributed new and distinct voices to the debate surrounding advances in medicine and health policy. While the emergence of these groups occurred roughly contemporaneously and in a somewhat interrelated fashion, each group is treated separately below in order to highlight its own unique perspective.

Minorities: A History of Distrust

The civil rights movement born in the 1960s brought institutional racism and entrenched social inequalities to the forefront of national attention. From the 1959 bus boycotts to the March on Washington in 1963, from the Freedom Riders to the Black Panthers, the movement chipped away at discrimination and instilled a collective consciousness and pride that coalesced African Americans into a powerful interest group (Branch, 1988; Garrow, 1989). While health care was not at the top of the movement's agenda, issues of distributive justice were; the 1963 March on Washington was not only about race discrimination, but also about poverty and economic opportunity. The movement provided impetus for President Johnson's "war on poverty," declared in 1964, which led to passage of Medicaid and other antipoverty programs; data show that after passage of Medicaid, utilization of medical services by the poor increased sharply (Starr, 1983).

Two events in the early 1970s highlighted the racism endemic to the U.S. health establishment and further entrenched the African American community's distrust of medicine: the Tuskegee Syphilis Study (see Chapter 1) and the African American community's experience with sickle cell anemia screening programs. The Tuskegee Syphilis Study has become the most potent symbol to African Americans and other minorities of racist exploitation by the public health community (Jones, 1993). Public outrage over the study was enormous and provided the impetus for the eventual crafting of federal regulations protecting human subjects. However, the study left another legacy that can still be felt today: a profound suspicion and distrust by the minority community of the motives of the U.S. medical establishment (Jones, 1992; Lex and Norris, 1994). Writes Jones (1992) about the exposure of the study in 1972,

> Confronted with the experiment's moral bankruptcy, many blacks lost faith in the government and no longer believed health officials who spoke on matters of public concern.

Ironically, the desire to respond to the historical neglect of the minority community led to another defining event that only reaffirmed this distrust: racial discrimination and stigmatization resulting from sickle cell anemia screening programs. These programs were spurred in the early 1970s by a perception that the disease, more prevalent in African Americans than in others, had been neglected, and by a desire to remedy the racial inequities brought to light by the civil rights movement. However, screening programs were undertaken with little public education, little counseling for those identified as carriers, and insufficient attention to clarification of the distinction between sickle cell traits and sickle cell disease (Fost and Kaback, 1972). Many of the 12 states that passed sickle cell screening laws required mandatory screening of infants and children, even though at the time the only valid scientific objective of the screening was to provide carriers with information concerning whether or not to have a child, since no treatment was available.

Fears that these laws would result in racial discrimination were borne out, with disastrous results for some in the African American community. Children with the disease were stigmatized; insurance carriers raised insurance premiums for sickle cell carriers; some corporations initiated screening programs; and most major airlines grounded or fired employees with sickle cell trait (Bowman and Murray, 1981; Duster, 1990). Indeed, the U.S. Air Force Academy decided to exclude candidates with sickle cell trait from 1973 until 1979 (when the policy was ended after a lawsuit), based on a National Research Council report that characterized its own evidence as inadequate (Duster, 1990). Such reactions to sickle cell disease tended to reinforce both racial discrimination and the suspicions of minorities that medical advances would be used to their detriment.

The legacy of distrust left by Tuskegee and sickle cell screening continues to shape the attitudes of minorities toward organized medicine. Fears of medical exploitation and racial discrimination have led some in the African American community to charge that AIDS was engineered as a program of genocide (Jones, 1993). Suspicions in the minority community have made it difficult to enroll minorities in AIDS and other clinical trials, despite a high level of infection among those populations (El-Sadr, 1992). Concerns remain that any racial differences found in the course of AIDS and other diseases will be used to justify discrimination against minority groups (King, 1992).

This persistent distrust of public health officials could thwart efforts to reverse the current decline in the health of minority groups. Indeed, the documented disparity between the health status of Americans based on race and class reinforces the view that current health policies are not responsive to the specific needs of these groups. These and other health inequalities likely reflect differences in access to and quality of health care services for minority and poor populations. While recent initiatives have been established to improve the health of minority groups (National Institutes of Health, 1991), the sad history of medical racism and the suspicion it engendered remains to be addressed.

Women: A Struggle for Control

The women's movement began to take shape in the late 1950s and early 1960s, on the heels of early successes in the civil rights movement. The first mainstream women's organization, the National Organization for Women (NOW), was organized in 1966 to focus on attainment of women's legal rights; other groups followed with a less traditional agenda. By the early 1970s, the "women's liberation movement" emerged full force, composed of both the more traditional groups and a younger, more radical, cohort. A slogan of the movement, "the personal is political," highlighted its concern not only with discriminatory legal barriers to women, but also with more subtle, pervasive cultural sexism (McGlen and O'Connor, 1983; Rosenberg, 1992).

The women's movement was unique in its concern, from the outset, with health-related issues—namely, the need for women to control their reproductive lives as a prerequisite for individual autonomy. Reproductive politics surrounding both abortion and contraception engaged feminists early on. Women exerted enormous pressure toward the repeal of restrictive abortion laws from 1968 to 1973. Women's groups were also instrumental in facilitating access to illegal abortions; one group in Chicago organized an underground abortion clinic where abortions were performed by self-trained women (Petchesky, 1990). Access to contraception, previously the purview of the population control movement, arose as another leading demand of the women's movement, centering on theories of self-determination, sexual discovery, or "sexual liberation" (Gordon, 1976).

These reproductive issues became the catalyst for the formation of a distinct women's health movement in the early 1970s. As restrictions on reproductive freedom came to be seen as an issue of male domination over women's sexuality and autonomy, the movement expanded to encompass a broader challenge to the male-dominated medical profession's authority to dictate women's health in many other areas. With the first publication of *Our Bodies, Ourselves* by the Boston Women's Health Book Collective in

1973, the women's health movement expanded throughout the country as a campaign by women to reappropriate control over their own medical experience, particularly by means of medical self-help and self-awareness training groups and women's medical clinics. The movement focused on issues such as demedicalizing women's routine health care and childbirth practices, sterilization and surgical abuses, and self-help gynecology (Ruzek, 1978).

In addition to its objections to and concerns with traditional medical practice, the women's health movement also grew distrustful of the drug and device industry over what it perceived to be inadequate drug and device safety measures for drugs marketed to women. Women became concerned over the dangers of the birth control pill, which frequently were not relayed to them by physicians; a book on this subject geared toward the lay reader set off a series of events that finally led the Food and Drug Administration (FDA) to require warning labels for oral contraceptives (Seaman, 1969). Women's suspicion of the drug industry was heightened further by revelations that diethylstilbestrol (DES), a synthetic estrogen prescribed to millions of women between 1945 and 1970 to prevent early miscarriages, caused vaginal cancer in some of their daughters. When concerns were raised about the health complications of IUDs, women's health advocates were instrumental in pressuring the FDA to recall Copper-7 IUDs and halt the manufacture of the Dalkon Shield; further protests eventually led to the regulation of such devices by the FDA (Ruzek, 1978).

More recent developments illustrate women's continued concern with the safety of drugs and devices prescribed for them, and a perceived lack of responsiveness to women's unique health needs by the medical establishment. The recent scandal over the safety of silicone breast implants sparked outcries by some feminists that women's health was being exploited for profit (Wolf, 1992). Allegations that there has been a historical lack of research attention to breast cancer, as well as cardiovascular disease and AIDS in women, has also sparked a wealth of efforts by a wide range of women's organizations to ensure that these areas of investigation are adequately addressed.

Despite increasing numbers of women entering careers in medicine, women continue to be underrepresented in the medical profession, and some within it have observed an entrenched bias against women (Komaromy et al., 1993). Women's health advocates were also instrumental in calling for the review and revision of existing NIH and FDA policies that routinely excluded women of childbearing age from research trials. This had led to revised policies at both agencies, reflected in the NIH Revitalization Act of 1993 (P.L. 103-43), which requires promulgation of guidelines to ensure that women and minorities are included in NIH-funded research.

A myriad of pressing issues continues to confront women in health care, including a renewed battle over abortion rights and access to RU-486 (Charo, 1991), disparate treatment of women in medical management of illness (Steingart et al., 1991), violence against women as a public health threat (American Medical Association, 1992), the growing population of women infected with HIV (United Nations Development Programme, 1993), and complex questions surrounding the maternal–fetal relationship, fetal diagnosis, and the control of pregnant women (Rothman, 1987; Mattingly, 1992). Despite these continuing concerns and problems, however, there is no doubt that women have become a viable, forceful interest group, challenging sexism in medical practice and research and calling attention to medical problems unique to women.

Gays and Lesbians: A New Activism

Gay rights, like minority and women's rights, have long been a part of U.S. political debate, but gays and lesbians emerged as a powerful, distinct interest group in the 1970s. The Stonewall riots in New York City in 1969, following a police raid on a gay bar in Greenwich Village, led to a decade of organizing, fundraising, and consciousness-raising among gays and lesbians throughout the country, modeled on the civil rights and feminist movements. The late 1970s saw renewed efforts in reaction to a backlash that resulted in the repeal of gay rights ordinances in Dade County, Florida, and other cities. In 1978, riots broke out in San Francisco after Dan White, the killer of gay supervisor Harvey Milk and mayor George Moscone, received a sentence of only seven years in prison (D'Emilio, 1983; Cruikshank, 1992).

As with minorities and women, the history of the gay community's relation with the U.S. medical establishment is characterized by suspicion and distrust (see background paper by Bayer). A decade before the AIDS epidemic, gay men began to form their own health clinics in response to perceived discriminatory treatment for sexually transmitted diseases. The American Psychiatric Association classified homosexuality as a mental illness until 1976; but even until 1990, the Public Health Service was responsible for enforcing a ban on immigration by homosexuals based on that mental classification (Levi, 1991). But as with other rights movements, the gay liberation movement focused its initial energies not on health issues, but on legal and social stigmatization and discrimination in housing, jobs, and other areas.

In the early 1980s, the general public's erroneous perception that AIDS was a disease affecting only gay men lent momentum to gay activism. The labeling of AIDS as a "gay" disease transformed what should have been a mass mobilization of public health resources to combat a critical health problem into the politicization of public health agencies. Former Surgeon General C. Everett Koop notes in his 1991 autobiography that "the Reagan revolution brought into positions of power and influence Americans whose politics and personal beliefs predisposed them to antipathy toward the homosexual community." Conservative politics, Koop adds, both slowed the understanding of AIDS and thwarted his attempts to educate the public about the disease. In the face of an establishment that failed to rise to the challenge of the AIDS epidemic, gays began to organize their own community health clinics and treatment networks, seeking to redefine the notion of AIDS as a disease rather than divine retribution (Shilts, 1987; Padgug and Oppenheimer, 1992).

Gay health advocates introduced a new level of activism and self-help to the previous endeavors of health interest groups. For example, in response to what was perceived as a sluggish federal drug approval process, gays organized an "AIDS underground," a network of illegal drug buyer clubs. In 1987, the AIDS Coalition to Unleash Power (ACT-UP) was organized in New York City as a more activist alternative to existing gay health groups. ACT-UP repeatedly caught the attention of federal and state policymakers by relying on dramatic modes of civil protest and disobedience borrowed from the civil rights movement (Arno and Feiden, 1992).

The development of a parallel track policy at the FDA, arising from the introduction of dideoxyinosine (ddI) as a potential AIDS therapy, exemplifies an unprecedented involvement by gays and other consumer groups in federal health policy-making, even though the outcome of this policy has yet to be evaluated. Extending the basic tenets of the patients' rights movement concerning participation in treatment decisions, gay activists succeeded in negotiating with federal officials and drug manufacturers to speed the availability of unapproved but possibly effective treatments for AIDS (Levi, 1991).

The activism of gays in response to the AIDS epidemic marks a significant turning point in the history of health interest organizations and their relations with the medical and research establishments. This activism may well inform the future efforts of other groups as well, perhaps changing the power dynamics between the medical community and patient groups.

HEALTH CARE AND SCIENCE: SHAPING THE SOCIAL CONTEXT FOR BIOETHICS

Patients, Employers, and Insurance Companies: Health Care Consumers

Substantial changes in the delivery of health care have transformed patients from trusting, relatively passive recipients of health care to a more skeptical and active group of informed consumers, voicing their concerns and challenging the previously unquestioned authority of physicians and other health care practitioners. In the past, a patient who wished to learn about advances in medicine would ask for information and guidance from a trusted health care provider and confidant, with whom a long-term relationship had been established. But as more Americans receive medical care in managed care settings from a series of specialists, and as patients/consumers must assume major responsibility for decisions about their personal health care, such close relationships no longer exist for many people. Health care consumers now express concern at the number of procedures to which they are exposed, and question whether these procedures are really necessary for the diagnosis or treatment of their illness. They are troubled by the apparent inability of the health care system to control spiraling costs for medical insurance and medical treatment, and wonder what type and level of basic research will provide relevant advances in medical care at an affordable cost to the public.

In considering patients' relationships to the health care system, employment-based health benefits and the role of employers have to be taken into account. The system of employer-based health benefits began in the early 1930s. It is a voluntary system, required by neither federal nor state law. The offering of health benefits to workers and their families is now almost universal in organizations with 100 or more employees. In contrast, only about one-half of employees in organizations employing less than 25 employees receive health benefits directly from their employer. At present, about two-thirds of all Americans under age 65 (about 140 million people) receive health benefits through the workplace. However, 35 million Americans are uninsured, and many other millions have inadequate or precarious coverage (Field and Shapiro, 1993).

Just as profit-making health conglomerates are concerned about health care costs, so too are increasing numbers of employers, who are alert to risk selection as a strategy to reduce the costs of their insurance. They may favor the hiring of individuals who are least apt to draw upon costly health benefits. They realize that any health plan that avoids providing coverage to high risk groups will have a competitive advantage. Thus, consumers and patients, particularly those with preexisting conditions or genetic diseases, may find that their problematic health status makes them less desirable as employees and, as a consequence, less able to secure adequate health benefits.

The government has provided some protection of health care benefits for vulnerable populations. In 1965, the federal government introduced Medicare for workers who were over 65 or disabled. Medicare separated coverage for hospitalization from that for the physician, in accordance with the pattern set by Blue Cross. For workers over 65 who are entitled to both

Medicare and employment-based health benefits, arrangements are generally made between employer and insurance company to charge Medicare first and leave the balance to the insurance company. This arrangement faces restructuring as the federal government moves to curtail Medicare benefits.

Until recently, insurance companies made profits by underwriting the cost of employer-based health plans. However, anticipating the advent of managed competition, they are now moving further into management as well as financing for a profit. Like hospitals, they are actively engaged in setting up networks, buying hospitals, and establishing a variety of diagnostic and therapeutic facilities and thus may be a powerful part of any future health care system.

Public discourse surrounding biomedical developments is affected not only by the activities of specific social groups, but also by the institutional landscape of hospitals, government and industrial research communities, and academic activities in bioethics. The interaction of public policies and structural changes has produced a vastly altered institutional setting for biomedical innovation, with major social and ethical ramifications.

Hospitals

Largely because of the resistance of physicians to national health insurance, the United States has a "system of private insurance for those who can afford it, and public welfare services for the poor" (Starr, 1983). The present system evolved gradually over 200 years, modified in large part by the changing role of the physician in the delivery of health care. Before the mid-nineteenth century, the public had little confidence in physicians. Health care was generally provided at home, by relatives and friends, often in consultation with professional healers. The practice of medicine was limited because physicians had few effective therapeutic interventions.

The tide turned for physicians in the mid to late 1800s, not only in their own practices but also in their relationships to hospitals. Five broad forces were responsible for this change: (1) urbanization, which concentrated patients in smaller areas; (2) improved transportation (the advent of the automobile in the 1890s); (3) growth in the application of science (e.g., bacteriology) to medical practice; (4) organization of physicians to resist competition from other health practitioners and to resist intrusions by government; and (5) educational and licensing reform. By the 1920s, the medical profession was a highly respected profession that controlled hospitals by controlling the flow of patients into these institutions. Increasingly, health care shifted from home to hospital.

Not until the 1970s did this costly, physician-dominated health system face serious challenge, when national health insurance was seriously debated as a desirable alternative. Thereafter, medical domination of hospitals began to yield to professional administrators (Starr, 1983). Increasingly, physicians offer the hospital professional skills, technology, and income; but in many hospitals their dominance was diminished with the increased control gained by administrators. Along with the change in control came a greater focus on the financial aspects of running a hospital.

Between 1850 and 1920, the American hospital was transformed from an asylum for the indigent—noisy, dirty, and in disarray—to a scientifically oriented institution for medical management and nursing care. The dramatic change was prompted largely by a combination of industrialization, urbanization, and immigration, as well as by advances in sanitation and medical treatment (Rosenberg, 1987). Not only did the hospital become clean and efficient, it became increasingly technological and interventionist (Stevens, 1989). It also assumed a dominant role in the training of physicians, shaping their interests, attitudes, behavior, values, and practice. In the process, it also became increasingly sensitive to political and societal pressures, cultural rewards, and economic incentives and disincentives, changing its scope, priorities, and structure as it accommodated to these influences. In this evolutionary process, the physician became less of a healer than an expert who provided access to the necessary technology; often, the nurse was charged with ministering to the patient's care and well-being.

For most of the nineteenth and early twentieth century, the health care system centered around the hospital and its inpatient activities. Surgery became its mainstay. More and more, its success and visibility depended on its ability to deliver up-to-date acute and specialized care. As the hospital's primary role as a charitable institution faded, however, it began to assume a more corporate mentality, and low occupancy became a major detriment to economic viability. In the 1960s and 1970s, with the advent of Medicare and employer-sponsored health insurance programs, admissions to hospitals rose; in the 1990s, due to AIDS and the rise in chronic diseases, they are increasing again.

At the same time, a growing emphasis on specialty medicine led to a decline of primary care medicine. Along with greater reliance on science and technological sophistication, specialists assumed a central role in the business of medicine. Some showed entrepreneurial instincts that verged on conflicts of interest. Physicians also became targets for those with products to sell (e.g., drugs) and for malpractice suits by those with failed expectations. All of these factors contributed to the rising cost of practicing medicine and of running hospitals. The term "hospital" refers today to short-term, acute care, general hospitals that include both medicine and surgery. Most are voluntary, not-for-profit organizations; these provide 70 percent of short-term beds in the United States.

Voluntary hospitals handled the financial pressures by becoming more aggressive, competitive, expansionary, profit-oriented, and income-maximizing. Access to health care became increasingly dependent on ability to pay. Some hospitals, faced with prospects of financial doom, merged with others; others fled to the suburbs where the payer mix was more favorable. This contributed to the growing problem of limited access to health care for the uninsured: the poor, the part-time worker without benefits, and the unemployed.

Currently, the voluntary hospital is a central part of the changing scene in health care delivery. The idea of "managed competition" is driving hospitals into health care networks. The tempo of competition among urban hospitals has become fierce as they strive to set up networks for managed competition. Insurance companies are prominently engaged in the struggle for a piece of the pie. Drug companies are resorting to novel strategies in order to maintain prized relationships with physicians and hospitals while the restructuring is under way.

A variety of influences is diminishing our society's traditional reliance on hospitals as independent entities:

- increased dissatisfaction of the public and of major political figures with the high cost of health care and the major role played by hospitals and their administrative costs in the genesis of this difficult burden;
- growing ability of and financial incentive for outpatient care to substitute for in-hospital care due to advances in medical management and technology (e.g., cardiac catheterization, renal dialysis);
- less need for hospitalization because of the development of non-invasive technologies for diagnosis and treatment (e.g., CAT scanning, MRI, or ultrasound);
- restructuring of health care (e.g., through HMOs, which discourage referrals to hospital-based specialists, and greater strictures on reimbursement by third-party payers);
- development of new effective therapeutic agents (e.g., antibiotics for cystic fibrosis);
- expanded use of living wills advance directives, which may limit interventions and expenditures for terminal disease; and
- greater effectiveness of preventive measures (e.g., education for AIDS, vaccines).

As the United States prepares itself for health care reform, it is important to recognize that in addition to unmet needs (e.g., preventive medicine), the aging of the population will introduce additional needs and related ethical questions. For example, disability from dementia, including Alzheimer's disease and stroke, will require research into etiology, medications, devices, and suitable treatment environments. The major causes of death have shifted from acute infectious diseases (e.g., influenza) to chronic diseases (e.g., heart disease and cancer), and death by these causes occurs later in life, after a period that includes limited functional capacity and impaired quality of life. In the course of a patient's dying, hospitals often provide a variety of expensive life-prolonging measures, even though the effect on survival time and quality of life is often small. Decisions have to be made concerning the availability of such measures.

The Health Care Industry

Health care is a big business with several components that are germane to our considerations of social and ethical issues: primary among them are health care services and the research, development, and use of drugs and devices. Health care costs include the money paid to physicians in managed care or private practice, to hospitals, laboratories, and other health care workers. Costs also include the money spent on the products of pharmaceutical and biotechnology companies as well as the money spent on health-related research to develop and produce these drugs and technologies. Some basic statistics illustrate the size and scope of this business and, hence, the stakes involved in changing any aspect through public policy. In 1991, according to Letsch and colleagues (1992), the United States spent a total of $751.8 billion for health care, or $2,868 per person. Approximately 88 percent of the health care expenditures paid for medical services or products such as hospital services, physician services, drugs, and nursing home care. Inpatient and outpatient hospital care comprised 43.7 percent of the total personal health care expenditures, but only 3.4 percent of this was paid directly by the patient, while private health insurance paid for 35.2 percent and public health insurance paid for 56.3 percent of the charges. Another $23.1 billion was spent on biomedical research and development, about half of it in federal funds.

Biomedical Research: The Federal Government and Private Industry

Since the end of World War II, a growing function of government has been sponsorship of biomedical research, primarily through the National Institutes of Health and the National Science Foundation (NSF). The idea that public investments in biomedical science should play a major role in improving the economic status of the country has become a recurrent theme and is prominently featured in the Clinton economic policy. A frequently cited analysis estimated 28 percent rate of return to society from funds invested in academic research (Mansfield, 1991).

Beginning in 1980, a series of laws and regulations have sought to benefit the economy through the commercial development of government-funded science. These laws have fundamentally altered the role of research scientists in relation to their discoveries. The Stevenson-Wydler Act (P.L. 96-480) of 1980 required that 0.5 percent of the R&D budgets of federal agencies be used for technology transfer activities. The Bayh-Dole Patent and Trademark Laws Amendment Act of 1980 (P.L. 96-517) assigned intellectual property rights to the institutions carrying out the government-funded research, allowing grantee institutions to patent and license their developments and collect and retain royalties. Also in 1980, the Small Business Patent Procedure Act (P.L. 96-517) reversed the federal policy of nonexclusive licensing by assigning patent rights to small businesses, universities, and some nonprofit organizations that were involved with government contracts. The Federal Technology Transfer Act of 1986 (P.L. 99-502), authorized government-operated laboratories to establish Cooperative Research and Development Agreements (CRADAs) with other federal agencies, state or local governments, and industrial and nonprofit organizations for the licensing of government-owned inventions, with inventors and their laboratories keeping part of the royalties received from these licenses. As a result of all of these actions, biomedical scientists began to benefit financially from their ideas by forming relationships with industry and by starting small biotechnology companies of their own.

The development of recombinant DNA technology, in combination with the change in government policies with respect to technology transfer, underlay the biotechnology industry that was created de novo during the 1980s. The number of new biotechnology companies soared during the 1980s, making the United States a world leader in the commercialization of biotechnology products. A June 1993 fact sheet from the Biotechnology Industry Organization (BIO) reports that there are 1,231 biotechnology companies in the United States, an 11 percent increase since 1991. Thirty-eight percent of U.S. biotechnology companies are involved in product development in therapeutic agents, while 28 percent are producing human diagnostics. Other companies are involved in agricultural, chemical, environmental, or service areas. The industry presently employs 79,000 individuals (BIO, 1993). By 1993, 21 approved drugs or vaccines and over 600 diagnostic agents had reached the market; another 16 agents are awaiting FDA approval, and 132 agents are in clinical trials. The biotechnology industry is predicted to grow to a $50 billion industry by the year 2000 (President's Council on Competitiveness, 1991). As was the case in the past decade, new technologies that alter existing practices and challenge traditional values and beliefs promise to accompany this growth.

Another site of biomedical innovation from which ethical and social quandaries are likely to arise is the pharmaceutical industry. The vast majority of new drugs have been developed by this industry, which has doubled its investment in R&D every 5 years since 1970. In 1993, the industry was expected to invest $12.6 billion in R&D—a 13.5 percent increase over 1992. This investment amounts to 16.7 percent of the industry's expected sales in 1993, four times the average of R&D investment for all U.S. industries that conduct research (Beary, 1993). Since 1988, the member companies of the Pharmaceutical Manufacturers Association (PMA) have supported more R&D than the NIH, with industry spending totalling $9.2 billion in 1991 (PMA, 1991). Although it is difficult to accurately estimate the costs of developing any single drug, DiMasi et al. (1991) estimated that the average cost of developing a single drug was $231 million. A more recent report by the OTA (1993) estimates that the average cost to a company for moving a single new medicine from laboratory to practice is presently $359 million.

The high cost of drug development is partly a result of the rigorous testing process that a new drug undergoes. It takes an average of 12 years for a new drug to reach the market, and for every 5,000 compounds that are evaluated, only 5 enter clinical trials in humans and only 1 is approved (Wierenga and Eaton, 1993). In spite of the huge investments of time and money required to produce a single drug, the pharmaceutical industry has been highly productive, commercially successful, and highly profitable to its investors. Kaitin et al. (1993) studied 196 new chemical entities that had been approved by the FDA between 1981 and 1990, and found that 181 drugs (92.4 percent) were developed by the pharmaceutical industry, 7 by academia, 2 by the government, and 2 by individuals.

As the biotechnology and pharmaceutical industries play an increasing role in the economic competitiveness of our society, industry needs new resources from various sectors of society. From the regulatory agencies, it needs clear guidance on what is expected in terms of safety and efficacy regarding the testing process, as well as an efficient approval process. The success of industry also depends on basic biomedical research in academic and government laboratories, a vital academic research enterprise that generates new scientific insights. Industry also looks to the academic research community for new skills and techniques, specific assays and reagents, personnel to conduct clinical trials, consultants and collaborators, individuals to provide expertise to regulatory agencies, and highly skilled scientists and technicians to work in industry. To facilitate cooperation between academia and industry, value questions related to ownership of intellectual property rights and conflicts of interest must be resolved.

A 1990 National Academy of Sciences (NAS) report on industrial perspectives on innovation and interactions with universities concluded that, in the early stages of large scientific breakthroughs, industry needs interaction with university scientists, who are at the forefront of scientific knowledge. As a breakthrough matures, however, incremental improvements (product- and process-oriented technical changes that are related to competitiveness) occur most often within industry only. Thus, primary roles for universities in academic-industry partnerships lie not in product development but in providing in-depth education about new and emerging concepts.

A cautious analyst of "technology transfer" from the university or the national laboratories to industry is John A. Armstrong, retired vice president for science and technology at IBM (1993). He holds industry responsible for poor management decisions, lack of attention to quality and cost in manufacturing, past high interest rates, and poorly trained workers. "The most effective technology transfer from universities in the short term is well-trained technical and scientific workers at many levels of sophistication and knowledge," he concludes. If universities become focused on technology transfer and economic competitiveness, he anticipates a variety of problems, including a shift in the amount and priorities of available funding, a distortion of the role of universities, and an increase in ethical issues such as potential conflicts of interest of research faculty. Universities could improve the rate of return on society's investment in basic research through the following actions:

• improve the training of scientists and engineers to make them more effective and enthusiastic participants in R&D exploitation with heightened interest in the challenges of manufacturing;
• make innovations in how universities and industry interact;
• rationalize university policy with respect to intellectual property rights;
• reexamine university conflicts of interest policies.

Harold Shapiro, president of Princeton University, echoes these concerns (Shapiro, 1992). He notes that technologic progress depends not only on new science and technology but also on cultural and social factors such as political stability, life expectancy, nutrition, attitudes toward risk, natural resources, property rights, religious values, demographics, and openness to change. The critical contributions from the university sector are education and advanced training, quasi-independent scientific agendas, and exploration of the human condition, through a broad set of historical, cultural, political, and value questions. In the final analysis, "[i]t is a society that is full of hope rather than fear, full of trust rather than alienation, full of knowledge rather than ignorance, full of honesty rather than cynicism, full of confidence rather than helplessness that will survive and progress."

Funding of Scientific Research

Since 1950, the federal government has been the main source of financing for scientific research and a principal shaper of the research agenda. One reason for growing public interest in scientific expenditures is the sheer size of the government-funded program of biomedical research. The NIH budget alone grew from $26 million in 1945 to over $10 billion in 1993, and the Clinton administration's budget request for FY 1994 is $10.668 billion. Almost 90 percent of the funding goes to extramural research. Additional matching funds are applied to the construction of biomedical research facilities. For its part, NSF has a FY 1994 budget request of $3.182 billion to fulfill its scientific mission.

The establishment and success of these premier scientific research agencies resulted partly from the early insights of Vannevar Bush, head of the wartime Office of Scientific Research and Development, who pointed out in his book, *Science—The Endless Frontier*, the importance of the uninterrupted flow of new scientific knowledge for both health and defense. To accomplish these purposes, Bush proposed a permanent governmental structure receiving funds from Congress to support basic research in the colleges, universities, and research institutes, as well as scholarships and fellowships for training. Bush specified that this proposed agency should recognize the importance of freedom of inquiry on the part of the individual scientist.

Today, it is precisely this unfettered freedom of the individual scientist to determine research priorities that is being questioned. Yet, who should be setting the priorities for science? Congress must respond to a variety of pressures from constituents, resulting in academic earmarks to fund "pork barrel," non-peer-reviewed science at levels that have grown from about $10 million in 1980 to almost $800 million in 1993 (*Washington Fax*, 1993). Congress also responds to the voices of special interest groups by specifying funding levels for specific diseases. Scientists as a group have not developed a way to effectively establish research priorities across the various fields of scientific endeavor. Unfortunately, Congress also seems to lack a mechanism for obtaining objective data to help to weigh scientific priorities across the spectrum of important diseases.

At the same time that the public demands greater accountability in the funding of biomedical science, it is generally optimistic about the ultimate outcome of its investments. A 1990 survey by the National Science Board showed that most Americans trust the motives of scientists; 80 percent of respondents agreed that most scientists want to make life better for the average person (National Science Board, 1991). The survey also showed that between 1979 and 1990, decreasing proportions of respondents agreed with the statement that "Science makes our way of life change too fast." Most respondents indicated that they believe that the benefits of scientific research had outweighed the harmful results; a majority perceived a strong link between advances in science and technology and improvements in their own daily lives.

How the public responds to developments in biomedicine is often influenced by the way such developments are presented in the media. In general, the media provide a valuable service by informing the public of developments in health-related research and biotechnology, not only the scientific advances but also the social, legal, or ethical impacts of these advances on the lives of all Americans. However, as the media strive to create a newsworthy story, the value of this service can be diminished. The 30-second soundbite conveys partial information but ignores crucial details. The limited success of an animal experiment can be reported in a manner that suggests an imminent breakthrough in human therapy; when the expected results do not immediately materialize, such stories can lead to public disillusionment.

These tendencies in the media compound the problems caused when politicians or scientists overpromise about expected breakthroughs. A salient example was the so-called "War Against Cancer" during the 1950s and 1960s (IOM, 1973). The funds that were expended under that program have contributed to advances in the diagnosis and treatment of cancer (and to the understanding of HIV disease), but the idea that cancer would be defeated by this program caused unfounded expectations on the part of the public, and resulting disappointment.

Research on the human genome is an area in which the media's influence has been more positive, however. There has been a concerted effort to deal with ethical, social, and legal issues related to the uses of new genetic technologies (see background paper by Hanna). Nobel laureate James Watson has been a central figure in expanding our understanding of the molecular structure of DNA and of the relationship between viruses and cancer. As head of the NIH Office of Genome Research (now the National Center for Human Genome Research), he responded to public and congressional concern by proposing to use part of the money allocated to the Human Genome Project to study the ethical, social, and legal issues that are raised by the information this research generates. Media coverage highlighted this effort and was partially responsible for encouraging public support for this initiative.

REFERENCES

American Medical Association (AMA), Council on Ethical and Judicial Affairs. 1992. Violence against women: Relevance for medical practitioners. *Journal of the American Medical Association* 263(3):3184–3189.

Armstrong, J.A. 1993. Research and competitiveness: Problems of a new rationale. *The Bridge* 23(1):3–10.

Arno, P., and Feiden, K. 1992. *Against the Odds: The Story of AIDS Drug Development, Politics and Profits.* New York: HarperCollins.

Beary, J.F. 1993. New Medicines: The Best Hope for Older Americans. In: *In Development: New*

Medicines for Older Americans. Washington, D.C.: Pharmaceutical Manufacturers Association.

Bellah, R.N. 1985. *Habits of the Heart.* Berkeley: University of California Press.

Biotechnology Industry Organization (BIO). 1993. U.S. Biotechnology Industry Fact Sheet (June). Washington, D.C.: BIO.

Bishop, L.J., and Coutts, M.C. 1994. Religious perspectives on bioethics. *Kennedy Institute of Ethics Journal* 4(2):155–183.

Boston Women's Health Book Collective. 1973. *Our Bodies, Ourselves.* Boston.

Bowman, J., and Murray, R. 1981. *Genetic Variation and Disorders in People of African Origin.* Baltimore, MD: Johns Hopkins University Press.

Branch, T. 1988. *Parting the Waters: America in the King Years, 1954–1964.* New York: Simon and Schuster.

Bush, V. 1945. *Science—The Endless Frontier.* Reprinted by the National Science Foundation. 1990. Washington, D.C.

Butler, J. 1990. *Awash in a Sea of Faith. Christianizing the American People.* Cambridge, MA: Harvard University Press.

Charo, R.A. 1991. A Political History of RU-486. In: *Biomedical Politics.* Institute of Medicine. Washington, D.C.: National Academy Press.

Cruikshank, M. 1992. *The Gay and Lesbian Liberation Movement.* New York: Routledge.

D'Emilio, J. 1983. *Sexual Politics, Sexual Communities: The Making of a Homosexual Minority in the United States, 1940–1970.* Chicago: The University of Chicago Press.

DiMasi, J.A., Hansen, R.W., Grabowski, H.G., and Lasagna, L. 1991. Cost of innovation in the pharmaceutical industry. *Journal of Health Economics* 10: 107–142.

Duster, T. 1990. *Back Door to Eugenics.* New York: Routledge.

El-Sadr, W. 1992. The challenge of minority recruitment in clinical trials for AIDS. *Journal of the American Medical Association* 267(7):954–957.

Field, M.J., and Shapiro, H.T. (eds.) 1993. *Employment and Health Benefits: A Connection at Risk.* Washington, D.C.: National Academy Press.

Fost, N., and Kaback, M.M. 1972. *Why Do Sickle Screening in Children: The Trait Is the Issue.* Pediatrics. Vol. 51(4):742–745.

Garrow, D.J. 1989. *Bearing the Cross.* New York: Vintage Books.

Gordon, L. 1976. *Woman's Body, Woman's Right: A Social History of Birth Control in America.* New York: Grossman.

Greenstone, J.D. 1975. Group Theories. In: *The Handbook of Political Science,* F. Greenstein and N. Polsby, eds. Reading, MA: Addison-Wesley.

Hartz, L. 1955. *The Liberal Tradition in America.* New York: Harcourt, Brace and World.

Institute of Medicine (IOM). 1973. *A Review: National Cancer Program Plan.* Washington, D.C.: National Academy of Sciences.

Jones, J. 1992. The Tuskegee legacy: AIDS and the Black community. *Hastings Center Report* 22:38–40.

Jones, J. 1993. *Bad Blood: The Tuskegee Syphilis Experiment.* Revised edition. New York: The Free Press.

Kaitin, K.I., Bryant, N.R., and Lasagna, J.L. 1993. The role of the research-based pharmaceutical industry in medical progress in the United States. *Clinical Pharmacology* 33:412–417.

King, P. 1992. The Past as Prologue: Race, Class, and Gene Discrimination. In: G. Annas and S. Elias, eds. *Gene Mapping: Using Ethics And Law as Guides.* New York: Oxford University Press.

Komaromy, M., Bindman, A.B., Haber, R.J., and Sande, M.A. 1993. Sexual harassment in medical training. *New England Journal of Medicine* 328(5):322–326.

Koop, C.E. 1991. *Koop: The Memoirs of America's Family Doctor.* New York: Random House.

Letsch, S.W., Lazenby, H.C., Levit, K.R., and Cowan, C.A. 1992. National health expenditures, 1991. *Health Care Financing Review* 14(2):1–30.

Levi, J. 1991. Unproven AIDS Therapies: The Food and Drug Administration and ddI. In: *Biomedical Politics*. Institute of Medicine. Washington, D.C.: National Academy Press.

Lex, B.W., and Norris, J.R. 1994. Health Status of American Indian and Alaska Native Women. In: *Women and Health Research, Volume 2*. Institute of Medicine. Washington, D.C.: National Academy Press.

Mansfield, E. 1991. Academic research and industrial innovation. *Research Policy* (June):295–296.

Mattingly, S. 1992. The maternal–fetal dyad: Exploring the two-patient obstetrical model. *Hastings Center Report* 22(1):13–18.

McConnell, G. 1966. *Private Power and American Democracy*. New York: Knopf.

McGlen, N., and O'Connor, K. 1983. *Women's Rights: The Struggle for Equality in the Nineteenth and Twentieth Centuries*. New York: Praeger.

Morone, J.A. 1990. *The Democratic Wish*. New York: Basic Books.

Morone, J.A. 1992. Hidden complications: Why competition needs regulation. *The American Prospect* (Summer):40–48.

National Academy of Sciences (NAS). 1990. *Industrial Perspectives on Innovation and Interactions with Universities. Summary of Interviews with Senior Industrial Officials, National Academy of Sciences Government-University-Industry Research Roundtable and the Industrial Research Institute*. Washington, D.C.: National Academy Press.

National Institutes of Health (NIH), Minority Health Initiative, Office of Minority Programs. 1991. *Healthy People 2000*. Bethesda, MD.: NIH.

National Science Board. 1991. *Science and Engineering Indicators*. 10th edition. Washington, D.C.: U.S. Government Printing Office.

Office of Technology Assessment. (OTA) 1993. Pharmaceutical R&D: Costs, Risks, and Rewards. Washington, D.C.: U.S. Government Printing Office.

Padgug, R., and Oppenheimer, G. 1992. Riding the Tiger: AIDS and the Gay Community. In: E. Fee and D. Fox, eds. *AIDS: The Making of a Chronic Disease*. Berkeley: University of California Press.

Petchesky, R. 1990. *Abortion and Women's Choice: The State, Sexuality, and Reproductive Freedom*. Revised Edition. Boston: Northeastern University Press.

Pharmaceutical Manufacturers Association (PMA). 1991. *PMA Facts at a Glance*. Washington, D.C.: PMA.

President's Council on Competitiveness. 1991. *Report on National Biotechnology Policy*. Washington, D.C.

Rosenberg, C. 1987. *The Care of Strangers: The Rise of America's Hospital System*. New York: Basic Books.

Rosenberg, R. 1992. *Divided Lives: American Women in the Twentieth Century*. New York: Hill and Wang.

Rothman, B.K. 1987. *The Tentative Pregnancy: Prenatal Diagnosis and the Future of Motherhood*. New York: Penguin.

Ruzek, S.B. 1978. *The Women's Health Movement: Feminist Alternatives to Medical Control*. New York: Praeger.

Seaman, B. 1969. *The Doctor's Case Against the Pill*. New York: Doubleday.

Shapiro, H.T. 1992. The research university and the economy. *The Bridge* 22:3–14.

Shilts, R. 1987. *And the Band Played On*. New York: St. Martin's Press.

Skocpol, T. 1992. *Protecting Soldiers and Mothers*. Cambridge, MA.: Harvard University Press.

Starr, P. 1983. *The Social Transformation of American Medicine*. New York: Basic Books.

Steingart, R.M., Packer, M., Hamm, P., Coglianese, M.E., Gersh, B., Geltman, E.M., Sollano, J., Katz, S., Moye, L., and Basta, L.L. 1991. Sex differences in the management of coronary artery disease. *New England Journal of Medicine* 325(4):226–230.

Stevens, R. 1989. *In Sickness and in Wealth.* New York: Basic Books.

United Nations Development Programme (UNDP). 1993. *Young Women: Silence, Susceptibility and the HIV Epidemic.* New York: UNDP.

Washington Fax. 1993. House SS&T Chair Brown continues effort to halt earmarking. (September 8):1–2.

Wierenga, D.E., and Eaton, C.R. 1993. The drug development and approval process. In: *In Development: New Medicines for Older Americans.* Washington. D.C. Pharmaceutical Manufacturers Association.

Wolf, N. 1992. Keep them implanted and ignorant. *Wall Street Journal* (23 January):A17.

3

Systematic Approaches to Bioethics

ACADEMIC BIOETHICS

Definitions

During the 1970s, scholars from several disciplines, principally moral philosophy, theological ethics, medicine, and law, began to study and write about the ethical issues of modern medical science and health care. Gradually, a discipline called bioethics began to emerge, with specialized faculty (usually located in schools of medicine), courses, conferences, and journals. What contribution can academic bioethics make toward public moral discourse about the biomedical sciences and health care practices and policies?

Academic bioethics is easier to describe than to define. Descriptively, the term refers to the scholarly activities of individuals, usually trained in an academic discipline that deals with ethics, such as theology, moral philosophy, or law, and usually working within institutions dedicated to teaching and research. These persons study a range of issues loosely arranged around the biomedical sciences and health care, apply the methods of their disciplines, and publish their conclusions in scholarly and semi-scholarly journals. In the 1980s, graduate programs in bioethics appeared; there are now about a dozen such programs offering higher degrees. Academic bioethicists, then, have scholarly and practical training that enables them to work in various settings: as faculty in medical and nursing schools or university departments, as hospital or organizational consultants, as government employees in policy or regulatory positions, and as members of public committees and commissions dealing with ethical issues.

Academic bioethics should be distinguished from what might be called *professional bioethics*, whose practitioners (such as physicians, nurses, and scientists) undertake to learn about the ethical standards and issues in their professional practices. They may utilize the work of academic bioethics and invite scholars to join their discussions as consultants, but their engagement tends to reflect the exigencies of their work more strongly than the theoretical and analytic features of academic bioethics. This is practical bioethics in the most commendable sense: individuals become competent—sometimes quite competent—in a subject, but work at it primarily as an adjunct to their primary occupation.

Academic bioethics can also be distinguished from *popular bioethics*, popular moral discourse that concentrates on issues in medicine, health care, and the biomedical sciences. Thus, public debate over genetic engineering or assisted suicide, carried out in many different forums and manifested in the media, constitutes popular bioethics. In this format, it is the story rather than the analysis that prevails. Participants in this "amateur" bioethics may become interested enough to learn something about ethical analysis, but do so casually and often without rigorous scholarship or argument. Sometimes, popular bioethics may be drafted into the service of strongly held ideologies and become quite sophisticated, although no longer impartial.

If public moral discourse is taken in the strictest sense, as the deliberately organized effort to marshall evidence and considered opinion with the purpose of formulating a broadly acceptable analysis or policy about an issue, then there must be an attempt to integrate these three sources, using each according to its appropriate contribution to the debate. What then is the proportionate contribution of academic bioethics, in relation to professional and popular bioethics, and indeed in relation to other forms of discourse in a democratic society, such as legal, economic, political, and religious? The primary task of any public body charged with providing a forum for public moral discourse is to orchestrate these various perspectives.

Origins

Academic bioethics came into being when persons other than physicians started to scrutinize the moral dimensions of the practices of medicine. There is a long history of physicians doing so, but only rarely did nonphysicians comment in a scholarly manner on the work of physicians. If a date is to be found for the earliest suggestion of an academic bioethics, it might be 1927. In that year, Chauncey Leake, a distinguished pharmacologist, but not a physician, published the first modern edition of Thomas

Percival's *Medical Ethics*, which originally appeared in England in 1803 and served as the model for the American Medical Association's Code of Ethics in 1847. In the preface, he noted that Percival, while using the term "ethics," had in effect written a book on medical "etiquette," describing the ways in which physicians dealt with each other and their patients. Leake suggested that a proper "ethics" would employ methods of moral philosophy, and he called on philosophers to examine modern medicine from the viewpoints of pragmatism, utilitarianism, and other ethical theories.

Leake's call was not heeded until 1953, when Joseph Fletcher, professor of moral theology at Episcopal School of Theology in Cambridge, produced *Morals and Medicine*, the first serious effort by a nonphysician academic to examine certain medical mores, such as euthanasia, truth-telling, abortion, and contraception. Fletcher, though a theologian, utilized the philosophical approaches of pragmatism and utilitarianism. Several years earlier, Williard Sperry, dean of the Harvard Divinity School, had published his reflections on similar questions, but without a discernable methodology or philosophical foundation.

In the mid-1960s, various academicians noted that the discoveries of modern medical science posed interesting moral problems. European theologians such as Karl Rahner and Helmut Thielicke ruminated about creative forces being put into the hands of fallible humans, either extolling their possibilities or warning about their misuse. In the United States, theologians James Gustafson and Leroy Augenstein and philosophers Hans Jonas and Martin Golding published reflective commentaries on similar themes.

These, however, were occasional essays, raising questions and testing approaches, rather than subjecting the world of biomedical science and practice to focused moral analysis. In response to the proliferation of ethical issues arising from developments in biomedicine, two centers for research were created almost simultaneously, the Institute for Society, Ethics, and the Life Sciences (now known as the Hastings Center) in 1969 and the Joseph and Rose Kennedy Center for Bioethics in 1970. These two centers can be seen as the principal source and stimulus for academic bioethics in the United States and they have, in the past two decades, been replicated in many forms and many places.

In the late 1960s and early 1970s, U.S. medical schools began to appoint faculty in medical ethics. These persons, surprisingly, were not physicians but philosophers and theologians. Gradually, these faculty positions generated scholarly work that, more often than not, was published in medical journals rather than in publications devoted to philosophy and theology. This required a change in style, moving away from the vocabulary and idioms common to those scholarly disciplines toward language and arguments used by health professionals.

The most important stimulus to the development of academic bioethics was the establishment by Congress of the National Commission for the Protection of Human Subjects of Biomedical and Behavioral Research. Because of the nature of its mandate, the National Commission was required to carry on moral discourse in a way that satisfied the criteria for formal ethics, met the exigencies of public policy and law, and responded to popular concern about the abuse of research subjects. Two of its eleven members were trained in theological ethics and a reputable philosopher was immediately hired as a consultant. During its four years of existence, the Commission asked a great number of philosophers and theologians to contribute essays on specific topics, and the preparation of its statement of the ethical principles that should govern research with human subjects was carried out with the advice of many scholars. The commission's work enlisted into the emerging field of bioethics many scholars who otherwise would have remained in the more speculative world of academic philosophy and theology. The subsequent President's Commission continued this endeavor.

Contributions

What did the early bioethicists, immigrants from other scholarly disciplines, contribute to the formation of this new field? Moral philosophy in the United States had been attracted, since World War II, to the methods of analytic and linguistic philosophy cultivated in British universities. This style emphasized the logic of moral discourse, attending to definition of terms and rigor of argument, and almost entirely ignored substantive moral questions. A new subtopic of moral philosophy called metaethics became the center of attention: it asked not what actions are right and good, but what do "right" and "good" mean.

The philosophers who did reflect on substantive moral problems did so in a remote manner, devoting their attention to the construction and defense of theories that could provide a moral foundation for particular moral claims. Thus, anyone trained in philosophy during the years after World War II was likely to have acquired skills in the analysis of moral language and the ability to defend or criticize utilitarian theory and its alternatives. R.M. Hare, one of the most prominent moral philosophers of the era, was asked to speak to the topic: Can the moral philosopher help in doing philosophical medical ethics? He responded:

> The main—perhaps the only—contribution of the philosopher to solution of these problems is the clarification of the logical properties of tricky words like wrong, and the establishment of canons of valid argument. It is my belief that once issues are thoroughly clarified in this way, the problems will not seem so perplexing . . . and, the philosophical

difficulties having been removed, we can get on with discussing the practical difficulties, which are likely to remain serious. (Hare, 1977)

Professor Hare's comment implies that those adept at clarifying "philosophical difficulties," which are mainly linguistic confusions, must bow out of the discussion when the serious "practical difficulties" are addressed. Or, at best, they enter this discussion with no more competence than any other person. This view leaves little place for academic bioethics in public moral discourse. At that time, the few philosphers interested in normative ethics were concerned to find ways in which moral views and arguments could be defended as objective, that is, based on some grounds other than the subjective personal attitudes and emotions of those expresssing the views. For example, one among many such efforts was R. Firth's theory called the "Ideal Observer," in which he proposed that the judgment "x is right" means "any person who is fully informed, impartial, and in a calm frame of mind would approve of x." This theory, and others like it, set a tone for the work of moral philosophers that gave them a larger place in public moral discourse than did Hare's clarification of tricky words. The Ideal Observer theory and its counterparts in the moral philosophy of that era defined the quality of mind and attitude that a moral philosopher should bring to public moral discourse.

This is not to claim that all moral philosophers employed Firth's Ideal Observer theory, or its variants, in the solution of moral problems. Rather, the theory implies that if public moral discourse is composed of popular moral concern and professional moral pronouncements, as suggested above, then the moral philosopher should approach the problem with an attitude that can correct the defects of both of these contributions. As noted in Chapter 1, the ideal of impartiality counters the pursuit of self-interest as well as the militancy of advocacy and contributes to the revelation of common interests and understandings. Popular moral concern is often not fully informed and is often not calm: it is the emotional response to what some perceive as a violation of rights. Professional moral pronouncements are likewise not necessarily impartial, since the professional group will advocate, often covertly and even unintentionally, for its own interests. Full information, impartiality, and a calm frame of mind must constantly be brought to bear on the discussion of contentious issues in public moral discourse. The experience of the National Commission, in which ethical analysis had to maneuver between public moral outrage over abuses and the values of scientific progress, provides a vivid example.

In addition, moral philosophy attends to one particular feature of moral discourse that is often neglected in popular and professional discussions, namely, the justification of ethical claims. Again, normative moral philosophy had provided the theories that provided ultimate justification, but at the same time it emphasized certain general features of justification that should be present, regardless of the preferred theory, namely consistency and generality. A good moral philosopher will be sensitive to inconsistency between positions or to the limited applicability of principles. These are significant virtues in public moral discourse, which is often highly particularist.

The moral philosophers of the 1960s were pulled out of their concern with the speculative questions of moral judgment into the world of practical concern over the rights and wrongs of such burning questions as civil rights and the justification of the war in Southeast Asia. Many serious moral philosophers initiated courses dealing directly with these questions, and a journal, *Philosophy and Public Affairs*, was founded to pursue these questions at the most rigorous intellectual level. Just as the questions of bioethics were emerging, moral philosophers were discovering the world of practical moral problems.

The moral philosophers who initiated bioethics brought to this new field certain virtues of intellect and attitude that improved the quality of discourse. They less commonly brought substantive moral positions. The moral theologians, on the other hand, often did speak from such substantive positions formulated within the ecclesiastical traditions from which they came. Many moral theologians, especially those from the Roman Catholic tradition, also utilized philosophical theory and method in their analysis of moral problems. Many others, however, were more skeptical of philosophy and relied on scriptural themes that they felt could be applied to contemporary problems. Thus, the theological concept of covenant was used to justify and refine the medical and research doctrine of informed consent. In addition, moral theology in that era had something of a prophetic mood: it was compelled to offer radical criticism of common life and accepted norms. Hence, the advances of biomedical science were to be viewed critically rather than accepted enthusiastically. Were these startling advances manifestations of God's creative power or examples of human hubris? Theologians who took this tone provided a cutting edge to public moral discourse.

Among the many theologians who discussed the issues, Paul Ramsey of Princeton University became the most prominent. Taking a stand firmly situated on biblical ethics of covenant and the faithfulness of God toward humankind, he trenchantly analyzed the new issues of the day—death by brain criteria, transplantation, research with human subjects—in ways that exposed their moral ambiguity and their threats to human dignity and freedom. His book, *Patient as Person* (1970), was a monumental contribution to the ethical analysis of biomedicine and, while written from a theological viewpoint, has been influential on all subsequent work in the field.

Neither philosophers nor theologians have been particularly successful at one feature of public moral discourse. Whenever ethical discussion rises to the level of public moral discourse, a variety of facts surround the topic under discussion. As philosopher Dan W. Brock (this volume) writes, "the consideration of economic costs, political feasibility, legal constraints, potentials for abuse, and so forth, all bear on and must be considered as part of the ethical case for a particular policy." Even though bioethics is remarkable for the concreteness with which it discusses its subjects, it remains unclear how these factual features "must be considered as part of the ethical case." In the experience of the President's Commission, philosophical arguments about the claims of individual research subjects that supported their compensation were countered by considerations of cost and feasibility. It was never made clear how all these facts fitted into a coherent philosophical argument (President's Commission, 1982). Currently, bioethics scholars are debating vigorously the relationship between principles and facts, a debate that is essential to the role of academic bioethics in public moral discourse.

Academic bioethics today has moved far beyond its beginnings. A number of academic programs prepare students for the field. These programs present students with a canon of topics and a variety of analytic methodologies. As the field grows, it incorporates the current trends in philosophy and theology. Feminist philosophy in particular is making its mark on bioethics and cross-cultural studies exert strong influence on younger scholars. Philosophers trained in these emerging approaches may be quite different from those in the earlier era: they may come with more substantive views, as did the earlier theologians, rather than with the Ideal Observer stance of moral philosophers trained after World War II. They will most likely be more sensitive to the distortions of argument due to differences in power or bias in the social construction of reality. They may be more deconstructionist than analytic. They are more skeptical of theory. Also, they are less likely than their predecessors to be uncritical heirs of the Western liberal tradition. The same can be said of students coming into bioethics from religious studies and theology. They too are now influenced by feminist, communitarian, and cross-cultural approaches; their theological commitments may be less doctrinal and ecclesiastical than in the past. The new generation of bioethicists, which is certainly more explicitly trained to deal with the complexities of the field, will probably bring different qualities to the public moral discourse about bioethics than did the early scholars in the field.

Contributions of Religious Ethicists to Biomedical Questions

Outside the field of academic bioethics, in which theologians have cooperated with philosophers, religious ethicists of many denominations have contributed to public moral discourse about developments in biomedicine. Clergy come into frequent contact with the wrenching moral dilemmas of life and death. Many clergy today have spent time in formal training programs in hospital pastoral counseling. Theological seminaries offer courses on bioethics and their faculty often contribute to the denominational literature on its topics. Several centers of theological and religious reflection on bioethics exist with church sponsorship, among them The Park Ridge Center for the Study of Health, Faith, and Ethics, supported by the Lutheran Hospital Association; the Loma Linda Center for Christian Bioethics, affiliated with the Seventh Day Adventist Church; and the Pope John XII Medico-Moral Research Center, operated under Catholic auspices. A research center that focuses on religious and theological aspects of the Human Genome Project has been funded by the ELSI program at the Graduate Theological Union in Berkeley. Many denominations have established committees and commissions to report on bioethical issues of relevance to their faith and doctrines. In these ways, theological insights enter into public discourse about bioethics.

Dangerous Ways to Present Religious Ethics

Even so, certain ways of presenting religious beliefs do not contribute to clear and sound ethical decision making. Many members of religious communities consider their ethical positions to be rooted in the divine will and religiously demanded. The problem comes when persons insist that these revealed positions *must* be accepted by everyone else. To refuse to allow others to see matters otherwise, and thus to be wrong, may be appropriate for one's coreligionists, but it is a dangerous position to take as a citizen. This impulse often arises when persons or groups locate evil in some distinct part of the world—certain groups, certain practices, certain ideas (see the background papers by Swezey).

Hopeful Developments

The rapid growth of multidisciplinary work on ethics is an immensely hopeful development. This development has its counterpart in religion, as in the production of periodicals like the *Journal of Religious Ethics* and the many institutes, commissions, and committees that confront questions of ethics. And in no area is this more the case than in the field of biomedicine and ethics. The essays produced for this study illustrate the point: such essays would hardly have been taken seriously by medical scientists and practitioners at an earlier time, but they are of much interest to many individuals and institutions of the medical world today.

Areas of tension remain and are probably inevitable. Religious views, precisely because they are religious, are likely to be held with great confidence and tenacity. But one should not suppose that the religious and ethical positions of any religious group are unchanging. One holds fast to what is central in one's religion, but the view of what is in fact central may and does change over time. American society faces many strains today, apart from those directly related to religion, and each of us lives within that ferment. The ferment demands attention, and urgently, and from many quarters. One thing is unmistakable: religious specialists and leaders want to be a part of the discussions, and many of them are qualified by temperament, learning, and experience to be valuable partners.

SCIENTISTS AND OTHER TECHNICAL EXPERTS

Do scientists as a community have any special contributions to make in decisions involving the social and ethical impacts of biomedicine? If so, what is the basis for their special status? Are there circumstances in which society inappropriately relies on science or scientists for help in making ethical decisions relating to biomedicine?

The American sociologist Robert Merton (1973) described science as a field of inquiry marked by unique ethical commitments (he called them "norms") that enhance its trustworthiness. The idealized view of science stresses its openness, its universality, its institutionalized procedures for self-criticism and self-correction. These attributes might be taken to support the argument that scientists as a group are more virtuous than other communities; their ethical judgments accordingly may be considered worthy of special deference.

Historical and sociological writing about science, however, undermines the notion of scientists as a community possessed of unique wisdom or virtue, even with respect to the social consequences of their own inventions. As Steven Shapin's background paper points out, we cannot deduce from the "truthfulness" of scientific claims that scientists themselves are virtuous. If anything, individual virtue and mutual trust have historically been preconditions for the production of scientific "truths" that are acknowledged as such within a community of researchers.

Apart from questionable claims about scientists' special virtue, there are three additional grounds that might be advanced for why scientists should be accorded a privileged place in ethical decision making:

• First, science, because of its openness and critical tradition, can be thought to provide a particularly appropriate discursive model for making ethical decisions in a pluralist society.

• Second, scientists, because of their closeness to the practice of medicine and the use of technology, may be expected to have special insights into ethical issues arising from their practice that would not as easily be apparent to other users or consumers of technology.

• Third, science can be counted on to remove certain issues from ethical debate because they are "facts" and hence are no longer open to social negotiation: there is only one correct way to see them. The possibilities and limitations of these arguments are discussed below.

Science as a Discursive Model

Arguably, U.S. political institutions have already incorporated some important aspects of science's discursive style into procedures for ethical deliberation. Openness and rational criticism, for example, are prized and deeply embedded features of our political discourse. Openness in particular is a feature that distinguishes our political culture from that of closely related polities like Britain's (Brickman et al., 1935; Vogel, 1986).

Science, however, shares the stage with law as one of the two dominant discursive traditions in America. These two traditions—the scientific and the legal—have consistently drawn on each other for legitimation and have in fact become closely intertwined over time. Judge David Bazelon of the D.C. Circuit Court, for example, defended the (ultimately ill-fated) notion of judicially imposed administrative procedures in the 1970s on the grounds that these would open up agency decisions to "peer review" (Bazelon, 1977). The Supreme Court in its recent decision in *Daubert v. Merrell Dow* cites peer review as a pertinent factor that courts should weigh in admitting scientific testimony (61 U.S.L.W. 4805, June 28, 1993). Equally, however, scientific bodies from the National Academy of Sciences to more specialized expert groups have adopted features of legal procedure—ideas of representation and due process, in particular—to give their opinions greater weight. Examples range from consensus development panels at NIH to the (successful) attempt by the California Medical Association to declare clinical ecology an "unscientific" theory (Jasanoff, 1991).

It may not be farfetched to argue that our public moral discourse is uniquely shaped by the confluence of scientific and legal norms of criticism. Science has supplied the authoritative model for determining what kinds of arguments may be advanced in public life, whereas the law has deeply influenced our thinking about who should be allowed to make these arguments and through what procedures. This marriage of technical rationality and political diversity sometimes produces authoritative results. Other times, however, rationality frays under critical attack from divergent viewpoints. Institutional design is the primary variable that can sway outcomes in one or the other of these two directions.

Some of the most robust institutions for addressing the ethical dimensions of biomedicine in the United States may be ones that combine the scientific tradition of rational criticism with the legal tradition of opening up expertise to scrutiny by non-experts or differently qualified experts.

"Successful" exercises in clarifying moral questions or establishing a moral consensus around biomedicine often reflect a deeper success in combining the critical resources of science and law. For instance, a hospital ethics committee may work because it opens up previously closed medical judgments to additional lay and expert viewpoints: those of nurses, administrators, religious counselors, and, of course, family members. The committee thus is an institution that democratizes expertise. At the same time, it is a forum that exposes lay values and assumptions that might otherwise have remained unexamined to questioning from other perspectives and frames of reference, including those of medical experts. Finally, it is a forum in which the specificity of the decision and the procedural rules of the game push parties toward making negotiated compromises.

Controversies about the work of ethics commissions (and public commissions more broadly) reflect our adherence to the ideals of due process as well as rationality. Thus, challenges to commissions often center on perceived violations of process values, such as inadequate representation of affected interests. As a recent reminder of the strength of these perceptions, we may recall that James Watt, former Secretary of the Interior, was forced from office because of disparaging remarks about the composition of an investigative commission. The legitimacy of commissions, in other words, seems to require the incorporation of recognized forms of political bias; to exclude relevant viewpoints—or to contest their inclusion, as Watt did—is to court public repudiation. Yet intellectual bias (with economic affiliations often taken as a convenient indicator of such bias) damages the credibility of commissions, perhaps because it negates the institutional commitment of such bodies to impartial discourse. Disqualification on grounds of intellectual bias may be the best way to describe the "voluntary" withdrawal of a member of the NAS committee on DNA fingerprinting who was felt to have inappropriately close ties to the biotechnology industry (Roberts, 1992).

The values of wide representation and technically grounded rationality are most likely to conflict in forums that employ overly formal processes of criticism. For instance, the structured, adversarial format of litigation has been shown to be considerably more effective in breaking down the bases for scientific claims than in reconstructing a set of shared factual beliefs. Accordingly, institutions that promote informal negotiation among competing viewpoints are more likely to produce consensus, or at least an unbiased airing of divergent positions, than are institutions that put their primary emphasis on conceptual clarification.

Scientists' Ethical Intuition

It is worth noting that scientists themselves have generally been eager to disavow any special sensitivity or predictive power with respect to new technologies or their social impacts. The idea that technologies are neutral at the time of their creation has many adherents in science and engineering. The corollary is the belief that it is society—not science—that imbues technology with moral overtones by deciding how inventions will be used. These beliefs may explain why suggestions by scientists like Robert Sinsheimer (1979) that certain lines of biological research may be intrinsically dangerous and should not be pursued were generally repudiated by fellow scientists.

Similarly, many geneticists and molecular biologists, including James Watson, have come to believe that the scientific community made a mistake at the 1975 Asilomar conference by seeking to prejudge the risks of recombinant DNA research. More politically sophisticated observers praise Asilomar as an important moment of self-examination but one that also happened to benefit science. The exercise was immensely effective in forestalling external regulation because it satisfied Congress for at least two decades that scientists can and do take responsibility for the consequences of their research. Yet, while many agree that Asilomar overstated the physical risks of laboratory-based recombinant DNA research, the realization has also grown that moral, social, and even environmental risks were underappreciated, possibly because of the relatively closed technical nature of the debate.

Recent scholarly writing in history, sociology, and politics has done much to dispel the notion of the neutrality of scientific discoveries and technological artifacts. In particular, we have grown used to the idea that technologies should be seen as products of social negotiation that necessarily incorporate trade-offs among competing values (Bijker et al., 1990). Technologies, particularly large and complex ones, are said to "have politics" in the sense that they presume the existence of particular social and cultural organizations for their management and control (Winner, 1986). Far from being rigidly bounded inanimate objects, modern technologies are regarded as systems in which things, people, skills, practices, institutions, and so forth are united in "networks" or "seamless webs" (Hughes, 1983; Latour, 1988). Technologies also have a fluid and changeable dimension, since they can be altered by the practices of their users. A simple example is the use of a drug that has been approved for one indication to treat another unapproved indication.

These new perspectives provide a basis for thinking that scientists may after all have special moral insights into the products of their ingenuity. By stressing features of social and cultural embeddedness, recent scholarly accounts help to read values back into science and technology. As central participants in the project of creating and applying expert knowledge, scientists necessarily participate in shaping the moral and political character of technological products. Participation in public moral discourse may help them to make their value commitments explicit, and then integrate these values into decision making. By contrast, preserving the fiction of scientific neutrality, and thus excluding scientists from full participation in ethical debate, may deprive society of an important avenue of moral criticism.

The difficulty, of course, is that the research community seems often not to be aware of the social and ethical judgments that are embedded in the practice of science or the design of technology. This is an area where feminist critiques of science have opened a discussion of the preconceptions of science (Keller, 1985; Haraway, 1989). For example, there is now general agreement that women's health issues have received disproportionately little attention in biomedical research and that study designs have often been insensitive to questions of gender and culture. One illustration is the case of clinical trials of contraceptives that assumed, inappropriately, that the characteristics of user populations in the developing countries would be the same as those in industrialized countries. Examples such as this suggest that, in order to play an effective part in public moral discourse, scientists may first need to develop a more reflective understanding of the ways in which they do science.

Facts and Values

Social and political institutions continue in hard cases to delegate to science the power to make binding ethical judgments. Such delegation often takes place in the guise of seeking a consensus on facts and then allowing these facts to dictate rules of action. Thus, medical expertise has variously been called upon to define "viability" for purposes of distinguishing lawful from unlawful abortions; to define "death" so as to guide the use of life-prolonging technologies; and to define "pre-embryos" in order to establish the limits of permissible research with the human conceptus. Building a scientific consensus around such morally loaded concepts can be a convenient way of ending disputes. Science then appears to draw a bright line that neatly separates permissible from impermissible social action. The facts provided by science constitute a seemingly objective basis for distinguishing right from wrong behavior.

Although this strategy of delegation may work well in terms of producing social harmony, we should keep in mind one or two caveats. First, as noted above, Americans are not in general given to unquestioning acceptance of the authority of science. Indeed, our legal system has been a powerful instrument for holding scientific experts accountable to lay members of the public. In part, the law accomplishes this result by making scientists speak in language that is accessible to nonexperts; this requirement has been particularly emphasized in the judicial review of agency decisions. Further, the adversarial processes of the law very effectively probe the basis for scientific claims and expose the assumptions and judgments that have gone into the production of alleged facts. Finally, our courts have in most cases refused to let legal outcomes be decided by technical consensus alone. Witness, for example, the judicial insistence that the expert's role in court is to assist the factfinder, not to make the ultimate factual assessment (see *Daubert v. Merrell Dow*, cited above).

Second, many studies of scientific controversies have called attention to the point that what passes for "fact" on either side is often a construct that incorporates clear elements of subjective judgment. The factual character of such "mixed" assertions can nevertheless be upheld through successful boundary drawing. For example, scientific advisory committees often effectively represent their views as "science" or as "fact" simply on the strength of their institutional role—which is to give factual or scientific advice (Jasanoff, 1990). If the boundaries are drawn tightly enough (e.g., when the experts are especially prestigious or closely knit), then others do not think of questioning the epistemological status of the claims advanced as "science." Accepting the boundaries that scientists draw in such instances, however, abdicates some degree of moral authority to experts. This insight has repeatedly caused U.S. policymakers to insist that important advisory bodies include lay opinions or, at the very least, a wide spectrum of scientific viewpoints.

Outlook

Summing up the three points discussed above, it is fair to say that scientists do have a special role in making ethical decisions at the frontiers of biomedicine. This role derives from their close involvement in the processes of discovery and technological innovation and their subsequent experience in monitoring and utilizing technologies in a health care context. Yet for scientists to play their ethical part most effectively, they need to be involved in forums that open up their perspectives and underlying assumptions to critical evaluation. Scientific advice will tend to be least ethically sensitive when it is offered as unexamined "fact." It may advance social decisions most in a context that forces scientists to become aware of their own value commitments. For such reflexivity to become routine among scientists working in changing areas of biomedicine, it may be necessary to broaden scientists' training to include formal work on the social and ethical foundations of scientific knowledge and practice.

HEALTH CARE PROFESSIONAL EDUCATION

Origins

Many of the improvements that make modern medicine so powerful in treating patients have resulted directly from the advances in our understanding of disease processes made possible by biomedical research efforts. These advances are rapidly incorporated into the education of health care professionals in science-intensive curricula. The pressure of the ever-increasing scientific content of the medical school curriculum, as well as the emphasis on a mechanistic, reductionist model of disease, important for the students' understanding of modern diseases, threatens to force the teachings about caring for the emotional and psychological stresses on the patients with the diseases into a back seat.

Although many health care professionals believed that the formal teaching of ethics was unnecessary, progress was being made to include ethics courses in the curriculum, frequently as an elective. The Society for Health and Human Values, founded in 1968, established a program through which consultations were provided to medical schools interested in initiating courses aimed at exploring the ethical and human values dimensions of the health care enterprise. Throughout the following decade, faculty trained in the humanities began to appear in gradually increasing numbers on medical school faculties.

In 1984, the Association of American Medical Colleges (AAMC) released a *Report on the General Professional Education of the Physician and College Preparation for Medicine* (GPEP), in response to what was perceived as a continuing and even accelerating erosion of the general education for physicians (Muller, 1984). This forward-looking report was aimed at helping the profession (and ultimately the patient) accommodate to the rapid advances that were occurring in biomedical science and technology, including the more complex and potentially more onerous treatments that were emerging. It also called attention to social, environmental, and life-style determinants of poor health status and increasing burdens of illness— issues that in the previous two decades had been overshadowed by medicine's focus on technology (Muller, 1984). GPEP's ethical dimension is captured in the introduction, written by chair Steven Muller:

> We believe that every physician should be caring, compassionate, and dedicated to patients—to keeping them well and to helping them when they are ill. Each should be committed to work, to learning, to rationality, to science, and to serving the greater society. Ethical sensitivity and moral integrity, combined with equanimity, humility, and self-knowledge, are quite essential qualities of all physicians.

It comes as no surprise that the first recommendation of the report was for a general professional education of the physician in which medical faculties emphasize the acquisition and development of social skills, personal values, and attitudes by students at least to the same extent as they emphasize the acquisition of technical knowledge. Unfortunately, the report had little early detectable effect on the medical curriculum.

Sociologist Renee Fox has noted the repeated, unsuccessful calls for such changes in medical education. In a penetrating article (1990), Fox explored the origins and possible remedies for the lack of broader social awareness among physicians. A highly analytic, logico-rational way of thinking and viewing the world, which produces a chain of dichotomies (mind versus body, thought versus feeling, objective versus subjective, self versus other, and individual versus social), is evident in the medical curriculum in, for example, considerations of biomedical versus psychosocial components. A second source of difficulty in developing caring competence in physicians is the "dehumanizing" and "brutalizing" effect of medical education on students. Medical students may experience these effects when they confront human suffering without sufficient mentoring, on exhausting schedules, and in the face of the scientific determinism and reductionism that characterizes molecular biology. Fox suggested several strategies for making medical education and, ultimately, medical care, more humanistic:

- more awareness of how biomedicine is imprinted with dichotomies that split competence from caring;
- more attention to the cognitive content of medicine;
- more attention to the defense mechanisms developed during training and their implications for humane competence;
- more effort to ensuring felicitous timing for training experiences; and
- a return by teachers to firsthand teaching.

As medical education has evolved to encompass ethics, a similar process has occurred in the other health professions. In 1983, for example, the American Dental Association (ADA) established a number of guidelines to serve as the ethical basis of the profession. The ADA Committee on the Future of Dentistry recommended that methods be designed to assess attitudes and interpersonal skills of dental school applicants and to identify values, preferences, and goals of recent dental graduates (ADA, 1983). In response to these two efforts, dental educator Muriel Bebeau designed a curriculum based on real-life ethical problems to help dental students identify, reason about, and adequately resolve ethical problems in the dental profession. Other schools have modeled programs using her insights.

Nursing schools have also developed educational programs in ethics. A 1986 report of the American Association of Colleges of Nursing (AACN) identified "essential" values to be addressed in the curriculum of nursing ethics: these are altruism, equality, aesthetics, freedom, human dignity, justice, and truth (AACN, 1986).

While some of the social and ethical issues facing doctors, dentists, and nurses are unique to their specific medical disciplines, the health professions share many of the same concerns. Possible goals of ethics education programs reflect those common issues:

- To promote understanding of one's own moral positions as well as understanding and tolerance toward views of others in our pluralistic society.
- To recognize ethical issues in medical practice and biomedical research, to improve skills for critical reasoning and analysis, and to influence in a positive manner the health care professional's moral maturity (Self, 1988; Bickel, 1991, 1993; Culver et al., 1985).
- To promote health care professionals' social responsibilities to patients and the public, in other words, to aid the individual professional in understanding his/her role within the rest of the society, thus encouraging individual professional activity within the legitimate constraints of social institutions and community values.
- To understand the relationship between ill health and the social context of disease (Tarlov, 1992; Maheux et al., 1990).

A 1987 AAMC survey of the medical ethics curricula, "Integrating Human Values Teaching Programs Into Medical Students' Clinical Education," examined 113 course descriptions from the 1984–1985 school year and 99 completed surveys from the 126 medical schools contacted. Ninety-five schools (84 percent) required students to complete a human values course in the first two years, while 38 schools (34 percent) required such a course in the last two years. Developments since 1980 included a reinforcement or addition of human values emphasis during clerkships, addition of one or more required human values courses into year one or two, enhancement of human values emphasis in existing preclinical courses, and improved integration of human values programs. The report finds that ethics education often becomes integrated into the traditional curriculum in definable stages, moving from preclinical courses given by humanities and/or social sciences faculty, to subspecialty conferences and ethic rounds, to more formal presentations and participation by the faculty in clinical education of clerks and residents, to more formal commitments from clinical departments and school administration. Barriers to integration of ethics education into the curriculum include funding constraints, emphasis on memorizing material rather than reflecting on it, competing faculty priorities, departmental segregation, nonoptimal inpatient teaching environment (e.g., shorter hospital stays), lack of role models, and the dehumanizing aspects of medical education. The report also notes the need to develop further mechanisms to improve human values education for residents.

More recent studies have attempted to define goals and basic curricula in medical ethics for medical students (Culver et al., 1985), for clinicians and ethics committee members (Thornton et al., 1993), and for internists

(ABIM, 1983). The Kennedy Institute has published a survey of the literature in this area (Coutts, 1991).

Contributions

Table 3-1 demonstrates the great number of medical schools that are teaching courses related to ethical and social concerns, as well as the diversity of curricular approaches to ethics-related topics. The variation in approaches may be related to the resources available at each school, as well as to the diversified subject matter, goals, and interests of the faculty.

Do such curricular additions have any impact on the individuals in training? The work of Lawrence Kohlberg (1980, 1984) supports the idea that moral reasoning ability is facilitated by exposing individuals to dilemmas that challenge one's current level of moral reasoning skills. Other studies reveal that moral development continues throughout formal education and can be dramatic in early adulthood (the time of professional training), and that well-developed educational interventions can enhance ethical consciousness and commitment (Rest, 1988; Blasi, 1980; Josephson, 1988; Leming, 1981).

TABLE 3-1 Number of U.S. and Canadian Medical Schools Teaching Selected Topics as Required Course Material (n = 139[a])

Topics	Part of Existing Course, Required	Separate Course, Required	Do Not Offer	Data Not Available
Computer applications in medicine	92	7	18	15
Cost containment	117	2	9	9
Death and dying	127	4	1	4
Domestic violence	95	0	23	18
History of medicine	53	10	38	25
Law and medicine (medical jurisprudence)	85	17	21	21
Literature and medicine	40	2	52	37
Long-term health care	105	7	9	17
Medical ethics	83	56	0	3
Physician–patient relationship	117	15	0	4
Termination of pregnancy	106	1	21	9

[a]Data for the four University of Illinois schools (Chicago, Peoria, Rockford, and Urbana-Champaign) were tallied individually. Six of the 145 (126 U.S., 16 Canadian, and 3 Puerto Rican) medical schools did not respond and are not included in this table.

SOURCE: Adapted from Association of American Medical Colleges (AAMC) Curriculum Directory, 1992–93 (21st Edition). Washington, D.C.: AAMC.

REFERENCES

American Association of Colleges of Nursing (AACN). 1986. *Essentials of College and University Education for Professional Nursing.* Washington, D.C.: AACN.

American Board of Internal Medicine (ABIM). 1983. Subcommittee on evaluation of the humanistic qualities in the internist. *Annals of Internal Medicine* 99(5):720–724.

American Dental Association (ADA). 1983. *Strategic Plan Report of the ADA Special Committee on the Future of Dentistry: Issue Papers on Dental Research, Manpower, Education, Practice and Public and Professional Concerns and Recommendations for Action.* Chicago, Il.: ADA.

Bazelon, D. 1977. Coping with technology through the legal process. *Cornell Law Review* 62:823.

Bebeau, M.J. 1985. Teaching ethics in dentistry. *Journal of Dental Education* 49: 236–243.

Bickel, J. 1991. Medical students' professional ethics: Defining the problems and developing the resources. *Academic Medicine* 66:726–729.

Bickel, J. 1993. *Promoting Medical Students' Ethical Development: A Resource Guide.* Washington, D.C.: Association of American Medical Colleges.

Bijker, W.E., Hughes, T.P., and Pinch, T., eds. 1990. *The Social Construction of Technological Systems.* Cambridge, MA: Massachusetts Institute of Technology Press.

Blasi, A. 1980. Bridging moral cognition and moral action: A critical review of the literature. *Psychological Bulletin* 88:1–45.

Brickman, R., Jasanoff, S., and Ilgen, T. 1985. *Controlling Chemicals: The Politics of Regulation in Europe and the United States.* Ithaca, NY: Cornell University Press.

Coutts, M.C. 1991. *Teaching Ethics in the Health Care Setting (Scope Note 16).* Washington, D.C.: National Reference Center for Bioethics Literature, Kennedy Institute of Ethics, Georgetown University.

Culver, C.M., Clouser, K.D., Gert, B., Brody, H., Fletcher, J., Jonsen, A., Kopelman, L., Lynn, J., Siegler, M., and Wikler, D. 1985. Basic curricular goals in medical ethics. *New England Journal of Medicine* 312(4):253–256.

Daubert v. Merril Dow, 61 U.S.L.W. 4805, June 28, 1993.

Fletcher, J. 1954. *Morals and Medicine: The Moral Problems of the Patients Right to Know the Truth, Contraception, and Artificial Insemination, Sterilization, Euthanasia.* Princeton, NJ: Princeton University Press.

Fox, R.C. 1990. Training in Caring and Competence. In: *Educating Competent and Humane Physicians.* H.C. Hendrie and C. Lloyd, eds. Bloomington, IN: Indiana University Press.

Haraway, D. 1989. *Primate Visions: Gender, Race, and Nature in the World of Modern Science.* London: Routledge.

Hare, R.M. 1977. Can the moral philosopher help? In: *Philosophical Medical Ethics,* S. Spicker and H.T. Engelhardt, eds. Boston, MA: Reidel.

Hughes, T.P. 1983. *Networks of Power- Electrification in Western Society, 1880–1930.* Baltimore, MD: Johns Hopkins University Press.

Jasanoff, S. 1990. *The Fifth Branch: Science Advisors as Policymakers.* Cambridge, MA: Harvard University Press.

Jasanoff, S. 1991. Judicial Construction of New Scientific Evidence. In: *Critical Perspectives on Nonacademic Science and Engineering.* P.T. Durbin (ed.). Bethlehem, PA: Lehigh University Press.

Josephson, M. 1988. Teaching ethical decision making and principled reasoning. *Ethics: Easier Said Than Done* (Winter):27–33.

Keller, E.F. 1985. *Reflections on Gender and Science.* New Haven, CT: Yale University Press.

Kohlberg, L. 1980. Stages of Moral Development as a Basis for Moral Education. In: *Moral Development, Moral Education, and Kohlberg.* B. Munsey, ed. Birmingham, AL: Religious Education Press.

Kohlberg, L. 1984. *Essays on Moral Development.* San Francisco, CA: Harper and Row.

Latour, B. 1988. *The Pasteurization of France.* Cambridge, MA: Harvard University Press.

Leming, J.S. 1981. Curricular effectiveness in moral/values education: A review of research. *Journal of Moral Education* 10:147–164.

Maheux, B., Delorme, P., Beland, F., and Beaudry, J. 1990. Humanism in medical education: A study of educational needs perceived by trainees of three Canadian schools. *Academic Medicine* 65:41–45.

Merton, R.K. 1973. The Normative Structure of Science. Reprinted in: *The Sociology of Science.* R.K. Merton. Chicago: University of Chicago Press.

Muller, S. 1984. Physicians for the twenty-first century: Report of the Project Panel on the General Professional Education of the Physician and College Preparation for Medicine. *Journal of Medical Education* 59(2):5–27.

Percival, T. 1927. *Medical Ethics,* C.D. Leake, ed. Baltimore: Williams and Wilkins.

President's Commission for the Study of Ethical Issues in Medicine and Biomedical and Behavioral Research. 1982. *Compensating for Research Injury.* Washington, D.C.: U.S. Government Printing Office.

Ramsey, P. 1970. The Patient as Person: Explorations in Medical Ethics. The Lyman Beecher Lecture. Yale University. Books Demand. Reproduction of 1970 ed.

Rest, J.R. 1988. Can ethics be taught in professional schools? The psychological research. *Ethics: Easier Said Than Done* (Winter):22–26.

Roberts, L. 1992. Science in court: A culture clash. *Science* 257:732–736.

Self, D.J. 1988. The pedagogy of two different approaches to humanistic medical education: Cognitive and affective. *Theoretical Medicine* 9(2):227–236.

Sinsheimer, R.L. 1979. The presumptions of science. In: *Limits of Scientific Inquiry,* G. Holton and R.S. Morison, eds. New York: W.W. Norton.

Sperry, W. 1948. Moral problems in the practice of medicine. *New England Journal of Medicine* 239:985–990.

Tarlov, A.R. 1992. The coming influence of a social sciences perspective on medical education. *Academic Medicine* 67:724–731.

Thornton, B.C., Callahan, D., and Nelson, J.L. 1993. Bioethics education: Expanding the circle of participants. *Hastings Center Report* (January–February):15–29.

Vogel, D. 1986. *National Styles of Regulation.* Ithaca, NY: Cornell University Press.

Winner, L. 1986. Do Artifacts Have Politics? In: *The Whale and the Reactor.* Chicago: University of Chicago Press.

4

The Spectrum of Societal Responses

Public moral discourse on bioethics has been fostered in a variety of ways in the United States. Some of the mechanisms described in this chapter entail the formation of a group of persons, as in grassroots organizations, while others relate to the activities of long-established social institutions, such as the legal system. Each mechanism offers distinctive capacities and limitations, and together they shed light from many perspectives on the complicated process of public deliberation of ethical issues. This chapter summarizes salient features and activities of some of the more prominent of these institutions.

Past social responses to ethical quandaries in biomedicine have succeeded in a variety of ways. For example, many public commissions, at the minimum, have enlisted outstanding scholars to contribute their insights on the issue of concern. Many of the products of these commissions have been viewed as authoritative and have had a substantial impact on policy decisions, as for example occurred in the cases of defining brain death and establishing standards for human experimentation. These and other similar examples are described later in this chapter.

Commissions and other deliberative bodies operate in a world where deadlines, personalities, and special interests converge. The necessity for compromise is unavoidable. Many products of these commissions have stood the test of time and continue to have a prominent role in education for health professionals and ethicists. Hospital ethics committees, for example, are often able to soften advocacy of patient interest in order to gain the willing participation of health care providers (Hoffman, 1991). While the committee does not attempt in this report to perform a comprehensive assessment of the performance of every social mechanism for deliberation of ethical issues, one of the background papers in this volume by Gray does assess some of the accomplishments, determinants of success, and views of participants in the National Commission and President's Commission. The accomplishments of other deliberative bodies described in this chapter are outlined in greater detail in Appendix A.

The social and institutional context within which bioethics deliberation takes place was described in Chapter 2. In this chapter, we are concerned with the vast array of specific responses and mechanisms that facilitate the public deliberation of ethical issues in biomedicine. Whether, and to what extent, the activities of these various groups and institutions have been effective is a separate question that receives attention in Chapter 5, where criteria for evaluating the effectiveness of the work of these bodies are set forth.

For organizational purposes, this chapter categorizes ethics bodies according to their source of sponsorship or authority: political and legal (e.g., federal commissions), professional and institutional (e.g., institutional review boards), or grassroots (e.g., individual and community initiatives). It will become obvious, however, that there is significant overlap in the functions served by the different mechanisms, an overlap that defies neat categorization. In some cases, there are functional similarities between mechanisms that have significant structural differences and operate in separate societal spheres. The mechanisms have been created to fulfill numerous functions—some very general, some quite specific, many interrelated—including the following:

- to bring to the larger public the opportunity and the responsibility (that previously belonged to elite groups) to define ethical issues;
- to identify ethical issues at stake in areas of societal controversy;
- to undertake a careful analysis of an issue;
- to develop and/or document areas of consensus;
- to expose and document areas of disagreement;
- to unify the expertise of authorities from a wide variety of relevant fields;
- to represent competing interests;
- to generate public awareness and debate;
- to be a lightning rod for public concern;
- to educate;
- to correct misunderstandings and errors in reasoning;
- to develop factual bases for public policy;
- to offer guidance for decision making;
- to develop recommendations for action;

- to recommend new legislation or changes or improvements in existing public policy;
  - to sanction delays or recommend unpopular policies;
  - to dignify and legitimize official action;
  - to overcome bureaucratic obstacles; and
  - to justify the expenditure of money.

The functions served by a particular mechanism or group may be dictated by a sponsor's mandate, or, as is frequently the case, be simply incidental. For example, a group convened to recommend legislation on a controversial issue may be unable to reach agreement on a plan of legislative action but, in the course of its work, may succeed at educating members of society and perhaps even at reducing controversy by clarifying various viewpoints. Finally, experience has shown that what is ultimately achieved through public deliberation often depends more on the particular issue and on societal circumstances than on the intended outcome of the deliberation.

POLITICAL AND LEGAL MECHANISMS

It is not surprising—at least in democratic societies—that governments should look for means to address the ethical and social consequences of biomedical research, since research is heavily supported and encouraged by government as a means of advancing human welfare. Yet during the 20 years following the Nuremburg tribunal, neither governments nor professional bodies paid more than glancing attention to the actual or potential problems inherent in the activities and discoveries of biomedical scientists. During this period, no framework existed for judging when, how, and for what reasons the government should get involved, nor was there a means for determining which developments in the life sciences might pose significant problems.

Beginning in the late 1960s, however, the first steps were taken toward sustained examination of the ethical and social effects of the processes and products of biomedical research. In 1966, for example, Surgeon General William H. Stewart promulgated rules for peer examination of the ethics of research protocols at Public Health Service grantee institutions (U.S. Public Health Service, 1966). In 1968, the Government Research Subcommittee of the Senate Committee on Government Operations held hearings on a joint resolution sponsored by Senator Walter Mondale to establish a National Advisory Commission on Health Science and Society (National Commission on Health Science and Society, 1968). After the Ad Hoc Task Force on Cardiac Replacement of the National Heart Institute acknowledged that this new technology had ethical and social implications that should be explored (1969), Dr. Theodore Cooper, then Director of the National Heart Institute, appointed the Artificial Heart Assessment Panel, which issued the first major government report on the ethical implications of new technologies (1973).

Commissions Established by Congress

When Senator Mondale initially proposed a commission, the first human-to-human heart transplants had just been performed, and his intention was for the commission to address ethical issues in biomedical developments and human subjects research. Over the next several years, further developments in human reproduction (such as in vitro fertilization), neuroscience, behavioral medicine, and control of lethal diseases underscored the need for a commission. Yet it was scandal in the research process rather than the worrisome products of research that apparently convinced the U.S. Congress to establish the first national commission on bioethics. In the wake of the revelation in 1972 of the Tuskegee Syphilis Study, the Senate Committee on Labor and Public Welfare held further hearings into research abuses in state mental facilities and prisons (Senate Committee on Labor and Public Welfare, 1973). The hearings were chaired by Senator Edward Kennedy, whose family has long been interested in issues affecting retarded persons and whose family foundation had recently established one of the first "bioethics" centers at Georgetown University.

National Commission

As a result of these hearings, provisions were included in the National Research Act of 1974 (P.L. 93-348) to create the National Commission for the Protection of Human Subjects of Biomedical and Behavioral Research (National Commission), as well as to require that Public Health Service (PHS) grantee institutions establish institutional review boards (IRBs) to review the ethics of research projects carried out by their employees. Although Senator Mondale's proposed examination of the ethical and social implications of medical developments was incorporated as a special study for the National Commission, the body's primary mandate was to make recommendations for the ethical conduct of research, including research that involved various vulnerable populations.

The National Commission, which functioned from 1974 to 1978, was appointed by the Secretary of Health, Education, and Welfare and operated within that department (DHEW). It was made up of 11 members, all from outside the federal government: three physicians (one of whom was elected chair of the body), two psychologists, three lawyers, two professors of ethics, and one civic leader. Their work was aided by a professional and support staff of 12 and further assisted by a number of consultants from medicine, philosophy, law, and the social and natural sciences. The public was allowed access to the commission's deliberations, as well as to draft papers; the commission also held several public hearings and made site visits. During its four years, the National Commission issued ten reports: five dealt with special groups of subjects (fetuses, prisoners, children, patients undergoing psychosurgery, and the institutionalized mentally infirm); two dealt with research review (reports on IRBs and on disclosure of information under the Freedom of Information Act); one provided ethical guidelines for delivery of health services by DHEW; and one reported the results of the "special study" (the implications of research advances, the topic inherited from the Mondale bill).

The best-known of the National Commission's reports was the *Belmont Report* (1978a), which abstracted the general principles for protection of research subjects that lay behind its other reports on particular aspects of biomedical and behavioral research. It set forth three comprehensive principles to "serve as a basic justification for the many practical ethical prescriptions and evaluation of human actions": (1) respect for persons, (2) beneficence, and (3) justice. Respect for persons requires that individuals be treated as autonomous agents, while persons with diminished autonomy are entitled to protection. Beneficence calls not only for protecting individuals from harm, but also for making efforts to secure their well-being.[1] Justice relates to fairness in distribution of the benefits and burdens of research. The commission's provision of these explicit principles for the analysis of ethical issues in language that was clear and accessible to a lay audience enabled the general public to engage in informed and effective discussion of such issues, and opened up a whole new field for public discourse.

The recommendations in the commission's report on fetal research were made in May 1975 and were quickly translated into proposed federal regulations. In that instance, DHEW's need for regulations was at least as important in provoking a rapid response as was the commission's statutory "action-forcing power" (i.e., the secretary had to either accept the commission's recommendations or make public the reasons for rejection). Not all of the commission's recommendations were as influential, however, and while its core points provided the basis for what are now government-wide regulations on human subjects research, several of the reports had little influence. For example, DHEW did not respond to the commission's report on the institutionalized mentally infirm (1978c). But in light of the novel nature of this enterprise, the work of the commission was impressive:

---

[1] While the *Belmont Report* did not employ the term "non-maleficence" (to do no harm), the language it employed makes it clear that it encompasses this notion in the discussion of beneficence.

its products met high standards of intellectual rigor, and the papers it commissioned from major scholarly figures catalyzed the study of bioethics as noted scholars became actively involved in addressing these issues.

President's Commission

The statute establishing the National Commission suggested that, at the conclusion of its term, a standing National Council for the Protection of Human Subjects would be established to carry its work forward. Instead, in 1978 the Congress authorized the President's Commission for the Study of Ethical Problems in Medicine and Biomedical and Behavioral Research (President's Commission), thereby combining Senator Kennedy's interest in elevating the National Commission above the departmental level with the desire of Representative Paul Rogers and his colleagues on the House Health Subcommittee that the successor body take on topics beyond research with human subjects (P.L. 95-622). In addition to requiring biennial reports on the latter topic, Congress mandated that the President's Commission also report on the ethical and legal aspects of determining death, informed consent, confidentiality and privacy, genetic issues, and disparities in access to health care.

While the National Commission had been quickly appointed, the President's Commission was not sworn in for 14 months after the passage of its authorizing statute. Like the National Commission, membership in the President's Commission was divided into several categories: three from biomedical or behavioral research (initially a professor of human genetics, a professor of psychiatry, and a molecular biologist), three from the practice of medicine (a general internist, a cardiologist, and a pediatrician), and five from other fields (a medical economist, a medical sociologist, a professor of law, a professor of ethics, and a lawyer who was appointed by the president to chair the commission). Two commissioners (the professors of ethics and law) had served on the National Commission, although one had to resign almost immediately when she was appointed to a high position in the federal government. Two other commissioners resigned later, and seven others were replaced as their terms expired, so that 21 people in total served on the President's Commission. The staff usually numbered about 20 (including 6 in support positions), but several of the professional staff (a total of 23 individuals over the life of the commission) served for only a year while on leave from academic positions. Additionally, 16 students (primarily from medicine, law, and philosophy) served as Congressional Fellows and interns.

Part of the delay in appointing the original commissioners apparently resulted from political friction between the White House and Congress. The executive branch was slow to choose the commissioners, and even after they had been named in the summer of 1979, the commission could not begin its work because no funds had been requested (or appropriated) for it in the FY 1980 budget. When pressed to "reprogram" monies from other activities, the leadership of DHEW eventually complied, but only after deciding that it would end operation of its Ethics Advisory Board (EAB) on the grounds that the President's Commission made the EAB redundant (see below) and then transferred the funds originally allocated for the EAB to the President's Commission (1983d).

The commission's statute included a "sunset" clause with a termination date of December 31, 1982. In 1982, Senator Kennedy proposed that the date be changed to 1984, but a provision of the December 1982 Continuing Resolution (P.L. 97-377) extended the commission only through March 31, 1983.

During its 39 months, the President's Commission issued 17 volumes, consisting of 10 reports (several with one or more appendix volumes), the proceedings of a workshop on policies and procedures for responding to reports of scientific misconduct (*Whistleblowing in Biomedical Research,* 1981), and a loose-leaf book (*The Official IRB Guidebook*). Five of the reports dealt with health care issues; four of these responded to the commission's statutory mandate: *Defining Death* (1981), *Making Health Care Decisions* (1982a), *Screening and Counseling for Genetic Conditions* (1983b), and *Securing Access to Health Care* (1983c). The fifth, *Deciding to Forego Life-Sustaining Treatment* (1983a), grew out of the studies on determining death, informed consent, and access to care. Four reports dealt with biomedical and behavioral research, including the subject of human genetic engineering (at the request of the president's science advisor) and compensation for research injuries (at the request of the EAB, shortly before its demise). Finally, on March 31, 1983, as it closed its doors, the commission issued a last report, entitled *Summing Up,* that provided an overview of its work and that addressed the one topic (privacy and confidentiality) in its original statutory mandate that had not been the subject of a separate report (1983d).

Biomedical Ethics Board

The third major congressionally chartered bioethics effort was less fortunate than its predecessors. Following 1982 hearings on the President's Commission report, *Splicing Life* (1982b), then-Representative Albert Gore, Jr., proposed the establishment of a presidential commission on genetic engineering, a proposal that was later broadened to include other bioethical issues. Because of differences in viewpoint between Senate conservatives and House liberals over what would result if another presidential bioethics panel were authorized (Cook-Deegan, 1994), Congress in 1985 chose to locate the successor within the legislative branch. A Biomedical

Ethics Board (BEB) was authorized through September 30, 1988, to be composed of six Senators and six Representatives (equally divided between the two major parties) (P.L. 99-158). The BEB was responsible for appointing a 14-member Biomedical Ethics Advisory Committee (BEAC) made up of experts from law, medicine, research, and ethics, as well as members of the general public. The BEAC was instructed to begin its work by studying three topics: human genetic engineering, fetal research, and food and fluids for dying patients (see Appendix A for a further description of the BEAC).

From the outset, politics—especially the sharp division in Congress over the abortion issue—complicated the operation of the BEB and the BEAC. It took nearly a year to choose the 12-member BEB and another 30 months of internal wrangling before BEB members could agree on 14 people for the BEAC; one of the 14 died before the BEAC could even hold its first meeting. Congress passed a two-year extension and an appropriation for FY 1989, but withheld authority to meet or to expend funds until the BEB agreed upon a new chair (which with the start of the 101st Congress had shifted from the House back to the Senate) and named a replacement for the BEAC member who had died. The BEB was unable to do so, and the BEAC had no further sessions after its second meeting in February 1989. It issued no reports, its staff departed by the end of FY 1989, and its mandate expired on September 30, 1990.

Ethics Bodies in the Executive Branch

Ethics Advisory Board, DHEW

Among the recommendations of the National Commission was the establishment of a group within DHEW to provide ethical advice regarding proposals that involved particularly sensitive types of research. This recommendation became a part of the department's regulations (45 C.F.R. 46), and in September 1977 Secretary Joseph Califano appointed a 14-member Ethics Advisory Board to review problematic protocols that required special scrutiny under the human subjects regulations (e.g., problematic protocols having to do with more than minimal risk for nonconsenting subjects). The group had a distinguished interdisciplinary membership (see Appendix A for further description of the EAB).

Between 1978 and 1980, the EAB's principal work was to produce a major report on *Research Involving Human In Vitro Fertilization and Embryo Transfer* (May 4, 1979), which came in response to an approved application for NIH support of research that would have used in vitro fertilization (IVF) in basic research. The EAB also conducted two inquiries in response to requests from NIH and the Centers for Disease Control for legislative recommendations that would provide for limited exemptions from the

Freedom of Information Act. At the time it was disbanded in 1980, it had also embarked on a study of another policy topic—compensation for research injuries—that had previously been examined by a DHEW task force (U.S. Department of Health, Education, and Welfare, 1977).

The EAB did creditable work, but for several reasons it remains at best a footnote in the history of public bioethics. First, its report on IVF was delivered to Dr. Califano's successor, Patricia Harris, who had little interest in the field. Neither she nor any of her successors have officially accepted or rejected the EAB's recommendations. Second, although the department's regulations continue to provide for the existence of an EAB, Secretary Harris disbanded the existing body due to what was perceived as duplication with the President's Commission, even though the EAB focused on intra-agency issues and the commission on broad, national issues. Finally, the lack of an EAB allowed the Reagan and Bush administrations to avoid approving any research with human embryos or tissues between 1981 and 1992, during some of which time explicit moratoria on such research were written into various congressional bills.

Recombinant DNA Advisory Committee, NIH

In 1975, the Director of NIH established a Recombinant DNA Advisory Committee (RAC). This committee and its implementing regulations were a response to the conclusions reached at a meeting held at the Asilomar Conference Center in California under the sponsorship of the National Academy of Sciences. The meeting addressed the concerns that had led several leading molecular biologists to call for an international moratorium on certain classes of laboratory research using newly developed methods of cutting and splicing DNA. As a result of the meeting, the scientists in attendance voted to lift the moratorium and adopted certain procedures for their research, including developing means to carry it out more safely. Since some members of Congress seemed to believe that these methods of self-regulation by scientists might be too self-interested, NIH Director Donald Fredrickson broadened the membership of the RAC to include nonscientists.

The primary concern of the RAC in its first years was laboratory safety; thereafter, it began to confront issues involved with commercial development of recombinant techniques and release of altered organisms into the environment. While ethical issues were inherent in such deliberations, the major focus was on technical concerns about the relative riskiness of particular microorganisms, with or without genetic alteration. In response to the 1982 report of the President's Commission, *Splicing Life,* the RAC decided to address ethical issues more intensely by appointing a task force on human gene therapy, subsequently modified into a standing Subcommit-

tee on Human Gene Therapy. This body eventually established the bench-
marks for review and approval of protocols to apply the techniques of gene
transfer to human beings in a set of "Points to Consider," which was first
issued in 1988 and subsequently modified on a number of occasions. For
several years, protocols were reviewed first by the subcommittee and then
by the RAC; by 1992, it was decided that, since the RAC was devoting most
of its own time to human gene protocols, the subcommittee's work was
redundant and all proposals would come directly to RAC. On all matters,
the RAC is advisory to the Director of NIH, who publishes the committee's
recommendations in the course of announcing which studies have been
approved for NIH funding or sponsorship.

The RAC is a multidisciplinary committee, a majority of whose members are physicians and scientists who work in some aspect of molecular
biology or genetics. The committee also includes lawyers, social scientists,
ethicists, and members of the general public with an interest in genetic
disease. Although traditionally chaired by one of its scientific members,
the current chair is an ethicist with long involvement in genetic engineering issues. As a federal advisory committee, its meetings are announced in
the *Federal Register* and are open to the public; when important new scientific projects are before the committee for review, media attention is often
intense and the group's recommendations are given extensive coverage.

At the present time, the protocols that come before the RAC usually
involve the transfer of genes to serve as markers on cells being administered in experimental therapies or to enhance the effectiveness of various
immunological methods of fighting diseases like cancer and AIDS; in addition, some studies involving gene transfer to treat single-gene diseases have
been approved. Beyond such somatic cell gene therapy, the "Points to
Consider" state that the RAC will not now entertain proposals for gene
transfers that would affect germ-line cells. In light of developments in
molecular genetics, it may soon become necessary to consider when (if
ever), under what conditions, and for what reasons it would be appropriate
to broaden gene therapy to germ-line cells, or for purposes of genetic
enhancement. No attention has been given to such issues because RAC
meetings for several years have been absorbed with protocols under the
existing guidelines. At its September 1993 meeting, however, the RAC
placed these issues on its agenda for the coming year (see Appendix for
further description of the RAC).

*Ethical, Legal, and Social Implications (ELSI) Working Group,
NCHGR and DOE*

The Ethical, Legal, and Social Implications (ELSI) Working Group was
founded in 1988 at the National Center for Human Genome Research

(NCHGR) of NIH. The U.S. Department of Energy (DOE) joined in support of the ELSI Working Group in 1989. Having recognized that the capabilities arising out of the Human Genome Initiative are likely to have a profound impact on individuals and society, NIH created the ELSI Working Group to explore such issues as fairness in the use of genetic information with respect to insurance, employment, and the criminal justice system; privacy of genetic information; and the influence of genetic information on reproductive decisions (see Appendix A and the background paper by Hanna in this volume for further descriptions of the ELSI Working Group).

Today, a sizable portion of the budgets for both NCHGR and DOE (from 3 to 5 percent) is formally designated to support studies on the identification and examination of these broader impacts of genetic science. This seems to be the first instance in which a portion of a science budget has been devoted specifically to the study of the ethical, legal, and social impacts of science. In all other instances, we have allowed the technology to develop and to be applied, and the resulting ethical, legal, and social dilemmas to arise, and then attempted to resolve them largely in retrospect.

The impact of the ELSI program is not yet clear. Arguments that it is overly academic and not adequately representative of society merit consideration (see Hanna, this volume). At the same time, however, many observers and even some critics seem to agree that the ELSI program is indeed stimulating effective ethical inquiries into genetic technologies and encouraging the molecular biology community to design their technological studies accordingly. Such an effect would be of great benefit to the genome project, and the success of this earmarked ELSI funding program could serve as a very useful model for other areas of science.

Human Fetal Tissue Transplantation Research Panel, DHHS

The NIH Human Fetal Tissue Transplantation Research Panel was convened in 1988 at the request of Assistant Secretary for Health Robert Windom. Following discussions with NIH Director James Wyngaarden about proposed research that involved the transplantation of human fetal neural tissue into patients with Parkinson's disease, Dr. Windom requested that a panel be formed to investigate the issue and formulated ten questions the panel was to address. Wyngaarden believed that the research was extremely important, but that it also had the potential to stir controversy and perhaps even to send a message to the public that NIH encouraged abortions (Childress, 1991). Windom responded to Wyngaarden's concerns by issuing a moratorium on the use of fetal tissue in federally funded transplantation research until NIH could convene a panel to deliberate the issue and offer recommendations.

In the summer of 1988, the 21-member Human Fetal Tissue Transplantation Research Panel was appointed. Nominations were submitted by members of Congress and the executive branch, and by other interested parties; categories for nominations included ethicists, lawyers, biomedical researchers, physicians, public policy experts, and clergy. The panel selection process was closely watched by outsiders on both sides of the abortion debate. Retired federal judge Arlin Adams, appointed as chairman of the panel by an internal NIH committee, was a Republican who was opposed to abortion.

When the panel met for the first time in September 1988, it was asked to respond to ten questions pertaining to the ethical implications of fetal tissue transplantation research. Concerns about the source of the tissue to be used in such research—elective abortions—figured heavily in these questions. For example:

- Is it morally relevant whether the source of tissue is from an induced or spontaneous abortion?
- Does the use of the fetal tissue in research encourage women to have an abortion that they might not otherwise undertake?
- Should there be and could there be a prohibition on the donation of fetal tissue between family members, or friends and acquaintances? (NIH, 1988).

In the course of this three-day meeting it became apparent that a single meeting did not allow sufficient time to address such complex and controversial issues. The panel had also intended to meet in executive session, but amidst vigorous public outcry it was decided that panel deliberations would be open to the public. At the September meeting, the panel heard from more than 50 invited speakers, as well as from representatives of various interest groups. The panel held a second meeting in October and a third in December, at which it prepared its final report to the assistant secretary. Volume 1 contained responses to the ten questions, along with panel members' votes on each question; a summary of the current scientific literature relevant to human fetal tissues transplantation research; three concurring statements; two dissenting statements; and a final dissenting letter. Volume 2 of the report contained text of the testimony submitted to the panel.

The majority of panel members (17 out of 21) voted in favor of permitting fetal tissue transplantation research, provided that a woman's decision to abort be kept carefully separated from research. The panel's report was unanimously approved by the Advisory Committee to the NIH Director, which urged acceptance of its recommendations, including the lifting of the moratorium on federal funding of fetal tissue transplantation research utilizing tissue from induced abortions, and the development of additional policy guidance by NIH as needed. The recommendations of the panel were not accepted, however, and the moratorium that had been declared prior to their meeting continued.

State Commissions

New York State Task Force on Life and the Law

Following a public outcry over apparent abuses of "do not resuscitate" orders in health care facilities, Governor Mario Cuomo of New York decided to appoint a multidisciplinary panel under the leadership of his Commissioner of Health, Dr. David Axelrod, to advise the executive and legislative branches on a range of bioethical topics. Because of the strongly held views of several religious communities in the state on some of these issues, the New York State Task Force on Life and the Law has had (in addition to the usual mixture of researchers, physicians, lawyers, and philosophers) a larger representation of religious leaders than the equivalent federal advisory commissions (see Appendix A and the background paper by Brody for further descriptions of the New York State Task Force).

In other ways, however, the New York group is quite similar to its federal counterparts. By 1993 it had issued eight reports on topics ranging from surrogate parenting to the determination of death, from health care proxies for incompetent patients to procuring and distributing organs for transplantation. Although the task force has attempted to develop a consensus position on the issues it addresses, its reports have sometimes contained dissenting positions. By holding its meetings in private, it does not use the meeting process itself to foster a consensus within the general community or to test its tentative conclusions by airing them before the community. Its reports are usually oriented toward practical recommendations for changes in state policy and hence are subject to public examination during the hearings held on any legislation proposed as a result. The task force operates with annual appropriations, and its small staff is supplemented by the volunteered services of consultants.

New Jersey Bioethics Commission

Beginning in 1983, an active grassroots group emerged in New Jersey to involve lay people and health care professionals alike in responding to the medical and legal developments reflected in such landmark cases as *In re Quinlan*. This group, the Citizens' Committee on Biomedical Ethics, encouraged the legislature to establish an official body in 1985 in the wake of the *Conroy* case regarding the withdrawal of artificial nutrition and hydration from an incompetent, dying patient. The State of New Jersey

Commission on Legal and Ethical Problems in the Delivery of Health
Care—known informally as the New Jersey Bioethics Commission—was
mandated to "provide a comprehensive and scholarly examination of the
impact of advancing technology on health care decisions" and specifically
to recommend policies to the governor, the legislature, and the citizens of
New Jersey (N.J. Public Law 1985, Ch. 363). The group was large (27
members) and included 4 legislators and 9 members designated from executive agencies and major statewide professional and health care organizations. Its membership, which included representatives from law, medicine, nursing, science, humanities, theology, health care administration,
and the New Jersey Citizen's Committee, was appointed by the governor,
the Senate president, and the speaker of the General Assembly (see Appendix A for further description of the New Jersey Bioethics Commission).

Within its broad mandate, the commission chose to focus its half-dozen
reports on three areas: surrogate motherhood (in light of the landmark
Baby M case), decision making about medical treatment (especially the use
of advance directives), and the determination of death. The commission
also established ad hoc task forces on other topics (ethics, AIDS, protection
of vulnerable subjects); these groups, which included noncommissioners,
made recommendations to the parent body. Besides obtaining consultants' advice and supporting research (to supplement the work of its small
staff of two to five professionals), the commission took testimony at public
hearings. Its work resulted in considerable public and professional education on its topics in New Jersey and in the adoption of two statutes (on the
determination of death and on advance directives for health care). However, conflicts within the commission and between the staff and commissioners (particularly the legislator members) brought its work to an end in
1991 after six years.

Analysis of Governmental Bodies

Experience with officially established and supported efforts to examine bioethical issues is too limited to justify definitive conclusions, but it is
sufficient to support some general findings. Since the broadest and best-
documented experience involved the National Commission and the
President's Commission, our analysis begins with them and then widens to
encompass other federal and state panels.

Comparing the Commissions

The two national commissions had several features in common: both
were made up of 11 people from a variety of fields (about half from medicine or research); they came from outside government; they met regularly

(on average, for two days nearly once a month) and in public; their work was carried out by a multidisciplinary staff; and they had "action-forcing power" (that is, although the commissions could not issue regulations, any federal agency to which they made recommendations was required to publish the recommendations and then respond within a specified time, either adopting the recommendations or explaining why they had been rejected).

There were also some marked differences between the two commissions: the mandate of the President's Commission was considerably broader, and it operated independently of any department or agency; no new members were added to the National Commission during its four-year life, whereas only three of the original members served throughout the life of the President's Commission; and the staff of the President's Commission—which began with much greater expertise in bioethics than the National Commission staff—was divided into working groups for the various reports, meaning that many worked only on specified topics with no involvement in other reports that concerned unrelated topics.

The President's Commission mandate was broader, more responsive to varied public concerns, and thus more publicly visible. Its first publication, *Defining Death (1981),* was eagerly awaited by various professional groups and legislators who had been involved in ongoing debate over policies that differed in only minor respects. The report presented a proposed resolution of the policy issues, and it also presented two very important consensus documents: (1) a new model statute that was endorsed by key professional groups (the American Bar Association, the American Medical Association, and the National Conference of Commissions on Uniform State Laws) and (2) a comprehensive statement of the criteria for the determination of death, which was endorsed by 56 coauthors, including virtually all of the physicians who had written about the subject in the United States. Thus, this publication eliminated the perception that the relevant professionals could not agree as to who should count as having died and what should count as a good statute, factors that had posed barriers to adoption of legislation in many states. The criteria for determination of death were also published shortly thereafter (AMA, 1981), which led to widespread awareness of the report itself.

Many of the later reports were awaited by engaged and eager audiences, although these concerned publics were smaller or less visible than the audience that welcomed *Defining Death.* In the last month of its term, the President's Commission published two reports that had broader appeal and receptive audiences: *Deciding to Forego Life-Sustaining Treatment* and *Securing Access to Health Care.* The former document had been circulated to hundreds of concerned citizens in draft and it included not only clear recommendations about practice but also extensive appendices outlining palliative care, statutes on advance directives, and policies on foregoing treatments. The *Deciding* report specifically addressed a series of troubling dichotomies (e.g., withholding and withdrawing, killing and letting die) and a series of troubling clinical settings (e.g., seriously ill newborns, orders to withhold attempts at resuscitation, decisions for adults who do not have decision-making capacity, treatment for patients who have permanently lost consciousness). Also, its prose and presentation was specifically designed to be accessible to any health care professional. By chance, the report was released just as the "Baby Doe" case and the federal response to it was unfolding, and it took a much more temperate tone than the official federal response. For these reasons, *Deciding* was one of the "best sellers" printed by the Government Printing Office, which made it available at cost. It remains a classic reference used in court cases professional literature, and education.

Securing also had an eager public, since allocation and equity were at least as central to public concern in 1983 as now. However, this report underwent many changes as the commission gained new members in its final months. The central ethical argument stayed largely intact, but many examples and much strong language were excised The report thus ended up being an academic discourse on the role and function of commissions, rather than affecting the public issue of access to health care.

The National Commission spoke primarily to federal officials responsible for human subjects regulations and to the biomedical research community (including members of IRBs). The President's Commission, on the other hand, chose to address many constituencies (which varied depending upon the topic). As a result, its reports on some subjects were virtually unknown to readers who were concerned solely with other topics, although specialists in bioethics generally kept abreast of—and commented on—the commission's work across the board, just as they had the work of the National Commission. Both commissions considered some reports more important than others, and these same reports were usually regarded as more influential and important by outsiders as well (see background paper by Gray in this volume).

The central characteristics of both commissions were that they undertook to study complex and sometimes quite highly charged topics; they were able to do so in a thoughtful way because they operated outside the usual political channels; and they were influential both because they operated with an official mandate and because they produced reports that were accessible to the intelligent lay person as well as the scientific or ethical expert. The ideal of impartiality, one of the primary characteristics of ethical discourse, may not have been met completely, but the work of these commissions was a serious approximation. They both attempted to examine all sides of the issues and to move beyond the limits of self-interest and advocacy to find broad grounds of agreement on controversial positions.

Location and Autonomy

Two other influential characteristics of these commissions also stand out: (1) national scope and (2) independence from political or ideological control. Ethics committees appointed by professional organizations and study groups established by bioethics centers have much to contribute, but the public and its representatives do not place any particular weight on the recommendations of these groups, which are neither accountable to the public nor burdened with obligations toward the broad and unbiased inquiry that is incumbent upon public panels.

Further, while state and local ethics committees (both those appointed by governmental entities and those established by institutions and professional groups) can play important roles, many of the most troublesome issues do not stop at state borders, and some process for national deliberation and formulation is needed. Not all states or localities have the resources (or interest) to mount an effective effort, but they may still be able to benefit from the conclusions and recommendations of a national commission. Many of the issues being studied are of greatest concern to the federal government, such as the ethics of various types of research supported by federal agencies. And even when the issues involve matters of state law and policy (such as the regulation of health care professionals and institutions or the rules of family law), a national inquiry avoids duplication and may have the added advantage of leading to uniformity among the states on issues where differences in policy or regulation can produce undesirable results.

The greater the visibility of a panel, however, the greater the danger that its work will be encumbered by bureaucratic, ideological, or political interference. In this sense, the sort of independence that the National Commission and especially the President's Commission enjoyed was critical to the work of these groups. The movement from departmental to presidential status and the freedom from the polarizing issue of abortion made the latter more independent and gave it greater visibility, higher prestige, and better access to sources of information and advice, both inside and outside the government.

The close relationship between an ethics panel and its appointing officer can also have beneficial results in terms of having its recommendations implemented. But there are other means of ensuring that the panel will be listened to; in the end, it is more likely to be widely influential because of the thoroughness of its inquiries and the soundness of its recommendations than because of its political connections. Moreover, the danger of too much entanglement with the political process (particularly when appointments are made by the legislative branch or involve legislators) is clearly evident in the experience of the Biomedical Ethics Advisory Committee and the New Jersey Bioethics Commission.

Courts, Regulation, and Legislation

Society can also handle the ethical issues related to developments in biomedicine through legal mechanisms such as courts, regulation, and legislation. Ethics commissions and other consensual mechanisms can be useful, but since these issues reflect choices among competing values, as well as assessments of available data, even groups composed of highly expert and well-intentioned professionals can produce markedly different decisions about bioethical questions. (See background paper by Gostin for further description of the ways in which courts, regulation, and legislation can impact such decisions).

Courts as Ethical Decision Makers

In our litigious society, courts often are the forum where ethical quandaries related to biomedicine first make their appearance and demand resolution. Courts therefore are necessary participants in the bioethics debate, although their special institutional features both facilitate and detract from their effectiveness in making health policy.

On the positive side, common law courts have developed for centuries a tradition of ethically relevant decision making that places a high value on reasoned explanation of judicial holdings. The practice of justification by precedent obliges courts to draw on settled legal principles, thereby reducing the likelihood of ill-considered or arbitrary judgments. Courts determine ethical issues in the context of specific cases; this heightens the immediacy of the questions, but, especially in the case of lower court decisions, also usefully limits the negative impact of poorly reasoned opinions. A dramatic case, such as *Quinlan* or *Cruzan*, provides a gripping narrative through which abstract ethical concerns are made concrete for varied publics. At the same time, the tiered structure of the court system, the existence of multiple jurisdictions, and the practice of writing dissenting opinions all serve to open up judicial reasoning to public criticism and improvement.

On the negative side, courts employ an adversarial process that is not necessarily conducive to dispassionate analysis or fact finding. Unlike legislatures, courts are compelled to resolve the issues related to specific cases and individuals that come before them, even if the basis for a principled decision has not been fully laid. Yet courts are fundamentally reactive, in that they cannot make policy unless decisions are put to them. This lack of capacity may be especially evident when courts are confronted with conflicts arising out of developments in biomedical science and technology. Finally, the decentralized nature of the court system leads to contradictory and confusing ethical pronouncements that may take years to sort out through legislation or an authoritative higher court ruling.

The institutional strengths and weaknesses of courts have been revealed in instances where new treatments raised ethical questions that were submitted to the courts. For example, judicial leadership on questions concerning the use of life-supporting technologies began with the New Jersey Supreme Court's decision about Karen Ann Quinlan's right to be disconnected from a life support system. Since then, a series of decisions by federal and state courts on refusing or withholding care have guided the nation's policy on these issues. Most significant was the Supreme Court's decision in *Cruzan,* which held that competent patients had a "liberty interest" in refusing treatment and provided an impetus for state legislation. Many state courts have extended this right of refusal to people who are incapable of making a decision by respecting the decisions of surrogates, particularly family members (see the background paper by Gostin in this volume).

In some cases, courts have turned to other bodies for guidance in defining the circumstances under which treatment can be terminated. The President's Commission report on foregoing treatment was instrumental in leading most courts to reject the distinction between withholding and withdrawing treatment, between ordinary and extraordinary treatments, and between terminal and nonterminal cases. In other cases, courts have acted independently to set out procedures and criteria for decision making, ranging from second opinions to the use of ethics committees or ombudsmen.

Many times state legislatures became involved in these issues; they acted only some time after court decisions and usually followed policies implicit in those decisions. The most recent national actions in this area came about when Congress passed the Patient Self-Determination Act, which was implemented on December 1, 1991. The law requires health care providers to inform their patients of the right to accept or refuse medical care, including the right to give advance directives on the use of medical means of sustaining life. Other times, state legislative action has preceded court decisions and set policy in this area, most notably in natural death acts, determination of death (which many states enacted before any court action as well), surrogacy, and, in recent times, reproductive decisions. An example is the California Natural Death Act of 1976, which preceded all court decisions, including *Quinlan.*

Courts have also been involved in a major way in the field of reproductive rights. Beginning with the landmark cases of *Griswold v. Connecticut* and *Roe v. Wade,* the courts for nearly two decades defined the reproductive rights of women. In the early cases, the Supreme Court found a constitutional right of "privacy" even though no mention of the concept appears in the Bill of Rights. In *Griswold* the Court used the newly identified right to privacy to prevent states from interfering with the sale and distribution of contraceptives. The Court explained that contraception concerns "the most intimate of human activities and relationships."

In *Roe* the Supreme Court stated that the constitutional promise of privacy protects not only the right to use contraceptives but also the right to decide whether to carry a fetus to term and the privacy of a woman's relationship with her physician (see the background paper by Gostin in this volume). In recent years, there has been a significant erosion of privacy rights. The Court has upheld the authority of the state to restrict the use of public employees and facilities for the use of nontherapeutic abortions (see Gostin). The Court also upheld a regulation prohibiting federally funded family planning clinics from counseling or referring women to abortions (the so-called "gag rule") (see Gostin). In *Planned Parenthood of Southeastern Pennsylvania v. Casey* (see Gostin), the Court changed the legal standard by which to evaluate restrictions on abortion. This rule may allow states to place new restrictions on access, timing, and information provision in abortion decisions.

In spite of these retrenchments, it has been argued that the extension of the right to privacy since 1965 has had profound and positive effects on reproductive policy (see Gostin). Prior to the Supreme Court's entry into the area, neither the legislative nor executive branch produced policies that adequately recognized the need to balance the interests of pregnant women against those of the state or the fetus. Current efforts to protect reproductive privacy use the same "fundamental rights" analysis that the Supreme Court employed in *Roe v. Wade*. State legislatures are also emulating thoughtful court rulings on related reproductive issues such as surrogate motherhood and artificial reproduction.

Courts will continue to play an important role in the deliberation of emotionally charged issues in health care and biomedical innovation where no formal policy is in place and where there is a fundamental claim of human rights by individuals and groups. If, as has frequently occurred in certain states, legislators have not proactively addressed issues of this character that flow from biomedical advances, the courts have been and will be required to take the lead in resolving the legal and ethical issues that arise in particular cases. For, while legislatures may choose not to act, courts cannot avoid this burden once a case is before them. For example courts have been involved in such issues as the right to die and the ownership of sperm in a sperm bank. If no statute provides a definite answer, courts must decide which precedents seem most helpful, whether the scientific aspects are supported by sound data, whether the common law provides guidance, and so on. Many court decisions in these areas read like laws—some even set up specific administrative procedures to handle future cases—and they provide a blueprint for subsequent legislation. Courts will also continue to play a significant secondary role through their power to review federal regulations.

Regulations can take several forms—instructions, findings, definitions of terms, and so on—but a prescribed set of actions, including solicitation of public comment, must take place before federal regulations become effective. It has become common for interested parties to pose legal challenges to regulations (in either their proposed or final form). These challenges may be made on several grounds—the law does not authorize them, they do not follow the law, the issuing process was faulty, and so on. Some of these issues also have strong ethical elements. For example, the Supreme Court has rejected challenges against several regulations issued by the Secretary of Health and Human Services that limited women's rights to abortion as established by *Roe v. Wade.*

Courts have to take the limited view imposed upon them by the case as presented and by precedent; legislatures are buffered by special interests and any legislation is inevitably marked by compromises. Public bioethical deliberation can provide the broader view that the courts, which are set up to focus on individual cases and circumstances, cannot easily provide and can attempt an impartiality that legislation cannot always achieve. The existence of bioethical opinion may inform the courts, as did the President's Commission opinion on foregoing life support in the Herbert case (California Court of Appeals, *Barber v. Superior Court,* 1983), and may influence the legislatures, as did the New York State Task Force on Life and Law.

International Perspectives[2]

Bioethics is generally regarded as a subject first developed in the United States. Until recently, a clear majority of books and articles in the field was published here, and the number of academic departments, courses, and conferences was far greater in the United States than abroad. Similarly, the U.S. government took the lead in investigating bioethical issues and in issuing regulations when it established the National Commission and President's Commission in the 1970s. In the past few years, however, bioethics has rapidly internationalized. Hospitals the world over have sprouted ethics committees, new journals are appearing in foreign languages, and regional and international bioethics societies have been formed.

While the United States has been notable for launching new initiatives and sponsoring numerous activities on bioethics in the academic world, it has not been as active in the support of governmental bioethics activity. Since the demise of the President's Commission in 1983, the United States has had no national bioethics commission, despite the still-increasing public and academic fascination with bioethical issues. In Europe, govern-

---

[2] This section is based on research by committee member Daniel Wikler while he worked as a consultant to the Office of Technology Assessment.

ments have taken the initiative in this area; elsewhere, development of bioethics is often prodded by governmental organizations. Multinational organizations also have begun to deal with bioethical issues. As the U.S. government considers the possible reestablishment of a bioethics agency or commission, these foreign bioethics groups are available as positive and negative models. A brief examination of the structure and agendas of some of these bodies may provide valuable guidance for future government-sponsored efforts in our own country.

A number of international organizations have been active in the field of bioethics. The Council for International Organizations of Medical Science (CIOMS) was established in 1949 by two United Nations agencies: the World Health Organization and UNESCO. In 1985, it constituted a steering committee on bioethics representing a variety of professional backgrounds and geographical areas, which in turn organized "international dialogues" on ethical issues arising in such subjects as battered children, human genome research, and family planning.

Over the years, CIOMS groups have offered international ethical guidelines on a number of topics, ranging from protection of human subjects of medical experimentation (1982 and 1993) to ethical review of epidemiological studies (1991). In addition, the Office of Health Legislation of the World Health Organization keeps track of bioethics actions of governments and multinational bodies, some of which are reported in its quarterly *International Digest of Health Legislation.* In 1993, UNESCO formed an International Bioethics Committee with 46 members, chaired by Mme. Noelle Lenoir, an attorney and member of France's Conseil Constitutionnel. Thus far this committee has held one meeting; another is planned.

The Council of Europe (CE), an organization created by European governments in part for cooperation in cultural and scientific affairs, has also become active in bioethics. Following a resolution presented by the French Minister of Justice to the European Ministerial Conference on Human Rights in Vienna in 1985, the CE created an Ad Hoc Committee of Experts on Bioethics (CAHBI) to further the interests of member states in bioethical issues. CAHBI's aim is "to fill the political and legal gaps that may result from the rapid development of biomedical sciences," but it must achieve the voluntary consensus of member states. In 1992, the CE elevated the group to full legal status and gave it a new acronym: CDBI, for Comité Directeur de Bioethique Internationale.

CAHBI/CDBI was given a proposal in 1989 to create a European Bioethics Committee; in 1992, it judged such a step premature. However, the committee recently held a Framework Convention for Bioethics, designed to present norms on a variety of issues for consideration by the European members of CE. The convention, which was open to nonmember states, considered general ethical principles related to organ transplantation, medical research on humans, including embryos, and the use of genetic information for nonmedical purposes.

Representatives of national bioethics committees, primarily but not exclusively European, have met three times under CAHBI/CDBI auspices. The council also empaneled a commission on ethical issues in reproductive technology, known as the Glover Commission after its chairman, Oxford philosopher and bioethicist Jonathan Glover.

The government of the European Community (EC), which is distinct both in members and in function from the CE, has not yet sought to establish a general European bioethics commission. In three instances, however, the EC has initiated working groups on specific topics: one on human embryos and research; a second on ethical, social, and legal aspects of human genome analysis; and a third on ethical issues in biotechnology. A fourth initiative involves the establishment of a research program in bioethics, offering grants to scholars on a competitive basis. This appears to be the world's sole general fund for investigator-initiated bioethics research. In addition, the European Parliament looks for technical advice to its Scientific and Technological Options Assessment (STOA) Programme, just as the U.S. Congress relies on its Office of Technology Assessment.

In the Americas, the Pan American Health Organization (PAHO, a regional office of the World Health Organization) has fostered the development of bioethics in Central and South America. PAHO's general counsel sits on the board of directors of the International Association of Bioethics, an international bioethics group founded in 1992. Planning is currently under way to establish a Pan American Institute of Bioethics, to be located at the University of Chile in Santiago. The institute, slated to begin its work in 1994, is charged to provide a "permanent place for . . . discussion of bioethical subjects." However, its chief mission will be support of research and training in bioethics for the region. Given the novelty of bioethics research and policy in Latin America, its prospectus does not suggest the kind of intergovernmental authority vested in the European organizations (PAHO, 1992).

Other international organizations dealing with bioethics include international medical specialty societies and international bioethics societies. The International Association of Bioethics (IAB) held its inaugural congress in 1992, hosted by the National Health Council of the Netherlands with the support of the EC. The IAB, headquartered in Australia, provides a forum for diverse views on bioethical issues but does not itself take positions on any of them. None of the other organizations has yet attempted to form an international bioethics commission.

Models of National Deliberation on Bioethics

Bioethics commissions have been widely used in other English-speaking countries. A number of federal and state bioethics commissions have contributed to health policy development in Australia, including the Law Reform Commission on Human Tissue Transplant, the Medical Research Ethics Committee, and the new Australian Health Ethics Committee (AHEC), a committee of the National Health and Medical Research Council (approximately analogous to the U.S. National Institutes of Health). Bioethical issues have been discussed in regard to potential legislation by Law Reform Commissions of both the Canadian government and the various provinces. A Human Subjects Research Ethics Committee advises Canada's National Research Council on issues arising in experimentation on human subjects.

Canada's Royal Commission on New Reproductive Technologies is a notably well-funded initiative that has only partially escaped the kind of political heat generated by abortion politics that doomed the Biomedical Ethics Advisory Committee in our Congress. It is charged with performing a comprehensive and authoritative review of Canadian laws and practices on present and forthcoming reproductive technologies. The commission has a large professional staff, has sponsored considerable research, and held hearings and open meetings around the country. Its reports were recently published in 1993.

Latin American countries are just beginning to establish bioethics commissions. In Mexico, a Commission Nacional de Bioetica, sponsored by the federal government and reporting to the Ministry of Health, was created in 1992. The commission's broad mandate includes oversight on environmental as well as medical issues. In December 1992, Argentina's National Ministry of Health and Social Welfare established a National Bioethics Commission for that country.

Despite the growing number of national bioethics commissions, few commissions make a visible and significant impact on national debate and policy. There is considerable diversity of approach among the well-established commissions, and the United States can learn from the experience of each of them. Three models of national deliberation on bioethics merit particular attention: the Danish commission, which stresses public education and participation; the French commission, distilling the considered judgment of an elite; and the current British approach, in which a private commission takes on a public function.

Denmark, A Populist Model. Denmark's national bioethics committee is notable for at least two reasons. First, the country has not one but two national bioethics commissions, with overlapping areas of interest. Second, one of these commissions has a uniquely active program of public education.

The Central Scientific-Ethical Committee (CSEC) has been in operation since the late 1970s. It was created in the wake of the Helsinki II declaration on human experimentation and has been chaired by one of its drafters. CSEC originally played its role through a voluntary arrangement of professional groups, but in 1992 it was given statutory authority. CSEC is at the apex of a system of human subjects review boards that covers the whole of Denmark; it acts on disputed proposals and in cases in which a matter of principle must be decided.

In 1988, Parliament created a second council, the Danish Council of Ethics, with a mandate to consider a broader range of bioethical issues. The council's 17 members are predominantly laypersons. Though the reports are written by the members of the council, it has a slightly larger staff than is common in Europe: three professionals, including a physician, as well as administrative support; it also takes on academics for short periods of service.

The council's public education efforts go beyond anything attempted by U.S. bioethics commissions. In considering the definition of death, for example, the council held public hearings and financed local debates. It produced a film that was shown not only on national television but also in movie theaters. The council produced booklets and brochures explaining the basic facts about the definitions of death and distributed them at public libraries. The council reportedly gathered the editors of 20 newspapers and induced them to carry articles and exchanges on the subject; 1,000 articles and editorials were published over three years, drawing hundreds of letters to editors. A competition for young people invited art works on the concept of death; the winner of a poster contest won the privilege of display as the cover of the council's annual report.

For the report *Protection of Human Gametes, Fertilized Ova, Embryos and Fetuses*, the council focused on schools (1990). It gathered educational materials and prepared teaching material for education on these ethical issues in the context of 17 subjects, ranging from biology and philosophy to drama, music, and literature. These were sent to every high school in the country. The council held a short-story contest, in cooperation with a newspaper, which drew hundreds of entries. Its film "Onskebarn" ("Wished-for Child") won a medal at the International Film and Television Festival in New York.

The Danish Council of Ethics appears to be closer to the grass roots than any other foreign commission, but it is not without its critics. Its findings on the definition of death rejected the current global consensus, which favors a brain death formulation, a step that drew criticism from members of the other Danish group, the CSEC. The two commissions also disagreed on the propriety of preserving brain tissue for research and teaching purposes. Moreover, the council's own surveys revealed widespread misunderstanding about brain death, not only before but also after the massive public education campaigns.

France, An Elite Model. A Comité Consultatif National d'Ethique Pour les Sciences de la Vie et de la Santé (National Consultative Ethics Committee on Life and Medical Sciences) (CCNE) was created by the President of the Republic in 1983. CCNE has over 40 members, drawn not only from scholarly specialties and professional groups but also representative of philosophical currents in France. The chair is appointed by the president, and half of the membership is renewed every two years. Members are not paid, and several have publicly complained about the lack of staff.

CCNE has issued over 30 reports thus far on topics ranging from the testing of drug addicts in employment to genetic fingerprints to reproductive technology. The committee also issues statements on topical questions, such as the introduction of RU-486 (the so-called abortion pill) and sex-determination procedures in the Olympics. The committee is housed at INSERM, which is analogous to NIH. Meetings are closed, and minutes, which are released to the public, do not reflect the identity of those making the remarks. However, a two-day public symposium is held each year (see the background paper by Charo for a further description of the CCNE).

Questions can be brought to the committee by members of the government, presidents of the two houses of parliament, or by public institutions involved in research. CCNE also takes up topics of its own choosing. The committee typically creates a subcommittee for each question or topic, which eventually reports to CCNE as a whole. The latter has occasionally rejected a subcommittee's report.

CCNE aims to play a central role in the country's deliberations over bioethical issues. Its unusually large size permits wider representation of views and interests. It attempts to enunciate general principles for the whole of French society (e.g., that body parts must not be traded in commerce). The committee not only carries out studies of the chief bioethical issues of the day, but also involves itself in day-to-day controversies arising in the hospitals and courts. High in visibility and prestige, its meetings have been addressed on several occasions by the President of the Republic. Its outgoing chairman has been venerated as a public sage, the more-or-less official national voice on bioethics. Its deliberations and findings are covered extensively by the press; the newspaper *Le Monde* covers the commission closely, providing reportage and commentary even on its philosophical deliberations. Thus, the French model, as opposed to the Danish one, might be characterized as prescriptive, elite, and centralized.

United Kingdom, A Private Model. Bioethics policy is developed in many ways and in many bodies in the United Kingdom. Its research councils, particularly the Medical Research Council, publish an ethics series that focuses primarily on human subjects issues. The British Medical Association has a medical ethics committee, and the Royal Colleges (e.g., of Psychiatrists) have issued numerous guidelines and position papers. Most prominent among the bioethics councils was the recent Warnock Commission on embryos and reproductive technology. Closely studied by academics as well as patients and physicians, its recommendations were largely embodied in new legislation.

However, the government has rejected suggestions that it create a national bioethics commission with a broader mandate. Explanations for this reticence vary; one reason seems to be the past prime minister's wish to avoid placing undue restrictions on scientists. In this respect, as in others, the United Kingdom is out of step with its fellow European states; prominent bioethicists have complained that without a national commission they are not able to identify and pursue the "British position" on these issues in pan-European councils and conferences.

With an interest in a national commission rising in the face of governmental refusal to go along, a private solution has been attempted. The Nuffield Foundation, an educational and charitable trust, was asked to consider the organization of a private body that would function like the governmental bioethics bodies in other European states. The new Nuffield Council on Bioethics was founded after elaborate soundings of professional, scientific, legal, and consumer groups. Its 15 members do not represent constituencies but are chosen for diversity. The council aims to stimulate coordination between the diverse groups now contributing to bioethics policy; to anticipate new problems, and to increase the public's awareness of the issues and of their importance. Several working groups have already been set up. The staff consists of an executive director and two administrative assistants.

The Nuffield Council on Bioethics, as a private advisory body, will have no regulatory role. Nevertheless, the foundation's initiative was welcomed by the government, and one of its staff is government salaried. The council seems to be fixed in the minds of British bioethicists as the national body. Indeed, in its makeup and procedures, the council is conducting itself just as it would if it were a creation of the national government. Whether it will achieve the same influence and authority in national deliberations over bioethical issues as its governmental counterparts abroad remains uncertain.

Dimensions of Bioethics Commissions

This brief survey of bioethics commissions abroad permits no firm judgments on relative successes and failures. However, the differences between national approaches suggest a number of questions that might be considered by the United States in designing its own mechanisms for deliberation on bioethics.

Scope. Until recently, most bioethics commissions abroad have been topical—i.e., devoted to one or a small number of issues—and temporary. Topics have been selected in advance by the sponsor. The French commission, however, is wide ranging and seemingly permanent, with the power to investigate topics of its own choosing. Other commissions established in Europe since the founding of the French commission, and perhaps in imitation of it, have also been general, self-generating, and open ended. Among the most influential commissions have been some single-topic efforts, such as the Warnock Commission in the United Kingdom.

Sponsorship. The independence of ethics commissions abroad has been regarded by most observers as essential to its moral authority. Whether based in the legislature or in the executive branch, all commissions but the U.K.'s are public. Most answer to, and are located within, the ministries of health. The U.S. President's Commission, which was administratively located outside the departmental structure of the executive branch, has not been seen as a precedent.

Public Access. Most of the commissions allow only limited public access. Meetings are generally closed. In some cases, members of the public may offer their views. Some commissions hold periodic public symposia. One reason offered for the lack of public access is that some commissions rule on particular cases and therefore require confidentiality.

Professional Dominance. All governments have striven to ensure lay membership on their commissions; in some cases, physicians and scientists are in a clear minority. No survey data exist regarding public perceptions of the commissions as independent or as "captured." Unsystematic opinion sampling suggests that, where separate boards or committees exist to oversee human subjects research, these tend to be perceived as protective of the interests of physicians and scientists, lay membership or majorities notwithstanding.

Evaluation and Soundness. Bioethics commissions may be evaluated in many dimensions such as productivity, influence, and soundness. Very little evaluation has been done in any country to date. In this sense, all countries are flying blind. Soundness is the most difficult of the criteria to assess, but it is among the most important. In responses to a survey conducted by OTA, the firmer the commentator's credentials in academic bioethics, the lower his or her opinion of the soundness of the bioethics commission reports. Complaints that commission's findings are poorly argued, or even not argued at all, are common. Only a few commissions have followed the

U.S. example of rotating professional staff recruited via paid leaves from academic departments.

A different perspective emerges in some of the solicited comments and in the literature: some believe that there is no such thing as expertise in ethics; the commissions' role is to act as forum, broker, and mediator for diverse points of view. Thus a finding that represents a compromise between conflicting commissioners representing diverse constituencies would be regarded as a successful one, even if none of the commissioners could (or would wish to) support the compromised conclusion with data or argument.

Role. National bioethics commissions differ in their basic purpose. In some instances, they are directly advisory to parliaments; their existence is justified by the need to develop legislation on complex technological and scientific issues that can go slower and deeper than the usual legislative process permits. In other cases, the commission exists to stimulate and educate the public. Still others take on the role of distilling and articulating the national sensibility on these matters.

Structure. All the commissions have a chair and numerous commissioners, though they vary in size by a factor of four. Large commissions can be more representative, but sacrifice working efficiency. More striking is the difference in the size of the staff. Most have hardly any, although in a few cases the staff is larger and well trained. Only Canada has provided to its bioethics commission a staff comparable to that of the National Commission or the President's Commission in the United States. As noted above, there is considerable complaining among commissioners over the lack of staff.

A National Voice? Particularly in international councils, the national bioethics committees are increasingly seen as defining their nation's position on bioethics issues. To this extent, they act as national spokesperson, even though few commissioners are elected to their posts. In the United States, commissions have not been regarded as bioethics policymakers except and until their recommendations have been adopted as law (e.g., the human subjects regulations of the National Commission, or the statutory definition of death of the President's Commission). As new entities multiply within and outside of government, the designation of a national voice will become more difficult, and the goal itself open to further question.

PROFESSIONAL AND INSTITUTIONAL MECHANISMS

When Americans are confronted with a change in the moral landscape arising from a change in our capacities to affect the world (e.g., a development in biomedicine), we often slip into an assumption that the relevant moral discourse need only address two questions: What should I do? And what should our government do? For example, when we worry about environmental degradation, we think of what each individual should recycle and what action the federal government should take with regard to environmental pollutants. When we worry about mapping the humane genome, we focus on the opportunities and risks for individuals afflicted with undesirable genotypes, and on the government's role in regulating the use and abuse of this information.

Between the isolated individual and the impersonal actions of government, however, lie numerous social institutions composed of deeply ingrained, patterned sets of behaviors that shape our expectations and opportunities (Bellah et al., 1991). Social institutions include both large-scale entities, such as the economy, the polity, religion, and the educational system, and small-scale entities such as the family and professional and voluntary associations. Voluntary and professional associations in particular often play active roles in changing policies and practices. For example, local citizens' groups, homeowners' associations, architects' and urban planners' professional associations actively participate in environmental decision making. Similarly, groups interested in possible effects upon the family, insurance pools and disability insuring, and the uses and abuses of genetic testing become active in shaping the ethical discourse and formulating guidelines and policies pertinent to genetic mapping.

Professional Societies and Voluntary Organizations

Professional medical associations and specialty societies [e.g., American Medical Association (AMA)], research institutes (e.g., RAND, the Hastings Center), and even individual health maintenance organizations (HMOs) (e.g., Group Health of Puget Sound, Harvard Community Health Plan) have responded individually and cooperatively to the changes introduced into the medical, legal, and ethical communities by biomedical technology. Medical associations in particular have long been involved in the formulation of clinical practice guidelines and ethical policies in an attempt to assist clinicians in the rendering of proper and appropriate care to their patients.

An impetus to these guidance efforts has been the frequent abdication by the federal government of responsibility for providing ethical guidance to clinicians in many of the fastest-growing areas of biomedical technology. In some cases, the guidance provided by professional societies is the sole source of up-to-date scientific, legal, and practical information available to practitioners. For example, the federal refusal to fund research on in vitro fertilization left both researchers and clinicians with no organized forum to consider practical and ethical issues presented by this technique. In response to this neglect, many medical associations have stepped up their efforts to provide ethical and practical guidelines to their members, and several associations have established subcommittees to explore the uncharted areas of biomedical technology and delineate practice options.

Medical associations have been in the forefront of the movement to guide physicians through the legal and ethical quagmire produced by the dual developments of greater technological advancement and government inaction. Four that have been influential, active, and prolific are the AMA, the American College of Obstetricians and Gynecologists (ACOG), the National Advisory Board on Ethics in Reproduction (NABER), and the American College of Physicians (ACP).

AMA

The American Medical Association has taken a lead in the attempt to guide its members through the ethical and legal dilemmas that surround medical treatment decisions and the use of new technologies. It has a long history of such guidance, beginning in 1847 with the establishment of a code of ethics. The nine-member Council on Ethical and Judicial Affairs addresses the moral and legal concerns that attend clinical practice, primarily through the issuance of regular reports containing opinions, guidelines, and relevant case law regarding a vast array of ethical and legal issues presented by the rapid advancement of biomedical technology. Periodic updates ensure that guidance provided to practitioners is based on the most current scientific and legal information.

Recent reports address a wide range of concerns and provide detailed advice to clinicians on topics such as:

- confidential care for minors, particularly those minors who may seek contraceptive information and/or abortions without parental knowledge or consent;
- the difficult issues to be resolved if a patient's AIDS status is to be kept confidential on autopsy reports; and
- complexities of treatment decisions for seriously ill newborns (AMA, 1992b).

Two groups within the AMA issue recommendations for clinical practice on specific technologies: the Council on Scientific Affairs and the Diagnostic and Therapeutic Technology Assessment Program. The AMA also promulgates guidelines and recommendations through the widely read *Journal of the American Medical Association*.

In addition, the AMA has been instrumental in fostering cooperation among specialized medical societies in order to provide professional guidance and forums for discussion of biomedical technology and clinical practice issues. The Practice Parameters Forum (PPF) is composed of nearly 50 volunteer specialty and state medical societies that attempt to devise criteria for judging the soundness of processes for developing practice parameters, define minimum standards of care, and set priorities for insurance coverage.

ACOG

The American College of Obstetricians and Gynecologists exemplifies the critical role that a medical specialty society can play in providing guidance to physicians. ACOG produces detailed reports and guidelines for a number of procedures that pose highly sensitive ethical and practical dilemmas for practitioners. Recent publications cover a wide range of issues, including the following:

- sterilization, and in particular the use of this procedure among the mentally retarded;
- multifetal pregnancy reduction, selective fetal termination, and the distinction between these procedures and abortion;
- surrogate motherhood;
- withholding or withdrawing life-sustaining medical therapy, which carefully explored the tension between the obligation to alleviate pain and suffering and prolong life;
- the potential for industry's financial and educational support of physicians to lead to conflict of interest and how best to avoid it; and
- the conflicts that arise when providing expert testimony in a trial and the need to distinguish between maloccurrence and malpractice when evaluating another physician's actions (ACOG, 1992).

NABER

Fetal tissue research is governed by state law and federal regulation. Department of Health and Human Services (DHHS) regulations, for example, require that all funding of in vitro fertilization research involving humans be reviewed by an officially constituted board that—with the disbanding of the EAB in 1980—no longer exists. Since 1980, the country has been without an officially constituted group to provide analysis and advice on ethically and socially controversial biomedical research protocols, and clinicians and investigators have been without much-needed guidance. Created in 1991 through the joint efforts of the American Fertility Society (AFS) and ACOG, the National Advisory Board on Ethics and Reproduction deals exclusively with the rapid growth in reproductive technology. NABER has two stated purposes:

1. To provide a public forum for informed and nonpartisan national debate over the ethical issues raised by modern reproductive sciences and technology.

2. To offer to the public, professionals, and policymakers sound, well researched, and nonpartisan counsel on the ethics of research and clinical practice involving reproductive services and technology (NABER, 1991).

The 12 members of NABER represent a variety of disciplines, including theology, pediatrics, biomedical ethics, law, public policy, and obstetrics and gynecology. NABER offers itself as an independent body for review of research protocols that have raised ethical problems difficult for local IRBs to resolve. It also conducted the initial work on the implications of fetal cell sorting and oocyte donation.

ACP

The American College of Physicians publishes the *American College of Physicians Ethics Manual*, now in its third edition (1992), which provides guidance to physicians in clinical and research settings. The newly revised manual treats a wide range of issues, including:

- end-of-life care;
- physician-assisted suicide;
- HIV and physician/patient susceptibility to infection;
- sexual contact between physicians and patients; and
- physician/pharmaceutical industry relations and potential conflict of interest.

The ACP also has an Ethics Committee that disseminates guidelines through the publication of background papers and policy statements in the *Annals of Internal Medicine*. ACP also has established a Clinical Efficacy Assessment Project that carefully evaluates the merits of medical interventions such as cardiac rehabilitation and certain diagnostic tests.

Other Medical Associations

A number of other medical societies has been actively engaged in providing ethical guidance to their members. The American Academy of Pediatrics (AAP) has developed influential guidelines for establishing hospital ethics committees and authored many papers on bioethical subjects such as informed consent, forced maternal treatment, research involving children, Baby Doe issues, religious exemption from child abuse laws, and organ procurement from anencephalic infants. The American Thoracic Society has developed guidelines on foregoing life-sustaining treatment (ATS, 1991) and on allocation within intensive care units.

A recently created organization called the American Association of Bioethics (AAB) aims to provide a forum for collaboration among varied professional societies in addressing ethical issues confronted in health science and health care. The AAB board is composed of representatives from the AMA, ACP, AHA, American Bar Association, and other professional organizations, as well as several bioethicists.

Health Maintenance Organizations

In addition to the efforts of medical associations, individual HMOs, motivated primarily by desires to reduce costs and simultaneously preserve a reasonable standard of care, have made several efforts to guide physicians and patients in their use of biomedical technology. Group Health of Puget Sound (GHPS) developed a preventive care manual for its primary care practitioners and has attempted to involve subscribers to the health plan in decisions about the allocation of resources. The manual includes, for example, risk-based guidelines for preventive services such as mammograms. Harvard Community Health Plan (HCHP) has also developed scientifically based clinical algorithms.

Challenges Presented by the Creation of Guidelines

All of these efforts to provide physicians with up-to-date information and guidance are welcome, particularly in light of limited governmental action in many areas. However, such efforts have not been without problems. Guidelines are devised by a variety of groups for a variety of purposes, and the resulting welter of guidelines can often be inconsistent and thus confusing. First, guidelines are sometimes not based on universally accepted scientific evidence. Second, they are sometimes haphazardly and inefficiently disseminated to their intended users. Third, they are sometimes offensive to physicians, who may not be receptive to guidelines that do not mesh well with their practice and experience. Fourth, the various guidelines may offer competing and contradictory advice, presenting practitioners with additional ethical problems (IOM, 1992). For example, AMA and ACOG offer conflicting guidance on the handling of surrogate motherhood: AMA disapproves of the practice and advises against involvement in it (AMA, 1992a), while ACOG regards it as a difficult but potentially acceptable pregnancy option (ACOG, 1990). Fifth, such guidelines often do not incorporate patient preferences. Finally, the professional self-interest of some groups may inadvertently inform and bias their specific recommendations.

IOM examined many of these issues in a 1992 report on the difficulties encountered by the Agency for Health Care Policy and Research (AHCPR) in its attempt to comply with the congressional mandate to facilitate the creation of clinical practice guidelines. As the importance of such guidelines becomes more apparent, however, greater care and increased attention are being devoted to rectifying these problems. As a result of such attention, more systematic, consistent, and scientifically grounded guidelines may be formulated by individual societies as well. Two specific cases illustrate the ways in which professional associations have dealt effectively with the challenges presented by technological change.

Seriously Ill Newborns. Between the mid-1960s and the early 1980s, an array of devices and interventions greatly improved our ability to sustain the lives of very small or seriously ill newborns. Lives were saved by these new interventions, but often at the cost of severe physical and developmental disabilities. Also, many lives were prolonged only to be lost after great suffering. Thus, neonatal intensive care became a laboratory for the ethical questions: should life always be saved, and at what cost? (see Jonsen, 1974).

In 1982, for example, a child was born in Bloomington, Indiana with treatable physical defects that threatened its life and with an untreatable genetic defect that predicted limited mental development. The parents chose not to correct the physical defect. Reports of this event reached President Reagan, who ordered DHHS to establish regulations to prevent such events in the future. The department ordered neonatal intensive care units to post conspicuous signs warning that children might be neglected and giving a hotline number to report alleged neglect. This crude effort was successfully challenged in court. Further efforts were made to regulate clinical practice, finally resulting in legislation passed by Congress. However, in a most unusual move, the American Academy of Pediatrics and the American College of Obstetricians and Gynecologists were invited to participate in drafting the language of the statute, allowing them to bring up considerations that reflected the bioethical discussions on such cases. The subsequent "Baby Doe Rules," issued in 1982, were far from perfect, but they were much improved by this contribution.

Artificial Nutrition and Hydration. Only a few decades ago, an elderly person with serious disabilities who lost the ability to eat would die. During the 1960s, advances in the use of feeding tubes allowed doctors to alter the timing and manner of death for these patients. Practitioners and scholars were among the first groups to question the advisability of such a procedure (Micetich et al., 1983; Lynn and Childress, 1983; Zerwekh, 1983). This new technology arrived without fanfare, without evaluation, and without significant direct cost (at least until the advent of total parenteral nutrition).

When the inevitable court cases arose, they were met with a surprising array of *amici* from professional societies. Briefs filed on behalf of the American Geriatrics Society (Lynn, 1984) and the members of the President's Commission (which had disbanded) were referenced in the *Conroy* opinion (1985). Throughout the discourse, various multidisciplinary and specialty groups, including the Hastings Center, American Nurses Association, and American Dietetic Association, issued guidelines designed to shape practice and public opinion. In the *Cruzan* case, for example, 19 health care provider associations supported the removal of the feeding tube.

These examples demonstrate that professional and voluntary societies, including HMOs, insurers, and research institutes, as well as medical associations, can play an impressive and central role in the response to biomedical advances. Without the intervention of these groups, practitioners would have little guidance in the proper employment of many new technologies and the ethical problems that their usage prompts. It seems reasonable to conclude that these associations can also influence the future course of policy and practice in the realm of biomedical technology.

Institutional Review Boards and Institutional Guidelines

The National Research Act of 1974 (P.L. 93-348), which mandated the establishment of institutional review boards in all research organizations receiving federal funds to support research using human subjects, also directed the National Commission to identify ethical principles relevant to human subjects research, develop guidelines for the conduct of such research, and examine IRB mechanisms for review of applications for human subjects research, particularly in the case of research involving vulnerable subjects. The National Commission described the purpose of an IRB as the balancing of the interests of society in protecting the rights of individual subjects with the developing of knowledge that can benefit not only specific subjects but society as a whole (National Commission, 1978b).

The commission recommended that IRBs include persons who are independent from the research process, so that objectivity is enhanced. It also recommended that IRBs be situated at the local level, since local committees would be more familiar with the conditions surrounding human studies research at particular institutions. The IRB protects the rights and the welfare of individuals who participate in research protocols at the institution that establishes the board. In reviewing human subjects research protocols, the IRB can approve or disapprove the proposed activity, or it can require modifications that will make the proposed research acceptable. Each IRB must have a minimum of five members with varying expertise, attitudes, and backgrounds, including racial and cultural heritage. Areas of expertise would include professional competence as well as understandings of institutional commitments, regulations, and law. The IRB is required to keep detailed records of its actions. Prior to conducting research on human beings, the institution must provide assurances to the funding agencies that it will comply with policy requirements. These requirements, the so-called Common Federal Policy, were adopted in 1991 by 16 federal agencies (not including the FDA, which has maintained its own regulations) that conduct, support, or regulate research utilizing human subjects.

Before endorsing a proposed protocol, the IRB reviews six basic areas of the protocol: the risks, informed consent procedures, equity, privacy, vulnerable subjects, and undesirable incentives.

1. *Risk.* The risks (defined in terms of probabilities or magnitude of harm or discomfort) and benefits (either providing new knowledge or improving the health of the individual) to subjects. These risks can be classified as physical, psychological, social, and economic (Levine, 1986).

2. *Informed consent procedures.* The human subject must clearly understand the proposed research, have the capacity to give consent, and voluntarily decide whether to participate. The kinds of information that must be presented include the nature, purpose, and length of the experiments; foreseeable risks and discomforts; potential benefits to the subject or to society; alternative procedures; the degree of confidentiality for the research records; whether compensation or medical treatments will be provided in the case of research-related injury; and a statement that the research is voluntary and refusal to participate will not result in any penalty.

3. *Equity.* The IRB must also consider whether the selection of subjects will be equitable so that burdens and benefits are fairly distributed.

4. *Privacy.* Will the proposed research assure that the subject cannot be identified in the research results and that the confidentiality of the information about the individual that is obtained will not be improperly divulged?

5. *Vulnerable subjects and undue influences.* Subjects classified as vulnerable include children, pregnant women, mentally disabled persons, prisoners, and economically or educationally disadvantaged persons. Distinct limitations on the use of research on fetuses, research on human in vitro fertilization, children, and prisoners are provided in the 1981 DHHS Common Federal Policy (45 C.F.R. 46).

6. *Incentives.* Finally the IRB considers whether the presence and kind of incentives provided to the patient present undue pressure limiting the voluntary nature of the participation decision. Payments can involve money, free health care, free contraception, or a variety of other benefits.

IRBs are an example of an innovative public mechanism for addressing social and ethical issues related to research involving human subjects. IRBs have been able to function with some efficiency because they have the guidance of the federal regulations that resulted from the work of the National Commission, especially from the principles established in the *Belmont Report*. In addition, the constant stream of bioethical literature on the ethics of research can provide insights about special problems that arise.

Although the presence of IRB review has seemingly avoided any new sensational transgressions in human investigation, at least three major problems remain to be addressed: (1) there has been little systematic study of the adequacy of the decision-making process; (2) uncertainty exists about the adequacy of balancing risks and benefits as used in IRBs; and (3) claims have been made that the IRB protects the interests of institutions and investigators over those of subjects (Levine, 1986). Another criticism is that, although IRBs are effective at using rights-based criteria that protect certain values such as autonomy, privacy, and justice, they are unsuccessful at protecting the welfare of subjects as defined in the federal regulations that call for the balancing of the risks and benefits of research (Williams, 1984). The reasons for this problem relate to the bias for approval in the DHHS guidelines, the composition of the committee, and the operation of committees (e.g., unwillingness to truly evaluate an investigator's competence, the unappealing dilemma of either having to reject or redesign the research, and the collective decision making that leads to greater willingness to countenance risks (Veatch, 1987).

An additional problem with which IRBs must contend is that patients may not adequately understand the scientific methodology used in a randomized clinical trial (Appelbaum et al., 1987). In spite of acceptable informed consent procedures, patients often distort or misinterpret the research so that the research is seen to benefit the person directly. This has been labeled the "therapeutic misconception." These concerns were also raised in an article concerning the deaths of participants in the NIH drug trial of Fialuridine, which raised questions not only about whether the consent form gave the volunteers enough information, but whether desperately ill patients involved in a study can truly be informed (Altman, 1993).

Another problem is the time, space, and effort required to deal with the paperwork generated by IRB review and monitoring. In the case of large-scale, multicentered clinical trials, the logistics of separate review by IRBs at all involved institutions, and responding to the concerns raised by each, are also problematic. Lynn et al. (1994) describe the many differences that arose in the proposed informed consent procedures in 50 applications for a health services research project sponsored by the Robert Wood Johnson Foundation. A similar diversity of institutional approaches to consent requirements and risk determination was found by Kavanaugh et al. (1979) when surveying genetic counseling centers.

Because of problems with the IRB system of review, NIH awarded a contract in 1992 to assess the status of the IRB system, in order to ensure that the criteria for the protection of human subjects is still adequate in light of the many changes that have occurred in biomedical, behavioral, and social science research in recent years. This study is designed to examine the costs and burdens borne by IRBs, and to make recommendations to improve the review process.

Hospital Ethics Committees and Physicians

Historical Development of Hospital Ethics Committees

In the last two decades many hospitals have instituted ethics committees charged with providing the institution and its staff with ethical guidance in policy and practice. The development of the hospital ethics committee (HEC) parallels the history of medical ethics and, more particularly, its rise as a clinical discipline (see the background paper by Heitman in this volume). HECs evolved as physicians and other health care professionals, hospital administrators, legal authorities, clergy, and patients and their families struggled to make good decisions about applying resuscitative and life-sustaining technologies. Hospital ethics committees constitute an evolving mechanism for sharing power that traditionally has belonged to physicians. The existence of HECs confirms that others also have the standing to define, discuss, and intervene when significant ethical problems interrupt the continuum of patient care. While most of the work on and by HECs has reflected developments in academic medical ethics, the constraints and practical nature of clinical ethics and institutional policy have sometimes led to significant divergence from theoretical ideals.

In 1990, the Joint Commission on Accreditation of the Health Care Organizations (JCAHO, formerly JCAH) proposed new accreditation standards on patient rights that included a requirement for "mechanism(s) for the consideration of ethical issues in the care of patients and to provide education to caregivers and patients on ethical issues in health care" (JCAHO, 1992). These standards took effect on January 1, 1992, making the existence of an ethics committee (or a similar body or process) a requirement for accreditation and eligibility for Medicare payments for all hospitals in the United States.

The actual prevalence of HECs has been difficult to determine, although there has clearly been remarkable growth in the last decade. The President's Commission survey of 602 hospitals found that in 1982 only 3 percent had an HEC or similar structure, all of them in hospitals with over 200 beds (President's Commission, 1983a). In 1983, 26 percent of hospitals responding to a national survey conducted by AHA's National Society for Patient Representatives reported having an HEC; in a repeat survey in 1985, that number had risen to 60 percent (*Hospitals*, 1985). Large teaching hospitals were much more likely than others to have an HEC, and the proportion of nonteaching hospitals with an ethics committee dropped almost 10 percent in the two years between the surveys.

Despite the fact that over three years have passed since JCAHO's patient rights standards were proposed, some hospitals—particularly small private hospitals and those in rural areas—still do not have formal mechanisms in place, and many are scrambling to determine what is required of them. Even in many hospitals that have established HECs, committee members remain uncertain about their roles, true purpose, and the adequacy of their knowledge in ethics, law, or medicine (Hoffman, 1991; Ross, 1991; and Cohen et al., 1992).

Roles of the HEC

As described in the extensive literature on clinical ethics, the HEC has three typical roles:

1. the creation or recommendation of policy on ethical issues in patient care;
2. the education of hospital staff, patients, family members, and the community on ethical issues and the institution's policies; and
3. deliberation and consultation on specific questions in the treatment of identified patients.

Not all HECs engage in all three activities, and some have additional responsibilities. JCAHO standards call only for committees to provide education on ethical issues and to provide a forum for the discussion of those issues. However, these three aspects of clinical ethics are complementary and mutually sustaining.

The membership of the HECs ultimately reflects the question of who the committee is intended to serve: the hospital, the physician, the staff, the patient and family, or some other entity. Diversity of discipline and professional expertise expands the HEC's ability to recognize and understand the medical and medically related problems and options that particular issues and cases may entail; the need for such diversity is widely appreciated and addressed in practice. Less well addressed in practice is the need for diversity of age, race, gender, ethnicity, and socioeconomic status.

In the past five years, networks of HECs have appeared across the United States as individual committees consult with one another in an effort to improve themselves (Kushner, 1988). Typically, members of networks share institutional policies and general advice with newly developing committees, coordinate educational efforts, and review the handling of particularly troublesome cases, real or fictional. Such administrative umbrellas may become increasingly important with the implementation of health care reform, both to facilitate the integration of allied HECs and to ensure that managed competition does not compromise the ethical quality of care.

As some HECs enter their second decade, many others are just getting started. A tremendous amount remains unknown about the future of ethics committees. A few issues on the horizon include the development of HECs in nursing homes and other long-term care facilities, the liability of HECs and their members for advisory opinions, the role of HECs in cost containment, and the need for careful evaluation of HECs in their many capacities.

In the more than 10 years that professional organizations and licensing and accrediting bodies have recommended or required the establishment of HECs, there have been many calls for substantive evaluation of their effects (Levine, 1977; President's Commission, 1983a; Rosner, 1985; Craig et al., 1986; Hosford, 1986; Ross et al., 1986; Lo, 1987; van Allen et al., 1989; McCloskey, 1991; West and Gibson, 1992). To date, assessment has been limited to a few academic articles (primarily on their effects on do-not-resuscitate orders and limiting intervention), workshops at professional meetings, and the informal shoptalk of clinical ethicists.

IOM and OTA

The Institute of Medicine (IOM) and the Office of Technology Assessment (OTA) have also from time to time engaged in bioethics deliberation. An arm of the National Academy of Sciences (NAS), IOM is a private, nonprofit organization, associated with the government by virtue of the 1863 NAS congressional charter to advise the federal government on matters pertaining to science. OTA is a branch of the U.S. Congress, established to advise congressional committees on technical issues in all areas of science and technology. Both IOM and OTA have issued reports on a variety of ethical issues over the past 20 years.

Institute of Medicine

IOM was chartered by NAS in 1970 to enlist distinguished members of the medical and other professions in the study of issues and problems that affect human health. IOM's principal resource for carrying out its mission is its elected membership of nearly 1,000 professionals from the fields of basic science, clinical science, behavioral and social science, and health care. As mandated, at least 20 percent of IOM members are drawn from fields outside of medicine, including law, economics, engineering, and the physical sciences, lending to the membership a diversity that ensures a breadth of perspective and multidisciplinary approach to IOM activities. Other distinguished professionals who are not IOM members also contribute greatly to the work of IOM through service on committees and advisory boards and through scholarly review of IOM reports.

IOM addresses health issues through a variety of mechanisms, including workshops, roundtable sessions, forums, and symposia. Most frequently, however, IOM convenes committees of persons with relevant expertise to conduct comprehensive studies of specific issues. Conducted in response to requests from the federal government and other public and private agencies, these studies usually last between 6 and 24 months and result in independently reviewed, published reports with policy recommendations. A large majority of the studies are funded by governmental agencies; a smaller proportion are funded by foundations, voluntary organizations, and industry representatives. In some cases, ideas about issues that merit study are generated within IOM and funded either from outside sources or from IOM/NAS internal sources. Reports and other products of IOM are disseminated to sponsoring agencies, interested professionals, and the public.

IOM has a long-standing interest in bioethics, which was a new discipline when IOM was founded. It seems evident from the wording of the IOM charter and from some of its initial activities that its establishment was prompted by some of the same concerns that pushed bioethics into the limelight as a discipline in its own right in the late 1960s and early 1970s. At that time, medicine was struggling (as it continues to do today) with new dilemmas brought on in large part by the development of new and expensive medical technologies. How should health care resources be allocated? When is it appropriate or inappropriate to use medical technologies to delay the end of life? These were some of the first questions that IOM attempted to answer in a 1973 conference on Health Care and Changing Values. The report that resulted from this conference, *Ethics of Health Care* (1974), examined such issues as the preciousness of life, the consumer's perception of health as a value, ethical problems in treating the chronically ill and aged, and the origin of professional values.

Throughout the 1970s, "ethical and legal aspects of health care delivery" remained an IOM program priority. A Division of Legal, Ethical, and Educational Aspects of Health was established in 1977 and subsequently published several reports, including *The Elderly and Functional Dependency* (1977) and *Beyond Malpractice: Compensation for Medical Injuries* (1978a), as well as commissioned papers such as *The Rights of Physicians: A Philosophical Essay* (1978c) and *Ethical Issues in Governmental Efforts to Promote Health* (1978b). Only one year after its establishment, a funding crisis stemming from changes in federal policy regarding indirect costs challenged the division's core funding and it was eliminated. Although several ongoing and newly initiated projects were shifted to other divisions and completed, the division itself—and IOM's only focused program on ethics—was not preserved.

IOM nevertheless continues to address social and ethical issues in the context of its reports. IOM has half a dozen of the leading bioethicists among its elected members. Other ethicists have been sought to serve as committee members and report reviewers, and social and ethical issues have been made the focus of report chapters in some cases, and integrated throughout reports in others (IOM, 1986, 1991a, 1991b, 1993). More recently, IOM's Division of Health Sciences Policy has taken on studies that explicitly address social and ethical issues. In 1989, the division published *The Responsible Conduct of Research in the Health Sciences,* a report that proposed ways to encourage high ethical standards in the conduct of research without harming the freedom and creativity that have traditionally characterized U.S. research institutions. In 1990, NIH's and Department of Energy's Ethical, Legal, and Social Implications Program commissioned an IOM study of the issues raised by new capacities in genetic testing. The report of this study committee, entitled, *Assessing Genetic Risks,* was recently published (IOM, 1994). In 1992, NIH also provided funding for an IOM committee to explore the legal and ethical issues relating to the inclusion of women in clinical studies. While both studies addressed some scientific issues, their primary focus was on ethical, legal, and social considerations.

How best to study ethical issues in medicine and health policy has been another recurrent concern. In June 1983, IOM convened a conference on strategies for deliberation of ethical issues at the national level. The President's Commission had expired at the end of March 1983, and the IOM conference was intended for discussion of the need for a new group to replace the President's Commission and of the role, if any, that IOM should play. Conference participants were unanimous in their belief that a new bioethics body was needed, but not in their opinions about whether IOM should have a role. In their debate about the role of IOM in national bioethics deliberation, they noted several advantages and disadvantages of IOM as a professional/institutional mechanism for deliberation of ethical issues.

Characteristics that enhance IOM's ability to address ethical issues carefully and credibly include the fact that IOM is a private organization and therefore less subject than a government agency or federal body to changing political winds. Its membership is large and diverse, and it frequently draws on the expertise of nonmember professionals when needed. Significant care is taken in the composition of IOM committees to ensure that diverse viewpoints on an issue are represented, that biases are disclosed, and that individuals with potential conflicts of interest do not participate in the development of recommendations in the area of conflict.

Other characteristics could be said to detract from IOM's ability to address ethical issues credibly. IOM has little stable funding and therefore has limited ability to direct its attention to issues that it deems important but for which funding might not be available from government or private sources. In addition, administrative complications arising from multiple sources of funding can delay the initiation of projects considerably, limiting IOM's ability to take on ethical issues or dilemmas requiring a prompt response. Recently, administrative reforms have enhanced IOM's capacity to conduct rapid studies on focused issues, once funding is secured.

IOM's effectiveness could also be called into question because it conducts the majority of its work in private. IOM is not subject to the Federal Advisory Committee Act of 1972, which requires federal advisory bodies to permit public access to their deliberations. Particularly in the American cultural context, people may be reluctant to embrace conclusions on value-laden ethical issues when they are reached behind closed doors.

Office of Technology Assessment

OTA was established by Congress in 1972 to respond to requests by congressional committees for analyses of emerging and complex technical issues in a wide range of fields. Governed by a 12-member Technology Assessment Board composed of six Senators and six Representatives, OTA organizes briefings, provides testimony, and conducts extensive studies, some requiring more than two years to complete. Participants include OTA staff, professionals from the private sector and the academic community, representatives from public interest groups and state and local governments, and citizens at large. Through these activities, OTA assists Congress in clarifying uncertainties, resolving conflicting claims, and explicating options in the vast arena of science and technology policy. As its name implies, one of OTA's foremost responsibilities is to assess the impact of new developments on future federal policy. While OTA frequently identifies the pros and cons of proposed policies or actions, however, it does not make policy recommendations.

OTA began to address ethical issues explicitly in the early 1980s, beginning with a 1983 report on the role of genetic testing in the prevention of occupational disease (OTA, 1983). The following year, OTA published a report on human gene therapy that specifically addressed the ethical acceptability of different kinds of gene therapy and their implications for society (OTA, 1984a). A series of reports followed that included chapters on ethical considerations or extensive discussions of ethical issues (OTA, 1984b; 1985a; 1986; 1987c; 1988b,c). Bioethicists were increasingly sought to consult on OTA projects related to health policy and biomedical research. At one point, each OTA report generally contained an ethics chapter, and, at times, OTA employed a resident bioethicist.

In the late 1980s and early 1990s, several more reports that gave primary emphasis to ethical considerations were issued by OTA: *Technology and Aging in America* (1985b), *Ownership of Human Tissues and Cells* (1987b), *Life-Sustaining Technologies and the Elderly* (1987a), *Infertility: Medical and Social Choices* (1988a), *Patenting Life* (1989), *Neural Grafting: Repairing the Brain and Spinal Cord* (1990), and *Summary: Evaluation of the Oregon Medicaid Proposal* (1992b). OTA continues to be involved in ethics today, having recently conducted studies of cystic fibrosis and health insurers (1992a) and ethics in U.S. public policy (1993).

Thus, while OTA has never had an explicit mandate to address bioethical issues, its efforts to assess the impacts of emerging technologies on society have forced it to confront complex ethical dilemmas on several occasions. Like IOM, OTA has inherent strengths and weaknesses as a deliberator of ethical issues in medicine and health policy. One of OTA's strengths is its ability to enlist the expertise of a wide range of persons representing different social and ethical perspectives to participate in working groups or to provide testimony. In addition, OTA has an informal policy that all of its activities are accessible to the public, a policy that enhances its ability to gather information as well as its credibility. Another strength is stable funding: OTA need not raise funds from outside sources to conduct its activities; all funding is provided by congressional allocation. This allows OTA to activate studies quickly and deliver reports in a timely fashion.

One of OTA's weaknesses as a deliberator of value-laden ethical issues is that, by virtue of its attachment to Congress, it is perceived as a highly political entity. When the President's Commission expired in 1983, OTA (like IOM) was considered as a possible locus for a replacement ethics body. Claims that an OTA-based ethics body would be "bureaucratized and inadequately buffered from the political process" and that "elected officials would retain direct control over OTA policy" in part kept this from coming to fruition (Abram and Wolf, 1984). Finally, while OTA is able to respond rapidly to direct congressional requests for studies, it is not well situated to respond quickly to needs that arise outside of Congress, whether in federal agencies or elsewhere. Federal agencies hoping to initiate an OTA study must work with Congress to have the study commissioned. In the case of ethical dilemmas requiring prompt resolution, delays in the commissioning of a study pose serious disadvantages.

Ethics Centers

Deliberation about ethical issues arising from developments in biomedicine also takes place at several research and educational centers throughout the world devoted specifically to the study of ethics. Described here are the Hastings Center and the Kennedy Institute of Ethics, two of the best-known ethics centers in this country. However, they are only two of a cadre of centers devoted to bioethics research and education that have experienced tremendous growth in the past two decades. Together, hundreds of bioethics organizations around the world comprise a remarkable new resource for policymaking, analysis, consultation, and education in medicine and the life sciences. Ethics centers such as Hastings and Kennedy influence policy development in the area of ethics through conferences, publications, and educational programs. In addition, staff from these centers are frequently called upon to serve on the boards of academic institutions, research centers, professional societies, and nonprofit organizations, as well as journal editorial boards. The Clinton administration's task force on health care reform provides a recent example of a public policy activity in which experts in ethics were called upon to participate.

Hastings Center

Founded in 1969, the Hastings Center is an independent, nonprofit, and nonpartisan research and educational institute for the examination of ethical and social issues in medicine, the life sciences, and the professions. The center is located in Briarcliff Manor, New York, and employs a professional staff of 13 persons with special interest and expertise in biomedical ethics. The center has three primary goals:

1. to raise the level of competence and research in the examination of the ethical and social problems arising out of advances in the life, behavioral, and social sciences;

2. to assist educational institutions in the development of programs designed to make a consideration of ethical problems an integral part of higher education; and

3. to bring the importance of the ethical and social problems to the attention of professional and policymaking bodies and to assist them, when requested, by supplying technical advice and by making available results of analysis, study, and research (Nolen and Coutts, 1993).

The Hastings Center strives to achieve these goals through sponsorship of conferences on topics in biomedical ethics and support of educational opportunities such as student internships, a visiting scholars program, and international fellowships. The center publishes the *Hastings Center Report,* a bimonthly publication that features articles, commentary, literature reviews, and announcements of conferences and educational and employment opportunities throughout the country and abroad. The center also publishes

IRB: A Review of Human Subjects, a bimonthly journal featuring articles of relevance to the work of institutional review boards.

Kennedy Institute of Ethics

The Joseph and Rose Kennedy Institute of Ethics was established in 1971 at Georgetown University in Washington, D.C., as a research and teaching center to offer moral and ethical perspectives on public policy issues (Nolen and Coutts, 1993). With 12 senior research scholars, 2 international scholars, and 29 senior research fellows, the Kennedy Institute represents the largest university-based group of scholars in the world devoted to research and teaching in biomedical ethics and other fields of applied ethics. Faculty members bring expertise from such disciplines as philosophy, religion, medicine, social science, and law. Bioethical issues such as in vitro fertilization, abortion, health resource allocation, use of life-sustaining technologies, organ transplantation, euthanasia, and gene therapy have been the focus of research.

In addition to activities in this country, the Kennedy Institute conducts an "Asian Bioethics Program" that, together with the Waseda University's Center for Human Sciences in Tokyo, has been organizing a series of U.S.-Japan Bioethics Conferences since 1985. These conferences have focused on cross-cultural aspects of both biomedical ethics and business ethics. The institute's European Program in Bioethics was established with the aim of developing and enriching moral awareness in the fields of business, environment, regulation, engineering, and medicine. Courses and symposia for this program are initially developed in Germany and subsequently in other European countries.

The Kennedy Institute also houses the National Reference Center for Bioethics Literature, the world's largest collection of books and articles related to ethical issues in health care and biomedical research. The reference center has several special collections, including collections on Jewish ethics, Christian ethics, and federal bioethics commissions. It also maintains and administers an online database of bioethics literature that is part of the National Library of Medicine's database system, which is accessible worldwide.

The Kennedy Institute produces several publications, including the quarterly *Kennedy Institute of Ethics Journal,* which contains essays and reviews; the *Bibliography of Bioethics,* an annual collection of citations to books, journals, court decisions, government documents, and other materials related to bioethics; and the *Encyclopedia of Bioethics,* a basic reference work containing information about ethical issues in the life sciences. A new edition of the *Encyclopedia of Bioethics,* first published in 1976, is currently being prepared.

Religious Groups

The connection between religion and health is as old as human culture. While conflicts have appeared along the way (traditional versus scientific medical practice, and the refusal of some religious groups to accept certain medical procedures, etc.), religion and medicine have developed a productive partnership over the past 100 years in most parts of the world. That partnership has been greatly enriched in recent decades.

Religion has made noteworthy contributions to medicine, especially in the area of patient care and in helping patients to understand and deal with disease and catastrophes. At the same time, religious beliefs have proved to be a formidable stimulus to the evaluation of some developments in biomedicine—especially contraception, birth control, and other aspects of human sexuality, as well as end-of-life issues.

Roman Catholic theologians have examined certain central questions about the ethical aspects of medical care for several centuries. They have written treatises in which they applied their principal ethical theory, natural law, to subjects such as abortion, sterilization, and the obligation to accept life-saving treatments. Similarly, Jewish law has for centuries attended to similar questions about life, death, health, and illness, and the acute analyses of the rabbinical scholars has become familiar to the orthodox. Thus, as the new issues of bioethics began to appear, two major religious traditions already had a stock of concepts and opinions on certain of these issues and scholars in those traditions began to apply them to the new questions.

In recent years, North American religious groups have produced some excellent, carefully researched reports for their national or regional bodies; the Presbyterian report on health care is a good example (Presbyterian Church, U.S.A., 1988). These documents have sometimes failed to gain full endorsement of the groups for which they were prepared, but as working documents available for study and reflection in the life of the religious communities, such documents have exercised great influence. And some of these documents produced by and for religious groups (churches, synagogues, religious societies) have become valued literature in the field.

As noted in Chapter 2, some twentieth century theologians and philosophers of religion were pioneers in reflecting on the import of religion for biomedical developments and in giving an entirely new character to the area in medicine called *medical ethics*. Theologians and clergy have continued to be important contributors to bioethics. The establishment of professorships at Georgetown University, the University of Notre Dame, and Vanderbilt University charged to deal directly with the relations of religion, law, and philosophy to medical sciences and practice has followed, giving further standing to the place of religion in biomedicine. Such work has been greatly furthered by separate institutions dealing with medical ethics described above. Work of this sort has also taken place in Great Britain and Commonwealth countries and is gaining ground in European nations.

Interfaith and ecumenical bodies have also begun to study the import for religion of developments in biomedicine. The World Council of Churches and the National Council of Churches have worked to develop guidelines dealing with such issues as population control, access to medical treatment, and ways to face life's end. Studies of this sort are particularly timely and valuable in light of today's widespread religious pluralism. Consensus is difficult on many of the issues in medical ethics that religious groups discuss, but religious pluralism itself may require of the leaders of religious groups not only more civility in dealing with opponents of their views but also greater understanding of positions different from their own. Some rapprochement may have developed in the summer of 1993 as the World Parliament of Religions sought common understanding on moral questions at its Chicago gathering.

On June 20, 1980, the General Secretaries of the National Council of Churches, the Synagogue Council of America, and the United States Catholic Conference addressed a letter to President Carter expressing concern over the ethical implications of genetic engineering. Their letter stated, "We are rapidly moving into a new era of fundamental danger triggered by the rapid growth of genetic engineering, albeit there may be opportunity for doing good; the term suggests the danger" and called upon President Carter to remedy the lack of "adequate oversight or control . . . by providing a way for representatives of a broad spectrum of our society to consider these matters and advise the government of its necessary role" (President's Commission, 1982b). President Carter passed the letter to his science advisor, who requested the President's Commission to consider it. The commission decided to undertake a special study, not included in its congressional mandate, that explored the questions raised by the religious leaders. This study, entitled *Splicing Life*, reviewed the religious and moral questions in light of the scientific possibilities and attempted to delineate with care the precise areas of concern to which public attention should be directed. Many of these areas now fall within the mandate of the ELSI Program of the National Center for Human Genome Research.

Religious groups often find it difficult to affirm their own stance and values without ruling out alternative views and visions. Intolerance is not, of course, restricted to persons of religious faith. But the sheer number of individuals and groups working on these issues offers some encouragement that more useful modes of discourse will be developed, and that religious controversies in the field of biomedicine will become more productive. Such a development would be a boon to religion, to medical science and practice, and to the public good.

INDIVIDUAL AND COMMUNITY RESPONSES

The widespread American tendency to initiate and develop voluntary associations around a whole range of social, moral, and political purposes has a long history. In the early nineteenth century (1835), visiting French social theorist Alexis de Tocqueville commented on the tendency for self-help groups to emerge in American communities. Indeed, Tocqueville appropriately characterized the proliferation of voluntary associations as a distinctly American phenomenon:

> In no country in the world has the principle of association been more successfully used or applied to a greater multitude of objects than in America. . . . The citizen of the United States is taught from infancy to rely upon his own exertions in order to resist the evils and the difficulties of life. . . .

While voluntary associations are hardly new to the American cultural scene, the self-conscious application of voluntarism and wider public participation in the medical sphere emerged most strongly out of the consumer and community organizing movements of the 1960s. For example, although self-care has always been an unacknowledged part of the informal health care system, the practice of self-care has increased dramatically in the past 20 years. Some have argued that the current embrace of self-help and health support groups, particularly by HMOs, reflects the transformation of a movement of consumers organized for themselves into an incorporated and co-opted component of the American medical establishment (DeFriese, 1989). Patient advocacy groups, family support groups, and disease-specific self-help groups, once considered radical for their aim of increasing individual control and responsibility over health, have become integral to the nation's dominant public health policy (Crawford, 1977; Stone, 1989; Taylor, 1986; Tesh, 1988). Such lifestyle changes and the public discussions they inspire touch the boundaries of important ethical issues concerning individual autonomy. Thus, activities that initially appear to be political and social in nature frequently have relevance to central ethical problems in biomedicine.

Grassroots Efforts

Individuals, groups, and communities are often spurred to action in the wake of changes wrought by developments in biomedicine. We have already seen the critical role that professional associations have played, primarily by providing ethical and practical guidance to physicians in the use of these technologies. Yet voluntary efforts are not confined to organizations with preexisting structures and stable numbers of professionally educated members. Some voluntary organizations are more loosely structured and come into being as a result of a perceived crisis, as did the National Abortion Rights League (NARAL) or in response to a particular condition or disease as did the AIDS Coalition to Unleash Power (ACT-UP). They often inspire the loyal support of individuals who have little else in common than their interest in resolving the crisis or managing the treatment for the disease. Others, such as the broad-based citizen-sponsored forums on health care that took place in Vermont, Maine, California, and Oregon, have devoted long hours to the examination of a wide variety of challenging issues in health care, attempting to provide both policy and personal guidance to legislators and fellow citizens.

Increasingly, patients actively participate in the delivery of health services, disease prevention practices, and health education. Contemporary "self-care" movements include participation in a variety of self-help groups from postoperative recovery groups, cancer support groups, support groups for those with a family member who has a chronic disease, and the various permutations in twelve-step recovery programs (from alcohol or drug problems to obesity). Practitioners, scholars, and ethicists justify the shift of responsibility to individuals on the grounds that it increases both patient control and the efficiency of care. Others argue that incorporating self-care improves health outcomes while increasing the experience of self-control and enhancing quality of life.

Such efforts and groups are best characterized as "grassroots," and, depending on their structure and purpose, sometimes are also known as community-based organizations (CBOs) (National Research Council, 1993). There are so many grassroots efforts and CBOs that it would be impractical to discuss all of them here; hence, the groups described in this section merely illustrate the wide variety of groups that exist. Some of these groups have had a significant impact on the research into and use of biomedical technologies, as well as public discussion of these issues. The impact of grassroots organizations has been particularly notable in the field of AIDS research and treatment, as well as in the areas of contraceptive technology and fetal tissue transplantation research.

AIDS Grassroots Organizations

Grassroots organizations have proliferated in direct response to the AIDS epidemic. It is estimated that more than 600 such organizations formed in the last decade alone (National Research Council, 1993). Many of these organizations had their roots in the gay community, which had created a network of medical self-help groups years earlier in response to perceived discrimination by the medical establishment. Such groups were flexible and quick to adapt to the needs of AIDS sufferers and their families. Their initial aims were to provide appropriate medical care and social support, but some extended their efforts into the political arena, challenging the way in which both the government and the medical community were responding to the AIDS crisis.

The AIDS Coalition to Unleash Power is one of the most visible and proactive of these groups, combining public protest, acts of civil disobedience, and media events with the more traditional political methods of lobbying and education to raise public awareness and change policies. ACT-UP is notable for its unprecedented success in changing federal drug development procedures to allow the early release of a promising new AIDS drug. Through careful organization, sustained contact with sympathetic elected representatives, and the acquisition of a well-deserved reputation for being knowledgeable and articulate on medical developments in AIDS, members of its Treatment and Data Committee gained standing to participate in pivotal discussions in NIH, FDA, and other forums. Their views influenced critical policy decisions concerning the research process for experimental drugs and set the stage for greater citizen involvement in the future in such decisions (Levi, 1991).

Abortion Grassroots Organizations

The National Abortion Rights Action League supports a woman's right to choose and has been vocal in its opposition to efforts to restrict that right. Although other women's organizations actively support the availability of abortion (e.g., National Organization of Women and the National Women's Health Network), no other has abortion as its raison d'être. NARAL publishes newsletters, rallies its supporters to public protests, lobbies representatives, and sponsors forums in which scientific, legal, and ethical scholars and legislators sympathetic to this cause present compelling arguments for policies that guarantee women's reproductive autonomy, including the continued availability of abortion and research into contraceptive technologies that make abortion less necessary. In 1991, NARAL sponsored a symposium on the federal ban on fetal tissue transplantation research at which participants decried both the policy itself and the tenuous linkage that DHHS had made between such research and a hypothetical increase in abortions (NARAL, 1991).

NARAL's antiabortion counterpart is found in the National Right to Life Committee (NRLC), a pro-life organization that opposes abortion, euthanasia, and infanticide. NRLC supports abortion alternative programs involving counseling and adoption, provides ongoing public education programs, lobbies before congressional committees, and conducts research. The NRLC was instrumental in preventing RU-486, a highly effective abortifacient, from being introduced into this country. Pharmaceutical companies have been very reluctant to conduct research on contraception, not only because of weak governmental support for such research but also because of the willingness of NRLC and other antiabortion groups to engage in public protests and threaten boycotts if they do proceed with such research. The history of the development and distribution of RU-486 in France confirms that these fears of reprisal are well founded. Because many drug companies are unwilling to become the target of controversial protests, they will avoid areas of research that may provoke such action. In the case of RU-486, and in the development of contraceptive technology in general, the grassroots antiabortion movement thus far has been largely successful in its goal (Charo, 1991).

Community Prevention

Sometimes entire communities (whether geographic, ethnic, or cultural) respond to the changes brought about by technological advances. The response of communities has been variable: weaker for general health initiatives, but often stronger for specific initiatives such as screening for genetic disease. Success in the latter enterprise has also varied widely depending on the particular community and the strategies of the agencies that initiate and organize the screening. In general, however, large-scale community-based health education and intervention programs—in such areas as heart disease, nutrition, smoking, and drugs—have either not worked or worked only within certain limited class, educational, cultural, and racially or ethnically distinct community segments. Few have succeeded in effecting lasting changes in health behavior (Mechanic, 1990, 1992). Their failure is increasingly recognized as a function of treating health behavior as an individual rather than a social and cultural phenomenon (Mechanic, 1990; Syme and Alcalay, 1982). One notable exception is the recent series of efforts to curb smoking by stepping up public education and by banning smoking in public places; these initiatives seem to have reduced smoking behavior in many sectors of society. A growing body of research shows that cultural factors are critical to understanding and modifying health-related behavior, including preventive action (Cruickshank and Beevers, 1989; Graham, 1984; Mascie-Taylor, 1993; Strauss, 1991; Helman, 1990; Biersecker et al., 1987; Armstrong, 1989).

Assessing Genetic Risks

Cultural issues are particularly salient in understanding responses to new genetic knowledge and screening possibilities, in part because genetic disorders, to a greater extent than other health problems, coincide with "risk populations" that are ethnically and racially demarcated. Thus, each disorder may exist in a different cultural context: Americans of African descent are at greater risk for sickle cell anemia; Americans of European descent are at greater risk for cystic fibrosis; Americans of Ashkenazi Jewish descent are at greater risk for Tay-Sachs disease; Americans of Southern Italian descent are at greater risk for beta-thalassemia (McKusick, 1988). Because genetic disorders are typically located in subsets of populations at greater risk due to ethnic and racial endogamy, because transmission is limited to offspring, and because there are no cures for any of these genetic disorders, the question of who screens whom and for what purpose is potentially charged and culturally loaded.

Genetic disorders are experienced not only by individuals and their families, but also simultaneously by risk populations that are culturally distinct, and these populations will have highly variable responses to "their disease." The variability will be linked to their social attributes, including the meaning of a genetic disorder in their respective cultural, racial, or ethnic groups. In the past, many community health interventions have not worked because they have not been articulated with the cultural meanings and constructions which are at the center of people's everyday life priorities (Syme and Alcalay, 1982). For example, important elements of genetic knowledge do penetrate into the popular culture, and people do use genetic explanations to account for maladies and odd traits in their families, but in most cases they do not use genetic information (through testing, screening, counseling) to guide their health-related behaviors. The exceptions to this pattern occur when the larger social context of a genetic disorder becomes either highly politicized, as with sickle cell anemia in the late 1960s, or when a community "takes over and possesses its own genetic disorder," as with Tay-Sachs disease during the early 1970s.

With respect to the latter, a community-based carrier screening program was initiated in the greater Baltimore/Washington area in the early 1970s. The program had the support of leading rabbis, and worked with a committee of committed lay people. Brochures from supportive physicians blanketed the Jewish community. Mass mailings and television and radio announcements were also used, all in support of a community-ratified voluntary screening program. Before the program, 98 percent of the Jews in the area that were surveyed had never heard of Tay-Sachs. Within a year, not only were 95 percent of those surveyed aware of the disorder, but thousands volunteered for screening (Stine, 1977). In the first year of the program, 7,000 adults, approximately 10 percent of the total eligible population, were screened (NAS, 1975). One of the key architects of this program, Michael Kaback, perhaps the world's leading specialist on the topic, had this to say about the issue of voluntary versus mandatory screening:

> An alternative approach, mandatory (or legislated) screening, although easier to implement perhaps, was regarded as unwarranted, unnecessary and ethically unacceptable (Kaback et al., 1974).

The estimated cost of the program was $65,000 to provide equipment, supplies, and personnel. All those screened were asked to contribute $5, and most did so. At-risk couples received counseling, and reports indicate that it was direct, careful, and sensitive (Stine, 1977). The success of the initial Baltimore/Washington project was such that scores of Jewish communities around the United States followed suit and were later joined by Jewish communities in five other countries. By the early 1980s, over 310,000 Jews around the world had been screened *voluntarily*, leading to the identification of 268 couples in which both partners were carriers. In New York city, Hasidic Jews developed a program, the Chevra Dor Yeshorim program, to deter the marriage of partners who were both carriers of the Tay-Sachs gene (Merz, 1987).

The history of screening for sickle cell was very different. Perhaps most significantly, many of the screening programs were developed without adequate consultation and education of the affected communities (IOM, 1994). Little could be offered to high-risk couples once they were identified and safe prenatal diagnosis of sickle cell disease was not possible at the time (as it was for Tay-Sachs). The failure of the Black Panthers (who were among the first to start and favor sickle cell screening) as well as the politically motivated whites, to recognize the technological limitations made the experience of sickle cell screening a very negative one for the African American community. Some have also suggested that, while many of those who were managing or recruiting for these screening programs were doing so for health and medical reasons, a sizeable proportion came from community-based organizations that had a political agenda, including urban poverty programs and methadone clinics (Duster, 1990).

Rationalizing Health Care Priorities

One of the side effects of advances in biomedicine has been skyrocketing health care costs, particularly of the elderly, premature infants, and those with rare disorders. In contrast, preventive medicine has sometimes gotten short shrift, despite the demonstrable cost savings to society. This situation has led to several attempts around the nation to "rationalize" the allocation of health care. The most famous case has been the work of the Oregon Health Services Commission, which expanded the notion of community responses to include well-organized, focused, volunteer-led group discussion of vital health care issues. The higher-level initiative brought together citizens from different geographical, socioeconomic, and cultural communities.

In the mid-1980s, Oregon was faced with a series of very difficult decisions about the provision of transplants for poor children. The cost for one liver transplant was so high that the same amount of money could provide prenatal care for poor women in the state for almost a year. As a result, Oregon ended funding for soft-tissue transplants. The rationale was simple enough: that it would be more cost-effective to transfer a projected $1.1 million per year from the transplants to prenatal care (Daniels, 1991). This action initiated fierce debate, but the debate itself provided neither the criteria for ranking health care procedures nor the process that would establish such criteria. It was not clear whether such a project should be entrusted to a group of medical experts, elected officials, the general public, or some combination thereof.

The solution was a major, statewide grassroots effort. Oregon Health Decisions, a private, nonprofit community educational group, sponsored citizen meetings throughout the state, encouraging serious thought about the proper allocation of Medicaid dollars through carefully led group discussions centering on specific difficult medical cases (Crawshaw et al., 1985; Garland, 1992; OTA, 1992b). The values undergirding a desirable health care system were enumerated by citizens, and included equity, quality of life, cost, functional independence, and community compassion (Garland and Hasnain, 1990). A summary document set forth these and other principles, one of which was that the poor should be guaranteed access to basic health care services, even if it meant that the range of services available to that same group had to be restricted. Thus, citizens favored the *breadth* of service provision (minimal services to many) over the *depth* of service provision (extensive services to a few). Because these fundamental principles were arrived at through an open and democratic process, they achieved a certain legitimacy that might not have been earned by alternative approaches (Welch and Dixon, 1991). The information provided by these discussions and the results of a parliamentary debate and vote taken by citizens chosen from these statewide discussion groups was part of the information used by the 11-member Oregon Health Services Commission to guide the ranking of health care services (Klevit et al., 1991).

In early May of 1990, the commission published a list of health care services, with each assigned a different level of priority; coverage would be restricted to those conditions assigned a high priority (Hadorn, 1991). The Oregon experience has generated considerable debate and controversy, in part because of particular rankings but primarily because it highlights the essential and enduring conflict between individual and collective interests. As health care is increasingly viewed as an issue in the public domain, this conflict—between expensive procedures to save the lives of a few and inexpensive preventive measures to save the lives (or improve the quality of life) of the many—will increase. Another set of issues raised by citizen-sponsored health forums in Oregon and other states and regions (e.g., California's Orange County, Hawaii, Maine, Washington, Idaho) is that of participatory democracy and its role in the allocation of scarce health resources, including the use and/or restriction of biomedical technologies (Jennings, 1988).

While political scientists have long argued that apathy pervades the democratic political arena (at least in the United States), this indifference has not been evident in the citizen-sponsored health forums (Jennings, 1993). On the contrary, citizens have been energized and active in these efforts, with minimal outside encouragement and no apparent rewards for their involvement other than the intrinsic satisfaction of participation. There was much variation among the states in their approach to these forums, but their successes had several critical elements in common:

• building a base of community support by utilizing existing community groups and recognized leaders;
• holding forums carefully structured to allow open discussion of competing views;
• relying on motivated, trained volunteers; and
• channeling the enthusiasm surrounding the discussions into constructive action (Jennings, 1988).

The success of these efforts suggests that true participatory democracy may play a unique and vibrant role in health care reform and practice. Not only does the process itself provide satisfaction to participants, it also confers legitimacy upon the decisions reached. Moreover, because biomedical advances are an integral part of the discussions concerning the allocation of health care, these forums set the stage for greater citizen monitoring of and influence in the development and use of biomedical technologies.

It is critical to note that these citizen efforts, while fruitful, are not without their limitations. Those who participated in these community discussions were more likely to be white, affluent, and better-educated than most Oregon residents. In some instances more than 50 percent of participants were health professionals. Only 9.4 percent of participants were persons without insurance. Given that the uninsured constitute 16 percent of Oregon's population, it is clear that this group was underrepresented. Medicaid recipients, too, were seriously underrepresented (Daniels, 1991). Thus, those least likely to attend these meetings—the poor, underemployed, elderly, minorities, and Medicaid recipients—were those most likely to be seriously affected by any rationing plan developed as part of health care reform. Without the input of these groups, the ultimate validity of such citizen proposals is seriously undermined.

Nearly every public issue requires moral judgment in its resolution. For some issues, however, consideration of moral ideas such as dignity, freedom, rights, justice, respect, and equality are especially critical to resolution. Scientific and social changes stemming from developments in biomedicine have raised such issues. These changes have exerted particular pressure on deep-rooted moral ideas acquired through experiences with one's family, church, and country, and have thus presented society with complex social and ethical quandaries. As we have seen in this chapter, debate about these quandaries is occurring in many places and in many ways throughout our society. Some of the debate has been conducted in an undisciplined fashion, in which the interests of particular interests groups have dominated. More constructively, however, the debate has involved open, informed, and impartial discussion, mutual respect, and rational moral deliberation. Given the impending changes in health care and the promise of continued scientific development, it will be important to ensure that there are places where this sort of deliberation can continue to take place so that the storm of debate can be picked up, channelled, made comprehensible, and perhaps even brought to bear on long-term solutions like the restructuring of institutions and laws.

REFERENCES

Abram, M.B., and Wolf, S.M. 1984. Public involvement in medical ethics: A model for government action. *New England Journal of Medicine* 310:627–632.

Altman, L.K. 1993. Fatal drug trial raises questions about "informed consent." *New York Times* (Oct. 5):C3.

American College of Obstetricians and Gynecologists (ACOG). 1990. *Ethical Issues in Surrogate Motherhood.* Committee on Ethics Opinion Number 88. Washington, D.C.: ACOG.

ACOG. 1991. News Release: New Board to Monitor Preembryo and Fetal Tissue Research Announced (4 September). Washington, D.C.: ACOG.

ACOG. 1992. List of Committee Opinions (December). Washington, D.C.: ACOG Resource Center.

American College of Physicians (ACP). 1992. American College of Physicians Ethics Manual, Third Edition. *Annals of Internal Medicine* 117:947–960.

American Medical Association (AMA). 1981. Guidelines for the determination of death: Report of Medical Consultants on the diagnosis death to the President's Commission. *Journal of the American Medical Association* 246(19):2184–2186.

AMA. 1992a. *Code of Medical Ethics: Annotated Current Opinions.* Chicago, IL: AMA.

AMA. 1992b. *Code of Medical Ethics: Reports of the Ethical and Judicial Affairs of the American Medical Association.* Vol. 3, No. 1 (January). Chicago, IL: AMA.

American Thoracic Society (ATS). 1991. Withholding and withdrawing life sustaining therapy. *American Review of Respiratory Diseases* 144:726–731.

Appelbaum, P.S., Roth, L.H., Lidz, C.W., Benson, P., and Winslade, W. 1987. False hopes and best data: Consent to research and the therapeutic misconception. *Hastings Center Report* 17:20–24.

Armstrong, D. 1989. *An Outline of Sociology As Applied to Medicine.* Third Edition. London: Wright.

Bellah, R.N., Madsen, R., Sullivan, W.M., Swidler, A., and Tipton, S.M. 1991. *The Good Society.* New York: Alfred A. Knopf.

Biersecker, et al. 1987. *Strategies in genetic counseling: Religious, cultural, and ethnic influences on the counseling process.* March of Dimes Original article series, March of Dimes Birth Defects: Vol. 23, No. 6.

Charo, R.A. 1991. A Political History of RU-486. In: *Biomedical Politics*. Institute of Medicine. Washington, D.C.: National Academy Press.

Childress, J.F. 1991. Deliberations of the Human Fetal Tissue Transplantation Research Panel. In: *Biomedical Politics*. Institute of Medicine. Washington, D.C.: National Academy Press.

Cohen, M., Schwartz, R., Hartz, J., and Shapiro, R. 1992. Everything you always wanted to ask a lawyer about ethics committees. *Cambridge Quarterly of Healthcare Ethics* 1:33–39.

Cook-Deegan, R.M. 1994. *The Gene Wars: Science, Politics, and the Human Genome*. New York: W.W. Norton.

Council for International Organizations of Medical Science (CIOMS) and World Health Organization. 1991. *International Guidelines for Ethical Review of Epidemiological Studies*. Geneva, Switzerland. CIOMS.

Council for International Organizations of Medical Science (CIOMS) and World Health Organization. 1993. *International Guidelines for Biomedical Research Involving Human Subjects*. Geneva. Switzerland. CIOMS.

Craig, R.P., Middleton, C.L., and O'Connell, L.J. 1986. *Ethics Committees: A Practical Approach*. St. Louis, MO: Catholic Health Association.

Crawford, R. 1977. You are dangerous to your health: The ideology and politics of victim blaming. *International Journal of Health Services* 7:663–680.

Crawshaw, R., Garland, M.J., Hines, B., and Lobitz, C. 1985. Oregon Health Decisions: An experiment with informed community consent. *Journal of the American Medical Association* 254(22):3213–3216.

Cruickshank, J.K., and Beevers, D.G. 1989. *Ethnic Factors in Health and Disease*. Oxford: Butterworth-Heinemann.

Daniels, N. 1991. Is the Oregon rationing plan fair? *Journal of the American Medical Association* 265:2232–2235.

The Danish Council of Ethics. 1990. Protection of Human Gametes, Fertilized Ova, Embryos and Fetuses: A Report. Copenhagen.

DeFriese, G.H. 1989. From activated patient to pacified activist: A study of the self-care movement in the United States. *Social Science and Medicine* 29:195–204.

Department of Health and Human Services. National Institutes of Health; Consultants to the Advisory Committee to the Director. 1988. *Report of the Human Fetal Tissues Transplantation Research Panel*, Vol. 1 (December). Bethesda, MD: National Institutes of Health.

de Tocqueville, A. 1835. *Democracy in America*.

Duster, T. 1990. *Backdoor to Eugenics*. New York: Routledge, Chapman, and Hall.

Ethics Advisory Board, DHEW. 1979. Report and Conclusions: Support of Research Involving Human In Vitro Fertilization and Embryo Transfer. Washington, D.C.

Garland, M.J. 1992. Justice, politics, and community: Expanding access and rationing health services in Oregon. *Law, Medicine, and Health Care* 20(1/2):67–81.

Garland, M.J., and Hasnain, R. 1990. Grassroots bioethics revisited: Health care priorities and community values. *Hastings Center Report* 20(5):16–18.

Graham, H. 1984. *Women, Health and the Family*. New York: Harvester Wheatsheaf.

Hadorn, D.C. 1991. Setting health care priorities in Oregon: Cost effectiveness meets the rule of rescue. *Journal of the American Medical Association* 267:2218–2225.

Helman, C.G. 1990. *Culture, Health, and Illness*. Oxford: Butterworth-Heineman Ltd.

Hoffman, D.E. 1991. Does legislating hospital ethics committees make a difference? A study of hospital ethics committees in Maryland, the District of Columbia, and Virginia. *Law, Medicine, & Health Care* 19:105–119.

Hosford, B. 1986. *Bioethics Committees: The Health Care Provider's Guide*. Rockville, MD: Aspen Systems Capacity.

Hospitals. 1985. Ethics committees double since '83: Survey. *Hospitals* 59:60–61.

In re. Conroy, 98 N.J. 321, 486 A, 2d 1209(1985).

In re. Quinlan, 70 N.J. 10, 355 A2d 647, *cert. denied*, 429 U.S. 922 (1976).

Institute of Medicine (IOM). 1974. *Ethics of Health Care.* Washington, D.C.: National Academy of Sciences.

IOM. 1977. *The Elderly and Functional Dependency.* Washington, D.C.: National Academy of Sciences.

IOM. 1978a. *Beyond Malpractice: Compensation for Medical Injuries.* Washington, D.C.: National Academy of Sciences.

IOM. 1978b. *Ethical Issues in Governmental Efforts to Promote Health* (by Daniel I. Wikler). Washington, D.C.: National Academy of Sciences.

IOM. 1978c. *The Rights of Physicians: A Philosophical Essay* (by Albert R. Jonsen). Washington, D.C.: National Academy of Sciences.

IOM. 1986. *For-Profit Enterprise in Health Care.* Washington, D.C. National Academy Press.

IOM. 1989. *The Responsible Conduct of Research in the Health Sciences.* Washington, D.C.: National Academy Press.

IOM. 1991a. *The Artificial Heart: Prototypes, Policies, and Patents* Washington, D.C.: National Academy Press.

IOM. 1991b. *Biomedical Politics.* Washington, D.C.: National Academy Press.

IOM. 1992. *Guidelines for Clinical Practice.* Washington, D.C.: National Academy Press.

IOM. 1993. *Veterans at Risk: The Health Effects of Mustard Gas and Lewisite.* Washington, D.C.: National Academy Press.

IOM. 1994. *Assessing Genetic Risks.* Washington, D.C.: National Academy Press.

Jennings, B. 1986. Representation and participation in the democratic governance of science and technology. In: *Governing Science and Technology in a Democracy*, M. Goggin, ed. Nashville, TN: University of Tennessee Press.

Jennings, B. 1988. A grassroots movement in bioethics. *Hastings Center Report* 18(3):S1–S16.

Jennings, B. 1993. Health policy in a new key: Setting democratic priorities. *Journal of Social Issues* 49(2):169–184.

Joint Commission on the Accreditation of Health Care Organizations (JACHO). 1992. *Accreditation Manual for Hospitals.* Oak Park, IL: JCAHO.

Jonsen, A. 1974. *Ethics of Newborn Intensive Care.* Berkeley, CA: University of California Press.

Kaback, M.M., Becker, M.H., and Ruth, M.V. 1974. Sociologic studies in human genetics, I: Compliance factors in voluntary heterozygote screening program. In: D. Bergsma, ed. *Ethical, Social, and Legal Dimensions of Screening for Human Genetic Disease.* New York: Stratton.

Kavanaugh, C.D., Matthews, J.R., Sorenson, and Swazey, J.P. 1979. We shall overcome: Multi-institutional review of a genetic counseling study. *IRB: A Review of Human Subject Research* 1(2):1–3, 12.

Klevit, H.D., Bates. A.C., Castanares, T., Paul, K., Sipes-Metzler, P., and Wopat, R. 1991. Prioritization of health care services: A progress report by the Oregon Health Services Commission. *Archives of Internal Medicine* 151:912–916.

Kushner, T. 1988. Networks across America. *Hastings Center Report* 18 (February/March):14.

Levi, J. 1991. Unproven AIDS Therapies: The Food and Drug Administration and ddI. In: *Biomedical Politics.* Institute of Medicine. Washington, D.C.: National Academy Press.

Levine, C. 1977. Hospital ethics committees: A guarded prognosis. *Hastings Center Report* 7(June):25–27.

Levine, R.J. 1986. *Ethics and the Regulation of Clinical Research.* New Haven, CT: Yale University Press.

Lo, B. 1987. Behind closed doors: Promises and pitfalls of ethics committees. *New England Journal of Medicine* 317:46–50.

Lynn, J. 1984. Brief and Appendix for *Amicus Curiae:* The American Geriatrics Society. *Journal of the American Geriatric Society* 32:915.

Lynn, J., and Childress, J. 1983. Must patients always be given food and water? *Hastings Center Report.*

Lynn, J., Johnson, J. and Levine, R.J. 1994. The ethical conduct of health services research: A case study of fifty institutions' applications to the SUPPORT project. *Clinical Research* 42(1):3–10

Mascie-Taylor, C.G.N. 1993. The Anthropology of Disease. New York: Oxford University Press.

McCloskey, E.L. 1991. The Patient Self-Determination Act. *Kennedy Institute of Ethics Journal* 1:163–169.

McKusick, V.A. 1988. Mendelian Inheritance in Man: Catologs of Autosomal Dominant, Recessive and X-Linked Phenotypes. 8th Edition. Baltimore: The Johns Hopkins University Press.

Mechanic, D. 1990. Promoting Health. Society (January/February):17–22.

Mechanic, D. 1992. Health and illness behavior and patient–practitioner relationships. *Social Science and Medicine* 34:1345–1350.

Merz, B. 1987. Matchmaking scheme solves Tay-Sachs problem. *Journal of the American Medical Association* 258:2636–2639.

Micetich, K.C., Steinecker, P.H., and Thomasma, D.C. 1983. Are intravenous fluids morally required for a dying patient? *Archives of Internal Medicine* 143:975–978.

National Abortion Rights Action League (NARAL). 1991. *The Politics of Abortion: The Impact of Scientific Research.* Report of a symposium held on 21 May. Washington, D.C.: NARAL.

National Academy of Sciences (NAS). 1975. *Genetic Screening: Programs, Principles, and Research.* Washington, D.C.: National Academy of Sciences.

National Advisory Board on Ethics in Reproduction (NABER). 1991. A Proposal for the National Advisory Board on Ethics in Reproduction. Washington, D.C.: NABER.

National Commission. (National Commission for the Protection of Human Subjects of Biomedical and Behavioral Research).1978a. *The Belmont Report. Ethical Principles and Guidelines for the Protection of Human Subjects in Research.* Washington, D.C.: U.S. Government Printing Office.

National Commission. 1978b. *Report and Recommendations: Institutional Review Boards.* Washington, D.C.: U.S. Government Printing Office.

National Commission. 1978c. *Research Involving Those Institutionalized as Mentally Infirm.* Washington, D.C.: U.S. Government Printing Office.

National Commission on Health Science and Society. 1968. Hearings on S. J. Res. 145 before the Subcommittee on Government Research of the Senate Committee on Government Operations, 90th Cong., 2nd Sess.

National Heart Institute, Ad Hoc Task Force on Cardiac Replacement. 1969. *Cardiac Replacement: Medical, Ethical, Psychological and Economic Implications.* Report by the Ad Hoc Task Force on Cardiac Replacement. National Institutes of Health, U.S. Department of Health, Education, and Welfare. Washington, D.C.: U.S. Government Printing Office.

National Heart and Lung Institute, NIH. 1973. *The Totally Implantable Artificial Heart: Legal, Social, Ethical, Medical, Economic, and Psychological Implications.* Report by the Artificial Heart Assessment Panel. Bethesda, MD: National Institutes of Health.

National Institutes of Health (NIH) Office for Protection from Research Risks. 1993. *Human Subjects Research Handbook.* Bethesda, MD: NIH.

National Research Council. 1993. *The Social Impact of AIDS in the United States. Economic and Psychological Implications.* Washington, D.C.: National Academy Press.

Nolen, N.A., and Coutts, M.C., eds. 1993. *International Directory of Bioethics Organizations.* Washington, D.C.: Kennedy Institute of Ethics.

Office of Technology Assessment (OTA). 1983. *The Role of Genetic Testing in the Prevention of Occupational Disease.* Washington, D.C.: U.S. Government Printing Office.

OTA. 1984a. *Human Gene Therapy: A Background Paper.* Washington, D.C.: U.S. Government Printing Office.

OTA. 1984b. *Impacts of Neuroscience.* Washington, D.C.: U.S. Government Printing Office.

OTA. 1985a. *Reproductive Health Hazards in the Workplace.* Washington, D.C.: U.S. Government Printing Office.

OTA. 1985b. *Technology and Aging in America.* Washington, D.C.: U.S. Government Printing Office.

OTA. 1986. *Alternatives to Animal Use in Research, Testing, and Education.* Washington, D.C.: U.S. Government Printing Office.

OTA. 1987a. *Life-Sustaining Technologies and the Elderly.* Washington, D.C.: U.S. Government Printing Office.

OTA. 1987b. *New Developments in Biotechnology, 1. Ownership of Human Tissues and Cells—Special Report.* Washington, D.C.: U.S. Government Printing Office.

OTA. 1987c. *New Developments in Biotechnology, 2. Public Perceptions of Biotechnology—Background Paper.* Washington, D.C.: U.S. Government Printing Office.

OTA. 1988a. *Infertility: Medical and Social Choices.* Washington, D.C.: U.S. Government Printing Office.

OTA. 1988b. *Mapping Our Genes—Genome Projects: How Big? How Fast?* Washington, D.C.: U.S. Government Printing Office.

OTA. 1988c. *New Developments in Biotechnology, 4. U.S. Investment in Biotechnology.* Washington, D.C.: U.S. Government Printing Office.

OTA. 1989. *New Developments in Biotechnology, 5. Patenting Life.* Washington, D.C.: U.S. Government Printing Office.

OTA. 1990. *Neural Grafting: Repairing the Brain and Spinal Cord.* Washington, D.C.: U.S. Government Printing Office.

OTA. 1992a. *Cystic Fibrosis and DNA Tests: Implications of Carrier Screening.* Washington, D.C.: U.S. Government Printing Office.

OTA. 1992b. *Summary: Evaluation of the Oregon Medicaid Proposal.* Washington, D.C.: U.S. Government Printing Office.

OTA. 1993. *Biomedical Ethics in U.S. Public Policy.* Washington, D.C.: U.S. Government Printing Office.

Pan American Health Organization (PAHO). 1992. *Progress Report on the Establishment of the Pan American Institute of Bioethics in Chile.* SPP19/5, 9 November. Washington, D.C.: PAHO.

Presbyterian Church, U.S.A. 1988. *Life Abundant: Values, Choices and Health Care. The Responsibility and Role of the Presbyterian Church.* Louisville, KY: Presbyterian Church, (USA)

President's Commission for the Study of Ethical Problems in Medicine and Biomedical and Behavioral Research (President's Commission). 1981a. *Defining Death.* Washington, D.C.: U.S. Government Printing Office.

President's Commission. 1981b. *Whistleblowing in Biomedical Research.* Washington, D.C.: U.S. Government Printing Office.

President's Commission. 1982a. *Making Health Care Decisions.* Washington, D.C.: U.S. Government Printing Office.

President's Commission. 1982b. *Splicing Life.* Washington, D.C.: U.S. Government Printing Office.

President's Commission. 1983a. *Deciding to Forego Life-Sustaining Treatment.* Washington, D.C.: U.S. Government Printing Office.

President's Commission. 1983b. *Screening and Counseling for Genetic Conditions.* Washington, D.C.: U.S. Government Printing Office.

President's Commission. 1983c. *Securing Access to Health Care.* Washington, D.C.: U.S. Government Printing Office.

President's Commission. 1983d. *Summing Up. Final Report on Studies of the Ethical and Legal Problems in Medicine and Biomedical and Behavioral Research.* Washington, D.C.: U.S. Government Printing Office.

Rosner, F. 1985. Hospital medical ethics committees: A review of their development. *Journal of the American Medical Association* 253:2693–2697.

Ross, J.W. 1991. What do ethics committee members want? *Ethical Currents* 3:7–8.

Ross, J.W., Bayley, C., Michel, V., and Pugh, D. 1986. *Handbook for Hospital Ethics Committees.* Chicago, IL: American Hospital Publishing.

Royal Commission of New Reproductive Technologies (Canada). 1993. *Proceed with Care. Final Report of the Royal Commission on New Reproductive Technologies.* Ottawa: Royal Commission.

Senate Committee on Labor and Public Welfare. 1973. *Quality of Health Care—Human Experimentation: Hearings Before the Subcommittee on Health,* 93rd Congress, 1st Sess., (February 21–23, March 6–8, April 30, June 28–29, July 10). Washington, D.C.: U.S. Government Printing Office.

Stine, G.J. 1977. *Biosocial Genetics: Human Heredity and Social Issues.* New York: Macmillan.

Stone, D. 1989. At risk in the welfare state. *Social Research* 56:3.

Strauss, A. 1991. *Creating Social Awareness: Collective Images and Symbolic Representations.* New Brunswick, NJ: Transaction Publishers.

Syme, L., and Alcalay, R. 1982. Control of cigarette smoking from a social perspective. *Annual Review of Public Health* 3:179–199.

Taylor, R. 1986. The politics of prevention. In: P. Conrad and R. Kern, eds. *The Sociology of Health and Illness.* New York: St. Martins Press.

Tesh, S.N. 1988. *Hidden Arguments: Political Ideology and Disease Prevention Policy.* New Brunswick, NJ: Rutgers University Press.

U.S. Department of Health, Education, and Welfare. 1977. *HEW Secretary's Task Force on the Compensation of Injured Research Subjects.* Bethesda, MD.: National Institutes of Health.

U.S. Department of Health and Human Services. National Institutes of Health Human Fetal Tissue Transplantation Research Panel. 1988. *Report on the Human Fetal Tissue Transplantation Research Panel.* Vol.1. Bethesda, MD. National Institutes of Health.

U.S. Department of Health, Education, and Welfare. U.S. Ethics Advisory Board. 1979. *Report and Conclusion: Health Education and Welfare Support of Research Involving Human In Vitro Fertilization and Embryo Transfer.* Washington, D.C.

U.S. Public Health Service. 1966. Clinical Research and Investigation Involving Human Beings. Memorandum of Surgeon General William H. Stewart to the Heads of Institutions Conducting Research with Public Health Grants, 8 February.

van Allen, E., Moldow, D.G., and Cranford, R. 1989. Evaluating ethics committees. *Hastings Center Report* 19(September/October):23–24.

Veatch, R.M. 1987. The Patient as Partner: A Theory of Human Experimentation Ethics. In: *Contemporary Issues in Bioethics,* Third Edition, T.L. Beauchamp and L. Walters, eds. Belmont, CA: Wadsworth Publishing Company.

Welch, H.G., and Dixon, J. 1991. Priortity Setting: Lessons from Oregon. Lancet i:891–894.

West, M.B., and Gibson, J.M. 1992. Facilitating medical ethics case review: What ethics committees can learn from mediation and facilitation techniques. *Cambridge Quarterly of Healthcare Ethics* 1:63–74.

Williams, P.C. 1984. Success in spite of failure: Why IRBs falter in reviewing risks and benefits. *IRB: A Review of Human Subjects Research* 6:1–4

World Health Organization and Council for International Organizations of Medical Science (CIOMS). 1982. *Proposed International Guidelines for Biomedical Research Involving Human Subjects.* Geneva, Switzerland. CIOMS.

Zerwekh, J.V. 1983. The dehydration question. *Nursing* 83(January):47–51.

5

Criteria for Success

How to evaluate the products and outcomes of public ethics bodies[1] using objective criteria has been a continuing question, not resolved by the work of this committee. For example, should they be evaluated relative to the specific mandate of each group or report or the particular public needs that the group or report addresses? Although certain general criteria can be articulated, their importance for evaluating a particular public ethics body may depend in large measure on the specific mission of that body. This is true not just for single-issue bodies, such as the Human Fetal Tissue Transplantation Research Panel, but also for bodies with a broader mandate, such as the President's Commission. The background paper written by Gray, who attempts to compare the "success" of the National Commission and the President's Commission, highlights many of the problems inherent in the evaluation and comparison of even two commissions, especially when the groups each have multiple functions and operated at different periods of time. Given the multiplicity of functions that public ethics bodies can serve (as noted early in Chapter 4) and the power of the societal context in which they operate to influence their outcomes (as described in Chapter 2), the committee did not believe that a complete, critical evalua-

---

[1] The term "public ethics body" is used in this chapter and in Chapter 6 to denote a group convened to deliberate about social and ethical issues stemming from developments in biomedicine. Such groups may exist at the level of the institution, community, state, federal agency, or federal government. Generally, these groups address public policy issues that involve moral ideas such as dignity, freedom, rights, fairness, respect, equality, solidarity, responsibility, justice, and integrity.

tion of all of the public ethics bodies discussed in this report was feasible. The committee instead sought to identify criteria that could be used as hallmarks (together with more wide-ranging exploration of social contexts) by individuals who are initiating or serving on such bodies, or attempting to evaluate the impact of their deliberations or reports.

Past social responses to ethical quandaries in biomedicine have succeeded in a variety of ways. For example, many public ethics bodies have enlisted outstanding scholars to contribute their insights on the issue of concern. Many of the products of these bodies have been viewed as authoritative and have had a substantial impact on policy decisions, as for example occurred in the cases of defining brain death and establishing standards for human experimentation. Many products of these bodies have stood the test of time and continue to have a prominent role in education for health professionals and ethicists. Hospital ethics committees, for example, are often able to soften advocacy of patient interest in order to gain the willing participation of health care providers (Hoffman, 1991). These and other similar examples are described later in this chapter.

Commissions and other public ethics bodies operate in a world where deadlines, personalities, and special interests converge. The need for consensus development and sometimes compromise is unavoidable. While the committee does not attempt in this report to perform a comprehensive assessment of the performance of every mechanism for public deliberation of social and ethical issues, it does explore some of the specific outcomes of this deliberation according to a set of criteria it identified as measures of "success."

Applying the criteria, the committee found, did not produce unqualified results. Among the criteria used for evaluation of public ethics bodies are items bearing on *integrity* of the reasoning process, *public education* (i.e., how well a report articulates the nature of a controversy, competing values, and alternative solutions, as well as how effectively the report is disseminated), and *effectiveness* (i.e., getting laws passed, forging a public consensus, etc.). Different reports of the same body, being aimed at different kinds of tasks, might well satisfy these criteria in different ways and to different degrees (see the background paper by Gray).

The President's Commission report on *Defining Death* (1981), for example, was intended to provide definitive resolution of a public policy problem. Viewed from this perspective, the report was a smashing success. Its recommendations regarding the Uniform Determination of Death Act were quickly accepted by the vast majority of states. The commission's reasoning in defense of its policy proposal has been a source of continuing controversy and even disparagement in the scholarly literature (Wikler, 1993; Veatch, 1993), and this might lead us to give the report a lower score on integrity and public education. But these scales may not be the most appropriate criteria, given this view of the primary mission of that particular report.

Conversely, the President's Commission report on *Splicing Life* (1982b) is most appropriately judged as an educational document. Seen as an attempt to calm the fears of religious leaders, and to separate morally positive work in somatic cell gene therapy from the unsavory specter of eugenics and germ-line manipulation, it would be judged a success. The report was clearly written; it deftly separated issues of genuine moral concern from ill-founded fears about "genetic engineering" and provided an excellent framework for future public discussion of the issue. The fact that this particular report did not generate new laws (as did *Defining Death*) or influence court decisions (as did *Deciding to Forego Life-Sustaining Treatments* [1983a]) would be relatively unimportant in its overall evaluation, given its predominantly educational mission. Another way of expressing this is to say that it was effective in educating the public, but not effective in pushing a regulatory or policy agenda because it was not meant to do so.

Few thorough evaluations have been done on the success of various other bodies covened to deliberate social and ethical issues in biomedicine—bodies such as HECs, IRBs, professional societies, grassroots organizations, or special interest groups.

In short, evaluative criteria and their specific weights depend crucially upon context, including the nature of the controversy, the specific tasks of the body, the social setting, legal environment, etc. (see the background paper by Brody in this volume). Notwithstanding this caveat, it is still possible to develop a number of important criteria that could be used in establishing, participating in, or judging the overall performance of public ethics bodies. The following discussion divides these criteria into three categories: intellectual integrity, sensitivity to democratic values, and effectiveness. As we shall see, however, there is a considerable amount of overlap and interplay among these categories.

One final caveat is in order before proceeding In offering a list and discussion of criteria for judging the success of public ethics bodies, we do not mean to suggest that the business of evaluating their performance might be reducible to some sort of perfunctory checklist. As Aristotle wisely reminds us in *Nicomachean Ethics* (Book 1), we must not expect more precision than the subject matter permits. There is no scoring system that will yield objective assessments that command universal assent. Often, public ethics bodies must grapple with extremely controversial and contested issues that implicate our most fundamental individual and social values. The judgments that we all bring to bear on the work of these bodies will naturally reflect our differing views on these fundamental controversies concerning life, death, and justice. Like evaluations of works of literature, art, or philosophy, our critical assessments of public ethics bodies and their products ultimately rest upon nothing more, and nothing less, than the quality of our reasoning and the soundness of our judgments. Consensus is possible, but controversy is to be expected.

INTELLECTUAL INTEGRITY

Logic

Logic is the first prerequisite of a successful report from a public ethics body. At issue here are the soundness of the reasoning and the overall coherence of the document. Does it describe the topics and issues clearly? Do the conclusions, including the policy recommendations, follow logically from clearly stated premises, or are they simply *announced* on the presumption that the authority or prestige of the body will carry over to its conclusions? Is the report characterized by consistency in standards, or is one standard used in one place and another used elsewhere in the report? Does the document present itself as a seamless web of argument and recommendations, all heading in the same direction, or is there a tension or perhaps outright contradiction between various parts of the report? Recall in this connection the President's Commission's *Securing Access to Health Care* (1983b): several commentators have noted the disparity between the report's liberal philosophical and factual premises, written by staff scholars, and the conclusion, dictated by the conservative moral and political stance of certain commissioners.

A related function of these bodies is to help clarify, through logical analysis, the terms and nature of the debates addressed in their reports. Frequently ethical decision making at all levels, from the bedside to legislative chambers, is confused by pervasive fuzziness in terminology and reasoning. For example, clinicians, journalists, judges, and ordinary people alike have tended to overlook important distinctions (e.g., between somatic and germ-line genetic therapies) or have based decisions and policies on distinctions of dubious merit (e.g., between so-called "ordinary" and "extraordinary" means).

Likewise, some debates are muddled by failure to attend to disciplinary distinctions and the resulting confusion of categories. The Ad Hoc Committee of the Harvard Medical School to Examine the Definition of Brain Death (1968), for example, mistook the *medical* criterion of "permanent coma" for an ethical and policy statement about the definition of death. Public ethics bodies should take care to identify separately the various disciplinary perspectives on an issue—e.g., theological, ethical, economic, political, legal, medical, biological, epidemiological—and to give each its due without mistaking one for another.

An important criterion for evaluating the efforts of a public ethics body, then, is the body's ability to advance the ethical discussion by means of logical analysis, including rigorous critique of definitions, arguments, and distinctions—what one committee member has labeled "logic policing."

Scholarship

Scholarship is another important dimension of intellectual integrity. The work of public ethics bodies must not only be coherent, it must also be *competent*—that is, based upon the soundest available scholarship. This means, first, that the body's "findings" must be grounded upon solid empirical facts pertaining to the relevant area of technological innovation. A report on fetal tissue transplants, brain death, or genetic screening and therapy must be premised upon state-of-the-art information regarding the current practice and future prospects of relevant technologies. If the membership of a public ethics body lacks this technical knowledge, it must consult with appropriate experts. Members and staff of public ethics bodies should be aware of empirical studies bearing on their topic.

Secondly, reports should reflect a thorough knowledge of the interdisciplinary field of bioethics. In addition to being factually accurate and well reasoned, such reports should be based upon an equally state-of-the-art understanding of the public and professional "conversation" surrounding a particular issue. The reasoning and conclusions of the report should reflect an awareness of "the best that has been thought" in the bioethical literature, journals of opinion, newspapers, etc.

When policy analysts, scholars, and teachers read an ethics body report that is scientifically and ethically "competent" in this sense, they are much more likely to credit its conclusions as being reasonable, thorough, and fair. In this way, the perception of competency helps to generate the moral authority of a commission. Those responsible for forming public ethics bodies must keep this point in mind as they select members and staff. Although it is reasonable to seek a broad range of cultural, professional, ethnic, and ideological diversity for membership, it is absolutely vital that all of the staff and many of the members of these bodies possess the required expertise in ethics, law, medicine, biology, and related fields.

Sound Judgment

Sound judgment complements logical analysis and scholarship in an overall assessment of intellectual integrity. Reports should be based not only on good facts, scholarship, and reasoning, but also on the less tangible (and more controversial) factor of judgment. Unlike logic or mathematics, ethics is not primarily driven by deductive reasoning. Ethical consideration is often "messy," complicated by uncertainty, lack of information, and conflicting values and principles. Ethical "skill" resides not so much in being able to apply a single ethical theory or principle to a set of facts as in the ability to discern the unique particularities of the problem in its social setting, to creatively reframe a question, to reason by analogy, to perceive and acknowledge the interests of affected parties, and to judiciously weigh and balance competing principles and considerations (Jonsen and Toulmin, 1988; Arras, in press).

These activities, while loosely connected to deductive logic, are crucial for the successful framing, debate, and resolution of moral problems. Just as individuals must display these skills in concrete moral reasoning, so too must public ethics bodies exhibit them in their reports (Jonsen and Toulmin, 1988). The sorts of judgments called for here can be exceedingly difficult and delicate, and thus very controversial. How heavily should economic efficiency weigh vis-à-vis equality of opportunity in structuring a health care policy? What will be the impact of the new reproductive technologies on women's identity and role in society, and how should this consideration be measured against the rights of women to do with their bodies as they wish?

Any group that comes to terms with such difficult questions, as any serious public ethics body must, will engage conflicting values and interests, and attempt to reach sound judgments. We call "judicious" those reports that strike an appropriate and fruitful balance between the relevant rights and interests, disciplinary perspectives, and cultural traditions of a given society. Unfortunately, there is no known algorithm for producing reports of this kind. In the final analysis, it is a matter of good judgment honed through years of experience.

SENSITIVITY TO DEMOCRATIC VALUES

Respect for Affected Parties

In addition to "the best that has been thought" on an issue, public ethics bodies should also be attentive to all the significant contributors to the public conversation about an issue. Rather than simply fixing on and advancing their own preferred approach to a problem, members and staff should make an honest attempt to hear all plausible, responsible views. This process is vital for two reasons. First, as John Stuart Mill wisely noted long ago (1859), seemingly marginal ideas may be true, or at least partially true; and even if they are false, the process of having to justify a received view in the face of dissenting arguments will usually strengthen and invigorate it.

Second, public ethics bodies should be attentive to minority or disenfranchised voices, not only because they can enrich our public discourse, but also because sometimes they may be attached to important individual rights or serious religious or cultural concerns that ought to be respected, so far as possible, by public policy. The New Jersey Bioethics Commission, for example, grappled creatively with the problem of Orthodox Jewish concerns over the definition of death.

Third, failure to attend to significant minority concerns in the process of policy formation may render implementation of a policy more difficult or even impossible if it requires the cooperation of the affected minority group. The experience of the city of Baltimore in distributing the long-term contraceptive, Norplant®, in the city's predominantly African American public schools is illustrative. Although the facts are in dispute, a number of vocal African American clergymen protested that the planned distribution of Norplant was decided upon without adequate consultation with the African American community, and that it violated the ethical and religious norms of that community.

Representation of Diverse Views

Concern for affected parties, including minorities, the disenfranchised, consumers, and public interest groups, should manifest itself not only in listening to the experiences and concerns of a wide variety of people, but also in the presence of representatives of such groups within the composition of the public ethics body itself. Some affected parties are difficult to recruit for membership on these bodies (e.g., psychotic individuals, drug users, and various persons suffering from serious addictions), so the bodies should seek not the affected parties themselves, but those who are known to be their dedicated advocates. Also, a seat at the table is sometimes demanded by persons who intend to champion a position and sway a deliberative body to accept it. This is undesirable for a public ethics body, which must be committed to impartiality and willingness to deliberate, yet the views of such parties deserve to be heard. Thus, advocacy should not have a seat, but appreciation and understanding of the advocates should, so as to guarantee that their interests and values will count in the body's deliberations (see the background paper by Bayer in this volume).

Open Versus Closed Meetings

An important question bearing on the process of a public ethics body's deliberations, as opposed to the substance of its recommendations, concerns the conditions under which meetings will be held. Specifically, the issue is whether these groups should operate in the 'sunshine"—that is, in open public sessions with everything on the record—or in the privacy and confidentiality of closed sessions. Important national-level bodies, including the National Commission and President's Commission, and one state-level commission (New Jersey) provide examples of open process, while the ethics work group of the recent Clinton administration health care reform task force and the New York State Task Force on Life and the Law have operated behind closed doors before disclosing their findings to the public. What are the implications for democratic values of these alternative approaches to process?

At first glance, it would appear that openness best reflects democratic values. The group is a public body, and its deliberations should be open for all to see and hear. Anyone with a stake in an issue under discussion may attend and, at appropriate times and places, speak his or her mind. Journalists may attend and write about what they see and hear, so that the public will know how the body it is funding conducts its business. Since the body deliberates before an attentive public, the members and staff must eschew the arcane jargon of their respective professions and speak in plain English. And with everything on the record, there will be no "smoke-filled rooms" and no secret deals that cannot be explained to an inquisitive public. The open meeting model is thus especially well-suited to the values of a democratic society.

In addition to expressing and reinforcing democratic values, the model of openness may also foster the effectiveness of public ethics bodies, which provide an open forum for all interested parties to witness the deliberations leading to public policy recommendations. Since the members' evolving views could be reported to the public in the print and electronic media, those with differing opinions will have a chance to be heard during this process and, in any case, will not be surprised by the resulting reports. Policy recommendations that pass through this crucible of publicity may be accepted more readily once they are finally published.

The virtues of the closed meeting model have more to do with collegiality and efficiency within a deliberative group than with democracy and public education. Perhaps the most common argument for privacy and confidentiality has to do with the fostering of mutual trust and openness among the commissioners and staff. Since these people come together to discuss and decide upon policy questions of great moment and difficulty, they need to keep an open mind. Indeed, they often require a good deal of intellectual elbow room in which to change their minds once confronted with compelling evidence and argument. Arguably, it is easier to do this in private than in public, where the virtues of flexibility and openness to new evidence might be wrongly interpreted as simple fecklessness and inconsistency.

Equally important, however, some members of public ethics bodies might be chosen in part because of their ability, not merely to think clearly about the issues, but also to represent various religious or secular view-points. A strong argument can be made that representatives from the clergy, labor, or civil liberties constituencies, for example, will have an easier time crafting inevitable, difficult, and highly sensitive compromises in private than in public. Thus, for example, a Catholic priest might be able to say things in private that he might not be able to say in public. ("As a Catholic and a priest I cannot countenance this kind of reproductive liberty, but as a citizen I will tolerate it.") Instead of spending much of their time "playing to the home audience," members can speak with one another in full candor, concentrating on the task at hand, and setting aside advocacy for calm impartiality.

The greatest disadvantage of closed meetings, still speaking on the level of efficiency and effectiveness, is that the public ethics body must do a thorough job of testing the waters with other groups most likely to be affected by or feel strongly about a policy, lest the public be surprised by the body's findings. Groups that feel excluded from the policy process are more likely to react in a spirit of opposition rather than mutual accommodation. Thus, if a body opts for closed meetings, it should make every effort to solicit the views of affected parties during the process of data gathering and policy formation.

In sum, it should be noted that closed meetings, while they do not directly advance democratic values, are not necessarily incompatible with them. When public ethics bodies do hold closed meetings, it is important that they also use mechanisms such as open hearings and public release of preliminary findings and recommendations. Conversely, the open meeting, while conforming outwardly to democratic norms, may in practice work around them. Recall that public ethics bodies, whether or not they hold open meetings, are not usually making the decisions; they are usually advisory in nature. In order for their recommendations to go into effect, they often must be acted upon by some publicly responsive and responsible body, like a state or federal legislature. Even if decisions are crafted in private, they remain *recommendations* that representatives of the people may still accept or reject as they see fit, following public discussion and debate.

The open meeting model, on the other hand, may outwardly conform to democratic norms of openness and publicity while deviating from them in private. Many of the issues dealt with by public ethics bodies pose problems of exquisite difficulty, problems generated in part by the presence of strongly held, conflicting views within society. Supposing that consensus is possible on a given question, it will often be achieved by virtue of the willingness of those on opposite sides to make reasonable but painful compromises. This delicate process of finding common ground through moral consensus building is much more likely to succeed in privacy and confidentiality than under the harsh glare of publicity. It may well be, then, that even within a model built upon the democratic value of openness, much of the real work of compromise and consensus-building takes place away from the public stage.

EFFECTIVENESS

Preconditions of Effectiveness

As noted above, judgments about the effectiveness of any particular public ethics body must be based upon a clear understanding of the group's purpose, the public need to which it responds, and the social context in which it deliberates. Notwithstanding the importance of purpose and context, we can note two preconditions of effectiveness for any group, no matter what its specific charge: communication and authority.

Communication

First, the body must communicate well with its audience. Its reports and recommendations must be clearly written, trenchantly argued, and comprehensible to as wide an audience as possible. Accordingly, drafters should be self-conscious about their writing style, avoiding wherever possible arcane jargon and academic prose. Since reports are all written in order to effect some change in the reader—either to change beliefs or to encourage alternative actions or policies—they should be written with the specific characteristics of their audience in mind. In a state with a very active and vocal religious presence, for example, drafters of reports should be sensitive, not only to the representation of religious views within the group's process, but also to the way these documents speak to members of religious communities. Reports that respect the sensibilities of their readers will be more persuasive, and hence more effective, than those that do not.

Even the most clearly written and persuasive reports can fail to be effective, however, if they are not disseminated to as broad an audience as possible. This means, first, that the reports themselves must be easily accessible to professionals and the general public alike. An adequate number should be printed and made available at reasonable prices to consumers, professional groups, and public libraries. In the future, public ethics bodies should take advantage of new information technologies, such as making documents available through computer networks and on CD ROM.

In addition to the documents themselves, members and staff of public ethics bodies should attempt to disseminate the main ideas behind their findings through a wide variety of media, including newspapers, editorial columns, book reviews, radio interviews, professional journals, and public and professional issue forums. If the body is proposing new legislation, its staff and members should attempt to educate members of the legislature about the issues and about the body's views.

Authority

The effectiveness or influence of a report is also in part a function of the extent to which the group itself is viewed as an authoritative body, i.e., a group whose recommendations carry weight with policymakers, professionals, and the general public. This kind of authority sometimes derives from the sponsoring body. A public ethics body appointed by the President of the United States or the Governor of New York, for example, automatically assumes a certain stature in the eyes of the community; this might, in turn, lend needed credibility to its recommendations. Authority can also be earned rather than bestowed, either through the individual reputations of members and staff, or through a successful track record of substantive accomplishment. The selection of well-known and respected academicians, community activists, and professionals can lend "clout" to a commission's findings, as can a succession of well-crafted reports, each building on the success of its predecessors.

Authority can also be a function of democratic representation. Not every group with a position on a particular controversial issue can be equally satisfied by a body's report, but its recommendations will nevertheless be perceived as authoritative to the extent that all sides have been heard and, ideally, represented in the body's deliberations. Conversely, groups whose voices have been excluded from the process will tend to view the result as a mere power play and, thus, as lacking legitimacy.

Different Goals, Different Yardsticks of Success

Achieving Consensus

The primary function of many public ethics bodies is to achieve consensus on issues that require some sort of public response. Thus, whatever may be the specific goals of a particular body, achieving consensus will usually be an explicit policy objective.

As Martin Benjamin explains in his background paper, consensus in public ethics bodies make take a number of forms. One such form is what Benjamin labels "complete" consensus, a term describing the situation in which members of a body agree unanimously on recommendations and on the reasoning behind these recommendations. Not surprisingly, complete consensus is an uncommon outcome for public ethics bodies because questions directed at these bodies are typically controversial and because the membership of these bodies tends to be broadly constituted so as to represent all points of view. A more common outcome for these bodies is "overlapping consensus," a term coined by political philosopher John Rawls to characterize a situation in which there is agreement on basic principles among individuals embracing different, and sometimes conflicting, outlooks. In the case of overlapping consensus, people appealing to different principles may agree on a recommendation and at the same time disagree about *why* they agree. Overlapping consensus is understandably more likely than complete consensus given a population as pluralistic as that in the United States.

Compromise, explains Benjamin, is another form of agreement that can occur in public ethics bodies. Central to the idea of compromise is mutual concession for mutual gain; people with opposing positions relinquish aspects of their positions to find some middle ground that is mutually satisfying. Compromise typically occurs in public ethics bodies when members value the body's speaking with one voice more than they value the body's endorsing of the view of a given individual at the price of continued impasse. Compromise is similar to consensus in that it entails a unanimous agreement that the collective body should recommend something rather than nothing. Another form of agreement that can also occur in such a situation is "majority rule." Majority rule represents "procedural" (as opposed to "substantive") consensus in that people have agreed to put forward the recommendation that most members agree on.

In all forms, consensus can be valuable to public ethics bodies. Most notably, consensus can be instrumental in obtaining external acceptance and implementation of a body's recommendations, especially (and, some may argue, only) when members of a public ethics body bring to the deliberations an array of different viewpoints on an issue. Observers with different viewpoints may be more likely to agree that a group's recommendation is valid if they perceive that their varied interests have been considered.

Consensus in all forms also presents dangers. For example, consensus can be used to obscure deep philosophical issues, in which case the public would be better served by discussion and reflection than by the false resolution provided by a consensus statement. Excessive pressure to reach agreement may also lead to underestimation of risks and objections, ignoring of unpopular viewpoints, failure to consider alternatives or to seek additional information, uncritical acceptance of secondhand information, or failure to exercise sufficient imagination or ingenuity in building consensus or devising compromise (Lo, 1987).

Social and political circumstances play a significant role in determining not only the value of consensus, but also the possibility of achieving consensus in any form. A particularly salient factor in public ethics deliberation is the "ripeness" of the issue in question for public resolution. In some cases, a body might merely have to place its imprimatur on a consensus that has been gradually building and is now more or less in place. A good example of this kind of "consensus articulation" might be the President's Commission report on informed consent and truth telling in *Making Health Care Decisions* (1982).

More frequently, however, public ethics bodies are faced with the harder task of actually forging a consensus that does not yet exist. In some instances, a report can help create a societal consensus in spite of some lingering opposition. A good example of this is provided by the New York State Task Force report on *Surrogate Parenting* (1988). The task force members were initially deeply divided on this issue, but through a process of intense and thorough discussion and debate, they eventually reached a unanimous decision to void surrogacy contracts in New York. Eventually, legislation premised on the task force's recommendations was passed, albeit over the objections of civil libertarians, the surrogacy industry, and some couples and prospective surrogates who wished to engage in this practice. It would probably be accurate to say that a consensus now exists in New York on this issue, although on many such issues consensus is subject to changes in public opinion over time.

Consensus has been more difficult to achieve on other issues, such as federal funding for research on fetal tissue transplants. The NIH panel that addressed this question achieved a clear majority in favor of funding such research, but it could not reach consensus. Try as they might to separate the question of fetal tissue research from the ethics and politics of abortion, the panel was ultimately divided on the question, reproducing within itself the divisions haunting the larger society.

Likewise, the President's Commission report on *Securing Access to Health Care* (1983b) faced the daunting task of attempting to create societal consensus on an issue that had divided Americans for decades. Forging ahead in spite of conflicting interest groups (doctors, hospitals, pharmaceutical companies, consumers, etc.), the commission was able to achieve internal consensus on the ethical principles that should govern the process of health care delivery and reform. The problem, according to some critics, was that this consensus was achieved by divorcing health care ethics from health care politics; the resulting consensus was, they claim, too abstract to be compatible with any live option for health care reform. The critics conclude that, in contrast to many of its other distinguished reports, this volume of the President's Commission has had virtually no impact on the public debate over health care reform (Bayer, 1984).

Achieving Specific Results

Apart from the global objective of forging a consensus on difficult bioethical controversies, public ethics bodies also seek to achieve more specific goals such as education, influencing of public debate, and stimulation of various government actions, including legislation. These disparate efforts, which may be pursued separately or in concert, must be evaluated according to a variety of different standards.

Starting with the obvious, public ethics bodies should successfully discharge the specific mandates that they are given. If a body fails to do what is asked of it, either because of political paralysis (e.g., the BEAC) or inadequate leadership and staffing, it cannot be judged a success.

Mandate is relevant to the overall assessment of a public ethics body in another way. Depending on the circumstances, some specific objectives may be more difficult to achieve than others. For example, articulating the contours of an emergent consensus for educational purposes, while a demanding and important task, is not nearly as difficult as drafting legislation on controversial topics for a population divided by fierce ideological and religious differences. Assessments of a body's accomplishments should thus resemble the scoring of a diving judge: assuming comparable quality, a greater number of points should go to the more ambitious and difficult projects. Neither public criticism of a work nor political opposition to its agenda are reliably reflective of inadequacies in its process or product; rather, they may simply represent the cost of doing very difficult business under contentious circumstances (see the background paper by Brody).

Assessing the effectiveness of a public ethics body's efforts at educating the public, influencing public opinion, or stimulating government action is a complex task. In large measure, judgments can be made based on criteria discussed above—e.g., intellectual integrity, respect for democratic values, and so forth—but they should also depend on criteria that reflect the nature of specific activities of the body. Thus, educational projects should be judged in part according to pedagogic standards, while judgment of legislative efforts should reflect the quality of the legal craft presented.

Examples of highly successful educational ventures include the Danish Council of Ethics, described in Chapter 4, and several of the President's Commission documents, including *Splicing Life, Making Health Care Decisions*, and *Deciding to Forego Life-Sustaining Treatments*. Successful legislative and regulatory efforts include the work of the National Commission and the respective reports of the New York State Task Force on Life and the Law and the New Jersey Bioethics Commission on the issue of advance directives. An example of a problematic legislative effort is the New York State Task Force's proposal for a statute on "do not resuscitate" (DNR) orders. While the task force's recommendations and the ensuing legislation can be credited with fostering greater dialogue among patients, families, and physicians, the law's apparent insistence upon emergency cardiopulmonary resuscitation (CPR) in the absence of a documented DNR order has given rise to unanticipated and vexing problems related to the

demands of some families for seemingly futile medical treatment. '
wise, many believe the President's Commission report on *Defining Dea..*
succeeded for the most part on the legislative front, but failed to advance a
cogent rationale for whole-brain death, thereby falling short in its efforts to
educate the public and shape public and professional opinion (Gervais,
1989).

Can Bioethics Be Disadvantageous?

Along with the advantages and benefits of public bioethical deliberation in many settings and at many levels, there are several potential risks.
Thus far, these are largely theoretical. No systematic research has looked
for the downside of bioethics, and this IOM study committee did not find
tangible evidence of their realization. Nevertheless, even hypothetical risks
deserve mention, if only as a suggestion for future research, evaluation,
and monitoring. We call attention to two concerns: the possibility of diversion and capture of bioethical deliberation by special interests and the lack
of proven methodologies and objective standards of evaluation.

Diversion and Capture

Bioethical deliberation could be useful to special interests in a number
of ways. Advocacy groups, for example, are usually perceived as partisan,
but, as mentioned at the outset of this report, bioethical deliberation aims
at impartiality. To the extent that an advocacy group could influence or
capture a body charged with the task of bioethical deliberation, it could
increase its influence by lowering the guard of the public. The same is true
for sectarian groups, religious or otherwise.

Financially self-interested parties are a particular cause for concern. In
the new era of health care reform the distinction between financing and
provision of care is likely to be further blurred. One result is that the
outcome of ethical disputes over clinical medicine affects the bottom line.
The current debate over the term "futile," which partly defines the authority of physicians to discontinue life-sustaining care, is a pressing example of
how an ethical definition impacts on the cost of medical care.

Special interests can subvert the process of bioethical deliberation at
every level described in this report. National and state commissions can be
lobbied by advocacy and sectarian groups, who can also exert pressure
when commission and staff are appointed. The ethics committees of professional societies have evident conflicts of interest when the interests of
their members hang in the balance; this presents a credibility problem, but
most importantly presents a danger that the ethical problems will be discussed first in terms of the management of risks to the members of the

society. Even at the grassroots level, there are risks of capture. Creation of seemingly-authentic grassroots organizations for the purpose of influencing legislators has become a new tactic in the public relations industry, and there are reports that this is occurring in the health care reform debate. It could also extend to bioethics.

The definition of "special interest" is itself a contentious issue. Are advocates for AIDS victims or the mentally ill, or defenders of civil liberties or human life, special interests? How about ethicists themselves, who receive public attention and even employment where bioethics is done? And what of the government itself? When the government is financially implicated, as with the use of "experimental therapies" in entitlement health care programs or in past research abuses where compensation may be due, the government is not a neutral party. Even when the state turns to grassroots bioethics for advice, there are risks: participation may serve a pacification function if the government controls the agenda and participants are confined to debating issues the outcomes of which are unthreatening to the government's interests. A state, for example, might set a low ceiling on health care expenditures and then involve grassroots bioethics groups in deciding how to ration within that budget.

None of these considerations demonstrates that the intimate involvement of "special interests" with bioethical deliberation is inherently undesirable or even suspect. Advocates and those with strongly held, sectarian views will be among the closest observers of groups engaged in bioethical deliberation. Their energy and knowledge can be an important asset to these groups and in any case can help to make up the public to whom these groups are accountable. Nevertheless, the need to avoid capture, diversion, and conflict of interest in bioethical deliberation will increase as these deliberations continue to increase in impact.

Methods and Evaluation

As the United States and other countries turn to applied ethics for enlightenment, a realistic appreciation of what academic ethics can contribute must be fostered. It is possible that some might expect bioethics to deliver something—answers, certainty, the morally correct view, etc.—that it is not equipped to produce. It must be clear that "ethical analysis" is not a single, straightforward method, like algebra or geometry. Different ethicists favor different approaches and methods and claim different philosophical antecedents. No school of thought, such as utilitarianism or contractualism, dominates the discipline. New views, such as feminist and narrative ethics, emerge constantly and even influence many who may not wholly endorse them. Thus, it is unwise to expect from ethicists a method all people would choose to use to unravel any ethical quandaries.

When academic ethicists have moved into the world of public moral discourse, they have often found that one of their skills as philosophers, seeking clarity of meaning in commonly used terms and logic in argumentation, has served better than their ability to explain ethical theory. They disavow the claim to provide answers and offer to help in identifying the assumptions underlying arguments and to point out inconsistencies in reasoning. These skills are often found useful by those struggling to make sense of an ethical problem. Even more useful is the ethicists' insistence that difficult and obscure terms, such as "dignity," "rights," and "justice," that are used constantly in ethical discourse be examined with care. If an ethical analysis is one that refers in significant ways to these concepts, as we have said, the ability to construct an argument in which they figure meaningfully and forcefully should be prized.

However, even if these skills are useful, an ethical argument is not merely logical; it is also substantive, arising from values and norms that are deeply held by individuals. These values and norms are colored by culture, religion, heritage, personal history, preferences, and tastes. Ethicists can often do little more than ask for clarification about the meaning of these values and norms in the minds of those who hold them and ask them to examine the consistency and consequences of holding them. Academic ethics cannot dissolve the differences that might exist between persons and groups at this level. At best, moral discourse can bring such differences to the surface, attempt to discover when they arise from misunderstanding, and invite those who hold them to find practical ways of living together. The best conclusion of an ethical analysis may be the description of alternative views. It may, in some cases, be folly to expect more. At the same time, in the process of examining alternative positions, many considerations are brought to light that illuminate and expand understanding of the moral problem. This, in public moral discourse, is an invaluable by-product of the bioethicist's presence.

It may not be possible to measure the success of this sort of activity with any indisputable standard. Nor is it possible to demonstrate that an ethics commission or committee has produced an analysis that meets some predetermined criteria for sound ethical argumentation. At best, we will rely on such imprecise indicators of success as those mentioned in Chapter 5. Thus, no one can prove that the public has gotten its money's worth out of such an enterprise. Given these difficulties, it may happen that ethics becomes the cover for ideology (as has often happened in history). The current favor in which ethics is held may make it possible, as we said above, for persons and groups with quite sectarian views to disguise their interests under the title "ethics", and it may be difficult for others to discern the difference, until the results are viewed. Even then, clever argumentation may persuade persons to accept a position that they would repudiate, had they been exposed to alternative reasoning. Thus, while this committee believes that more good than bad can come from public moral discourse, it also recommends prudent caution whenever an ethical analysis of a major problem is proposed. Broad representation of distinct opinions is probably the best antidote.

REFERENCES

Ad Hoc Committee of the Harvard Medical School to Examine the Definition of Brain Death. 1968. A definition of irreversible coma. *Journal of the American Medical Association* 205:337.

Arras, J. In press. Principles and particularity: The roles of cases in bioethics. *Indiana Law Journal.*

Bayer, R. 1984. Ethics, politics, and access to health care: A critical analysis of the President's Commission for the Study of Ethical Problems in Medicine and Biomedical and Behavioral Research. *Cardozo Law Review* 6(2):303–320.

Gervais, K.G. 1989. Advancing the definition of death: A philosophical essay. *Medical Humanities Review* 3(2):7–19.

Hoffman, D.E. 1991. Does legislating hospital ethics committees make a difference? A study of hospital ethics committees in Maryland, the District of Columbia, and Virginia. *Law, Medicine, and Health Care* 19:105–119.

Jonsen, A.R., and Toulmin, S. 1988. *The Abuse of Casuistry: A History of Moral Reasoning.* Berkeley, CA: University of California Press.

Lo, B. 1987. Behind closed doors: Promises and pitfalls of ethics committees. *New England Journal of Medicine* 317:46–50.

Mill, J.S. 1859. *On Liberty.* New York: W.W. Norton.

New York State Task Force on Life and the Law. 1988. *Surrogate Parenting: Analysis and Recommendations for Public Policy.* New York, NY: New York State Task Force on Life and the Law.

President's Commission (President's Commission for the Study of Ethical Problems in Medicine and Biomedical and Behavioral Research). 1981. *Defining Death.* Washington, D.C.: U.S. Government Printing Office.

President's Commission. 1982a. *Making Health Care Decisions.* Washington, D.C.: U.S. Government Printing Office.

President's Commission. 1982b. *Splicing Life.* Washington, D.C.: U.S. Government Printing Office.

President's Commission. 1983a. *Deciding to Forego Life-Sustaining Treatment.* Washington, D.C.: U.S. Government Printing Office.

President's Commission. 1983b. *Securing Access to Health Care.* Washington, D.C.: U.S. Government Printing Office.

Veatch, R.M. 1993. From forgoing life support to aid-in-dying. *Hastings Center Report* 23(6):S7–S8.

Wikler, D. 1993. Brain death: A durable consensus? *Bioethics* 7(2/3):239–246.

6

Conclusions and Recommendations

INTERPRETING THE COMMITTEE'S CHARGE

One motivating factor behind this report was the fact that little public bioethics activity took place in the 1980s when the country was sharply divided on several ethical issues. After the closing of the President's Commission, no mechanisms for public discussion and consensus building have been employed effectively. Ethical issues that have been left unresolved include: the nation's public health response to AIDS, research on fetuses and embryos, research involving RU-486, research on the sexual practices of teenagers and adults and their link to sexually transmitted diseases, and the wide range of implications by findings by the Human Genome Project.

The committee's initial charge was to analyze the nation's current capacity to anticipate, recognize, and respond to social and ethical issues arising from advances in biomedical science and technology. Part of this analysis was a survey and evaluation of the mechanisms that have been used in the past—at national, state, and local levels—to resolve such issues. Where such mechanisms are needed but no historical models exist, it was the committee's task to make recommendations regarding processes and structures by which the functions of anticipation, recognition, and response could be established.

During its discussions, however, the committee decided that "anticipating" social, legal, and ethical problems associated with as yet unknown discoveries was not practical, given the difficulty of accurately foreseeing the future. In retrospect, most of the ethical dilemmas generated by innovative technologies in the past would have been impossible to predict.

Furthermore, it seems impractical to spend time and energy imagining *potential* dilemmas when we are already faced with so many. Hence, the concepts of "anticipation" and "recognition" were merged into "early recognition" for the purpose of the committee's deliberations.

Next, the committee was asked to propose processes and/or structures by which early recognition and response could be accomplished on an ongoing basis; the committee was not asked to resolve any particular issue or set of issues. This portion of the committee's charge reflects the idea that the need to anticipate new issues becomes less pressing if established processes exist to address issues promptly as they arise.

The committee was apprehensive about the wording of its charge, noting that not all scientific and technological "advances" are, in fact, advances. The word "advances" implies positive impact, which is not always the case for new technologies. With this in mind, the committee agreed that it was actually addressing "developments" in biomedical science and technology.

Spheres of Concern

Finally, the committee recognized that not all ethical quandaries that have confronted society in the context of biomedicine have resulted from a single radical change or the introduction of a unique new technology. Limiting discussion to single radical changes or unique technologies did not produce a useful boundary for the committee's mandate. Rather, it pointed to a need to define more carefully the variety of circumstances under which troubling social and ethical issues can arise. The committee identified four illustrative scenarios, which follow.

Novel Developments

Novel developments may raise unique ethical concerns that did not exist prior to their introduction. The controversy provoked by the recently reported cloning of human embryos is illustrative (Kolata, 1993). So too are developments in genetics, which raise new questions about the interplay of free will and genetic determinism in generating behavior and about the value of information about future health status.

Innovations Already Integrated into Practice

Innovations may diffuse into medical practice more rapidly than related ethical issues can be resolved. Last year's innovations sometimes become this year's practices, with application far outpacing our capacity as a society to cope with the ethical dimensions raised by these new practices.

When doctors routinely employ a procedure, and when insurance companies reimburse for that procedure, we tend to think that ethical quandaries raised by that procedure have been resolved. This is not always the case. For example, in vitro fertilization is no longer regarded as new in many quarters, yet the ethical dilemmas it raises have never been satisfactorily addressed in the United States. Along with other new reproductive methods (such as surrogate motherhood), in vitro fertilization continues to challenge widely accepted understandings of parenthood and the legal status of the embryo/fetus.

Aggregate Effect

Some technical changes or developments, considered individually, may not raise substantial ethical issues. Yet an accumulation of such developments can present a novel circumstance that alters existing practices and beliefs, triggering a sense that the developments as a whole require deeper examination because they raise unexamined ethical questions. For example, the accumulation of developments in health care, such as immunizations and antibiotics that prevent or cure infectious disease and arterial bypasses that avert death from heart disease, have made it possible for people to live longer than ever before. Longer life spans, however, have increased the incidence of chronic disease, which in turn has provoked reflection on social and ethical issues related to death and dying, the rationing of medical care, and the ends of medicine.

Organizational Innovation

Organizational changes can also raise new ethical concerns. Our society is about to undergo significant change in the delivery of health care services, including both established and new technologies. This raises new ethical quandaries related to equity. It is likely that health care reform will necessitate explicit ordering of priorities regarding health resources as well as new judgments about rationing of expensive medical technologies. The empowerment of distinct social groups, discussed in Chapter 2, is also illustrative of an organizational change that can engender new social and ethical quandaries. For example, the success of women's health advocates has compelled NIH, the scientific community, and others to address questions of justice and self-determination in health care and health care research.

Limitations in Scope

As illustrated in Chapter 4, the committee recognized that efforts to address the sorts of social and ethical quandaries described above can take a variety of shapes, from community groups to hospital ethics committees to state and national ethics commissions. The committee also recognized that the way in which our society responds to such quandaries is influenced significantly by actions that take place in the context of the legal system, sometimes through individual landmark cases such as *Roe v. Wade* or *In re Quinlan,* and sometimes through more subtle accumulations of legal decisions. The role of the legal system in influencing the atmosphere for social and ethical quandaries in biomedicine is fascinating and complex. Given resource and time limitations, however, the committee chose not to address the legal system in a comprehensive fashion. In order to introduce readers to the role played by courts, legislatures, and other lawmaking bodies in bioethics deliberation and policymaking, a background paper by Lawrence Gostin is included in this volume.

CRITERIA FOR EVALUATION

Potential Yardsticks

The committee worked to develop a series of criteria by which past efforts—public ethics bodies and the products of these bodies alike—could be evaluated. These criteria were described in Chapter 5.

Other criteria can and frequently have been used. In his background paper for this report, for example, Bradford Gray evaluated the President's Commission and the National Commission by examining the frequency with which the work of these bodies has been cited in court cases, the *Federal Register,* medical journals, and law reviews. He also solicited the opinions of former commissioners and staff of the two groups. In a recent publication entitled *Biomedical Ethics in U.S. Public Policy* (1993), the Office of Technology Assessment (OTA) judged public ethics bodies and their products as successful on the basis of prevailing sentiment among OTA study participants and advisors, as well as on the basis of whether or not the recommendations of a particular body stimulated legislation.

Several problems arose in attempting to apply the criteria identified by the committee in a uniform, checklist fashion. First, although one can list what might be valued about a public ethics body or its products, the committee recognized that such bodies operate in complex situations in which some of these values necessarily come into conflict, or at least tension, with other values. For example, the committee believes that the practice of holding open meetings enhances the effectiveness of ethics bodies because openness is consistent with the democratic orientation of our country. Yet in some situations, as with the New York State Task Force on Life and Law, closed meetings may enhance internal collegiality, efficiency, and consensus building—also important considerations.

Another complexity arises from the fact that public ethics bodies operate in a pluralistic society where citizens' values vary greatly. For example, agreement on issues that involve abortion is extremely difficult, if not impossible, due to the deep divisions in our society on this subject. In fact, partisan adherence to strongly held opinions on abortion played a major role in the failure of the Biomedical Ethics Board (BEB) and the Human Fetal Tissue Transplantation Research Panel (HFTTRP), as well as the failure of efforts to reestablish the Ethics Advisory Board (EAB).

The mandate given to a public ethics body will also affect the way in which the success of that body or its products are judged. One reason that the National Commission has been judged a success by many observers is that it led to revised regulations for human subjects research (OTA, 1993). However, that success might have been impossible without the action-forcing clause in the original law, which forced the Department of Health, Education, and Welfare either to accept the commission's recommendations or publicly state its reasons for not accepting them. Conversely, the HFTTRP was charged to respond to ten specific questions—a charge that stimulated the majority of panel members to develop responses to the individual questions rather than to provide comprehensive and consistent justifications for all of its conclusions (King, 1991.) Some observers believe that the report of this panel would have been more persuasive had it developed an analytical framework for considering the issue that took account of existing norms, methodologies, and cultural perspectives (King, 1991).

Baruch Brody in his background paper in this volume maintains that both context and mandate were important factors in the effectiveness of the three New York State Task Force reports, *Do Not Resuscitate Orders, Life-Sustaining Treatment: Making Decisions and Appointing a Health Care Agent,* and *When Others Must Choose,* as well as that of the President's Commission report, *Deciding to Forego Life-Sustaining Treatment.* The three reports of the New York State Task Force on the topic of life-sustaining treatment occasioned more controversy because they were focused on the development of proposed legislation—an activity that is frequently accompanied by conflict.

Finally, some public ethics bodies serve functions that they were not specifically mandated to serve. For example, a body convened to draft legislation may be unsuccessful in that regard but may increase public awareness of an issue through its deliberations. Consequently, the evaluation of the success of a particular public ethics body may be more meaningful if it also takes into account achievements that are incidental to or unrelated to a group's mandated function. It is also necessary to ask whether public ethics bodies are to be judged on the basis of overall effect or on the basis of their particular products. When evaluating the overall effect of an ethics body, factors such as the authority of the appointing body, the esteem in which its members are held by society, the adequacy of the staff and resources available, and the impact of previous products issued by the group, in addition to the criteria outlined in Chapter 5, may be influential.

Applying the Yardstick

Although the criteria for success cannot be reduced to a checklist, the committee members believe that—with the appropriate scholarly analysis—general agreement on the success of public ethics bodies often can be obtained.

As noted in Chapter 4, the Ethics Advisory Board, established in 1978 by the Secretary of DHEW as a permanent advisory body, met frequently for two years and produced four documents, marking a degree of success. However, the EAB was disbanded in 1980 and the recommendations of its principal report were never acted upon by DHHS. Moreover, since DHHS regulations require that all research involving human in vitro fertilization or embryo transfer be reviewed by such a board, work in this area has virtually ceased. Disbanding the EAB might be considered a success by individuals who wish to block controversial research. The committee disagrees and considers the demise of the EAB to have left unmet a critical need for bioethical deliberation and decision making. Without the EAB, the country has had no officially constituted group of national scope to provide analysis and advice on ethically and socially controversial biomedical research protocols or guidance to the research community. Human in vitro fertilization has nevertheless become a standard accepted form of medical practice, but without what many would consider sufficient scientific, social, and ethical underpinnings to optimize clinical practice (IOM, 1989; OTA, 1988).

The HFTTRP, also described in Chapter 4, was convened in 1988 by the NIH and concluded that the use of human fetal tissue in transplantation research was acceptable public policy if certain guidelines were in place (Childress, 1991). Although the panel's report lies within the range of an international consensus (Walters, 1988), the Reagan and Bush administrations did not accept the panel's recommendations and the moratorium on the funding of research using fetal tissue from induced abortions remained in effect until rescinded by the Clinton administration in 1993. Some analysts believe that the continuation of the moratorium stemmed from the report's failure to make clear how persons holding radically different views about abortion could nonetheless agree that use of fetal tissue from induced abortion could be acceptable public policy under specific conditions (King, 1991).

The National Commission is an example of an advisory body that was housed within the agency it advised and had an action-forcing mandate. The commission published several effective reports on specific topics and summarized its thinking in *The Belmont Report* (1978), which clearly enunciated the underlying ethical principles that should guide research involving human subjects. Whether or not due to National Commission reports, the incidence of gross abuse of research subjects appears to have diminished subsequent to their publication. The requirements that the commission's recommendations be published in the *Federal Register* and that DHEW respond in writing within 180 days proved useful in the implementation of the recommendations.

The President's Commission, on the other hand, is an example of a commission convened to examine issues that spanned the concerns of several agencies—not only human subjects research, but also aspects of medical practice. With a prodigious output of reports, many of which have influenced thought in ethics, law, and subsequent legislation, the President's Commission can be considered overall to have been an effective societal mechanism for deliberation about social and ethical issues in biomedicine.

A MULTILEVEL APPROACH TO BIOETHICS DELIBERATION

After considering all of these factors, the committee concluded that the most effective method for dealing with complex ethical and social quandaries would be a capacity for response at multiple levels of society. The committee therefore proposes strengthening the multitiered system of public deliberation at local, institutional, professional, community, state, and national levels, and particularly recommends filling a key gap through reestablishing a supra-agency ethics commission at the national level. The recommendation for a multitiered system rests on the conviction that capacities for public ethical deliberation (through academic experts, health professionals, religious communities, secular agencies, and an increasingly informed and interested public) have blossomed in all regions of the country. At the same time, certain contemporary ethical quandaries, including many ramifications of molecular genetic research, can best be considered for the nation as a whole through a supra-agency national commission. Two supra-agency models presented by the committee are a single national commission with a broad mandate and a set of national commissions, each with a more focused charge. The recommendations elaborate on the elements proposed for the multitiered system and the features the committee deems desirable for any new national commission. In general, the committee believes that decisions about public policy should occur as closely as possible to the levels at which relevant actions are taken, and must involve those likely to be affected by the policy. The committee is not proposing a new policymaking authority, but a system, separate from existing political structures, for reflecting on and informing public policy decisions at all levels.

In considering issues related to genetic technology, for example, some questions will require resolution on the level of the individual, the family, health care workers (such as physicians and counselors), and other trusted advisors such as ministers. Many of these scientific, social, and ethical issues will also require examination during the training of the professionals who aid in the decision-making process. Professional societies will need to provide their members with guidelines and educational materials to ensure that patients receive accurate medical advice as well as appropriate and empathetic treatment and guidance. As the process of genetic screening moves out of the research laboratory and into the primary care arena, a consensus must be developed on the kinds of information needed by physicians and patients (IOM, 1994).

At the level of the institution, hospital ethics committees will confront issues relating to provider–patient interactions in the case of patients with genetic conditions. Within institutions that conduct research on humans, institutional review boards will have to determine the appropriate risks and benefits for research subjects as genetic testing and screening move into wider use. Should research subjects involved in the development of genetic tests be provided with preliminary diagnostic information, and if so, when? When should such testing or screening procedures become part of medical practice?

Social and ethical issues related to genetics must also be addressed at the state level. States, which regulate many aspects of medical practice, form the locus for legal decisions concerning not only what genetic screening should be done at various stages of life, but what information, counseling, and quality assessment will accompany each step of the processes.

Several federal agencies are also involved with research and practice relating to human genetic disease. One example is the Health Care Financing Agency, which is responsible for laboratory quality assurance in genetic testing; it must assure that the information given to the individual is accurate, since crucial decisions are often made on the basis of this information. The NIH Recombinant DNA Advisory Committee assures that present and future gene therapy research involving human subjects is undertaken appropriately. The Ethical, Legal, and Social Implications Working Group provides a funding mechanism for ethicists, social scientists, lawyers, and health care professionals to describe, analyze, and educate professionals and the public concerning the many issues this new technology raises (see the background paper by Hanna in this volume).

To date, however, the ELSI Working Group has not developed an effective mechanism for translating the work being done in various professional communities into public policy.

Governmental agencies have also solicited advice from groups such as OTA (OTA, 1993) and IOM (IOM, 1994) on issues related to research in human genetics. The issues raised by what has been called the "genetic revolution" are so ubiquitous that it may be appropriate to appoint a commission charged with oversight of issues related to human genetics and situated so as to span the various agency concerns. Issues of individual privacy and confidentiality of medical information, employment and insurance discrimination, and various eugenic implications are national in scope.

The recommendations made by the committee are divided into nongovernmental, state, and national levels for ease of description. The committee recognizes and applauds the growth that has occurred over the past several decades in our nation's capacity to deliberate social and ethical issues. The committee envisions a strengthening of this capacity to fulfill the broad array of functions (understanding, education, analysis, and debate) necessary to facilitate the development of consensus in our pluralistic society. In facing contemporary social and ethical quandaries stemming from developments in biotechnology, society now has a richer capacity for deliberation and a deeper pool of expertise than was available as few as 10 to 20 years ago. The modern bioethics movement is now in its fourth decade. Since its origins in the 1960s, it has grown and matured in several ways. Paralleling the growth in bioethics, there has been a growing body of literature in the social science arena. Academic experts, members of the public, government officials, and health care professionals with basic knowledge and genuine interest in bioethics and social concerns can be found in every region of the country.

RECOMMENDATIONS

Since much of the structure for dealing with the impacts of biomedical developments is already in place at the local level (e.g., IRBs, HECs, and professional organizations) many desirable actions might be taken at this level. The committee addresses these recommendations to consumers of biotechnology and biomedical research, as well as professional organizations at all levels, recognizing that their members and staffs have unique capabilities for dealing with some of these impacts. In addition, hospitals and IRBs have particular opportunities and responsibilities to confront issues and problems presented by biomedical developments. Many of the social and ethical impacts of developments in biomedicine are better addressed at the state or national level, for reasons indicated below. The committee presents its recommendations for state or national response, noting the advantages that state-level action can have. Finally, the committee describes the value that national advisory bodies would have and recommends establishing a national bioethics commission at the supra-agency level.

A Multitiered Response

The committee envisions multitiered response to social and ethical issues arising from developments in biomedicine, with deliberations and decisions occurring as close as possible to the level at which relevant actions should be taken. These efforts should be democratic in nature, with a capacity to combine individual and community preferences and values, practical experience in biomedicine, the academic knowledge of bioethicists, as well as the expertise of other disciplines in which ethical discourse is prominent (e.g., law, philosophy, and religion), into its operational procedures. The committee envisions these efforts taking place at locations at which social and ethical policy decisions related to health science and health care are being made.

The matching of deliberation to the level at which the decisions are made could be achieved through the creation of deliberative capacity* at levels within the health care system where decisions are jointly made among consumers, providers, payers, and policymakers. The committee is not proposing a new focus of policy-making authority, but a deliberative capacity, separate from political structures, for reflecting on and informing public policy decisions at all levels.

Given the growth in the discipline of bioethics over the past 20 years, and the growth in public interest in social and ethical issues in health and health care, the "infrastructure" for such a diffuse capacity seems to be already largely in place. This capacity can be further strengthened to provide for greater consideration of the social and ethical issues that almost invariably accompany technologies and organizational developments in biomedicine. The committee believes that many ethical decisions are best made by the affected individuals and families, with the help of advisors such as health care professionals and ministers. However, some issues will require communal levels of decision making about quandaries that may affect every citizen of the community.

Ongoing changes in the structure of the health care system, in combination with focused national efforts at health care reform, are creating new

---

*By "deliberative capacity" the committee means some formal assignment of persons and resources that can make possible the gathering of persons to deliberate in an impartial and informed way on specific ethical issues. This can be inside or outside of an agency, it can be public or private, it can be an office or committee.

opportunities to address social and ethical issues in public policy decision making. The mechanisms for addressing these issues should be consistent with the structure of health care in each state, and if health care reform brings central authorities, they too should be supplemented by an ethics deliberative capacity. If health alliances are established, an ethics capacity should be built into the alliances at those points where major allocation decisions are made. Some states might prefer a freestanding ethics commission to advise on a broad range of bioethical issues. State committees, in turn, could communicate with a national bioethics committee, one of whose functions would be to help coordinate the activities of state committees and bring together individuals to deal with national issues that require special attention.

Ethical deliberations will be particularly important in the case of decisions about allocation of health care resources so that health care plans, at whatever level, balance ethical and social considerations with considerations of cost. Health care reform is entering unknown and uncharted territory characterized by an explicit focus on health care costs and financing. The system is presently in flux and the future will bring major changes in the way health care services are delivered. Traditional ways of making decisions will also change.

It seems likely that a local ethical deliberative body can best balance the competing interests of individual needs and desires for intervention and the economic burdens borne by the institution or community. However, deliberations at the local level should not replace consideration of related issues at higher levels.

The committee notes that there are large disparities among the citizens of this country with respect to income, wealth, and power. Concerns about social justice, which drive some of the present efforts to explore the social and ethical impacts of developments in biomedicine, point to a need for national deliberations. One advantage of a national deliberative capacity is the authority and credibility with which it is imbued, and which make it better able to reflect on and account for the interests of the disadvantaged in these deliberative efforts.

Nongovernmental Organizations and Individuals

The committee considered the current and potential roles of individuals and nongovernmental organizations—grassroots efforts, hospitals, institutional review boards, professional societies, and health professional educational institutions—in responding to social and ethical issues raised by biomedical developments. The committee believes that those people who play major roles in the generation and proliferation of new biomedical capabilities bear an ongoing obligation to consider the potential impacts of their work on the general public and on the particular individuals and groups to whom innovation is targeted.

The committee recommends that the people or organizations that conduct, fund, and commercialize research, as well as those medical providers who apply new technologies, establish a formal capacity whereby they can participate in public moral discourse about the ethical implications of developments in their field. They should attempt to anticipate how these developments may affect society for better or worse and to prepare ways in which adverse effects on social values can be prevented.

The committee recommends that the National Institutes of Health provide funding mechanisms to support (1) the exploration by individual investigators of social and ethical aspects of biomedical technologies as they are developed and (2) the creation of a social and ethical knowledge base for all of biomedical science (e.g., extend the ELSI program to other institutes and programs within the NIH).

Based on letters solicited from scientists and practitioners in a variety of fields, the committee noted that those who discover, develop, or apply new technologies in biomedicine are often well positioned to recognize the potential for adverse social and ethical consequences of these technologies (although sometimes they do not). One of the most efficient ways to initiate deliberation of and responses to such consequences may therefore be to call upon researchers, commercial developers of technologies, and medical providers who use new technologies to share their special knowledge of these technologies in ways that could facilitate awareness of these consequences. Such avenues might include publications and professional presentations; perhaps inquiry about such consequences could even be made part of grant applications. The more that it becomes the norm for consideration of these issues to be part of scientific investigation, the greater the likelihood that our society would identify problems in their early stages and address them more effectively.

Professional Organizations

The committee believes that professional societies, such as organizations of health care providers or scientists within a field, have an obligation to provide professional guidelines for practitioners and patients dealing with new technological or organizational developments.

The committee recommends that organizations of biomedical professionals establish ethics committees that can be easily mobilized to respond to social and ethical issues as they are identified. Collaboration

among professional associations dealing with related issues is to be encouraged.

Professions exist as part of a societal contract that grants learned experts a certain latitude and self-control in return for the expectation of service to the public. In addition, the resources used to support biomedical innovation and development are generated by the community, largely through governmental support of research. These economic considerations support a role for professional organizations in bioethics deliberations; so too does the good track record of professional organizations in advising on these issues. In the court cases adjudicating the foregoing of life-sustaining treatment during the last 20 years, professional organizations have participated as *amici* (e.g., *Cruzan* and *Conroy*) and as parties (Baby Doe cases involving the American Academy of Pediatrics and the American College of Obstetricians and Gynecologists). More recently, the American College of Obstetricians and Gynecologists and the American Fertility Society, finding no publicly authorized forum for resolution of some of the complex issues that repeatedly confront their practitioners, established the National Advisory Board for Ethics and Reproduction, a privately funded, and now separately incorporated, forum for discussion of ethical issues in reproduction.

> **The committee recommends that professional associations, including those for health care providers and biomedical scientists, recognize their special obligation to investigate the ethical implications of biomedical developments and advocate for the interests of the public and of patients, especially when those adversely affected by changes are unable to advocate for themselves.**

Professional organizations may often be among the first to note the potential for adverse effects for some patients or clients. Especially when these adversely affected persons are already disadvantaged, they may lack sufficient resources to advocate for themselves. As part of the promise to serve the public that is fundamental to professional standing, this circumstance creates an obligation to advocate on behalf of those at risk of even greater disadvantage. This may well be a difficult mandate, but the committee notes that professional societies, as representatives of professionals themselves, have derivative obligations to speak out, and especially if developments that offer advantage to some actually worsen the lot of others who are already seriously disadvantaged.

Hospital Ethics Committees

> **Preliminary evidence indicates that hospital ethics committees provide many useful support functions for staff, patients, and their families**

relating to the handling of social and ethical issues that arise from developments in biomedicine. The committee nevertheless recommends that formal studies of the optimum roles, use, and outcomes of HECs be undertaken by such groups as the Office of Technology Assessment, Institute of Medicine, and foundations interested in health care issues.

As has been described in this report, HECs were originally proposed as a mechanism for sharing responsibility for morally charged treatment decisions by hospital staff, patients, and their families. However, a tension exists between the HEC as a forum for professionals and as a vehicle for fostering the rights and interests of patients and their families (Wolf, 1991, 1992). HECs constitute one way in which medical decision making has been democratized by being opened to input from nonphysicians (e.g., nurses, administrators, clergy, and family members).

The Joint Commission on the Accreditation of Health Care Organizations (JCAHO) requires that hospitals have a HEC or a similar body or process as a condition for U.S. hospital accreditation (which is tied, in turn, to eligibility to receive Medicare payments). The JCAHO also requires accredited hospitals to provide education on ethical issues to staff, patients, and families. It has been suggested, but not required, that HECs assume additional roles such as developing patient rights standards; formulating and/or reviewing institutional policy and procedural guidelines on decision making for medical care; reviewing diagnoses, prognoses, and treatment decisions made for specific patients by doctors and surrogates; and mediating conflicts that might arise over treatment decisions. Although HECs seem to be potentially useful bodies to help patients, families, surrogates, and other decision makers deal with ethical and social issues, it is unclear at present how many HECs exist, how they function, and what the outcomes are of the various ways in which they can operate.

The committee believes that HECs or similar committees operating across health plans could help patients and health care professionals deal with social and ethical issues that arise from developments in biomedicine. Little is known about the range and characteristics of effectiveness of these committees; this knowledge needs to be expanded. This sort of knowledge will aid in the design and evaluation of similar ethics committees that may accompany health care reform.

Institutional Review Boards

As discussed elsewhere in this report, the committee believes that past experience with IRBs has been important and salutary, but that the present structure and role of IRBs should be evaluated and, if necessary, modified.

This includes IRBs that review research sponsored by all federal agencies as well as that sponsored by industry. IRBs are known to be variable in their application of federal rules and local prerogatives Where one IRB might approve a particular research proposal with little question, another might question many components of the same proposal. Some IRBs uniformly require written documentation of consent, irrespective of risk or feasibility; others do not. Some irregularity among IRBs can be positive since it can reflect appeal to local understandings and values. However, these irregularities also point to a need to understand the reasons for diversity and to correct diversity that arises from bias. Moreover, since research is blocked by an IRB's rejection, due process seems to require that IRBs develop some method for appeal of their decisions and for identification of error or prejudice.

The committee believes that the NIH, in conjunction with other federal agencies (such as the Food and Drug Administration) to which IRBs relate, need to carefully examine the IRB system and assess whether it is functioning well. Some questions that could be assessed include:

1. Are IRBs successfully representing the interests of human subjects in research and not merely those of their sponsoring institution?

2. Do IRBs generally fulfill their goals?

3. What lessons can be learned about effective IRB function from the wide variation in actual IRB practices, and should greater uniformity be encouraged?

4. Would communication among different IRBs facilitate effective functioning?

5. Are there adequate forums for the appeal of institutional rulings or for resolution of issues that an individual IRB cannot easily address?

6. How do freestanding IRBs operate, especially with respect to conflict-of-interest considerations?

Health Professional Educational Institutions

As part of the remarkable growth in numbers of individuals trained in academic bioethics, the curricula of health professional schools have begun to reflect the critical role of social and ethical considerations in the education of health professionals. The committee is convinced that continued integration of these concepts into health professional education will ultimately help caregivers relate effectively to patients who are faced with difficult decisions stemming from technological developments. There is a developing literature on the integration and evaluation of some of the efforts to introduce social and ethical issues into the curriculum of health professional students.

The exposure of graduate students in basic and clinical sciences to ethical and social issues has lagged behind the exposure of health professional students by 10 to 20 years. Since individual integrity and mutual trust among scientists are preconditions for the production of scientific truths (see the background paper by Shapin), it is necessary for students to understand the importance of issues such as scientific responsibility and the roles of conventions and consensus in modern science. The NIH recently introduced a requirement that institutions applying for National Research Service Award training grants demonstrate the presence of a program for instruction on scientific integrity for all NIH-supported trainees. Since the requirement is new and still in the early stages of implementation, the degree to which this includes exposure to social and ethical issues related to developments in biomedicine is unknown. The committee believes that it is important for biomedical scientists to be part of the process of examining the social and ethical dimensions of science and technology because: (1) the tradition of openness and internal criticism found in science could fruitfully be extended to the deliberation of ethical issues; (2) biomedical scientists and medical practitioners, due to their understanding of the use of technology as part of the practice of medicine, might have special insight into related ethical issues; and (3) scientists may facilitate the discrimination between factual and value-laden components of scientific belief.

The committee recommends that an evaluation be undertaken of the process of education for graduate students in the health sciences on the social and ethical implications of technology as part of the current educational efforts on scientific responsibility. The committee also urges increased efforts to integrate social and ethical issues in biomedicine into the curriculum of undergraduate and graduate health professional programs.

The State Level

States need to play an active role in defining a capacity for ethical deliberation in biomedicine given their oversight of professional certification, medical practice, health care financing, and legal liability. Due to the number of roles that states play in the development and use of biomedical technology, the committee believes that each state needs to shape the method and scope of its commitment to finding these answers.

The committee recommends that states foster or participate in a public deliberative process for responding to social and ethical quandaries stemming from technological and organizational developments in biomedicine and health care.

In a democratic society such as ours, mechanisms should be in place for participation of the public in decision making about public policy. Such efforts may be designated as "public" either by virtue of their funding or governmental sponsorship (e.g., state-sponsored commissions or publicly supported "town meetings"), or merely by virtue of the fact that deliberations take place in open meetings. States should assume a special responsibility to establish or participate in such a process for several reasons, one being that states are responsible for administering programs that inevitably raise ethical issues (e.g., Medicaid, maternal and child health programs) and for developing health care regulations. For example, in response to the Patient Self-Determination Act, a number of states did solicit input from a wide variety of individuals and groups regarding how the Act should be implemented (Teno et al., 1993).

Because states are also the primary locus for family law, public health law, malpractice provisions, and criminal law, states should play an important role in stimulating public discussion and resolution of such issues as the use of reproductive technologies; laws and regulations concerning the "definition" of death and foregoing life-sustaining treatments; the practice of assisted suicide and active euthanasia; public health measures involving screening, contact tracing, and quarantining for infectious diseases; screening programs to detect either the presence of genetic disease or susceptibility to diseases such as cancer or heart disease; the procurement and allocation of organs for transplantation; and so on. State mechanisms can also channel consensus into the particular legislative form that is appropriate for and acceptable to citizens of a particular state.

The committee does not recommend a single specific mechanism for public deliberation of ethical issues at the state level, nor does it recommend a formal institutionalized response in each of the 50 states. Some states may want to establish their own ethics commissions, such as that in New York. Other states lacking the resources or breadth of representation for such undertakings may wish to cooperate with neighboring states to form regional ethics commissions and information exchange programs.

There are several advantages of having a commission operating at the state or regional level. State-level commissions, by virtue of their more restricted geographic domain (compared to national-level commissions) may be better able to target their deliberations to reflect local conditions, constituencies, historical traditions, and legal requirements.

Second, with respect to some controversial issues regulated at the state level, a state-level commission may be successful at achieving consensus. In some instances, reports based on national-level deliberations may fail to appear to a locally focused citizenry as being pertinent to meeting their needs. For issues on which nationwide consensus is unlikely at present (e.g., rationing health care), some states have managed to confront the issue in a more direct way. Oregon showed a willingness to deal with the complexities of prioritizing health care services; the state was also able to develop a public process that included grassroots input unlikely to be replicated at this time at a national level.

Third, no matter how well a national commission might frame its policy recommendations, these will in any case have to be implemented at the state level. A state-level commission can serve as a helpful mediator between a nationally articulated consensus and the particular demographic and legislative constraints of a given state or region. Particular religious constituencies or interest groups may exercise little influence at the national level but play pivotal roles at the local or state level. By working closely over time with a state legislature or by inviting the representatives of particular groups to participate in its deliberations, a state- or regional-level commission may find it easier to implement a policy consensus that has been forged at the national level.

Grassroots efforts may also be effective, as illustrated by efforts in Oregon, Vermont, and Colorado (Jennings, 1988). Assuming that some form of health reform is enacted, states may also wish to recommend or perhaps even require that each regional or corporate health alliance set up an ethics committee charged with forging policy on access questions. Still other states may wish to sponsor or encourage a wide variety of educational efforts in schools, museums, and other forums and via print and electronic media.

The committee acknowledges the possible objections to these recommendations. For example, all this activity on the state level could be construed as duplicative and different states could take different positions on controversial issues, as they once did regarding the definition of death. In addition, states may not choose to commit adequate funds for the kind of staffing and process that the committee recommends elsewhere in this report. It should be noted, however, that states have the right and responsibility to make these decisions. The fact that they will disagree, especially on highly contested policy questions, can and should be regarded as an advantage. The states provide a much-needed laboratory for social policy experimentation.

The New Jersey Bioethics Commission, for example, acknowledged the essentially philosophical and religious nature of the debate over brain death; it then took the bold step of allowing members of certain religious groups to define death for themselves, in accordance with their religious beliefs. New Jersey's experience with this legislation may provide the rest of the nation with an interesting counterpoint to the proposition, endorsed by the President's Commission and the New York State Task Force, that strict uniformity is a prerequisite of good public policy in this area.

The National Level

Agency-level Advisory Bodies

The committee recommends the establishment of a deliberative capacity within relevant government agencies and departments to provide advice on issues relating to biomedical research and applications of biomedical technology. The committee strongly recommends that as a first step, the Ethics Advisory Board or a similar body within the Department of Health and Human Services be reestablished.

The committee perceives a need for a permanent ethics staff within governmental agencies. Ethics panels located within, and related to, specific agencies have provided valuable advice to these agencies in the past. Specific examples of advisory bodies located within agencies have been the National Commission, the NIH Recombinant DNA Advisory Committee with its Subcommittee on Human Gene Therapy, and the Ethics Advisory Board. All three of these bodies provided advice to their sponsoring agencies regarding research ethics. The committee strongly supports the reestablishment of an EAB-like body, because the tasks assigned to it in its originating regulation are not being accomplished at present and constitute a national need and a missed opportunity for leadership in this area. Comparable bodies, often located in ministries of health, have been established in many countries in the past 10 years.

A Supra-agency Commission

For certain issues of broad national interest, the committee believes that it would be highly desirable to have a national-level commission address these issues as they concern multiple governmental agencies. Some complex issues are better examined and analyzed in a disciplined fashion at a national level, because they affect people throughout the country. In addition, some issues may be ripe for a broad social consensus. The committee believes that at the present time there are several such issues that might be incorporated into the mandates of one or more national commissions:

1. issues related to scientific advances in genetics, including new possibilities for shaping future generations in unusual and unexpected ways, and the impact of genetic knowledge on peoples' insurability and employability;

2. issues related to confidentiality and privacy of medical information, especially in light of health care reform;

3. the interplay of serious disability and life-sustaining treatment, as well as discrimination on the basis of disability;

4. the principles to be used for allocation of medical services and integration of costs with social and ethical considerations into clinical and allocation policy decisions; and

5. issues related to reproduction and research and medical treatment of embryos and fetuses.

A high-level commission has several institutional advantages over efforts at a lower level, including greater visibility, higher prestige, greater capacity to address a broad mandate, and more independence. A centrally situated body would be readily available to work on complex issues and give coherent responses. A national body can more readily call upon the national and international expertise that is required for complicated and difficult issues; experts can function as commissioners, staff, witnesses, and/ or authors of background papers. A national body is also in a better position to formulate and represent distinctively American views on bioethics, at a time when issues relating to biomedical research and applications are becoming increasingly internationalized.

National professional bodies may have the expertise to deal with social and ethical issues, but may lack the authority and legitimacy that comes from being authorized and appointed by the federal government. The National Commission and President's Commission demonstrated the effectiveness of federally appointed bodies in dealing with ethical issues.

The committee recommends that the federal government establish a public deliberative body (or bodies, depending on the breadth of the mandate to be addressed) for a limited term at the supra-agency level to consider social and ethical issues stemming from technological and organizational developments in biomedicine that are of concern simultaneously to several governmental agencies or are nationwide in scope.

The experience of BEAC should not be forgotten, however, in any vision of a national-level commission and the sorts of issues it might address. BEAC has been described as having "crashed on the shoals of abortion politics," an idea that raises the question of how another national-level commission might navigate through some of the issues that BEAC was convened to address. As Hanna and colleagues describe (1994), issues in which abortion is a factor may be issues of which public bioethics deliberation must simply steer clear. They suggest that abortion and issues involving abortion are issues that simply cannot be productively engaged at the present time because they elicit "strongly held incompatible views that rational people reach from different moral premises." Even if competing biases were equally balanced on a commission, opinions about abortion are usually so strongly held that it is unlikely that significant movement toward a middle ground could occur. At some time in the future, bioethical issues that touch on such divisive issues as abortion may be ripe for some form of useful explication or consensus, but they are decidedly unripe now.

In the event that one or more national ethics commissions are established, the committee recommends that each have the following attributes:

Mandate. **The body must have a broad yet clearly defined and coherent mandate, as well as the ability to add additional related topics as they become salient.**

The committee was unable to reach consensus regarding the appropriate breadth of a national commission's mandate. The majority of committee members believe that it is not feasible for a single national commission to address *all* social and ethical issues in biomedicine, since the expertise and experience required by such a broad mandate could not be encompassed in a membership of reasonable size. These committee members propose that a national commission's mandate include a set of related social and ethical issues. This proposal reflects a perception that some of the topics in the mandate of the National Commission were quite removed from the central issues of that body and hence were less well handled by the group. Examples of such topics include the study on *Psychosurgery* and the *Ethical Guidelines for Delivery of Health Services by DHEW*. Commissions with a mandate to address interrelated issues will ordinarily have an easier time studying and resolving subsequent issues after they have reached conclusions in one area.

A second group of committee members believed that a national commission with a broad mandate was preferable, so long as it had sufficient time and funding to hire staff and commission background papers to encompass all of the appropriate expertise needed. In this case, commission members—who could be generalists—would evaluate background papers and staff research in order to reach conclusions. One advantage of a commission with a broad and general mandate is that knowledge gained by commissioners and staff in one area may be applied to the subsequent study of other areas. Furthermore, if the group is effective in resolving issues, the credibility of its conclusions on subsequent topics will—and should—be enhanced.

When Congress or the president identifies issues in special need of attention, they could ask for a national commission's advice on these topics. Yet it is also desirable to permit the commission to add extra topics to its mandate, as its time and resources allow and as dictated by the urgency and importance of such additional topics. This prerogative was usefully exercised by the President's Commission in its reports on *Deciding to Forego Life-Sustaining Treatment* and *Splicing Life*.

Sponsorship. **National commissions could be appointed by the president or Congress. Wherever located, each national commission should operate autonomously.**

Appointment by the president enhances a commission's prestige and may also increase its access to government and other information. In addition, if the appointing power is vested in the president, it can be made subject to certain categorical requirements that would ensure that members reflect the range of views relevant to the topics under study. Congressional power over appropriations may encourage responsiveness to statutory expectations. Both the perception and reality of independence are important to the credibility of a commission's recommendations. In spite of appointment by the president or Congress, a national commission needs insulation from self-serving, narrow political interests at the same time as it needs strong ties to affected or vulnerable groups.

Membership. **Each national commission should have a diverse membership in order to represent the points of view of all those concerned with or affected by the social and ethical issues to be considered. The composition of the body should enhance the qualities of impartiality.**

All of the national-level public ethics bodies convened in the past have been composed of experts in a range of relevant disciplines, including academic bioethics, the health professions, biomedical science, social and behavioral sciences, law, philosophy, and religion. Some have also included members representing the general public. Given the logistical desirability of limiting the group to a relatively small size (11 to 20 members), care must be taken to ensure that the group reflect not only disciplinary expertise but also the diversity of views and personal characteristics relevant to the topics under study. Members should be able to rise above their representation of groups or constituencies.

The appointment procedure needs to strive for a delicate balance among the needs of such a body. While the committee recommends that the membership represent a diversity of interests, members should be chosen in order that they may be free to consider issues independently, to deliberate, argue, and reach conclusions based on the information presented, without fear of being removed from or disappointing any particular constituency. Efforts need to be made to include people with formal or informal training in bioethics or who are willing to read and discuss the literature of bioethics seriously.

Membership on federal ethics bodies has traditionally been restricted to persons not employed by the federal government—a restriction that has helped to ensure independence from political influences. There may be reasons in some instances to deviate from this pattern through the appoint-

ment of executive or legislative branch personnel Given the volatility of
some issues in bioethics, however, any arrangement that ties the appointment process directly to the president or Congress, or to a governor or
legislature, can engender a struggle over ideological "balance." This can
result in a group that is potentially polarized, with at least some members
who regard themselves (and are regarded by others) as "representatives" of
the groups or organizations that lobbied for their appointment. Such a
group does not serve one of the most useful functions of a commission,
which is to remove sensitive topics from the political arena and consider
them in a more neutral atmosphere, allowing individuals who come with
differing views to discover common ground, as issues are fleshed out and
relevant data are collected. Ideological polarization was responsible for
the failure of BEAC.

> *Public Access.* **To the extent possible, a national commission should
> deliberate in public. If such public deliberation is not possible, means
> need to be found to gain input from all persons and groups with inter-
> ests in the deliberations. A national commission must reach out to
> segments of the population whose voices are less regularly heard.**

Public media coverage can help to educate the public about the deliberations of a national commission. Public meetings can also facilitate broad
public involvement. The National Commission and President's Commission did not find that public meetings interfered with full and frank exchange of views.

> *Advisory Role.* **A national commission should provide advice not only to
> its authorizing body but to all concerned parties, including the bio-
> medical community; federal, state, and local governmental bodies; and
> the public.**

The commission could be required to report to the president, to Congress, and to any departments or agencies affected by its recommendations, but commission reports should also be disseminated to all interested
parties outside of the government. Some findings and recommendations
of a national commission may lead to federal legislation or regulation;
others may be of primary importance to individuals, as patients or professionals, or to state legislators, judges, and officers of health care institutions. A national commission might well address topics of interest to all
these groups. Local bodies (e.g., HECs and IRBs) can also benefit from
national advice. The experience of the President's Commission demonstrates that conceiving of a commission's audience broadly encourages
better communication and wider dissemination of findings. Commissions
at all levels should therefore take specific steps to assure that the results of
their deliberations are made accessible to the public. In addition to the

use of newspaper and radio, thought needs to be given to how newer methods of information transmission (e.g., electronic means such as computer bulletin boards) might be utilized to communicate commission conclusions.

Action-forcing Powers. **Although a national commission should be advisory, its recommendations should be published, and relevant federal agencies should be required to respond to those recommendations within a defined "comment period" (e.g., 180 days), either by adopting the recommendations or by explaining why they are not being adopted.**

For recommendations that are addressed to federal departments and agencies, action-forcing authority is highly desirable, as the positive experiences of both the National Commission and President's Commission and the negative experiences of the HFTTRP demonstrate. However, such authority is not self-executing, and agency officials who want neither to act nor to explain their inaction may sometimes disregard the statutory requirements. This is especially easy for them to do once the commission goes out of existence.

Having action-forcing powers means that deliberations will be approached more thoughtfully by all, including members of the commission itself. National commissions of the past have worked more effectively in reaching their recommendations when they knew that the recommendations would be responded to by others and would potentially have a direct regulatory impact.

Funding and Staff. **A national commission should be given adequate resources and staff to accomplish its task. It should be funded by direct appropriation to ensure its independence. It should have authority over its own budget and the hiring and firing of its staff.**

The cost of running a national commission depends on the breadth of the group's mandate, the estimated number of commissioners and staff needed, the number and location of the anticipated meetings, and the cost of printing and disseminating the reports that will be produced. The President's Commission was authorized for $5 million per year for four years; in operation, it expended under $5 million over its entire lifetime (39 months), meeting 28 times (generally for 2 days) and publishing a total of 17 volumes. The ability to bring highly qualified experts to the staff for one- and two-year terms of service has several beneficial results: it accelerates a commission's work, because of the experts' knowledge of their fields; it enhances the quality of the work, because such staff members want to produce work they can be proud of when they return to their home institutions; and it helps to avoid bureaucratization of the commission.

Duration. **The commission should have a defined term that is adequate to allow for achievement of assigned tasks.**

There are important reasons to limit a national commission's term, one of which is that limited terms enhance members' ability to maintain energy, focus, and timeliness. The committee considered two possibilities: (1) the term of the commission could be approximately 3 years, with commissioners serving for the entire term, or (2) the commission could have a longer term, with rotating appointments so that one-third of the membership would be replaced every 2 years. As the experience of both the National and President's Commissions indicates, the existence of a date by which work must be completed can result in a high level of productivity. Furthermore, time-limited commissions are less likely than standing commissions to become overly bureaucratic in their approaches. Arguments for longer terms (up to 6 years, with staggered terms for members) include considerations of consistency, credibility, and efficiency of group interaction.

The majority of the committee favored a commission with a defined lifetime as well as a mechanism for initiation of new commissions to consider future issues as they arise (see next recommendation). Some committee members favored the idea of a fixed-term national commission with a "sunset clause," which sets an initial date for termination while still making it easy to extend the commission's term if the issues it is addressing merit further attention and if the quality of its work justifies, in the eyes of the Congress and the president, the commission's continuation.

If a national commission has a limited term, then the value of continuity and the "learning curve" favor a fixed membership. If the group is constituted as a longer-term body (subject to periodic review and renewal), then a rotating membership with staggered terms seems advisable, both to ensure diversity of views and to avoid bureaucratic narrowing of the group's collective vision.

If a term-limited national commission is appointed, the committee recommends that responsibility be located within some existing government locus for ongoing monitoring/reporting on social and ethical issues in biomedicine and for recommending the appointment of new commissions as serious issues of national scope emerge. This responsibility could be located in the Office of Science and Technology Policy, the Office of the Secretary of Health and Human Services, or at some other location chosen by the president or Congress.

The committee believes that, during times when no national commission is functioning or when issues arise at an agency level but remain unaddressed, there should be a continuing surveillance mechanism to identify developing unsolved problems that require more focused attention. A governmental locus for such monitoring could provide several specific functions: it could initiate/prepare a biennial report to be published in the *Federal Register* on social and ethical issues emerging from biomedical technology; it could serve as a receptor for the input of local communities, individuals, institutions, and states that identify issues that need to be addressed in a broad fashion; it could facilitate networking among the various groups addressing social and ethical issues; and it could advise the executive branch about special social and ethical issues that need immediate attention. At the same time, by virtue of its location, it would allow the solution to be part of the political process.

Most of the committee members felt that this function could be accomplished in an existing governmental office, without increasing the bureaucracy by creating a new office. A few of the committee members favored having an external advisory committee, related to the governmental locus, that is charged with identifying issues to be dealt with at a departmental or interdepartmental level, developing mandates, and nominating commissioners.

REFERENCES

Childress, J.A. 1991. Deliberations of the Human Fetal Tissue Transplantation Research Panel. In: *Biomedical Politics*, Institute of Medicine. Washington, D.C.: National Academy Press.

Hanna, K.E., Cook-Deegan, R.M., and Nishimi, R. 1994. Finding a forum for bioethics in public policy. *Politics and the Life Sciences* 12:205–219.

Institute of Medicine. 1989. *Medically Assisted Conception: An Agenda for Research.* Washington, D.C.: National Academy Press.

Institute of Medicine. 1994. *Assessing Genetic Risks: Implications for Health and Social Policy.* Washington, D.C.: National Academy Press.

Jennings, B. 1988. A grassroots movement in bioethics. *Hastings Center Report* 18 (June/July):Supplement S.1–S.16.

King, P. 1991. Commentary (on Human Fetal Tissue Transplantation Research Panel article by J.A. Childress) In: *Biomedical Politics*, Institute of Medicine. Washington, D.C.: National Academy Press.

Kolata, G. 1993. Cloning human embryos: Debate erupts over ethics; some see nightmare, but others hope to begin. *New York Times* (October 26):A1.

National Commission for the Protection of Human Subjects of Biomedical and Behavioral Research. 1978. *The Belmont Report. Ethical Principles and Guidelines for the Protection of Human Subjects in Research.* Washington, D.C.: U.S. Government Printing Office.

Office of Technology Assessment (OTA). 1988. *Infertility: Medical and Social Choices.* Washington, D.C.: U.S. Government Printing Office.

OTA. 1993. *Biomedical Ethics in U.S. Public Policy.* Washington, D.C.: U.S. Government Printing Office.

President's Commission for the Study of Ethical Problems in Medicine and Biomedical and Behavioral Research. 1983. *Deciding to Forego Life-Sustaining Treatment.* Washington, D.C: U.S. Government Printing Office.

Teno, J.M., Sabatino, C., Pariser, L., Rouse, F., and J. Lynn. 1993. The impact of the Patient Self-Determination Act's requirement that states describe law concerning patients' rights. *Journal of Law, Medicine, and Ethics* 21(1):102–108.

Walters, L. 1988. Statement. In: *Human Fetal Tissue Transplantation Research Advisory Committee to the Director.* Bethesda, Maryland.

Wolf, S.M. 1991. Ethics committees and due process. *Maryland Law Review* 50(3):798–858.

Wolf, S.M. 1992. Toward a theory of process. *Law, Medicine, and Health Care* 20:278–290.

PART II
COMMISSIONED PAPERS

The second part of this report presents a series of essays commissioned by the committee on various aspects of the social and ethical dimensions of decision making in biomedicine. Altogether there are 12 essays; they are ordered according to the scope of the issues they address. The first several essays explore broad questions while the later essays are more narrowly focused on a specific aspect of decision making or a particular bioethics effort.

Moral Epistemology

Thomas Nagel provides a definition of moral knowledge, examines mechanisms for acquiring such knowledge, and considers the possibility of arriving at moral knowledge through some kind of intellectually defensible process. He relates these issues to the challenges faced by public ethics bodies in contemporary, pluralistic America as they seek to explain and justify their views to their fellow citizens.

Public Moral Discourse

Dan W. Brock describes some of the features of the nature of public ethics bodies—the different goals they pursue, their typical charge and composition, and the role in public policy that they typically play. He argues that the method by which ethics bodies have tended to address and reason about moral issues is fundamentally similar to the methods of moral philosophy, and explains why the substantive conclusions that public ethics bodies reach by this process are justified.

The Value of Consensus

Martin Benjamin examines the nature, value, and limits of consensus in bioethical deliberation. He describes various types of consensus, as well as notions such as compromise and majority rule, and raises normative and methodological issues to be explored by ethics bodies as they consider what role consensus should play in their deliberations.

Bioethics Commissions: What Can We Learn from Past Successes and Failures?

Bradford H. Gray provides an analysis of the lessons to be learned from the experiences of two earlier ethics commissions—the National Commission and the President's Commission—both of which are generally cited as successes. From a survey of the members and staff of these commissions, he draws conclusions about the senses in which these two commissions were successful and the reasons behind their successes and failures.

Limiting Life-Prolonging Medical Treatment: A Comparative Analysis of the President's Commission and the New York State Task Force

Baruch A. Brody compares the accomplishments of these two ethics bodies, one at a national level and one at a state level, in their different approaches to one issue: limiting life-prolonging medical treatment. He explains why the nature of their successes differed and explores the important connections between the role of an ethics body and the context in which it operates, and the structure and process of that body.

The Formulation of Health Policy by the Three Branches of Government

Lawrence Gostin explores the role of government in formulating health policy. He considers the kinds of health policy questions that different government bodies are best equipped to solve, the data that they need to do so, and the mechanisms for making that data available to decision makers.

The Role of Religious Participation and Religious Belief in Biomedical Decision Making

Charles M. Swezey provides a framework for understanding the complex relationship between religion and bioethical decision making. He identifies significant dimensions of religious belief, sketches the elements of decision making, and traces the interactions between the two to illuminate the impact of religious belief on the practice of modern medicine.

Trust, Honesty, and the Authority of Science

Steven Shapin explores the moral authority of scientists by way of an historical inquiry into their credibility. He describes how the credibility of scientific claims and the moral standing of those who make the claims have been intertwined in the past. He points to the modern disengagement of virtue and expertise—the weakening of trust relationships in science—as problematic to science.

Institutional Ethics Committees: Local Perspectives on Ethical Issues in Medicine

Elizabeth Heitman examines the historical development of institutional ethics committees and describes the roles of these committees in policymaking, education, and consultation on ethical issues in medical care. She provides a comprehensive account of the administrative aspects of institutional ethics committees and identifies issues that these committees will confront in the future, such as cost-containment, liability, and long-term care.

The Ethical, Legal, and Social Implications Program of the National Center for Human Genome Research: A Missed Opportunity?

Kathi E. Hanna provides a comprehensive history and description of the Ethical, Legal, and Social Implications Program of the National Center for Human Genome Research. She explores the program's role in policy debate about genetic technology, analyzes its strengths and weaknesses, and considers strategies for reshaping the program so that it can more effectively achieve its intended goals.

AIDS, Ethics, and Activism: Institutional Encounters in the Epidemic's First Decade

Ronald Bayer examines the role of consultation between ethicists and those at risk of HIV in the confrontation of critical policy questions raised by the HIV epidemic. He explores how the distinctive political context of this consultation—the intensity of the discussion, the political forces called into play, and the demands made and solutions sought by activists—have fostered an unusual series of institutional efforts to engage activists in the process of establishing guidelines for AIDS policy.

"La Pénible Valse Hésitation": Fetal Tissue Research Review and the Use of Bioethics Commissions in France and the United States

R. Alta Charo compares and contrasts the roles and experiences of bioethics commissions in France and the United States, focusing on both countries' efforts in the area of fetal tissue research. She explores the political and historical context for bioethical deliberation in the two countries and points to significant social conditions to which commissions may have to be responsive in order to succeed.

Moral Epistemology

THOMAS NAGEL, Ph.D.
Professor of Philosophy and Law, New York University

If our interest is the public evaluation and control of advances in biomedicine or other technologies, the problem of moral knowledge has to be closely connected with the conditions of political legitimacy. The issue is not just, "What are the grounds and methods of moral thought in general?" but "What methods can be used to justify conclusions that are fit to serve as the basis for public policy and public restraint?" There may be grounds of moral belief which can serve legitimately as a basis for personal conduct, but which it would be inappropriate to rely on in justifying the actions of official bodies, taken in the name of a public which comprises a wide range of conviction.

I shall return to this point later. But for most of this discussion I won't distinguish between the morality of public and of private choice, but will talk about the foundations of moral judgment in general. Because of the essentially public concerns which prompt the discussion, however, I shall leave aside the morality of individual virtue, which may have some bearing on the conduct of particular public officials but has little to do with technology assessment.

Epistemology, or the theory of knowledge, is a function of the subject matter. How to arrive at conclusions, how to justify or criticize them, and the pitfalls along the way, all depend on what kind of thing you are trying to make up your mind about. So the first question to answer is: What is morality about—what kind of thing is a moral belief? What is it, in other words, that moral epistemology must investigate our knowledge of?

The minimal answer has two elements: (1) Moral conclusions are practical, which means that they are about what to do rather than about what is the case (even though they may be based partly on what is the case); (2) they are not merely individual but represent a possible area of interpersonal agreement. The most general concept of morality, shared by those who may differ widely about its substantive content or foundation, refers to standards of individual or collective conduct which permit people to agree in the determination of what ought to be done in a given case or under given circumstances.

There is difference of opinion over how wide the range of possible agreement should be—whether morality should seek answers that permit convergence only among members of a particular community or culture, or among all human beings or even all rational beings (a class which could in principle include nonhumans). But however we answer that question, the main point is that such standards, if they exist, are supposed to give the same result whoever in the moral community is trying to answer the question. If you are trying to decide what to do, and if there is a moral answer to the question of what you ought to do, that answer should be available not just to you but to anyone else informed about your situation. It should be independent of the point of view of the individual making the judgment, and in that sense objective. If such an answer is available, it should permit you to justify your conduct not only to yourself but to others.

So the search for moral knowledge is the search for a basis for objective judgments about what people ought to do—judgments on which they can agree and which allow them to offer justifications to one another for their conduct. Such justifications will have to appeal to something independent of the differences in point of view that ordinarily divide us, and that are generally so important in motivating our actions—something we can rely on in common. What this is, or whether such a thing can be found at all, is the central issue of ethical theory. But most theorists would recognize, as characteristic of morality, the aim of convergence by individuals with diverse and conflicting points of view on standards of conduct and choice which all can see as justified. Morality, if there is such a thing, requires us to transcend in the practical domain our individual perspectives, and by means of this collective transcendence to converge on a common standpoint of evaluation. It aims to supply a framework of potential agreement or harmony within which the remaining differences can operate without doing harm.

There is in this sense a loose analogy between the aims of moral and of factual knowledge: Both are concerned with convergence on results all parties can recognize as correct, and both require transcendence of a purely personal point of view to one that is more shareable and objective. But the convergence sought by moral thought is practical and motivational, whereas the convergence sought by factual and scientific thought is convergence of belief—convergence on a true account of how things are, or a common picture of the world. The pursuit of moral knowledge, therefore, must proceed by the development of our motives and practices, not of our beliefs and descriptions.

Because our personal desires are so individual and conflicts of interest and attitude are often so severe, the question whether moral objectivity is possible is more serious than the comparable question about other fields. Nonevaluative subjects like mathematics, science, and history don't provide models for a conception of moral knowledge: In trying to determine how to live together, we are not talking about abstract timeless structures or about the observable external world. To reach a common standpoint that is practical rather than merely theoretical, as morality requires, we must modify our motives and attitudes by some process of coordination that is suited for the purpose.

The first step, common to many moral theories, is to put yourself in other people's shoes, with sufficient imagination to be fairly sure that you understand their point of view and their preferences, experiences, and interests. An appreciation of the antecedent divergence that creates the conflicts to which morality seeks a solution is essential in pursuing convergence. The other effect of putting yourself in other people's shoes is to induce the sort of impartiality and escape from egocentricity which is needed to reach a common standpoint. Whatever the moral solution, it should have an appeal that is the same for everyone, even if it also impinges unequally on their nonmoral interests.

But to get further, we have to decide what to do with all these points of view, how to generate some kind of unity out of them. And to say any more than this about moral epistemology, we must move to the level of substantive moral argument. The methods of thought in this field, as in others, are revealed in the way one thinks about particular hypotheses. It is no more possible here than elsewhere to specify a pure, content-free method that can be used mechanically to produce results. If we look instead at the disagreements among leading theories of moral justification, and the way in which criticism of general principles can emerge from particular counterinstances or counterarguments, we will get a better picture of the process.

I am going to begin by tracing the disagreements among several representative theories of how this is to be done—theories which have made an enduring contribution to our understanding of moral knowledge, even if none of them captures the whole truth about it. Each of them offers a different account of the basis of convergence, as follows: collective self-interest (Hobbes), natural rights (Locke), general benevolence (Hume), and universalizability (Kant).[1] Though they are associated with classic authors, each of these approaches has its contemporary representatives.

The Hobbesian approach to moral argument is motivationally the simplest. It assumes that the motives which produce conflict, notably self-interest and the desire to survive, must also be relied on to resolve those conflicts, because no other motives of comparable power are available to override them. Hobbes therefore identified the content of morality with those rules of conduct that it would be in everyone's interest for everyone to follow. He also recognized, however, that this by itself was not sufficient to give any individual a self-interested reason to follow those rules himself. (In effect, Hobbes was the first thinker to describe the prisoner's dilemma.) To bring collective self-interest into accord with individual self-interest, thereby making its achievement motivationally possible, it was necessary to change the external circumstances by setting up an enforcer of the moral rules, the sovereign. Only in that way would it become safe for individuals to adhere to the rules that each of them has a reason to want everyone to adhere to. According to Hobbes, the realization of morality, though not its content, depends on political institutions.

However, the important point for our purposes is that Hobbes thought moral discovery did not depend on any modification of human motives. Rather, the convergence on common standards of conduct characteristic of morality was the result of social and psychological theory, on the basis of a single principle of motivation. The problem was, how to create the conditions of convergence and harmony on the basis of the most reliable motive, self-interest. The reasoning to that end was essentially instrumental: An analysis of human interactions and conditions of trust and distrust suggests a method of overcoming the destructive effects of self-interest and fear not by altering human motives, but only by changing the means of their expression. We are not, on this theory, led to accept moral constraints on our conduct by a concern for the good of others.

While Hobbes's recognition of the gap between individual and collective self-interest, and his proposal for closing it, are among the most important insights of moral and political theory, his conception of the motivational basis of ethics seems too narrow. Intuitively, there seems to be some reason to refrain from harming others which derives from *their* interests, and not just from your own.

When Locke tries to express this recognition, he appeals both to the Golden Rule and to the equality of mankind in the sight of God; but the idea can be understood in completely secular terms—indeed in terms of the imaginative step already mentioned, of putting yourself in other people's shoes. The most basic moral argument, 'How would you like it if someone did that to you?" can be given either a Hobbesian or a Lockean interpretation. In the former sense, it is an appeal to self-interest, through an implied reference to general practices and conventions whose imposition would serve everyone's interest, yours included. In the latter sense, it is a direct invitation to imagine the situation from the point of view of the other, in order to induce a recognition that what happens to him matters in itself, and should matter not only to him but to you. Thus it is designed to evoke motives which are in a broad sense altruistic or other-regarding.

This is an example of the sort of appeal to intuition that is as indispensable in moral thinking as appeals to observation are in empirical thinking, and appeals to self-evidence in logical thinking. Moral intuitions are not infallible, but they provide the only data we have to support or discredit general hypotheses. Some moral intuitions can be explained away as illusions or prejudices, but even then the alternative is generally supported by other intuitions, at some level. In the case of Locke, the anti-Hobbesian intuitions are not limited to a general consideration for the interests of others, but take the form of a system of equal natural rights, essentially rights against interference, which are said to constrain us in our dealings with others even in the absence of a legal enforcement system.

This type of conception has been very prominent in subsequent moral and political theory. The idea is that morality requires us to accord everyone an equal status in some sense—the same status we claim for ourselves in their treatment of us—and that this status should be defined as a kind of inviolability. Each of us is protected by a moral boundary which accords us a degree of freedom to act in pursuit of our personal aims without interference by others, provided what we do does not violate the identical boundary protecting anyone else. While there has been much disagreement over what should be included in this category of equal rights, as a form of moral thought it continues to be very much alive.

However, it has also provoked an equally important reaction, the tradition of utilitarianism, stemming from the work of Hume. Rights are supposed by Locke to be natural and morally basic. That is, they are not merely legal or conventional creations which serve an instrumental purpose. This contrasts with Hobbes, who had held that property rights, for example, serve the common interest but are brought into existence only with the creation of the state; Locke believed that property rights were prepolitical. Hume, by contrast with both of them, held that the motivational foundation of morality was a single sentiment of impartial benevolence, or concern for people's well-being, but that it did not express itself directly in the recognition of equal rights. Rather, rights of property, obligations of contract and promise, and other strict moral boundaries are in his view conventions—sometimes legally enforced—which are justified by the contribution of their strict application to the overall or general welfare of persons living under them: justified, in other words, by their utility.

So Hume differs from Hobbes in believing that morality can rely on a motive other than self-interest—a motive of benevolence that arises when we view the lives of all persons, ourselves included, from a detached and sympathetic perspective. But he differs from Locke in believing that this is the only fundamental moral principle, and that all others, specifically the various individual rights, are derived from it. The sole criterion of the correct moral rules, on this view, is whether they promote utility or the general welfare of all persons added together. (Note, this is different from the Hobbesian standard of the *common* interest, or the simultaneous interest of each person taken separately.) This position is known as rule-utilitarianism, and it holds that while some moral assessments of policies and actions depend on their direct contribution to overall utility, many of the most important assessments are indirect—placing an act like respect for property or contract under a rule or convention that serves utility not act by act, but only as a whole.

The controversy between natural rights theory and rule-utilitarianism illustrates an important type of theoretical controversy in ethics. The disputants may agree roughly in their substantive moral judgments of central cases, but they disagree over what is fundamental and what is derivative: They disagree, in other words, about the correct moral *explanation* of those substantive intuitions in which they agree. And this may in turn be connected with disagreements about less obvious substantive questions, which will be decided differently by the extension of different justificatory principles. For example, the answer to the question of how much discretion people should have over the use and disposition of their property will depend significantly on whether property rights are, as Locke thought, an aspect of a natural right to equal liberty, or, as Hume thought, a set of conventions designed to promote security, stable long-term expectations, and the general welfare—in which case their appropriate scope will vary with contingent circumstances.

In its development by Bentham and Mill[2] and later writers utilitarianism became the clearest example of a moral theory based on only a single purely moral intuition, with everything else following from it with the help of nonmoral, factual premises. The moral principle at the top is that the only measure of good is the sum of the welfare of individuals, and the only measure of right is how effectively an act or policy contributes to that good. Determining how we should live, how societies should be organized, and what laws and policies they should adopt is then entirely a matter of instrumental reasoning about what will maximize expected utility (the utility of the possible results combined in proportion to their relative probabilities).

Many moral theorists are drawn to this structural feature of utilitarianism. It seems cleaner and more reliable to depend on a single, simple principle that seems intuitively certain, rather than having to rely on moral intuition over and over again in judging different principles and different choices. With a single principle like the principle of utility, one can derive results using only the data of empirical natural and social science, plus quantitative calculation. The application of morality to life is thus provided with a well-defined *method,* often called cost–benefit analysis, and the only remaining uncertainties or vaguenesses are factual. Most of moral epistemology becomes factual epistemology.

However, this outlook attracts strong resistance from those who believe that moral thought is far more complex and autonomous, and that the structure of values and moral requirements is normative throughout, rather than just consisting of the deductive and empirical consequences of a single normative premise. According to this alternative view, morality is general in the sense that its reasons treat like cases alike, and morally relevant differences must be found to justify treating different cases differently—but this generality cannot be captured in a single, simple principle.

Probably the most important representative of this position is Kant, in spite of his claim to be able to derive all of morality from a single principle, the Categorical Imperative. What makes the Categorical Imperative logically different from the principle of utility is that it cannot be applied without substantive evaluative judgment all along the way to the conclusion, whereas the principle of utility requires only factual and mathematical judgment for its application. Kant formulates the Categorical Imperative in more than one way, but the most famous version is the principle of universalizability—that one should govern one's own conduct only on principles that one could will to be universal laws applying to everyone. The derivation of particular moral conclusions from this formula is anything but straightforward, and the words "could will" conceal a demand for further normative judgment.

In contemporary theory, this approach is usually identified with a contractarian method of resolving the conflicting interests and values of different individuals. The method has something in common with traditional social contract theory, but it attempts to place the different points of view to be combined on a footing of greater equality, by making the contract a hypothetical rather than an actual one, to avoid the influence on its outcome of differences in power or threat advantage. What equally situated individuals *would* agree to or converge on as a common standard is offered as a justification for accepting it as morally correct.[3] But here again, the process of justification seems normative "all the way down."

This raises a particularly vexed issue in moral theory: whether the reliance on evaluative or normative judgment in deriving particular moral conclusions from general moral principles makes the whole process circular and the system empty. Rawls, who is a contemporary representative of the Kantian tradition, has defended the method of moral complexity under the heading of "reflective equilibrium."[4] We suppose that our moral sense is the imperfect apprehension of a complex structure of principles and justificatory reasons, and we try to refine our understanding of this structure by exercising moral intuition both at the level of plausible general principles and at the level of particular substantive judgments of action or policy. We proceed by trying through mutual adjustment to produce the best fit between persuasive principles, plausible specific consequences that follow from them, and general theoretical accounts of the overall structure and motivational foundation of moral constraints. The reasoning is moral at every point, but the partial independence of the points creates a kind of check, and the possibility of confirmation, disconfirmation, and revision.

Apart from method, the opposition between the Kantian and utilitarian traditions is also one over the right way to count everyone equally in moral thought. Utilitarians count everyone equally by counting everyone's welfare impartially as a contribution to the total, whose maximization then serves as the criterion for all other moral requirements. According to utilitarianism, therefore, all other forms of equality (of rights, opportunities, status, or resources) are morally favored only if they serve as instrumental means to the maximization of that total.

According to the Kantian tradition (which in this respect has something in common with Locke), there are independent values of equality, not derivative from the maximization of utility, which in fact limit the way it is permissible to treat people even in order to advance the general welfare. Certain rights to equal treatment, equal liberty, equal inviolability, and equal opportunity are not, in other words, merely instrumental to the promotion of the good, but are morally basic. This is a very deep disagreement about the form of equal regard for everyone that underlies morality. The issue is whether certain minimal protections for each individual have a privileged position which cannot be overridden by a greater aggregate balance of benefits to numbers of other individuals. There is no reason a priori to think that counting people's interests equally as input to the total is the only adequate form of moral respect. Obviously the issue is not going to be easy to resolve. It can be understood in broader perspective as the opposition between two conceptions or models of impartiality: the model of collective sympathy and the model of individual identification.

If one wishes to give substance to the idea of impartial respect for everyone, which is the essence of an ethical system, two psychological models offer themselves. The first is that of an impartial sympathetic spectator, who cares equally about the happiness and unhappiness, fulfillment and frustration, of all persons. The solution to a typical moral problem in which individual interests conflict would then be the one this spectator would be motivated to choose by his sympathy for all the affected parties. Such a method of decision tends toward maximizing the total balance of happiness over unhappiness; so the sympathetic spectator model has a natural association with utilitarianism, which accords to everyone equal status as a potential contributor to that total—but not equality in the outcome, as such.

The second psychological model of impartiality does not employ a spectator at all, but imagines someone who instead of remaining outside, *identifies* himself with each of the persons whose conflicts give rise to the moral problem—as if each person's interests and attitudes were his own, but separately. This model of simultaneous multiple identification is much harder to imagine,[5] but the point of the method is to discourage the kind of blending together of everyone's happiness and unhappiness that is encouraged by the sympathetic spectator model. If one identifies separately with each individual, those interests cannot be so easily combined.

This is an attempt to build the distinction between different persons more deeply into the interpretation of impartiality from the start. It calls for an alternative method of dealing with conflicts of interest and of combining advantages and disadvantages to yield a solution. The method suggested by this model, as an alternative to maximizing the aggregate total welfare, is that of a system of *priorities*. To express one's identification with each individual, one tries to identify an order of priority among needs, interests, benefits, and harms, and meets higher priority needs before less urgent ones in case of conflict—even if more people would receive the lower priority benefit. This different method of according people equal respect requires us to focus on urgent matters of survival and basic capacities for a minimally decent life before going on to the provision of benefits higher on the scale of well-being. That will mean resisting the method of aggregation which allows the accumulated weight of sheer numbers of better-off people to override the more urgent needs of a minority. (An example would be the costly provision of education, assistance, and access to the handicapped, which is hard to justify in utilitarian terms.) Similar reasoning may assign priority to the protection of certain basic individual rights, whose violation can't then be justified by appeals to the general welfare.

The present state of moral controversy reveals a high level of uncertainty about both methods and conclusions, but at the same time there is clearly a lot of value in the three primary standards I have described: common interest, overall utility, and equal rights. On some questions these standards will give the same answer: All of them justify the most obvious rules against killing, assault, coercion, theft, and breach of promise, and all of them are plausible justifications for the evaluation of policies, even if none of them can be the whole truth. It is also important that all of them try to count everyone the same, in the evaluation of policies and measures, even though the way interests are counted and combined is different from one method to the other.

For an individual or a group wishing to justify policy in the public forum, it would be a mistake to think there was some standpoint of pure moral epistemology, above the level of moral disagreement, from which that can be done. One cannot, in other words, move to a domain outside of moral controversy to find objective grounds for settling it. However general the principles one appeals to, the arguments must be substantive, for that is where the problems arise and where their solutions have to be found. In this respect morality is no different from anything else. There is no abstract rule for discovering the right answer to every historical, medical, or economic question either: If there are objective justifications in those fields, they show themselves at the level of substantive argument, where alternatives are proposed and evidence is evaluated.

I have described some methods of moral thought which to one degree or another carry conviction, but those engaged in a task like technology assessment have to actually employ such arguments, and make first-order judgments as to their relative cogency when they yield conflicting results. In the exercise of public responsibility, those judgments cannot be merely personal, but must attempt to express a moral outlook that the public in whose name the decision is being taken can reasonably be expected to adopt, in light of the reasons offered. This doesn't mean that the acceptable justifications have to be discovered by surveys of antecedent moral opinion, since carefully reasoned decisions about public questions should attempt to supply the grounds for their own acceptance. But it does mean that new decisions should aim to cohere with a publicly available moral understanding, and to form part of its natural evolution. In this respect the task has something in common with that of a court deciding a difficult and morally loaded case.

It is not easy to identify a public moral philosophy for the United States, since we are such a pluralistic society. However, I think it is safe to say that the quasi-consensus is not Hobbesian, and not utilitarian either. Rather it is a qualified priority view, in which (1) the guarantee to everyone of certain individual rights against interference (justified partly but not entirely on rule-utilitarian grounds) limits the methods that can be used to pursue the general welfare; (2) there is also a prioritized understanding of welfare itself, with (3) greatest importance being assigned, from the point of view of public policy, to things that are in everyone's interest, like defense, security, and the environment (a Hobbesian element), and (4) also increasingly to the most basic or urgent human needs; (5) above that level a utilitarian standard is supposed to be roughly approximated by the balancing of interests in democratic politics, though of course the system doesn't often work as it should. But the identification of standards and arguments has to be carried out, in good faith, by those who make decisions and offer reasons for them. It is only by actual argument that we can find objective standards, whether we are talking about ethics, biology, or anything else.

In dealing with controversial cases, there is no substitute for the familiar process of formulating general hypotheses and testing them by the credibility of their implications in other cases where intuitions may be clearer. If two people disagree about the right thing to do in a particular situation, they should be able to find reasons for their different opinions, and those reasons will reveal principles which in turn imply other decisions in other cases, permitting the justifications to be compared. Of course the whole system of justification is quite involved, and various principles may interact, but progress can often be made on this basis—at least to produce greater understanding of the grounds of disagreement, if not to resolve it finally.

Even if morality is ultimately to be based on a single axiom like the principle of utility, the defense of that claim must involve more than an appeal to the self-evidence of the principle: It must be shown by detailed argument and consideration of actual and hypothetical cases to provide the best way of justifying the moral conclusions that, on reflection, prove most convincing. This doesn't mean a moral theory has to preserve the intuitions we start out with, only that if it does not, it must genuinely persuade us of something else. That is not a matter merely of drawing logical consequences from a formula, but of changing our values and motives.

As regards the motivational and attitudinal developments involved in moral thought, there are two ways of interpreting the process, as we have already seen. According to the conception common to Hobbes and the utilitarians, the basic motive stays the same—self-interest or benevolence— and the details of morality are developed by attaching that motive to different policies, institutions, and courses of action, on the basis of information about what will actually promote either the common interest or the aggregate general welfare. According to the other conception, characteristic of the modern Kantian tradition, moral thought involves the development of more complex, morally influenced motives, as our sense of what is and is not a sufficient reason for action is altered by changing conceptions of equity, fairness, responsibility, cruelty, desert, and so forth.

On either conception, the aim of moral thought is to discover justifications which can produce convergence in what people find acceptable in one another's conduct. Often it will involve breaking a fairly wide existing consensus on the way to finding a new, firmer foundation for agreement. The aim of convergence has nothing essentially conservative about it. Accepted orthodoxies cannot so easily be overthrown in ethics, as in science, by the discovery of new empirical evidence, but they can be overthrown by new arguments and new appeals to the moral imagination—as has happened conspicuously in the recognition of traditional social inequalities as morally arbitrary.

Let me close by commenting on two related issues, the question of expertise and the place of moral considerations in political decision.

The first issue naturally arises in connection with anything like technology assessment, because scientific expertise is indispensable with regard to the facts, the risks, and probabilities, and often there is no way of making the full grounds of such expert judgments generally accessible. Only someone with years of training and experience can evaluate them, and others, including politicians and most of the affected public, just have to try to find grounds for deciding whom to believe. Even where specialists disagree about the likely effects of an advance, those charged with public decisions can't really expect to arrive at an independent view of their own.

By contrast, there is much less room for expertise with regard to the moral and evaluative aspects of policy. Moral judgments are everyone's job, and while some people are better at them than others, the reasons behind them ought to be made available, for the purposes of public choice, in a way that those responsible, and eventually the public at large, can find directly persuasive. Moral grounds for public decisions, unlike scientific grounds, should be at least potentially part of public rather than expert knowledge. As I said earlier, this doesn't mean that they have to be familiar in advance; but if they break new ground, they should nevertheless aspire to offer reasons which can command assent not only from specialists—even if those who spend more of their time thinking about these things may be better able to come up with plausible proposals. Morality's ambition is, or at least ought to be, to provide a system of conduct under which everyone can live, with a sense of mutual justifiability. This follows from the conditions of political legitimacy: We do not live in a theocracy, where some people are thought to have a privileged and direct line to the moral truth.

That brings me to the second issue, which was also mentioned at the start of our discussion: the modification of moral argument for political purposes. In a democracy, the aim of procedures of decision should be to secure results that can be acknowledged as legitimate by as wide a portion of the citizenry as possible. Even those who personally disagree with a result, or whose interests are harmed by it, should ideally be able to recognize as legitimate the methods by which their preferences and opinions were overruled by others. This means that in a democratic polity, there may have to be some restriction on the types of moral grounds on which it is legitimate to base policy decisions. Those that are too particular to be generally authorized may have to give way to more public grounds.

Our society is not only democratic but richly pluralistic. Many different religions and systems of ultimate value coexist here, and it is important to their coexistence that they be able to find terms for living side by side, and dealing with potential conflicts, that do not require them to convert one another. The cost of conflict resolution and cooperation cannot be the total elimination of disagreement. It may therefore often turn out that principles of conduct that serve as moral justifications within a community of belief or practice are not suited to serve that role for political or policy decisions made in the name of the society as a whole. This is conspicuously true of moral requirements rooted in a specific religious faith, but it may also apply more widely.

It can affect not only the rules of conduct one accepts, but also the correct measure of individual well-being for the purpose of calculating benefit, harm, and overall utility. For example, the fact that someone cares more about spending money on a religious pilgrimage than on basic medical care may provide a good reason for that person to decide how to use his own resources, but it is a poor reason for a program of public assistance to support his religious rather than his medical expenditures—because the value of medical treatment can command public recognition and the religious claim cannot. While someone's preferences are ordinarily a good basis for deciding what is better or worse for him, a less individual standard of value may be needed for purposes of public justification.[6] The pluralism of our culture requires that public choices be made on a leaner and more universalistic basis than private ones.

The extent to which universality is itself a necessary aim of moral theory is a matter of controversy. There are those who believe that the ambition of traditional theories to search for the correct principles for persons as such is misplaced—even if that is not an inappropriate aim for mathematics and science. I am not sympathetic with this view, but even if one thinks that morality is by its nature more local than logical or factual thought, the ambition of universality at least within the community concerned with the decisions—the community in whose name they are taken, if not all those affected—follows from the function of moral argument in supporting convergence and mutually acceptable standards of justification.

To go beyond this would involve deeper epistemological questions which cannot be adequately treated in a discussion of this sort. I would say only that although the aim of moral thought is to provide a basis for agreement, the bare empirical appeal to community consensus where it exists is never in itself a moral argument. It can serve only as the starting point for the examination, and criticism or endorsement, of the reasons underlying that consensus.

NOTES

1. Thomas Hobbes, *Leviathan* (1651); John Locke, *Second Treatise of Government* (1690); David Hume, *Enquiry Concerning the Principles of Morals* (1751); Immanuel Kant, *Foundations of the Metaphysics of Morals* (1785).

2. Jeremy Bentham, *An Introduction to the Principles of Morals and Legislation* (1788); John Stuart Mill, *Utilitarianism* (1863).

3. See John Rawls, *A Theory of Justice* (Harvard University Press, 1971); T. M. Scanlon, "Contractualism and Utilitarianism," in Amartya Sen and Bernard Williams, eds., *Utilitarianism and Beyond* (Cambridge University Press, 1982).

4. Rawls, op. cit.

5. Something corresponding to it has been proposed by Rawls in his hypothetical social contract model called the Original Position.

6. See T. M. Scanlon, "Preference and Urgency," *Journal of Philosophy*, Vol. 72, 1975.

Public Moral Discourse

DAN W. BROCK

Professor of Philosophy and Biomedical Ethics, Brown University

What is the nature of public moral discourse as it is done by ethics commissions charged with addressing ethical or moral issues in medicine and biomedical science and technology?[1] In what ways does it differ from the methods of moral philosophy and moral philosophers when they address such issues? Can public ethics commissions provide reasoned solutions to these ethical issues, and if so how? I shall first discuss some features of the nature of ethics commissions—the different goals they pursue, their typical charge and composition, and the role in public policy which they typically play. These features distinguish the processes they employ in some respects from moral reasoning as it is done by either moral philosophers or ordinary citizens. But I shall argue that these differences are relatively superficial and that how ethics commissions address and reason about moral issues is not fundamentally different from the method, when it is properly understood, of moral philosophy in addressing substantive moral issues of practice and policy. I shall show as well the respects in which this method can provide solutions to moral issues in public policy, or more specifically the respects in which an ethics commission's process of public moral reasoning warrants the claim that the substantive conclusions reached by that process are justified.

SOME FEATURES OF PUBLIC MORAL DISCOURSE
AS DONE BY ETHICS COMMISSIONS

Goals of Ethics Commissions

What are some of the different goals or aims that public ethics commissions typically have? First, they often are charged with developing relatively discrete legislation to deal with a particular ethical issue. For example, the President's Commission for the Study of Ethical Problems in Medicine and Biomedical and Behavioral Research (hereafter President's Commission) addressed in its first study the definition of death and developed a proposal for a uniform statutory definition, which has subsequently been adopted by nearly all states. Even with this relatively narrowly focused outcome, the President's Commission evaluated alternative definitions of death, for example, the "whole brain" account, which it supported, and the "higher brain" account, which it rejected, and offered philosophical and policy arguments in support of its choice of the whole brain formulation.

Second, ethics commissions are sometimes charged with addressing specific unethical practices and recommending governmental responses to correct those practices. For example, the National Commission for the Protection of Human Subjects of Biomedical and Behavioral Research (hereafter National Commission) was established in large part as a response to a number of well-publicized examples of abuses of human subjects in research and to an influential article detailing such abuses.[2] A central component of the National Commission's recommendations was the establishment of Institutional Review Boards whose task is to assure that human subjects are properly protected. The National Commission also developed detailed guidelines and recommendations governing the use of specific populations in research. Here, too the National Commission offered arguments in defense of its recommendations, and indeed in its *Belmont Report* developed the general moral principles on which its recommendations rested.

Third, an ethics commission may seek to have a broad and diverse influence on policy and practice with regard to a particular moral issue. For example, the President's Commission in its report, *Deciding to Forego Life-Sustaining Treatment,*[3] sought a multifaceted impact on such practices and policies as institutional, especially hospital, policies that guide practice within particular health care institutions; court decisions that set the legal framework of permissible practice; and the beliefs and practices of physicians and other health care professionals. A part of the influence of the President's Commission's work on this issue derived from its prestigious nature as a nationally constituted body, as has no doubt been true of other ethics commissions. But the influence of its recommendations also derived importantly from the force and persuasiveness of the moral reasoning the commission offered for its conclusions and recommendations.

Finally, an ethics commission may sometimes have aims rather less focused on public policy. It may see its role more as influencing ongoing public debates on specific moral issues. In doing so, it may seek to have quite different kinds of influence on different occasions, for example, on the one hand sharpening the issues in dispute or on the other hand seeking to forge a consensus on those issues. These roles too, of course—whether sharpening the issues or forging consensus—require providing the ethical analysis and arguments which either sharpen the issues or on which a new consensus might rest.

Consensus building, broadly understood, is an important part of each of these four different aims of ethics commissions. In part, this is simply because in a democratic society public policy is forged in political processes requiring majority, or at least broad, support of a proposed policy. However, there are deeper reasons why consensus is seen as especially important in the work of an ethics commission. For many public policy issues, that a majority of policymakers, reflecting a majority of citizens support a particular policy position, is reason enough to warrant its adoption (for example, decisions to expend public resources on particular projects like public parks or medical research). It is not that supporters and opponents will have no reasons for their respective positions on such issues, which of course they will, but that we consider it appropriate to settle the disagreement by some form of majority rule decision process; within limits, the position that should be adopted is what the majority supports. On a moral question, however, it would be at the least odd or problematic for a commission to declare that it found by a vote of 6 to 5 that, for example, patients have a moral right to forego life-sustaining treatment. Many political questions and legal disputes may be reasonably decided by majority decision procedures, whether in legislatures or courts, but whether a public policy is moral or just is not settled by counting votes. In some sense, the moral question can only be settled by the quality of the arguments that can be offered for different positions on it. There are no authoritative bodies to settle moral questions and disputes such as exist in politics and the law for settling political and legal disputes. It is in part for this reason that the development of moral arguments and positions is common to all the diverse goals of ethics commissions noted above. The nature of the argumentation that commissions should employ is therefore at the heart of understanding their work.

Typical Scope of Ethics Commissions' Concern

Ethics commissions are typically charged with addressing the social, ethical, and legal issues concerning a particular topic like genetic screening or informed consent. To the extent that moral philosophy addresses only the moral or ethical issues, the scope, and perhaps in turn the methods, of ethics commissions' work will have apparently to be different from moral philosophy. However, I believe it is a mistake to see this typical charge to ethics commissions as instructing them to go beyond the moral or ethical issues and to take up independent social and legal issues as well. Instead, this charge is usually best understood as instructing the commission to address the moral issues of public policy in their broader social and legal context, rather than to engage in social and legal analysis independent of the moral issues. This typical charge reflects as well a widespread confusion as to just what the domain of the moral or ethical is in the context of public policy, a confusion which has contributed in turn to two views—both of them, I believe, mistaken—which assign a more restricted scope to ethics commissions' proper concerns. The first view understands ethical analysis to be addressed to individual actions, whereas policy analysis applies to many cases and institutional practices, and so must in some way extend beyond ethical analysis. The second view understands moral considerations, as well as the method of moral reasoning employing those considerations, to be only a part of the overall considerations relevant to evaluation of public policy. In this latter view, moral philosophers and the methods of moral philosophy may analyze the morality of some policy, but overall policy analysis and evaluation must take into account additional nonmoral considerations such as economic costs, political feasibility, legal constraints, and so forth. Consequently, the distinctly moral or ethical analysis of an ethics commission would not yield "all things considered" judgments or recommendations about public policy. To do that the ethics commission would have to consider these additional nonmoral economic, political, and legal considerations as well, which it has no special expertise to do. On the other hand, if these nonmoral economic, political, and legal considerations are part of the proper province of ethics commissions and ethical analysis, then it seems all policy analysis has been collapsed into ethical analysis, an unwarranted ethical aggrandizement of the policy field. I shall address each of these related, but, I believe, mistaken, views in turn.

In the first view, ethical analyses and judgments apply only to particular cases, not the general practices that are the province of public policy. This view is sometimes expressed by a distinction between when one is "doing ethics" and when one is "doing policy." This putative ethics-policy distinction rests on what can be called the one-many assumption about the relation of ethics to policy. Policy evaluation, in this view, is not ethics because it must address policies that apply to many cases. In the evaluation of what action is ethically justified or permissible in a particular case, it is natural to believe that only the particulars of that case are relevant, though those particulars will include the social context in which the case takes place, the social and professional roles of the different involved parties, the causal impact of what is done in that case on what will be done in future cases, and so forth. For example, if the case concerns a dying patient suffering from pain that has proved impossible to relieve adequately and who requests euthanasia from her physician, it would appear that it is only the particulars of this case which are morally relevant to its moral evaluation. Different people will disagree about which features of the case are morally significant or important, and about what moral principles or reasons bear on it. For example, some people might hold that euthanasia would be morally wrong in this case because it would be the deliberate killing of an innocent person, which they believe is always morally impermissible; others might see it as morally permissible because it is an exercise of an individual's moral right to self-determination. Still others of more consequentialist or utilitarian leanings may evaluate the act by its impact on the well-being of all affected by the action. If doing it would make the physician more likely to perform euthanasia in other similar cases as well, then that too is a consequence of this particular action. But these are all differences about how the act in question should be morally evaluated.

The moral evaluation of a social or legal policy, for example, permitting euthanasia, is, of course, not unrelated to the moral evaluation of particular instances of euthanasia.[4] But a person's moral position about such a policy need not follow directly from his or her moral position about a particular case. Many people who grant that there are individual cases in which euthanasia would be morally justified nevertheless oppose a public or legal policy permitting it because of worries about how that policy might or would be abused, leading to other wrongful performance of euthanasia. Because the policy must apply over time, in many circumstances and to many persons, the policy's effect in these other cases is relevant to its moral evaluation as well. Many of the differences in the substantive moral principles and reasons different people applied to the individual case will resurface in the moral evaluation of policy as well. But both evaluations—of the particular case and of the general policy—can be equally and fully moral evaluations to which one's moral principles and reasons apply. The typical object of moral evaluation by ethics commissions, namely one or another public policy, does not entail a fundamental difference in the moral principles or reasons used in making the evaluation, or in the methodology of moral reasoning and argument employed.

There is reason then to remind ethics commissions to attend to the broader social and legal context of the ethical issues they address. The general practices which are the proper province of concern of ethics commissions exist in a social context, often in diverse social contexts involving individuals with diverse motivations and knowledge. These actions and practices are also often regulated by law. Although the law is only one form of influence on and regulation of practice, public policy, as opposed to forms of private regulation of behavior and practice, is often distinguished by the presence of legal or quasi-legal oversight. Because ethics commissions typically address policy and general practices, not individual actions, various empirical questions regarding practice are relevant to their deliberations: What is the nature of current practice in the area under consideration? What are the possible means of policy and institutional change? What are the means of enforcement of specific policies? What would be the economic and other costs of different policy alternatives? The answers are relevant and integral to an ethical analysis of the policy issue.

This ethical analysis must also address questions like the following: What ethical principles and values bear on the ethical evaluation of current practice in the areas of behavior in question? What would be ethically more desirable practice in the areas of behavior in question? What means are available to shift practice in those desirable ways? Thus, the consideration of economic costs, political feasibility, legal constraints, potentials for abuse, and so forth, all bear on and must be considered as part of the ethical case for a particular policy. But this brings us directly up against the second mistaken view noted above about the proper scope of ethics commissions' concern. That view rejects a conception of ethical analysis which encompasses these economic, political, and legal considerations, and restricts the ethical analysis only to the distinctly ethical considerations. It follows from this that the ethical recommendation on policy in a particular area cannot be an "all things considered" recommendation regarding the policy, what John Rawls claimed for justice in characterizing it as the "final court of appeal" in practical reasoning.[5] Instead, in this second view of the restricted scope of ethics commissions' concern, the ethical analysis takes account of only some considerations relevant to what policy should be. This implies that when the ethical analysis is completed, additional relevant considerations will remain that have not yet been taken into account, but which must be, before drawing a conclusion about what, all things considered, practice and policy ought to be. Why is this view mistaken?

It is certainly correct that moral philosophers are not experts on the economic, political, and legal considerations about which economists, politicians, lawyers, and social scientists are typically consulted. Consequently, an ethics commission will still have to consult with these experts when economic, political, and legal considerations form a significant part of its policy analysis and recommendations. But why should an ethics commission be burdened with these additional concerns which apparently go beyond its ethical expertise? In part, because ethics commissions are asked to make public policy recommendations, "all things considered" recommendations about what policy should be, not just restricted recommendations about what would be ethical in some restricted sense. To fulfill this role, they cannot restrict themselves only to the considerations that most people would intuitively identify as ethical. But this common intuitive distinction between ethical and nonethical considerations is itself misleading. Perhaps a very simple example will most clearly make the point. If you promise to meet a friend tomorrow at 3:00 p.m., that promise gives you a moral reason to do so. But then tomorrow, quite unpredictably, it turns out that you must finish some project or take some action to avoid a very substantial financial loss. Doing so will prevent you from meeting your friend whom you cannot now reach. Ought you morally to keep your promise at very substantial and unexpected financial cost to yourself? If we apply the intuitive distinction assumed above between ethical and economic considerations, then the promise is ethical and the financial cost is economic. Could the ethical analysis concern only the ethical consideration—the promise? It should be clear that this would make no sense. The moral question just is the "all things considered" question of whether you must keep the promise in the face of the very substantial unexpected financial cost to you of doing so. The moral analysis must weigh these two considerations against each other; it cannot consider only the ethical consideration of keeping promises. The same is true of policy analysis. It is not that the common intuitive distinction between moral considerations, such as promise-keeping, and nonmoral considerations, such as financial costs, is mistaken. The mistake is in thinking that moral judgments can avoid weighing the two when they come into conflict; when that occurs, the financial cost becomes a morally relevant consideration in the moral judgment about whether the promise ought to be kept. The same will be true of moral judgments about the public policies that ethics commissions address; for example, apparently nonmoral considerations (financial costs) are morally relevant to the moral question of how much equality of opportunity (the moral consideration) requires society to do to improve opportunities for the handicapped. Does this account make "all things considered" policy evaluations and recommendations ethical, and so result in unwarranted aggrandizement of the policy realm by ethics or morality? And why are only some policy questions then seen as ethical and given to an ethics commission? My view here does not lead to ethics swallowing up policy. Many policy choices remain essentially nonethical because ethical considerations are not significantly affected by them and so are not relevant to them. For example, on the policy questions of what rate of growth of the money supply and what economic stimulus packages are compatible with holding inflation to a three percent level, the economic analysis is appropriately sought from bodies such as the Federal Reserve and the Council of Economic Advisors, not an ethics commission. (This is not to deny, of course, that there are ethical implications of policies to control inflation, but that is a different policy question.) If there is no neat and clear division of labor for ethical and nonethical considerations, which policy questions should go to an ethics commission for analysis and which should go elsewhere? Very roughly, policy questions are appropriately referred to an ethics commission when the considerations commonly and intuitively considered ethical have a significant role or impact in the policy question. But the ethics commission cannot then do its job of analysis and recommendation without weighing those considerations quite appropriately considered ethical against other considerations with which they come into conflict, but which are intuitively seen as nonethical.

Membership of Ethics Commissions

The principal ethics commissions in the United States in recent decades were deliberately established with widely diverse members. Typically, only a small minority of members are professional ethicists or moral philosophers with extensive professional training in ethics and moral philosophy. But this does not mean that what an ethics commission does when it addresses moral issues, nor how it does so, is different in kind or method from how professional ethicists would or do address the same issues. Professional ethicists and other commissioners will be engaged together in ethical reasoning on the issue at hand. Ethical reasoning and argument is done in the ordinary circumstances of everyday life by ordinary persons without academic or scholarly training in moral philosophy. It is not an esoteric subject like cell biology or quantum mechanics, accessible only to experts. Ordinary people make ethical judgments when they morally evaluate different states of affairs, different individuals' actions and character, and different social and political institutions. We employ such judgments in morally justifying our own actions to ourselves and to others, as well as in moral evaluations of the actions of other people.

Professional ethicists and moral philosophers, who are typically at least represented among commissioners and staff members on ethics commissions, do bring a certain expertise to the work of ethics commissions—typically, at least the results of having studied ethical reasoning and alternative ethical theories in a full-time, formal, and rigorous manner. They should be trained in the careful, critical evaluation of the soundness of arguments. They should have systematically studied and evaluated arguments for and against different moral theories, principles, reasons, and positions. Nevertheless, the methods by which professional ethicists or moral philosophers address substantive moral issues do not differ in kind from the methods used to address those issues by ordinary persons unschooled in the formal study of moral philosophy. Ethics commissions typically have diverse membership in order to ensure diverse experience, training, and viewpoints required by the diversity of considerations noted above that bear on their overall recommendations, not to represent diverse approaches or methods of doing ethics. I will have more to say about the role of this diversity below.

METHODS OF MORAL REASONING—IN MORAL PHILOSOPHY AND IN ETHICS COMMISSIONS

One reason some believe that moral reasoning as done in moral philosophy is different from public moral reasoning as done by ethics commissions is what I consider a mistaken view about the nature of moral reasoning in moral philosophy or in public ethics commissions, or in both. Understanding the respects in which these accounts are mistaken or confused will help clarify the appropriate common method which both moral philosophy and public moral reasoning can and do employ.

Deductivism

Some believe the method of reasoning by which public ethics commissions address ethical issues in public policy is different from the method of moral reasoning in moral philosophy from a mistaken view about the latter. In this view, which I shall call deductivism, the philosophical approach to moral reasoning in applied and policy contexts ideally consists in employing the true or correct moral theory and principles, together with the empirical facts relevant to their application, to deduce logically the correct moral conclusion for the case or policy in question. When the issue is not what it is morally correct to do in a particular case, but instead what public policy should be on an ethical question like whether voluntary euthanasia should be permitted, the moral calculus will be more complex. Assume for the sake of illustration that the correct moral theory is some form of consequentialism or utilitarianism, according to which an action is morally right just in case it has at least as good consequences for human well-being as any alternative action open to an agent. When the moral issue is about the evaluation of a public policy, the calculation is much more complex since it is then necessary to estimate the effects over time of alternative policies on the well-being of all who would be affected by the alternative policies. In the case of voluntary euthanasia, the possible effects to take account of would include positive effects like the relief of suffering and giving people control over the circumstances of their dying, together with negative effects like possible abuse of the policy for purposes of controlling costs or possible erosion of trust in the medical profession. The empirical determination of the consequences would be difficult, complex, and controversial, and there would be much ineliminable uncertainty. But deductivism provides a method of moral reasoning that at least in principle yields right answers to the moral problems of policy that ethics commissions face.

Once the likely effects on the well-being of the various affected parties are determined, the consequentialist moral principle can be used straightforwardly and deductively to determine which alternative policy is morally right or justified. The truth or correctness of the consequentialist theory would solve the problem of justifying the commission's policy recommendations by transferring its truth to the conclusion that whichever alternative policy will best promote well-being is morally right or correct. Nothing about the general method of deductivism depends, of course, on the correct theory being consequentialism. If instead the correct moral principle, is that the intentional killing of an innocent person is always wrong, that principle, together with the premise that euthanasia is the intentional killing of an innocent person, deductively yields the conclusion that euthanasia is morally wrong.

Is deductivism a feasible and defensible account of how moral reasoning is and should be done either in policy contexts or in moral philosophy? One obvious problem is that it does not seem an accurate account of how ethics commissions in fact function. Most people, including most members of such commissions, have no relatively comprehensive, or even more limited, moral theory that they know, or even believe, to be true or correct, and so it is hardly a surprise that we do not find them using and applying one in practical contexts. Most people are largely ignorant of philosophical work in developing general moral theories and principles, and yet they nevertheless do reason and have moral views about concrete moral issues like euthanasia. So deductivism is certainly not an accurate description of the moral reasoning that real people typically do in applied or policy contexts. Defenders of deductivism might, nevertheless, respond that it is the method used in moral philosophy and is how people ought to do moral reasoning. Is deductivism a defensible account of moral reasoning?

The central difficulty with deductivism is that there is no single comprehensive moral theory, nor even theories or principles of more limited scope, which is agreed to be true or correct and so could be deductively applied to policy issues. For example, even if there were agreement that the overall effects on human well-being of permitting voluntary euthanasia would be positive, some people nevertheless would still believe that because euthanasia is the deliberate killing of an innocent person, it is morally wrong and should not be permitted. What began as a specific disagreement about what public policy should be about euthanasia has shifted to a more fundamental disagreement about whether consequentialism is the correct or true moral theory, or whether instead duties to protect innocent

human life are paramount. Those who disagree on the policy will frequently do so because they do not agree about which moral principles or
theories are correct. Consequently, so long as the different moral principles and theories are being correctly applied, moral disagreement about
a particular policy will be reproduced in disagreement about the correct
general broader principles or theory. So if moral reasoning should begin
with the correct general moral theory and its principles, which are then
deductively applied to the particular policy in question, we face the embarrassment of having no agreement about what are the correct theory and
principles to employ. To make matters worse, if a moral theory or moral
principles can be true or false, correct or mistaken, as deductivism requires, then even were there agreement about which principles and theory
are true or correct, this would be compatible with all parties to that agreement being mistaken.

The existence of disagreement about which general moral principles
and theory are true or correct would not be an insuperable barrier to
deductivism if there were agreement about the criteria for determining
which principles and theory are true or correct. Disagreement about which
principles and theory are correct then might only reflect a mistaken application of those criteria by one party to the disagreement. I will not canvass
here the different views on this issue, but will only note that there is no
agreement in philosophical ethics, or in ordinary morality, about the criteria which would establish general moral principles or a general moral
theory to be true or correct. A final important barrier to deductivism is
that, even if there are basic moral truths, there is no agreement or assurance that they are to be found or established at the level of general moral
principles or theories, which through application could then transfer their
truth to conclusions about particular policies which ethics commissions
address.

Deductivism as a method of moral reasoning takes a position on how
the justification of moral judgments is secured that is commonly called
foundationalist. A foundationalist account of justification in moral reasoning requires that some moral beliefs, which might be at any level of generality—the most general moral principles (like the consequentialist principle), very specific judgments about concrete cases, or moral beliefs at any
level of generality in between—can be established to be true or correct.[6]
These foundational moral truths, as we might call them, have foundational
status in moral reasoning in the sense that all other moral judgments gain
their justification by being derived through sound reasoning from them.
Foundationalism assigns privileged epistemic status regarding truth or correctness to some moral beliefs—foundational status—with the justification
of all other moral beliefs coming from their being deductively derived
from the foundational beliefs.

Deductivism is the particular version of foundationalism which assigns this foundational status to general moral principles or to a general moral theory. Deductivism fails as an account of moral reasoning and justification not only because we lack any agreement either on the true moral principles or theory, or on any method for determining the true general moral principles or theory, but also because foundationalism more generally is a mistaken account of the nature of justification in ethics. No version of foundationalism is a correct account of justification in ethics, as I shall argue shortly, and that includes deductivism, which accords foundational status to general principles or theories.

One further problem with deductivism should be mentioned. Consequentialism, in the very simple form specified above, appears to be a comprehensive and fully determinate theory for the moral evaluation of both actions and social policies—all are justified to the extent they promote human well-being. But in fact there are many possible versions of consequentialism depending on how some key terms are interpreted. Assuming a single determinate interpretation, however, there should always be, at least in principle, a correct answer to the moral evaluation of any action or policy. This simplicity and comprehensiveness is bought, however, at the unacceptably high cost of sharp conflict with many important components and complexities of most people's considered moral judgments. Moral principles and theories that incorporate these other components and complexities, however, have their own costs. They typically have significant indeterminacies in their content which tend to occur at just the points of significant moral conflict and intrapersonal and interpersonal controversy—for example, where different moral rights, duties, or important values within the theory come into conflict.

In the absence of strict priority rules or other determinate methods for resolving these conflicts and the moral issues in which these different moral considerations come into conflict (essentially all the interesting or hard moral cases), deductivism will be impossible to apply in just the cases in which we most need it.

Particularism

The polar extreme position about moral reasoning and moral knowledge or justification I shall call particularism. It holds that moral reasoning in practical and policy contexts begins and remains with the specific concrete case under consideration. If some moral judgments are true or correct, and so others false or mistaken, moral knowledge is achieved only at the level of particular cases. Some particularists hold that there is no standard for evaluating our moral judgments external to the particular judgments themselves. Others hold that moral knowledge resides at the level of particular paradigm cases, with moral reasoning in new cases then consisting of fitting the new cases to the paradigms closest to them.[7] Thus, in the example of the commissioners' policy dispute about euthanasia, reasoning remains at the level of a particular case, or a particular paradigm case, of euthanasia, with no external appeal to moral principles or theory from which, in foundationalist fashion, a conclusion could be derived and justified about euthanasia.

One problem for the particularist is moral disagreement, illustrated in the example about euthanasia. If moral reasoning remains only with the particular case, with no external appeal to moral theory or principles, then we will have no external appeal by which the disagreement might be resolved. Moreover, if two conflicting judgments about a paradigm case of euthanasia cannot both be true, then particularism seems to provide no standard by which we might determine which position is true or correct. Because particularism locates moral knowledge only at the level of particular judgments and confines moral reasoning only to the particular case, it seems to provide no standard for determining which particular judgments are true when they cannot all be true. But the most serious difficulty for particularism is that it is incompatible with the very process of giving reasons for moral judgments at all. It is important to see why this is so.

Moral judgments are unlike some judgments of taste, and moral disagreements are unlike some disagreements over matters of taste, because moral judgments must be backed by reasons. If you like vanilla ice cream and I like chocolate, we can just accept this as a difference in taste—there is no correct preference about flavors of ice cream and if asked why I prefer chocolate, I may only be able to repeat that it tastes better to me. Unlike matters of taste, moral judgments, for example about whether voluntary euthanasia is wrong, must have reasons backing them. A moral discussion between a proponent and opponent of euthanasia might only begin, not end, with claims that it is right or wrong. An opponent of euthanasia might challenge its proponent by arguing that the deliberate killing of an innocent person is wrong. A proponent might respond that voluntary euthanasia is different from most killing because the victim wants to die and consents to being killed.

And so their discussion might continue. Their initial disagreement quickly turns into a process of giving and clarifying reasons for their respective moral views about why euthanasia is or is not morally justified. Their discussion rapidly moves to more general issues about when killing is wrong, and for what reasons. This is inevitable. Their discussion could not remain at the level of a particular instance of euthanasia. *Whenever* we offer reasons in support of a particular moral judgment, we do so by picking out properties of the object of the judgment that support or are the basis for the moral judgment. Any feature of an object of moral evaluation which is offered as a reason supporting a positive or negative moral evaluation of it will be a property which on another occasion could be a property of other objects of evaluation. Being an innocent human being, or having consented to be killed, are each properties that can apply in other possible cases—to other innocent human beings and to other persons who consent to be killed.

Now clearly neither the proponent nor the opponent of euthanasia need appeal to a comprehensive moral theory in supporting his or her position about euthanasia, but both appeal to moral principles or reasons with some degree of generality—they can be applied to other particular actions, that is, other possible killings, as well. Indeed, if one of the two was a consequentialist and was then pressed about why killing human beings was wrong, she would respond that it is wrong when, and only when, it has worse overall effects for human well-being than not killing the person in question. And then she would have been driven to appeal to her most basic moral beliefs, her comprehensive moral theory, in providing her reasons for supporting or opposing the particular case of euthanasia. Of course, most people are not consequentialists and would stop the process of offering reasons for their moral position about euthanasia well short of any comprehensive theory, if for no other reason than that most people do not have any explicit, comprehensive theory that they accept; they might stop instead with appeal to a basic moral duty not to kill, or a basic moral right not to be killed. But while not a comprehensive theory, a principle specifying a general moral duty or right of this sort can be thought of as a potential part of a broader theory, or a theory fragment.

The central and fatal problem for particularism then is that it is incompatible with the very process of having and offering reasons for our moral judgments, which is the principal feature distinguishing morality from mere expressions of simple taste or preference. Some, at least partial or fragmentary, moral theorizing is an unavoidable part of moral reasoning, of making and offering reasons for moral judgments in practical and policy contexts. What level of generality the reason-giving process in fact reaches on a particular occasion of moral reasoning or disagreement will depend both on theoretical factors, such as how deep and general the parties' reasons for their positions are, and on practical factors, such as how deep one's own uncertainty or another's challenge goes on the issue in question. Even if a person's reasons for a particular moral judgment are so many and complex that as a matter of fact they fully fit few if any other real cases, the reasons must be such that they at least in principle can apply to other cases. Particularism, which locates moral reasoning and knowledge only at the level of the particular judgment regarding an individual case, is not a feasible alternative.

JUSTIFICATION WITH CONSIDERED MORAL JUDGMENTS

A Critical Screening Process

Neither deductivism, which gives a foundational role to general moral principles or theories in moral reasoning, nor particularism, which purports to give no role to general moral principles or theories in moral reasoning, is a plausible account of the nature of moral reasoning and justification. We need an account of moral reasoning that is neither too ambitious in the role it gives to moral principles and theories, as deductivism is, nor too dismissive of their role, as particularism is. One grain of truth in particularism is that people's moral thinking does typically begin with particular practical moral choices and cases. A discussion of euthanasia, for example, usually would begin with a particular instance of it, but proceed with the participants providing reasons in support of their positions. But how might their different moral judgments and positions be evaluated in order to determine which are true or false, correct or mistaken, or justified or unjustified? I want now to address the problem of justification more directly. If not deductivist or particularist, what method or process of moral reasoning could ethics commissions use that would warrant a claim that their conclusions are morally justified?

John Rawls introduced the notion of "considered moral judgments," which can be of use here, though I shall add features to it beyond those Rawls specified.[8] The idea is to characterize an idealized process at which both individuals and an ethics commission could aim in their moral deliberations. How do considered moral judgments differ from simply moral judgments? What does *considered* add? In answering this question, I will develop what I will characterize as a critical screening process through which individuals can put their moral views and judgments. Considered judgments generally, not just considered moral judgments, are, first, judgments that are not made in conditions that we know from experience often lead to mistakes. Here are some examples of such conditions: when we have insufficient time to consider the matter carefully; when we lack significant, relevant information bearing on the question at hand; when we have a relatively fixed commitment to a particular position on the question at hand that makes us inadequately open to a fair consideration of other positions; when the question at hand requires technical knowledge or training that we lack; when we must make a decision while distracted or emotionally overwrought; when we lack sufficient relevant experience to appreciate fully some considerations and to integrate them adequately into our decision making; and so forth. Notice that none of these are features in any way special to *moral* judgments—they are features that, if present, should equally weaken our confidence in judgments about empirical matters of fact. There is in addition at least one important feature which should likewise weaken our confidence specifically in our moral judgments, a condition that experience tells us often leads to moral judgments we later come to believe were mistaken. It is that what we decide morally to believe or do will importantly affect our own interests—this often leads us to rationalize in the pejorative sense, that is, to find some purported rationale for why *we* are not morally required to do a burdensome or unwanted action that we would have no trouble concluding others morally must do. Of course, when our interests are importantly at stake this often leads us to give more careful attention to the issue at hand. This condition does not rule out considered moral judgments, but warns us to look carefully for this form of rationalization. With this qualification, considered moral judgments then are, first, judgments made in the absence of conditions like those just noted that we know from experience often lead to mistakes.

There is a second aspect of considered moral judgments that needs to be brought out. With empirical judgments about matters of fact, our confidence in a judgment is increased, other things equal, the more fully we have been able to consider all relevant evidence that bears on the issue. While disputes about empirical matters of fact often bear on moral questions as well, moral judgments have specifically moral reasons which support them. Considered moral judgments then are also judgments made as a result of having fully considered the reasons that support them. In the ideal or limiting case, this would involve fully considering to the deepest level possible the nature of the reasons to which one would appeal in attempting to justify one's judgment. In the example above of voluntary euthanasia, this would involve fully probing one's moral views about killing and any factors that bear on one's views about killing in the context of euthanasia. Any example like this in which different people disagree brings out another important feature of evaluating the reasons in support of our moral judgments—this evaluation involves not just exploring as fully as possible the reasons in support of one's own judgment or position, but also considering all possible reasons and arguments *against* one's own position and in support of alternative positions. Until one has examined what can be said both for and against all plausible alternative positions on a particular issue, one will not have fully considered all alternatives, and all that can be said for and against all alternatives, to one's own position.

A third aspect of considered moral judgments and the critical screening process which produces them is that the process of considering alternative positions and evaluating the reasons that support them on any issue typically has both an intrapersonal and an interpersonal component. It will often begin as an intrapersonal process as one initially thinks about the issue oneself; but then it should expand to an interpersonal process as well, because we know from experience that our moral vision is often enlarged by discussion and reasoning with others and by confronting the positions and arguments of others, either in discussion or in print. Thus at the limits, arriving at one's considered moral judgment about a particular action or policy will involve considering all the reasons that can be offered by anyone for and against any alternative position, choice, or decision on the matter at hand. A practical implication for ethics commissions is that having diverse membership helps ensure a process in which diverse moral perspectives, experience, and views are brought to bear in the commission's deliberations.

Reflective Equilibrium

In criticizing particularism, I argued that it is impossible to give reasons for moral judgments while at the same time restricting the implications of judgments solely to the particular case at hand. By their very nature, moral reasons can apply to other cases beyond the specific case in which they are being employed. Sometimes these reasons have substantial scope or generality and so potentially apply to many other moral choices and evaluations that people face. We might therefore say that people's moral beliefs, and in turn their considered moral judgments which have survived the critical screening process I have just sketched, come at all levels of generality. Now a substantive or normative moral theory can be briefly characterized for my purposes here as a small body of relatively general principles applying to the objects of moral evaluation in a given domain. While the domain of a maximally comprehensive moral theory would be all possible objects of moral evaluation, most people at best hold less comprehensive theories, or what are partial theories or theory fragments from the more comprehensive perspective. This means that, although deductivism may be mistaken in holding that moral reasoning and justification begin from a moral theory already and independently established as true and which then could be somewhat mechanically applied to particular cases, it is correct that at least parts or fragments of moral theories are either implicitly or explicitly appealed to in reasoning about particular cases. It is this scope of moral reasons—that they always can apply to cases beyond the one at hand—that gives considerable force to the requirement of consistency in moral reasoning: consistency requires accepting the implications of the reasons or principles to which one appeals in a particular case for the other cases to which they also apply. A few important additional aspects of the appeal to general moral principles need to be emphasized.

Since our considered moral judgments and beliefs include general moral principles, these principles can often be appealed to in reasoning about particular cases or policies. For example, some principle of equality of opportunity is an important component of American moral and political culture, and can be used to help decide what kind of inequalities are morally acceptable in access to health care. This much is true about deductivism—sometimes we may have greater moral conviction about a general moral reason or principle than we do about a particular judgment concerning a concrete case or policy, and so we largely form or revise our moral judgment about the case or policy to fit the more general reason or principle that applies to it. Our moral conviction about the case or policy is then principally derived from our conviction about the more general reason or principle. Different moral judgments about particular cases or policies as well as different general moral principles are held with different degrees of conviction by any individual, even at the end of the critical screening process. This is important for understanding how internal conflicts within an individual's moral views should be resolved.

When there is conflict between our moral judgments about particular cases or policies and our moral principles, as often occurs, no systematic priority can be assigned either to the judgments about the particular cases and policies or to the general principles regarding which should be retained and which revised or abandoned in the attempt to eliminate the inconsistency in our moral views. In removing the inconsistency in order to reach what Rawls has called "reflective equilibrium" between an individual's particular judgments and general principles, the revision should be made so as to leave the individual with a consistent view that retains as much overall conviction as possible. Sometimes the initial judgment about the particular case or policy will be revised or abandoned, sometimes the more general principle. When an ethics commission is seeking interpersonal consensus among its members, or in the broader society, the resolution of conflicts will be more complex than, but in some respects similar to, this intrapersonal process. Compromises between individuals should be sought which require different individuals to make concessions at points of least conviction, scope, and importance in their views, and with a presumption for some rough equality in the concessions that individual members make to the others.

Foundationalist accounts of justification, of which deductivism is one instance, hold that some moral beliefs have privileged status regarding truth and/or justification, and so are not subject to revision in the case of conflict with other judgments lacking this privileged status. In the different account of justification sketched here, usually called coherentist, no judgments are assigned such privileged status that they never should or could be abandoned or revised. In any instance of conflict between particular judgments and general principles, it is an empirical matter, to be determined on a case-by-case basis, which carries least conviction and could be revised with least cost to a particular individual's other moral convictions. To seek reflective equilibrium is to seek the consistent, comprehensive set of considered moral judgments at all levels of generality, including both judgments about particular cases and general moral principles, which carries for the individual the greatest overall conviction.

Besides this role in reflective equilibrium, general moral principles and theories also play a more direct role in justifying moral judgments about particular cases or policies which is analogous to how scientific theories provide explanatory force to a domain of phenomena. A central function of theories in natural and social science is to provide order and structure to a body of observations or data about the world that would otherwise be merely a large set of unconnected data. Scientific theories thereby produce gains in understanding: by displaying a structure and order in the data, they show us the variables and causal relations that explain what would otherwise be a disordered and unrelated mass of observations or phenomena. In this respect, it is the same with moral theories. In morality, the analog to the observation statements and data that a scientific theory explains is the particular moral judgments about some range of cases which the more general principles of a moral theory, or of a partial moral theory, explain.

Because the principal role of moral judgments is to guide action, unlike both data and theories in science whose principal roles are to guide belief, moral judgments are subject to a special worry. The worry is that they may be no more than a hodgepodge of thinly veiled rationalizations and biases reflecting our own self-interest, prejudices, and arbitrary preferences. General moral principles or theories can help allay this worry by explaining these judgments: they are shown to fit, and to be derivable and made from, a coherent, unified moral conception. We come to see that our particular moral judgments have a coherent, identifiably moral source, heretofore likely only implicit, and are not just a cover for our prejudices and self-interest. The principles and theory display those judgments as recognizably moral and make the moral basis lying behind them subject to explicit critical evaluation. This can in turn increase our conviction in particular judgments because we come to see that they fit within or have the same basis as, other judgments about which we may have additional and/or more confidence. In this coherentist account of justification no particular part of a person's overall moral beliefs or conception has any privileged status with regard to truth, correctness, or justification. Instead, each component of the comprehensive moral conception gains part of its justification from all the rest of the moral conception of which it forms a part.

Fully coherent and comprehensive general principles or theories covering all of one's moral judgments are more than most people can in fact achieve. For most of us, there is no single, unified moral framework from which all our particular moral judgments are made or can be shown to follow. In fact, I believe that for most people there are multiple different and independent sources of moral value, or parts of their overall moral view, with no single deeper unified account of those parts. One of the central problems for applied ethics and practical moral thinking and deliberation is giving an intelligible account of how the unity of moral deliberation and action is possible, even for a single individual, in the face of this lack of unity or full coherence in the individual's moral beliefs or overall moral conception created by these different, independent components of the person's morality.[9] Of course, if we look across a culture or society, this diversity of sources of moral value is greater still—and is one of the greatest challenges public ethics commissions face.

This process of reaching one's considered moral judgments in reflective equilibrium is an ideal which in practice can only be more or less approached. Besides the obvious limitations of time and effort, there are always limitations at any point in time on the alternative positions on any issue that we and others can imagine, as well as on the arguments that we and others can think of for and against any alternative. So even if this ideal were fully realized at any point in time, we could never be sure that in the future we or others would not think of new alternatives and/or arguments, perhaps on the basis of new experience, that would change our minds. This critical screening process, even in its ideal form, never warrants absolute certainty about any particular moral judgment that could put it beyond further question. While this ideal of considered moral judgments in reflective equilibrium is never fully achievable in practice, it is useful nevertheless because it specifies an ideal process by which all possibly relevant reasons and arguments available to anyone and bearing on a moral issue can be given due consideration; the shortcomings and more restricted focus of moral reasoning in the real world can be measured against this ideal.

There is one important respect in which the ideal process of moral reasoning at which a public ethics commission should aim differs from what I have just sketched for individuals. It will rarely, if ever, be appropriate for an ethics commission to seek, much less present in its reports, a single fully comprehensive and determinate moral conception in support of its analyses and recommendations, even if it thought that possible. It will usually be enough to present the principal reasons and arguments that bear on and support the specific policy recommendations it makes. Often this will require criticizing alternative positions and/or responding to natural objections to its own positions and recommendations. In the example of euthanasia discussed above, the commission might at most offer a general analysis and argument on the wrongness of killing, and the kinds of cases, if any, in which killing can be morally justified which bear on euthanasia. Exploring the implications of the commission's argument and position for other cases of killing, for example, killing in war or capital punishment, would be unnecessary, indeed undesirable, because a source of unnecessary controversy and a diversion of attention from the commission's policy focus on euthanasia. For the same reasons, presenting an entire moral theory or a complete set of moral principles would be all the more unnecessary and uncalled-for given the policy focus. Nevertheless, the process of moral deliberation in which the commission engages, together with the results of that process which it presents to the public in its reports, is properly understood within this broader account of moral deliberation, reasoning, and justification.

We noted above that one respect in which general principles and theories help justify particular moral judgments is by showing them to be made from a coherent and unified moral conception. There are two further respects in which moral judgments that have survived the critical screening process and reflective equilibrium are justified. First, they are justified because they are made in relatively ideal conditions for judging, that is, in the absence, to the extent possible, of conditions that we know from experience often lead to mistakes; as noted above, these will include conditions leading to mistakes in judgments generally, as well as conditions leading to mistakes in moral judgments in particular. Second, they will have survived a process of critical examination in which all arguments both for and against them, as well as in support of and against alternative conflicting positions, have received due consideration. In both of these respects, considered moral judgments in reflective equilibrium are justified because they have survived a maximally broad critical screening process. To repeat, this is not to say that we may not later come to change our view, and/or come to believe that our earlier conclusions were mistaken. Even when our moral judgments have been maximally subjected to arguments for and against both them and other alternative positions, there are limitations in our and others' moral thinking at any point in time. Thus, just as with justified empirical beliefs, justification does not provide any guarantee of the truth or correctness of our moral beliefs.

Some readers may object that this account of moral reasoning and justification, which begins from the moral beliefs we happen to have at any point in time, is unduly conservative. Our moral beliefs are a result of our experience and the socialization process to which we have been subject. Consequently, those beliefs will likely reflect the values and moral beliefs predominant in our culture and society, and be biased in favor of the status quo. But this objection is misplaced. The critical screening process for reaching considered moral judgments, which describes an ideal of considering all arguments for and against both the particular moral judgment or position with which one began, as well as all judgments or positions which are alternatives to it, asks us to consider all criticisms of and alternative perspectives on the status quo, no matter how radical. Failures to consider sufficiently radical criticisms or alternatives will be failures of our critical and moral vision or will, to some degree unavoidable, but not failures fostered by the method of moral reasoning that I have described.

Relativism and the Subjectivity of Moral Judgments

Is the method of moral reasoning that I have sketched for use both by individuals and by public ethics commissions objectionably relativist? Moral relativism is usually understood as the view that different incompatible moral beliefs can be true for different individuals, groups, or societies. In this view, whether a moral judgment is true or correct will depend on who is making it. One of the central problems of moral methodology is how the justification, rather than the truth or correctness, of the moral judgments of either an individual or a group, such as an ethics commission, can be established. From the standpoint of justification, the problem of relativism is whether incompatible moral judgments can each be justified for different individuals or groups. It is a familiar point that even in the case of judgments that most people believe are noncontroversially capable of being either true or false, or correct or mistaken, such as empirical judgments about matters of fact, one individual may be justified in accepting a judgment as true that another individual can be justified in rejecting as false. This is because different people may have different evidence available to them bearing on the judgment in question, and an individual's justification for accepting a belief depends on the relevant evidence he or she has, or should have. If evidence tending to confirm or disconfirm a particular belief is available to one individual but unavailable to another, they can each be justified in holding beliefs both of which cannot be true.

So the question about the relativism of moral judgments is whether different individuals with all the same empirical or factual information and beliefs relevant to a moral issue can be justified in holding incompatible moral judgments on that issue. Another way of putting this question is whether some moral disagreement can be in principle, not just in practice, rationally irresolvable. Much moral disagreement is in practice irresolvable when people cling irrationally to beliefs in the face of evidence of their falsity, make mistakes in their reasoning that cannot be corrected, and so forth. Moral disagreement that is irresolvable in principle is clearly a more serious problem for any account of public moral discourse because it means that even when different people fully conform to the standards for that moral discourse, there may in the end be no way of resolving their moral disagreement.

It should be clear that the account of moral reasoning and justification sketched above, which employs a critical screening process together with reflective equilibrium, does allow for the possibility of moral disagreement that is in principle rationally irresolvable, and for the possibility that different individuals may each be justified in holding incompatible moral judgments; we can call this justificatory relativism. Of course, we will not know that any particular moral disagreement, such as among members of an ethics commission, is in fact irresolvable, either in principle or in practice, until their different views have gone through the critical screening process and achieved reflective equilibrium. Any conclusion that a particular moral disagreement is in principle irresolvable should only come at the end of a full, but failed, attempt to resolve the disagreement. The possibility that moral disagreement can be even in principle irresolvable is compatible with moral disagreements rarely, or even never, in fact turning out to be such. Some moral disagreement does, I believe, turn out to be irresolvable even in principle, but not as often as many people today suppose. Very often disagreement that initially appears to be moral turns out on closer analysis to be empirical disagreement about matters of fact.

Justificatory relativism implies that moral judgments are correctly understood to be in one sense subjective. Claims about the subjectivity and objectivity of morality and moral judgments are commonly so poorly defined and used in so many different senses that they often bring more confusion than clarity. What I have in mind here by the claim of subjectivity is this. At the end of the day, so to speak, after the process of moral reasoning and justification that I have sketched here has been completed, a particular individual's moral judgments, principles, or theory will depend on what that person is prepared on reflection to accept, to try to live by, and to judge him- or herself and others by. The same is true for groups of people living together in a society, and for bodies they establish like ethics commissions to help them address moral issues of public policy. Choice of and commitment to a way of life in this broad sense cannot in the end be avoided, and different individuals can choose and pursue different ways of life. But this hardly implies, as R.M. Hare pointed out long ago, that such choice is ungrounded or arbitrary; the choice I am describing here is choice after everything of relevance to the choice has been given due consideration, which is exactly the opposite of arbitrary choice understood as choice for which we have no basis.[10]

The Appeal to an Overlapping Consensus

One important qualification must be put on the account of moral reasoning I have sketched above for its use in public moral discourse in contexts in which identifying or forging a consensus about public policy, or making recommendations about public policy, is the goal. In more recent development of his theory of justice, John Rawls used an "overlapping consensus" to capture the idea that people who hold quite different comprehensive moral, religious, philosophical, and cultural views might share an overlapping consensus about principles of justice and about the political reasons that support those principles.[11] If people appeal to their comprehensive moral conceptions, including the full moral, religious, philosophical, and cultural underpinnings of those views, they will often give different and conflicting reasons or support for particular substantive positions on which they agree. The "fact of pluralism"—that different citizens hold different comprehensive moral, religious, and philosophical conceptions—is a permanent feature of free liberal democracies. It implies that the ethical and political bases that all citizens can reasonably accept for public policies in a liberal democracy cannot rest on these full comprehensive conceptions. The task of ethics commissions is often to try to find a common public moral discourse that can yield a consensus on which public policy can be formed among individuals and groups otherwise in disagreement on many important matters.

The role of an overlapping consensus for policy raises complex and controversial issues that cannot be explored here, but one point needs at least to be mentioned. In a liberal democracy, public policy which requires everyone to act in specific ways should not be based on sectarian views reasonably rejected by substantial segments of the population. This is a goal that cannot always be realized for all policy, certainly in practice, but I believe in theory as well; still, it is an important goal nonetheless. It implies, for example, that public policy should not be based on specific religious beliefs that many do not share. Not just public policies themselves, but the reasons that are offered in their support in policy debate, whether in ethics commissions or other settings, should not be reasons that others can reasonably reject as a basis for public policy in a pluralistic society. The common agreement to search for an overlapping consensus in public policy, a search in which an ethics commission can sometimes play a significant role, should be understood to mean not only that we seek to find or forge a consensus on particular policy issues, but that we also seek consensus on the kinds of reasons that we will offer in support of policy positions. One crucial aspect of this latter is the consensus on what reasons are appropriate for policy debate.

This is a qualification on the account of public moral reasoning on policy questions sketched above for ethics commissions, since the full exploration of one's reasons for one's moral positions and judgments will take one deeply into the details of one's comprehensive religious, philosophical, and moral views. To appeal to those comprehensive views is to go beyond what should be the basis of public policy. This restriction on reasons that are appropriate in the policy debates of an ethics commission is an implication of wanting public policy in a liberal democracy to be justified as far as possible by shared reasons that all could accept as reasonable.

CONCLUSION

I shall emphasize only two general points in conclusion. The first is that the process of public moral discourse in which an ethics commission engages is not fundamentally different in its nature from the moral reasoning in which individual members of the society engage in public and private contexts. The second point is that while the process of public moral discourse, even properly carried out, does not guarantee the truth or correctness of the conclusions it yields, it can provide us with a warrant for accepting them as a justified basis for public policy.

NOTES

1. While some people make a distinction, although usually not a clear one, between "ethics" and "morality," I shall use them interchangeably in this paper.

2. D. Rothman, *Strangers at the Bedside: A History of How Law and Bioethics Transformed Medical Decision Making.* New York: Basic Books (1991); Henry Beecher, "Ethics and Clinical Research," *New England Journal of Medicine* 74 (1966) 1354–1360.

3. President's Commission for the Study of Ethical Problems in Medicine and Biomedical and Behavioral Research, *Deciding to Forego Life-Sustaining Treatment.* Washington, D.C.: U.S. Government Printing Office (1983).

4. Brock, D.W. "Voluntary Active Euthanasia," *Hastings Center Report* 22 (March–April 1992) 10–22, and reprinted in Dan W. Brock, *Life and Death: Philosophical Essays in Biomedical Ethics.* Cambridge University Press (1993).

5. Rawls, J. 1971. *A Theory of Justice.* Cambridge, MA: Harvard University Press.

6. Foundationalists differ on how this privileged truth status can be secured for some moral judgments, as well as on what the privileged status is, e.g., contingent or necessary truth. Intuitionists like H. A. Prichard and W. D. Ross both held that some moral statements are necessary truths, although they disagreed about whether the moral statements that had this privileged truth status were concrete, all-things-considered moral judgments about particular actions, or general principles specifying moral duties such as to keep promises and not to deceive, which could be overridden in some particular circumstances.

7. Jonsen, A.R. and S. Toulmin. *The Abuse of Casuistry: A History of Moral Reasoning.* Berkeley: University of California Press, 1988. To what extent Jonsen and Toulmin are examples of what I call Particularists is unclear. They do endorse a "stronger claim—namely that *moral knowledge is essentially particular* so that sound resolutions of moral problems must always be rooted in a concrete understanding of specific cases and circumstances. . . . The stronger account sees the primary locus of moral understanding as lying in the recognition of *paradigmatic examples* of good and evil, right and wrong." p. 330 (Italics in original) This suggests that they do accept the epistemic aspect of what I call Particularism that moral truth or knowledge is to be found at the level of particular cases, their *"paradigmatic examples."* It may be that their account of the actual *process* of moral reasoning, which is centrally a matter of fitting specific actual cases to the paradigmatic examples, does make room for general principles in the manner of reflective equilibrium discussed below, although I am unsure of this. But it is unlike Rawlsian reflective equilibrium in giving judgments about particular

cases privileged epistemic status, and that is the only respect in which I am interpreting them to be Particularists here.

8. Rawls, *op. cit.*

9. Thomas Nagel has stressed this point in "The Fragmentation of Value," in *Moral Questions.* Cambridge: Cambridge University Press (1979).

10. Hare, R.M. *Freedom and Reason,* Oxford: Oxford University Press (1963)

11. Rawls, J. *Political Liberalism.* New York: Columbia University Press (1993).

The Value of Consensus

MARTIN BENJAMIN, Ph.D.
Professor of Philosophy, Michigan State University

In 1988, a group of 33 physicians, bioethicists, and medical economists from ten different countries met at Lawrence University in Appleton, Wisconsin, to formulate guidelines for stopping medical treatment. Apart from minority dissents on two matters of detail, the guidelines were endorsed by the group as a whole and subsequently published as "The Appleton Consensus: Suggested International Guidelines for Decisions to Forego Medical Treatment" (Stanley et al., 1989). What, if anything, is added to the value of such guidelines by the inclusion of "consensus" in the title? Does consensus give special credence or authority to this and similar outcomes of group deliberation? Should members of such groups be encouraged to strive for consensus? Or is preoccupation with consensus likely to obscure important differences, leading in many cases to recommendations so general or abstract as to be practically useless?

These and related questions have assumed greater importance as governments and health care institutions turn to ad hoc or standing committees or commissions for guidance on perplexing bioethical issues. In what follows I examine the nature, value, and limits of consensus in bioethics. I begin by identifying different types of consensus and their relations to notions like compromise and majority rule. I turn then to a variety of normative and methodological issues that must be addressed by ethics committees and commissions as they consider whether, and if so to what extent, their deliberations should be directed by a search for consensus.

FORMS OF AGREEMENT

Agreement among members of bioethics committees and commissions may take a number of forms. At one end of the spectrum is full agreement on both the substance of a recommendation and its supporting arguments. At the other is vote-taking and the group's endorsing the will of the majority. In between are "overlapping consensus" and compromise.

Complete Consensus

A consensus is, most generally, an agreement—a collective unanimous opinion—among a number of persons. If, for example, members of an ethics committee immediately agree on a recommendation and its supporting values or principles, consensus is predeliberatively complete. The entire position—argument and conclusion—of each member is, at the outset, congruent with that of the others.

Predeliberative complete consensus will, for two reasons, be uncommon. First, questions directed to such committees are usually contested. Ethics commissions or committees are created when the larger group they represent must speak with one voice on complex ethical questions to which members or clients of these groups give uncertain or conflicting answers. Issues likely to elicit complete consensus at the beginning of a group's deliberations are, as a result, not often addressed to ethics committees. Second, committee members usually represent differing social or ethical viewpoints or differing areas of biomedical, social scientific, or other types of expertise, or both. It is, in part, the diverse and representative composition of such committees that lends special authority to whatever agreement emerges from their deliberations. At the same time, this diversity is unlikely to produce predeliberative complete consensus.

Yet if complete consensus rarely emerges at the beginning of a group's deliberations, it will, more often, develop toward the end. Consider, for example, questions so novel or puzzling that committee members have, at the outset, no firm positions on them. "This is not to say," as Jonathan Moreno puts it, "that they come with no views or principles in relation to the matter at hand, but rather that they do not hold them in such esteem that they are prepared to insist that their essence be represented in the solution" (Moreno, 1990a, p. 43). Here, open-minded, informed, mutually respectful, give-and-take discussion aimed at well-grounded agreement may produce convergence on both reasons and conclusion—complete consensus.

Still, such consensus will not be frequent. Committee members often bring differing moral outlooks or principles to the deliberations that affect their reasoning or conclusions. Moreover, individuals representing differing areas of expertise are likely to emphasize different aspects of complex, multidimensional questions in their thinking, leading to differing arguments, if not differing conclusions. If, however, committee members agree in their conclusions, but come to these conclusions in different ways, the result may still be consensus, though not complete consensus.

Overlapping Consensus

The term "overlapping consensus" has been coined by political philosopher John Rawls to characterize agreement on basic principles of justice among individuals embracing a plurality of different, occasionally conflicting, comprehensive moral, religious, and philosophical outlooks (Rawls, 1993, pp. 15, 133–72). As different premises may lead to the same conclusion, different comprehensive outlooks, Rawls argues, may support the same conception of social justice. There is, in this event, overlap among those parts of different individuals' comprehensive moral, religious, and philosophical views that include a particular conception of social justice, but not among their moral, religious, and philosophical views as a whole. Thus, for example, one person may situate his or her support of a particular conception of justice within certain religious convictions, while another may find a place for the very same conception within either Kant's or Mill's comprehensive (secular) moral theory (Rawls, 1993, p. 145).

Agreement among members of an ethics committee or commission may also be a type of overlapping consensus. Individuals arguing from different moral, religious, philosophical, and empirical premises may nonetheless reach the same conclusion with respect to positions or policies in bioethics.[1] Stephen Toulmin observed this sort of consensus in his role as a staff member with the National Commission for the Protection of Human Subjects of Biomedical and Behavioral Research. Although commissioners were usually in agreement about their recommendations—"even about quite detailed recommendations"—the consensus did not, Toulmin writes, extend to the arguments or principles supporting these recommendations:

> When the eleven individual commissioners asked themselves what "principles" underlay and supposedly justified their adhesion to the consensus, each of them answered in his or her own way: the Catholics appealed to Catholic principles, the humanists to humanist principles, and so on. They could agree; they could agree what they were agreeing about; but, apparently, they could not agree why they agreed about it [Toulmin, 1981, p. 32].[2]

Consensus in societies acknowledging a plurality of conflicting comprehensive moral outlooks will often be overlapping. The wish for complete consensus on all moral issues is, as I will show below, utopian. I want now to compare consensus—complete and overlapping—with compromise and (what may be construed as a special kind of compromise) majority rule.

Compromise

Compromise bears more than a superficial resemblance to consensus, but it is also importantly different. Central to compromise is the idea of mutual concession for mutual gain. Consider, in this connection, the deliberations and conclusions of the Warnock Committee of Inquiry into Human Fertilization and Embryology (Warnock, 1985b). Among the issues addressed by this group of British physicians, lawyers, theologians, social scientists, and ordinary citizens, chaired by philosopher Mary Warnock, was the question of the permissibility of research using human embryos. Moral opinion on this matter was at the time (and still is) deeply divided. At the root of the controversy are opposing views of the moral status of the embryo. Those who believe that human life protected by laws against murder begins at conception consider the embryo to have the same status as an adult human being, and are thus strongly opposed to any research of this kind. Those who regard the moral status of the human embryo as significantly lower than that of an adult are heavily influenced by the undeniable utilitarian advantages of such research with respect to inquiries into infertility, miscarriage, congenital defects, and related matters. The Warnock Committee was charged with making a recommendation at the national level on this highly controversial question. Although moral views on this matter were divided, a policy embodied in law would necessarily be singular and binding on all.

The most basic recommendation of the majority of the committee's members on the question of embryo research seems to have been a compromise between the two polar positions. Such research would be permitted, but only for up to 14 days from fertilization. It would, after this, be categorically forbidden. As Warnock puts it,

> in the end the Inquiry felt bound to argue, *partly* on Utilitarian grounds, that the benefits that had come in the past from research using human embryos were so great (and were likely to be even greater in the future), that such research had to be permitted; but that it should be permitted only at the very earliest stage of the development of the embryo [Warnock, 1985a, p. 517].

Thus, each polar position to the disagreement (that representing an extreme conservative or "pro-life" view of the moral standing of the embryo, and that representing a considerably more liberal, or utilitarian, view) received part, but not all, of what it was after. Members of the committee holding either of these positions who nonetheless agreed to the compromise must be presumed, for one reason or another, to have valued the committee's speaking with one voice on this matter more than they valued the committee's endorsing their own view at the price of continued impasse.

Compromise in this and similar situations resembles consensus insofar as the group speaks with one voice in making and supporting a particular recommendation.[3] There is consensus, in these circumstances, on what position ought to be adopted by the group. Compromise differs from consensus, however, insofar as those supporting the compromise retain personal moral views that are more or less at odds with the position they endorse in their roles as committee members.[4] Each party to the compromise makes concessions for the sake of agreement on a single recommendation that seems to have some independent validity and to capture as much of one polar position as it does of the other. The matter is not, however, fully settled; there is no closure, no final harmony, no complete or overlapping consensus. Moral compromise is not, strictly speaking, resolution. It makes the best of what contending parties regard as a bad situation. Individual committee members may subsequently try to persuade those with whom they disagree of the superiority of their initial position with an aim to its eventually being reconsidered and endorsed by the group as a whole.

Majority Rule

Occasionally a committee will be unable to reach complete or overlapping consensus on a particular issue or to devise a satisfactory compromise. Still, each member may believe that the group's making either of two recommendations on the issue would be better than its making no recommendation at all. In this event a consensus may emerge from taking a vote between the two alternatives, then endorsing, as a committee, the recommendation receiving a majority of votes.

A resort to majority rule under such circumstances includes elements of both consensus and compromise. There is, first, consensus on the procedure to be followed in determining the group's substantive position—what we might call procedural—as opposed to substantive, consensus. Second, agreeing to abide by the outcome of this procedure is a type of compromise. A committee member favoring position A over position B would rather have the entire committee recommend A on its merits. But since this will not occur and efforts to find a compromise position between A and B have been unsuccessful, the committee member agrees to the vote because he or she believes the possibility of B's winning a majority of votes and becoming the committee's recommendation is from an ethical point of view better than the committee's remaining deadlocked. If those favoring position B follow *mutatis mutandis* the same chain of reasoning, the result may be characterized as a procedural, as opposed to a substantive, compromise.

Though less desirable than substantive consensus or substantive compromise, employment of majority rule under such circumstances is fair to all committee members. What would be unfair, however, is resorting to vote-taking without the consent of all committee members and then attributing the results to the committee as a whole. A majority position, under such conditions, is attributable only to those who voted for that position, and not to those who were opposed to settling the matter by vote-taking. Where a resort to vote-taking is a product of procedural consensus and represents procedural compromise, however, the outcome is endorsed by and attributable to the group as a whole.

Following customary usage, I have to this point restricted the term "consensus" to pre- and postdeliberative complete consensus and overlapping consensus. But because both compromise and majority rule contain elements of consensus and are sometimes employed by ethics committees and commissions, I consider them as forms of consensus in what follows.

STRATEGIC CONSIDERATIONS

Arguments for consensus may be either strategic or normative. Strategic considerations emphasize the instrumental value of consensus. The principal value of consensus is, on this view, its contribution to obtaining external acceptance and implementation of a group's recommendations. Normative arguments center on a more direct connection between consensus and moral rightness; consensus is regarded as adding substantive value or weight to the recommendations of an ethics committee or commission. I discuss strategic considerations in this section and normative considerations in the next.

In an article describing and defending the structure and operation of the President's Commission for the Study of Ethical Problems in Medicine and Biomedical and Behavioral Research, Commission Chairman Morris B. Abram and attorney Susan M. Wolf emphasize the practical importance of virtual unanimity or consensus among the commission's members:

> A Commission such as this one has only the power of persuasion. A group performing ethical analysis with no coercive powers cannot be persuasive without internal agreement. Unlike a court or legislature, which is structured to have effect as long as a majority agrees, a commission requires agreement that is as close to unanimity as possible, to have any effect at all. Without such virtual unanimity, the commission members simply voice possible arguments; with it the commission can persuade. The commission method thus forces the commissioners to find areas of common accord [Abram and Wolf, 1984, p. 629].

The provisions governing membership on the commission, Abram and Wolf add, mandated that commissioners have diverse backgrounds and represent a variety of ethical viewpoints. Though making agreement more difficult to achieve, this same diversity contributes to the persuasive power of any consensus emerging from such a group. The more dissimilar their backgrounds and viewpoints, the more likely it is that positions on which they achieve consensus (or even well-grounded compromise) will be endorsed by legislators and public.

Yet stressing consensus for strategic reasons may weaken the substantive power or coherence of a group's recommendations. Consider, for example, criticisms of the President's Commission's volume on access to health care. Ronald Bayer, in a well-documented review of the commission's deliberations on this matter, identifies and sharply criticizes the "kinds of compromises that were necessary to bring the Commission's work [on this topic] to a successful conclusion" (Bayer, 1984, p. 314). Agreement between the commission's staff, who favored the language of rights, and most commissioners and the staff's executive director, who did not, required replacing the notion of a right to health care with the weaker notion of a societal obligation to provide access to care. This was, to Bayer's mind, an unfortunate concession. "The concept of positive or social welfare rights," he argues, has emerged in recent American history as the most potent political language for those seeking to make claims against a nonegalitarian social structure. By explicitly rejecting the concept of a right to health care, thus breaking with recent public discourse on this matter, the commission deprived those poorly served by the current health care system of a language with which to express their discontent. In so doing, the commission implicitly adopted a perspective that views social change as the consequence of the recognition of moral obligations by the socially powerful, rather than as a result of demands pressed from below as a matter of right (Bayer, 1984, p. 320).

This charge has been echoed by John Arras, who argues that the commission's "retreat from the right to health care" represents "a significant retrenchment of our public commitment to provide health care for the needy" (Arras, 1984, p. 322).

In a different but related vein, Baruch Brody criticizes the commission's work on access to health care for failing to come to grips with underlying philosophical questions about distributive justice. "The Commission," he maintains, "needed to delve more deeply into the philosophical issues in order to show the extent to which we lack an appropriate social policy about access because we lack a social consensus about distributive justice" (Brody, 1989, p. 376f). A number of deep and divisive philosophical questions were papered over in the interests of maintaining a strategic consensus. Yet this served no purpose and may even have hampered subsequent efforts to address the important underlying questions. "By failing to delve into the philosophical problems about justice in the allocation of resources," Brody concludes,

> the Commission failed to provide a coherent approach to the difficult problems of securing access to health care. It would have done better, I submit, to be more philosophical, to present a series of alternative theories of justice and their implications, and to call upon society to make some choice among them [Brody, 1989, p. 383].

Where deep philosophical differences underlie conflicts about policy, a committee or commission does better to identify these differences and urge further reflection than to obscure them with a shallow strategic consensus on what proves to be an empty or incoherent substantive recommendation.

In a revealing account of the complex workings of a hospital ethics committee, Ruth Macklin charts one group's struggle to reach consensus on a difficult philosophical question. Charged with developing policy for blood transfusions involving Jehovah's Witnesses, the committee was unable to agree on guidelines for transfusing pregnant Witnesses. The issue was whether these patients should have the same right to refuse lifesaving transfusions as other adult Jehovah's Witnesses. On the one hand, some members of the committee believed that pregnant Witnesses should have the same rights to control their bodies as other Jehovah's Witnesses. On the other hand, some physicians maintained that the presence of what they considered a "second patient"—the fetus—would not permit them to accede in good conscience to any refusal of a lifesaving transfusion by a pregnant Witness. After two years of deliberation and numerous reversals of position, the committee eventually determined that it could not reach a consensus on specific guidelines for pregnant Witnesses. "Reluctantly," Macklin reports, "the committee adopted the suggestion that it not even attempt to dictate a policy but limit its task to describing the competing principles, leaving the decision-making process to the patient and clinician" (Macklin, 1988, p. 20).

NORMATIVE CONSIDERATIONS

Abram and Wolf do not ask whether consensus can have normative as well as strategic or persuasive value. Does consensus add moral weight to a position in bioethics? Philosophers have long argued that the mere fact of agreement does not make a position morally right (Moreno, 1990b). Still consensus may, in some circumstances and under some conditions, contribute to the normative significance of a group's recommendations. To show how this is so I must say something about (1) the nature and extent of moral pluralism; (2) the distinction between rationality and reasonableness; (3) the extent to which questions of biomedical ethics generate genuine uncertainty or reasonable disagreement; (4) the importance of agreement, both in health care institutions and in national policy, on some of these questions; and (5) the likelihood that informed, unforced agreement on a particular issue or policy among members of a conscientious, well-constituted ethics committee or commission will respect, if not incorporate, all reasonable positions on the matter.

Moral Pluralism

Moral pluralism, as I use the term here, is the view that moral disagreement cannot be eliminated by appeals to abstract impersonal principles. Our positions on particular issues are usually grounded in our comprehensive moral, religious, and philosophical outlooks and there is no single comprehensive outlook that should be embraced by all insofar as they are informed and rational. The comprehensive, identity-conferring outlooks that we bring to ethical reflection include a variety of conflicting, often equally reasonable, world views and ways of life.

A *world view* is a complex, often unarticulated (and perhaps not fully articulable) set of deeply held and highly cherished beliefs about the nature and organization of the universe and one's place in it. Normative as well as descriptive—comprised of interlocking general beliefs about knowledge, reality, and value—a world view so pervades and conditions our everyday thinking that it is largely unnoticed (Luker, 1984, p. 158). Among the elements of a world view are one's deepest convictions about: (a) God—that is, whether there is a God and, if so, God's nature; (b) the nature and purpose (if any) of the universe and human life; (c) the nature, justification, and extent of human knowledge; (d) the nature of human beings (including, for example, their capacities for free will, goodness, compassion, selfishness, and, in certain world views, sin and redemption); (e) the best way(s) to structure human relationships (including sexual and familial relationships, friendship, political institutions, and obligations to strangers); (f) the nature and status of morality, especially injunctions and principles having to do with the taking of life, the nature of equality, respect for liberty, and so on; and (g) the moral standing of nonhuman animals and the intrinsic value (if any) of the natural environment. A world view, as this list suggests, may be theistic or entirely nontheistic.

Closely related to a particular world view is a corresponding *way of life.* "Ways of life," writes Stuart Hampshire, "are coherent totalities of customs, attitudes, beliefs, institutions, which are interconnected and mutually dependent in patterns that are sometimes evident and sometimes subtle and concealed." Ways of life include "repeated patterns of behavior, . . .

admired ideal types of men and women, standards of taste, family relationships, styles of education and upbringing, religious practices and other
dominant concerns" (Hampshire, 1983, p. 5). A person's world view and
way of life are dynamically interrelated. A world view helps to structure a
way of life; a way of life presupposes and embodies a particular world view.
Deep changes in one are likely to occasion related changes in the other.

A distinctive and easily recognized world view and way of life is that of
the Amish. Most world views and ways of life are, however, more difficult to
delineate in rapidly changing complex societies like ours which permit, if
not encourage, the exercise of individual choice. A complex amalgam of a
wide variety of beliefs, attitudes, values, ideals, and practices, a contemporary world view and way of life is often highly customized. This is not,
however, to say that these more individualized world views and ways of life
are less significant to those who identify with them than a distinctively
Amish world view and way of life is to those who identify with it. A world
view and way of life gives shape and meaning to a person's life, providing
the basis for his or her identity and integrity as a moral being.

World views and ways of life come into conflict because they are, for
the most part, based on local and particular, rather than more general and
universal, aspects of human life. Their perspectives are historically conditioned, contingent, and sometimes fiercely personal and parochial. Loyalties to particular institutions, practices, projects, and persons are often
regarded as essential to one's way of life; they constitute much of one's
identity and set one off from others as a particular person.

Not all world views and ways of life are, however, worthy of respect. A
world view and way of life may be criticized for inconsistency or instability,
or for clearly and systematically violating the principle of utility or the
second formulation of Kant's Categorical Imperative ("So act as to treat
humanity, whether in thine own person or in that of any other, in every
case as an end withal, never as a means only"). Though unable fully to
determine our world views and ways of life, these well-grounded principles
serve as important constraints on them.[5] Each centers on a morally significant feature of human beings that cuts across social, cultural, national,
religious, racial, and sexual differences: sentience (for the principle of
utility) and the capacity for rational self-direction (for the Categorical Imperative). World views and ways of life systematically indifferent to or
contemptuous of the principle of utility or the Categorical Imperative must
be rejected (or at least constrained) regardless of their historical roots or
their importance to the identities of those holding them. It is thus that
world views and ways of life endorsing what clearly amounts to wanton
cruelty and neglect, human sacrifice, and slavery are widely and rightly
condemned. Campaigns to reform world views and ways of life incorporating more subtle violations of these principles are now being undertaken.

Some—for example, those that have added "racism" and "sexism" to our vocabularies—have already achieved a measure of success. Others—for example, those attempting to raise our consciousness about homophobia and speciesism—still have a long way to go. But the general point remains: World views and ways of life that clearly and systematically violate these more abstract and general principles are *unreasonable* and may be restricted.

A world view and way of life is reasonable to the extent that it satisfies well-grounded, widely shared standards and principles of reason. The problem is that there are a number of reasonable world views and ways of life that occasionally engender differing answers to moral questions, especially questions of biomedical ethics. This diversity of *reasonable* comprehensive moral outlooks, as Rawls points out, "is not a mere historical condition that may soon pass away; it is a permanent feature of the public culture of democracy" (Rawls, 1993, p. 36). So long as people enjoy a certain amount of liberty of thought and action they will embrace a variety of reasonable world views and ways of life that will occasionally yield conflicting answers to moral questions. Agreement by all on a single world view and way of life can be maintained, as Rawls adds, only by "the oppressive use of state power" (Rawls, 1993, p. 37).

Rationality and Reasonableness

Rationality is, for the most part, an intellectual virtue having to do with the selection and pursuit of the most effective means to a set of carefully selected ends. "I behave irrationally," W. M. Sibley writes,

> when I do not bother to ascertain the true nature of the ends I set myself; or when I heedlessly sacrifice one end to a second, which when attained I find to be of less worth to me than the first would have been; or when I select unrealistic means; or when, having reached a rational enough decision, I fail to implement that decision in practice [Sibley, 1953, p. 556].

One's ends as a rational agent need not, however, be egoistic. Consider, for example, a paternalistic physician whose world view and way of life places a premium on improving other people's health and saving their lives. Insofar as this physician is rational he will do what he can to pursue this end. But he is not, simply as a rational agent, required to give equal respect and concern to the conflicting reasonable ends of his patients. Rationality requires that the physician take his patients' ends into account only insofar as doing so is instrumentally necessary for effectively furthering those of *his* ends (which incorporate, in this instance, *his conception* of their welfare) that may be distinct from or opposed to theirs. If, therefore, the physician's obtaining consent to what he regards as beneficial treatment from a competent adult patient requires that he deceive the patient and he knows he can get away with it, the physician will, insofar as he is rational, be deceptive.

Reasonableness, on the other hand, requires giving equal or fair consideration to the reasonable ends or viewpoints of others for their own sakes. A person can therefore be rational without being reasonable, as shown by the example of the paternalistic physician. Reasonableness is a moral virtue, not simply an intellectual one. To be reasonable is to seek reasons for one's conduct that respect the reasonable ends and points of view of those affected by it.

It is therefore, in the light of moral pluralism, unreasonable to suppose that there is one and only one right answer to all moral questions. Insofar as I acknowledge that a disagreement between another person and myself is rooted in a conflict between reasonable world views and ways of life and I am committed to respecting the (reasonable) ends and points of view of others, I must admit that abstract, impersonal reason cannot, at least at this point, provide a resolution (Benjamin, 1990a, Ch. 4).

Bioethical Questions

Questions of biomedical ethics place unusual strain on our moral frameworks and traditions. In some cases, advances in medical knowledge and technology create choices and possibilities so complex or radically new or unprecedented that neither particular world views and ways of life nor abstract general principles provide much in the way of firm or direct guidance. The questions, we know, are important, but we are not quite sure what to think or do about them. We feel a need to learn more about the complex clinical, scientific, social, and ethical aspects of them before coming to a decision.

In other cases, these new choices and possibilities—especially those involving procreation, childbirth, childrearing, the nature of the family, and the termination of life—elicit clear and firm responses rooted in different world views and ways of life. Not only do we have ethical positions on these choices and possibilities, but they are deeply held and identity-conferring. Yet they conflict with ethical positions rooted in other (reasonable) world views and ways of life that we cannot, insofar as we are reasonable, simply dismiss. Although we are clear about what we, as individuals, believe to be right, we are not quite sure what should be done by a health care team, a hospital, or a society when those directly affected hold conflicting, yet not unreasonable, positions.

Need for Agreement

It is the need for some sort of agreement or consensus in the light of the genuine uncertainty and reasonable disagreement characteristic of many questions in biomedical ethics that has prompted the development of ethics committees and commissions. The complexity of modern medicine often requires the close cooperation among members of a health care team, patients, and patients' families. Though some of these individuals may, at least initially, be uncertain about or hold conflicting positions on bioethical issues, they often need to agree on a single treatment plan. Respect for reasonable moral differences requires that this agreement be informed and uncoerced rather than imposed by deception or force by those with a monopoly on power. If parties to a particular conflict are unable to come to such an agreement by themselves, they may seek assistance from an institutional ethics committee.

The same is true of questions of hospital or national policy. Though different individuals and organizations may, for example, have conflicting, reasonable views on how transplantable organs ought to be allocated in the United States, a national system requires agreement on a single set of principles and criteria binding on all. Here, too, respect for reasonable moral differences requires that this agreement be informed and uncoerced rather than imposed by force or deception.

Value of Consensus

Suppose we find ourselves in a situation requiring a single policy on a complex bioethical question characterized by genuine uncertainty or reasonable disagreement. A committee or commission is constituted to examine the situation and recommend a policy. The committee members represent or have access to all relevant aspects of biomedical, social scientific, cultural-religious, legal, and bioethical expertise on the matter, with emphasis on patient-citizen viewpoints. The group makes a concerted effort to identify all reasonable positions on the issue and to give them fair consideration. Moreover, no committee member or coalition of committee members is able to dominate the group's information-gathering, deliberation, or decision-making. Finally, after considering all actual or imagined reasonable arguments and positions on the matter, the group comes to an informed, uncoerced agreement on what, for institutional or social purposes, is regarded by each member as the best answer to the question. This agreement may take the form of complete consensus, overlapping consensus, compromise, or even consensus to endorse the outcome of a vote between two or more reasonable positions, each of which is regarded by everyone as superior to the group's coming to no agreement on the matter.

A consensus *meeting these conditions* carries moral weight or adds normative significance to the group's recommendation because it respects both the depth of genuine uncertainty or the extent of reasonable disagreement on the matter and the need for informed, uncoerced agreement. This is not to say that the recommendation must be accepted without question. Yet the burden is on those who disagree to show why, for purposes of reasonable agreement in a pluralistic society, it is defective.

An Illustration

Consider, as an illustration, a statement of general principles for allocating transplantable organs and tissues developed by the 1991 Ethics Committee of the United Network on Organ Sharing (UNOS) (Ethics Committee, 1992).[6] The Ethics Committee identified three principles governing most allocation decisions: (1) Utility (interpreted as net medical benefit); (2) justice (requiring fair or equitable treatment to all those awaiting organs); and (3) autonomy (respecting informed, self-directing patient choice, even if this does not in certain instances maximize utility or promote equitable distribution). The group then acknowledged possible conflicts between the three principles and addressed means of resolving them.

One strategy is to establish a fixed ranking of the principles—to prioritize or lexically order them in some way—and to always follow this ranking. One might, for example, propose that autonomy is prior to and, in cases of conflict, overrides justice; and that justice is similarly prior to and, in cases of conflict, overrides utility. This was, however, rejected as overly rigid. Whatever ranking one established ahead of time, it is always possible to imagine situations in which the consequences of adhering to it would be unacceptable. A second strategy is to address conflicts case by case, appealing to moral intuition. The problem with this is that people's intuitions differ widely on these matters, resulting in deadlock or a lack of uniformity from one transplant center to another and within centers from one person to another.

A third strategy, which the committee endorsed, is to acknowledge the complexity of the situation and seek some sort of compromise or accommodation among the three principles. With regard to conflicts between utility and justice, for example, the committee states:

> While [individual] members of the Committee hold diverging positions regarding the ethically correct relations between utility and justice, a *consensus has been reached for purposes of policy relative to organ and tissue allocation:* utility . . . and justice (or fairness in distribution) should be given equal status. This means that it is unacceptable for an allocation policy to single-mindedly strive to maximize aggregate medical good without any consideration of justice in distribution or for a policy to be single-minded about promoting justice at the expense of the overall (medical) good [Ethics Committee, 1992, p. 2229, emphasis added].

In cases of conflict, the committee proposed, justice and utility require equal consideration:

We make this proposal fully realizing that it may not square with the personal morality of many people. Some would insist on higher priority for utility; others for equity. In fact, whole classes of people might be so inclined invariably to favor one of these principles or the other. The fact that one group would give very heavy weight to one or the other of the principles cannot, for public policy purposes, settle the matter. Inasmuch as: (1) neither side can provide conclusive arguments for its position; (2) each side can provide plausible arguments for its position; and (3) ours is a pluralistic society in which individual views cover the entire spectrum from pure utilitarianism to extreme egalitarianism, we believe that giving equal consideration to each is *a fair and workable compromise* [Ethics Committee, 1992, p. 2230, emphasis added].

Apart from minor differences in wording, this line of reasoning closely resembles the one developed in this section.

Though the committee's compromise might be rejected as the best moral position by a number of individuals as *individuals*, it cannot, the Committee suggests, be *reasonably* rejected as a basis for public policy by individuals *as citizens* for whom informed, unforced reasonable agreement on such principles is of great importance.[7] While a person may reasonably reject a policy that ignores or violates his or her personal moral position, he or she cannot reasonably reject a coherent policy that (1) acknowledges reasonable disagreement on the matter; (2) incorporates important elements of his or her personal moral position; and (3) respects as many different reasonable positions as any workable alternative.

Finally, we should note that this Committee, like the hospital ethics committee described above by Macklin, was unwilling to reach consensus at any cost. The subcommittee drafting the initial document could not, for example, agree on whether (carefully screened, abstinent) alcoholic end-stage liver disease patients should be able to compete equally with non-alcoholic patients for access to the limited supply of transplantable livers. After considerable discussion and a 3–2 straw vote, subcommittee members concluded they could not, in good conscience, answer this question *as a group*. The final document states that "the Ethics Committee has not at this time reached a single position regarding the nonpunitive use of this factor [organ-damaging patterns of behavior] in allocation of organs" and then identifies arguments for and against the alternatives (Ethics Committee, 1992, p. 2234).

PROBLEMS AND LIMITS

A consensus among members of an ethics committee or commission may be questioned in a number of ways. Doubts may be raised about a particular group's composition, its deliberations, and its substantive recommendations.

Composition

Recall the "Appleton Consensus" (Stanley et al., 1989). One might reasonably ask whether a group consisting only of physicians, bioethicists, and economists has given adequate consideration to all relevant, reasonable views on questions of foregoing medical treatment. Were, for example, the possibly differing, reasonable viewpoints of patient-citizens, nurses, and allied health professionals given the same weight as those of the committee members? Were the committee members aware of, and capable of adequately representing, these other viewpoints? Consensus among members of a bioethics committee or commission has normative significance only if the group is broadly constituted. The group forming the Appleton Consensus, though it may in fact have identified and considered all reasonable positions, appears to fall short on this ground.

Yet it is one thing to urge that such groups be broadly constituted—having access to all relevant aspects of biomedical, social scientific, cultural/religious, legal, and bioethical expertise as well as knowledge of all reasonable ethical positions on matters that come before it—and quite another to actually constitute such a committee while retaining workable size. There is no mechanism or formula for putting together an effective, broadly constituted bioethics committee or commission. If, however, we are to attribute normative significance to any consensus it may reach, we must pay careful attention to the breadth of its membership (Fleetwood et al., 1989; Lo, 1987).

Deliberations

The deliberations of well-informed, broadly constituted committees or commissions may go wrong in a number of ways. First, such groups may be co-opted to serve the partisan interests of those who appoint them (Callahan, 1992). Second, the view of powerful or charismatic chairpersons, individual members, or subgroups may be given more weight than they deserve. Third, pressure to reach agreement may lead to avoiding controversial issues, underestimating risks and objections, ignoring unpopular or powerless viewpoints, failing to consider alternatives, failing to seek additional information, uncritically accepting secondhand information, or failing to exercise sufficient imagination or ingenuity in building consensus or devising compromise (Lo, 1987, p. 43). A problem endemic to committee deliberations is "groupthink," defined by Irving L. Janis as "a mode of thinking that people engage in when they are deeply involved in a cohesive in-group, when the members' strivings for unanimity override their motivation to realistically appraise alternative courses of action" (Janis, 1972, p. 9).

To be forewarned of these and other pitfalls of group dynamics is, however, to be forearmed. "Ethics committees that recognize the dangers of groupthink can," as Lo points out, "take steps to avoid them":

> First, committees can guard against premature agreement. The chairperson may explicitly ask that doubts and objections be expressed or may appoint members to make the case against the majority. Second, committees can scrutinize any secondhand information they receive. . . . Third, the committee can look for innovative ways to settle disputes [Lo, 1987, p. 48].

Recommendations

That a broadly constituted, well-informed ethics committee or commission has reached consensus on a particular recommendation is reason for giving serious, but not uncritical, attention to it. The presumption is that such multidisciplinary groups have examined all aspects of a bioethical question characterized by genuine uncertainty or reasonable disagreement and, after considering all reasonable alternatives, conscientiously come to informed, unforced agreement on the best position for institutional or social purposes. This is, however, only a presumption. Given the many ways in which a group's deliberations can go wrong, a morally autonomous individual must critically examine the group's reasoning before endorsing its conclusions.

CONCLUSION

Advances in medical knowledge and technology together with moral pluralism create a variety of bioethical questions about which we are genuinely uncertain or deeply divided. The problem is aggravated by the fact that the complexity of modern medicine requires close cooperation among members of a health care team, patients, and patients' families who may, as individuals, have differing, but not unreasonable, positions on bioethical issues. The question, then, is whether it is possible to obtain unforced, informed agreement on ethical issues requiring joint conduct among individuals who are either genuinely uncertain or committed to conflicting positions. The same is true, at the policy level, for hospitals and other health care institutions and for society as a whole.

In response, governments and health care institutions have turned for guidance to various more or less broadly constituted, multidisciplinary committees or commissions. At their best, such groups represent or have access to all relevant expert knowledge and moral perspectives. They strive to identify all reasonable moral positions and give them fair consideration. Avoiding "groupthink" and related pitfalls, the committee or commission may then come to informed, uncoerced agreement on what, for institutional or social purposes, is regarded by each member as the best (or most reasonable) answer to a certain question. Agreement may take the form of complete consensus, overlapping consensus, compromise, or endorsing the results of a vote.

The ultimate test of such a recommendation is whether it is specific enough to be of practical value and, at the same time, unable to be *reasonably* rejected by the larger population as the basis for informed, uncoerced agreement (Benjamin, 1989, Scanlon, 1982). These conditions, as indicated above, cannot always be satisfied. In such cases committees or commissions do better to identify difficulties and problems than to paper them over (Brody, 1989; Fleetwood et al., 1989; Macklin, 1988). In other cases, however, the deliberations and recommendations of a well-constituted ethics committee or commission may be able to meet these conditions. Both the Warnock Committee's recommendation on embryo research (Warnock, 1985b) and the UNOS Ethics Committee's recommendation on principles for organ allocation (Ethics Committee, 1992) seem to me to be sufficiently specific and, given the need for broad societal agreement, difficult for anyone to *reasonably* reject. These groups succeed, in part, because they explicitly acknowledge various conflicting positions, together with the need for reasonable agreement (Warnock, 1985a; Ethics Committee, 1992). More important than a committee's achieving consensus among its members is its ability to stimulate and guide the development of an informed, uncoerced agreement in the larger society. Broadly constituted groups that aim at this end may not always reach consensus. But when they do, it is more likely to be of genuine value.

NOTES

1. This should not be unfamiliar to bioethicists who can often construct both utilitarian and Kantian arguments for the same conclusion.

2. Toulmin himself might be reluctant to characterize such situations in terms of "overlapping consensus" or different principles leading to the same conclusion. He is prompted to question the value of principles in ethical reasoning: "So, by the end of my tenure with the Commission I had begun to suspect that the point of 'appealing to principles' was something quite else: not to give particular ethical judgments a more solid foundation, but rather to square the collective ethical conclusions of the Commission as a whole with each individual commissioner's other *non*ethical commitments."

3. There were, however, dissenters and a minority report on this issue in the case of the Warnock Committee.

4. The discrepancy between an individual's personal moral position and the compromise position he or she endorses as a member of the committee raises questions of personal integrity. I cannot pursue these questions here. Elsewhere I have argued that compromise may, in such circumstances, be integrity-preserving (Benjamin, 1990a, 1990b).

5. One must distinguish between the principle of utility and the Categorical Imperative, on the one hand, and utilitarian*ism* and Kantian*ism*, on the other. The principle of utility

and some form of the Categorical Imperative are likely to be part of any reasonable, comprehensive moral outlook. Utilitarianism and Kantianism, however, are particular comprehensive outlooks that derive or subordinate all other ethical considerations to the principle of utility and the Categorical Imperative, respectively.

6. "Members of the committee were purposely selected to represent diverse fields of expertise and varying perspectives. Physicians, ethicists, clergy, lawyers, transplant coordinators, nurses, patients, and individuals from other fields are included on the committee" (1991 Ethics Committee, 1992, p. 2226). I was a member of this committee.

7. This formulation draws on the contractualist criterion of moral justification developed by T. M. Scanlon (Scanlon, 1982).

REFERENCES

Abram, M. B., and Wolf, S. M.: 1984, "Public Involvement in Medical Ethics," *New England Journal of Medicine* 310, 627–32.

Arras, J. D.: 1984, "Retreat from the Right to Health Care: The President's Commission and Access to Health Care," *Cardozo Law Review* 6, 321–45.

Bayer, R.: 1984, "Ethics, Politics, and Access to Health Care," *Cardozo Law Review* 6, 303–20.

Benjamin, M.: 1989, "Value Conflicts in Organ Allocation," *Transplantation Proceedings*, 21, 3378–79.

Benjamin, M.: 1990a, *Splitting the Difference: Compromise and Integrity in Ethics and Politics*, University Press of Kansas, Lawrence, Kansas.

Benjamin, M.: 1990b, "Philosophical Integrity and Policy Development in Bioethics," *Journal of Medicine and Philosophy* 15: 375–89.

Brody, B. A.: 1989, "The President's Commission: The Need to be More Philosophical," *Journal of Medicine and Philosophy* 14: 369–83.

Callahan, D.: 1992, "Ethics Committees and Social Issues: Potentials and Pitfalls," *Cambridge Quarterly of Health Care Ethics* 1, 5–10.

Ethics Committee of the United Network on Organ Sharing: 1992, "General Principles for Allocating Human Organs and Tissues," *Transplantation Proceedings* 24: 2226–2235.

Fleetwood, J.E., Arnold, R.M., Baron, R.J.: 1989, "Giving Answers or Raising Questions?: The Problematic Role of Institutional Ethics Committees," *Journal of Medical Ethics* 15: 137–42.

Hampshire, S.: 1983, *Morality and Conflict*, Harvard University Press, Cambridge, MA.

Janis, Irving L.: 1972, *Victims of Groupthink*, Houghton Mifflin, Boston.

Lo, B.: 1987, "Behind Closed Doors: Promises and Pitfalls of Ethics Committees," *New England Journal of Medicine* 317: 46–50.

Luker, K.: 1984, *Abortion and the Politics of Motherhood*, University of California Press, Berkeley and Los Angeles.

Macklin, R.: 1988, "The Inner Workings of an Ethics Committee: Latest Battle over Jehovah's Witnesses," *Hastings Center Report* 18: 15–20.

Moreno, J. D.: 1990a, "What Means This Consensus? Ethics Committees and the Philosophic Tradition," *Journal of Clinical Ethics* 1: 38–43.

Moreno, J. D.: 1990b, "Getting to 'Maybe'," *Bioethics Books* 2: 41–43.

Rawls, J.: 1993, *Political Liberalism*, Columbia University Press, New York.

Scanlon, T. M.: 1982, "Contractualism and Utilitarianism," in Sen, A. and Williams, B.: 1982, *Utilitarianism and Beyond*, Cambridge University Press, Cambridge.

Sibley, W. M.: 1953, "The Rational Versus the Reasonable," *Philosophical Review* 62: 554–60.

Stanley, J. M. and 32 others: 1989, "The Appleton Consensus: Suggested International Guidelines for Decisions to Forego Medical Treatment," *Journal of Medical Ethics* 15: 129–36.

Toulmin, S. E.: 1981, "The Tyranny of Principles," *Hastings Center Report* 11:31–39.

Warnock, M.: 1985a, *A Question of Life: The Warnock Report on Fertilisation and Embryology*, Basil Blackwell, Oxford.

Warnock, M.: 1985b, "Moral Thinking and Government Policy: The Warnock Committee on Human Embryology," *Milbank Memorial Fund Quarterly* 63: 504–22.

Bioethics Commissions: What Can We Learn from Past Successes and Failures?

BRADFORD H. GRAY, Ph.D.

Professor, Institution for Social and Policy Studies, Yale University

Who will live and who will die? Who decides, and on what grounds? Are there certain characteristics—when "defining" life or setting the boundaries of permissible genetic experimentation—that are essential for "humanness"? In distributing risks and benefits, when should choices be left to the consciences of individuals and when should they be constrained collectively—by expert or lay groups, legislators, administrators, or judges? [From *Summing Up* (1983), the final report of the President's Commission for the Study of Ethical Problems in Medicine and Biomedical and Behavioral Research.]

Developments in biomedical and behavioral research, and changes in medical practice and the health care system, have raised many challenging ethical and policy problems in recent decades. Policymakers, the courts, scientists, medical practitioners, patients and their families, and the public at large have been presented with new dilemmas (and new versions of old problems) that involve conflicts between deeply held values. When faced with problems that involve such conflicts, factual disputes, or complicated technical issues, policymakers often create commissions (or turn to commission-like bodies at the Office of Technology Assessment and the Institute of Medicine) for advice.

The question of whether a new bioethics commission is needed is again on the policy agenda. The Office of Technology Assessment is nearing completion of a new report to Congress called "Biomedical Ethics in U.S. Public Policy." The Institute of Medicine's Committee on Social and Ethical Impacts of Developments in Biomedicine is also considering the question.

TABLE 1   Reports of the National Commission for the Protection of
Human Subjects of Biomedical and Behavioral Research and the
President's Commission for the Study of Ethical Problems in Medicine
and Biomedical and Behavioral Research

National Commission Reports	President's Commission Reports
Research on the Fetus, 1975	*Defining Death*, 1981
	Protecting Human Subjects, 1981
Research Involving Prisoners, 1976	
	Compensating for Research Injuries, 1982
Research Involving Children, 1977	*Making Health Care Decisions*, 1982
Psychosurgery, 1977	*Whistleblowing in Biomedical Research*, 1982
Disclosure of Research Information	
Under the Freedom of Information	*Deciding to Forego Life-Sustaining Treatment,*
Act, 1977	1983
	Implementing Human Research Regulations,
Research Involving Those Institutionalized	1983
as Mentally Infirm, 1978	*Screening and Counseling For Genetic*
Institutional Review Boards, 1978	*Conditions*, 1983
The Belmont Report, 1978	*Securing Access to Health Care*, 1983
Ethical Guidelines for the Delivery of	*Splicing Life*, 1983
Health Services by DHEW, 1978	*Summing Up*, 1983
The Special Study (Implications of	
Advances in Biomedical and Behavioral	
Research), 1978	

This paper is written at the request of the IOM committee, which asked for an analysis of the lessons to be learned from the experience of two earlier commissions that are both generally cited as successes[1]—The National Commission for the Protection of Human Subjects of Biomedical and Behavioral Research (the National Commission) and the President's Commission for the Study of Ethical Problems in Medicine and Biomedical and Behavioral Research (the President's Commission). The National Commission issued ten reports between 1975 and 1978; the President's Commission also issued ten reports (plus a summary report) between 1981 and 1983. (These reports are listed in Table 1.) This paper will explore the senses in which these two commissions were successful and the reasons behind their successes and failures.

WHAT MAKES A COMMISSION SUCCESSFUL?

The question of what makes a commission successful is far from straightforward.[2] A report that helps to break a policy impasse may be viewed as successful by advocates of one policy option and as a disaster by their opponents. Contemplating the same report, a philosopher or legal scholar might judge its success largely by the intellectual quality and rigor of its analysis, a matter that is distinct from its success as a political document. (*Defining Death* by the President's Commission is a case in point, having had a widespread impact on state laws while leaving some philosophers unsatisfied.) Although it is certainly fair to judge a report by the quality and weight of the evidence it assembles and logic of its analysis, a commission's influence may depend as much or more on its prestige[3] and the skill with which it attends to political considerations.

Even a report whose conclusions or recommendations are rejected in the political process might be considered a success if it becomes the starting point for future discussions of the topic. In terms of its legislative impact, the Commission on the Cost of Medical Care in 1930 failed. Nevertheless, its work is discussed in health policy circles to this day. (Indeed, its final report, *Medical Care for the American People* [1932], is still in print.) This suggests that the evaluation of a commission's success may depend not only on the criteria that one applies, but also upon one's time horizon. One report's "success" in resolving an issue may prove to be quite temporary, while another report's significance may grow over time.

None of this should be surprising. After all, commissions are established under many auspices for a great diversity of purposes—to marshal facts to explain an event, to assess the evidence on a controversial topic, to call attention to (or increase understanding of) a problem, to clarify policy options and make recommendations for action, or to substitute for action when politicians need to do something but cannot agree upon what. A commission may be created either to play up or play down an issue. All of these considerations create perplexing problems for the evaluator of "success." At the very least they suggest that different criteria might be applied to different commissions and to different reports.

THE TWO ETHICS COMMISSIONS

Table 2 summarizes the similarities and differences between the National Commission (1975-1978) and the President's Commission (1980-1983). Both were established legislatively to deal with ethical issues in research. Both sets of commissioners were selected through a process that reflected both substantive and political considerations. Appointees did not necessarily have expertise in the matters assigned to the commission, although some certainly did, and many had connections with key politicians.[4] Whether or not this is desirable—arguments can be made either way—it is probably inevitable, since officials responsible for appointments may pick particular individuals either as an expression of appreciation or respect or because their views on the issues are seen as congenial.

TABLE 2 Key differences between the National Commission and the President's Commission

National Commission	President's Commission
Was the first bioethics commission	Had National Commission as a model
Research involving human subjects was core mandate, but several other topics were involved	Research involving human subjects was one of several major responsibilities; commission had a more diverse mandate than the National Commission and had power to add topics to it
Eleven members appointed by Secretary, DHEW; law required them to be "to be distinguished in the fields of medicine, law, ethics, theology, the biological, physical, behavioral and social science, philosophy, humanities, health administration, government, and public affairs," with five (and no more than five) engaged in biomedical or behavioral research involving human subjects	Eleven members appointed by President; all to be distinguished—three in biomedical or behavioral research; three in medicine or provision of health care; and five in ethics, theology, law, the natural sciences, the social sciences, the humanities, health administration, government, and public affairs
Members served for life of commission; except for loss of two commissioners through death, no membership changes occurred	Commissioners appointed to two-, three-, or four-year terms, resulting in complications of changing commission membership; a total of 21 commissioners served
Located at NIH; achieved independence by discharging initial Executive Director, an NIH official	Independent agency
Budget negotiations internal to NIH, but budget limitations were not problematic and did not jeopardize commission's independence (though the potential was present)	Had annual budget authorization of $5 million; was subject to budget negotiations with OMB and through the congressional appropriations process; potential threat to commission's independence did not become a problem; total expenditures were less than $4 million
Staff director/initial staff selected by NIH official	Staff director selected by commission chair and hired other staff
Staff director served primarily management and quality-control functions	Staff director was key intellectual leader of the enterprise and primary author of several reports

TABLE 2 *Continued*

National Commission	President's Commission
Issued homely self-published reports available from the commission	Issued professionally designed, glossy reports through the U.S. Government Printing Office
Most staff did not begin as specialists in ethics	Many staff defined bioethics as their primary professional activity before working for the commission
Most staff served for the life of the commission and participated, to a greater or lesser extent, in the entire mandate (though most were identified primarily with particular topics)	Many staff worked only on particular reports and had little or no involvement with others
Commission created for 24 months, later extended by one year	Commission created for four years, later extended by three months

There were other similarities in the two commissions. The professional mix of commissioners was specified legislatively and included scientists, ethicists, lawyers, and others. Commissioners maintained their regular positions outside of government, while attending regular (usually monthly) commission meetings. Both commissions had full-time staffs, which prepared background materials and drafted reports, under the guidance of the commissions. Both staffs were headed by lawyers. In both instances the staff was a combination of full-time employees (some were long-term federal employees; others were hired from the outside), part-time employees, and consultants. Some staffers worked on numerous reports; others were specialized. In the aggregate, the commissioners and staff represented a complex mix of bureaucratic savvy, interest in law and ethics, concern to reform or defend the status quo, and political and academic values.

Both commissions held hearings, commissioned many papers, and sponsored major empirical studies.[5] Both were covered regularly by major newspapers and the trade press, and both issued ten reports, though the President's Commission also issued a very useful summary report.

The fact that each commission issued many reports provides an opportunity to understand better the complicated nature of commission success. As we will see, neither commission was uniformly successful across all of its reports.

There were also many differences between the two commissions. These differences pertained to the crucially important matters of mandate and the role of commissioners and staff.

The Commissions' Mandates

The National Commission's core focus was clearly on ethical issues in research involving human subjects. It was directed to issue reports on four types of subject populations (the fetus, children, the institutionalized mentally infirm, and prisoners), on institutional review boards that review the ethical acceptability of proposed research, and on the basic ethical principles that should underlie research involving human subjects. However, the National Commission was also asked to report on several other topics: psychosurgery, ethical issues in DHEW-supported health services programs, and the applicability of the Freedom of Information Act to research proposals submitted to NIH. Finally, the commission's mandate included Senator Walter Mondale's idea for a "Special Study" of the implications of new developments in biomedical and behavioral research.

The President's Commission had a more diverse mandate, which eventually included almost every burning bioethical issue (except abortion itself) on the policy horizon. Certain topics were assigned to the commission by the legislation that created it: informed consent in research and medicine, the definition of death (particularly for patients whose brain function had ceased but whose other major organ systems were still operating, often with mechanical assistance), genetic testing and counseling, differences in access to health services, and issues of privacy in research and medicine. It was also directed to report biennially on the adequacy of federal policies (and their implementation) for protection of human subjects. In addition, the authorizing statute gave the commission the mandate to "undertake an investigation or study of any other appropriate matter which relates to medicine or biomedical or behavioral research . . . and which is consistent with the purposes of [the legislation]." As a result, the commission studied and issued reports on genetic engineering in humans (at the request of the White House), compensation for injuries to research subjects, and decision making for terminally-ill patients and seriously defective newborns. Significantly, as we shall see, this last topic, undertaken on the commission's own initiative, became the commission's most successful report.

The Roles of Commissioners and Staff

The commissions also differed with regard to bureaucratic location, who appointed the commissioners, and the ways the chairs and staff were selected. These differences, in turn, help account for some more subtle differences in the functioning of the two bodies. Both of these commissions issued reports that were innovative, well-documented, carefully argued, persuasive, and influential. But the relative strengths of the membership and staff of the two commissions were quite different from each other. The strength of the National Commission lay in its membership and chair. The President's Commission's strength lay in its staff.

The difference between the commissions was not a simple matter of credentials and intellectual strengths of their members. Like the National Commission, the President's Commission had distinguished members, particularly the original set of appointees. The differences lay in other areas.

The National Commission's membership strength came from several factors. The first was its commitment and continuity. The commission had the same membership, except for the death of two members who were not replaced, throughout its existence. With its first report—on fetal research—due four months after the members were installed, the National Commission established a pattern of meeting monthly on a Friday and Saturday. Under time pressure and with considerable attention from national media and trade publications (meetings were public), the commissioners struggled intensively to find ways to reconcile their differences, particularly their deep moral division over the abortion issue. They held hearings, commissioned and discussed background papers, and had extended, passionate deliberations.

The divisiveness of the issues and the differences between the commissioners—not only regarding abortion but also in their professional backgrounds (ranging from the chairman of obstetrics/gynecology at Harvard, Kenneth Ryan, to deeply anti-abortion law professor, David Louisell)—could have destroyed the possibility of respectful working relations among the commissioners. The chemistry worked in another way, however, and the pattern was established of members taking each other's views very seriously and seeking common ground on which to base recommendations. (Also contributing to the working relationships among commissioners and staff was a practice, established at the very beginning, of a social occasion or dinner on the Friday night of the commission's two-day meeting. Bonds and a group history developed that would be hard to match.)

One other early development in the National Commission's life set the tone for the relative roles of the commission itself and its staff. Under the legislation that created the commission—the National Research Act of 1974—members were appointed by the Secretary of Health, Education, and Welfare and the commission was located administratively in the National Institutes of Health, even though several of the topics assigned to the commission fell outside of NIH's jurisdiction. NIH appointed Charles U. Lowe, M.D., a career employee, as executive director, and he hired the staff director and staff, which included two members of his own staff. Lowe took an active role in managing the work of the staff and the perception grew that there was a conflict between his role as an NIH official and the commission's need to independently examine ethical issues in NIH-sponsored research. The tensions grew quickly in the first few months of the commission's life and culminated in the commission's decision to request Dr. Lowe's resignation.

These events dispelled any doubt regarding whether the enterprise belonged to the commission or the staff, and left the staff in the hands of staff director Michael Yesley, a career government lawyer who had been hired from the Department of Commerce. Yesley devoted himself to making sure that the staff was doing what the commission wanted. An important, regular staff responsibility was to convert the commission's discussions into draft material—the meeting transcripts that arrived in the staff office a few days after the meeting were reviewed very closely for guidance—that would be mailed ten days before the next monthly meeting. (The staff also engaged in many other activities, such as commissioning background papers requested by the commission, organizing hearings and site visits, and planning and overseeing empirical research in support of the commission's deliberations.)

All of this contrasted with the President's Commission. The President's Commission experienced enormous turnover of membership. Two of its initial 11 members had to be replaced during the first year because the enabling legislation did not allow federal employees to be members, and another was replaced the next year. Then, in 1992, eight of 11 commissioners were replaced in the last year of the commission's life as a result of the law's provision for a rotating membership and the election of Ronald Reagan. Thus, while a total of 11 individuals served on the 11-member National Commission, 21 individuals served on the 11-member President's Commission. Only three members of the President's Commission, including its chairman, served throughout the commission's life.

The President's Commission had no experiences parallel to the National Commission's intensive first few months on the topic of fetal research (the President's Commission's first report, *Defining Death*, was issued two years after the commission was appointed) or the National Commission's frequent social occasions. As one staffer noted, there was never a "family" feeling within the President's Commission.

There were also leadership contrasts. The National Commission's chair, Kenneth Ryan, M.D., was elected chair by the commission itself at its first meeting. He was the commission's own designated leader. As a physician and researcher from a prestigious institution (chairman of obstetrics/gynecology at Harvard Medical School and chief of staff at Boston Hospital for Women), he was able to speak with authority on the core topics in the commission's mandate. Ryan had extensive experience with many of the issues considered by the commission and was the clear leader of the entire enterprise through the commission's life.

By contrast, the chair of the President's Commission was appointed.

Although Morris Abram's appointment by the President unquestionably carried enormous prestige, it was understood that the appointment was a reflection of President Carter's gratitude for Abram's role in Carter's election. Abram's most pertinent experiences were as a patient who had received experimental treatments for a potentially fatal disease. Although this was valuable on certain topics (particularly those addressed in the report *Making Health Care Decisions*), Abram was essentially an informed layperson on most of the issues addressed by the commission. Perhaps in recognition of this, he selected a staff director, Alexander Capron, who was a nationally recognized expert on legal and ethical issues in medicine and science and who had published books and articles on many of the topics that were taken up by the commission. Abram worked closely with Capron for guidance about how the commission should address the issues on its agenda and was relatively distant from both the staff and other members of the commission. Capron, in turn, hired a strong staff made up primarily of professionals who had made career commitments (in law, philosophy, sociology, and medicine) to the issues on the commission's agenda. Individually and as a group, the President's Commission's staff probably had stronger professional credentials than did the commission itself.

So, the National Commission's staff was dominated by career governmental employees for whom the staff role was already familiar. The President's Commission staff was dominated by people from outside of government who identified primarily with their fields of professional activity and disciplinary work. As was evident in my survey in 1993, they continue to evaluate the President's Commission's reports primarily in terms of its scholarly quality. The National Commission was clearly more interested in finding a set of recommendations that they could agree upon than in laying out a rigorous line of reasoning regarding how they got there.

METHODS OF THIS INQUIRY

What does it mean when the National Commission and the President's Commission are said to have been successful? And how and why did this success vary across their various reports? I approached these questions by using objective measures of influence as well as seeking the views of former members and staff of the two commissions. For each commission, the major variable across reports was the topics themselves.[6] I sought lessons about the success of these two commissions by seeking to understand the differences in impact from report to report.

Two methods were used. The first involved searches of on-line databases (Nexis, Lexis, and Medline) for citations to the reports of each commission. The second involved a survey of former members and staffers of the two commissions to obtain their assessments of their work and of differences in the success of the reports issued by their commission. (I should note that I served on the staff of the National Commission and was a long-term consultant to the President's Commission. My views about the two commissions and their reports are not among those reported later in this paper, but my experiences no doubt influence my interpretations.)

Citations to Commission Reports

In April and May of 1993, searches were done of pertinent databases for citations to the two commissions and their reports. Table 3 shows citations to both commissions in the news media covered in the Nexis on-line service. Table 3A shows cites to the two commissions in the National Library of Medicine's Bioethicsline database. It snows a similar number of cites for the two commissions. Tables 4, 5, and 6 respectively, show citations to each National Commission report in court cases and the *Federal Register*,[7] medical journals (including the ethics journals included in the National Library of Medicine's Medline database), and law reviews. Tables 7, 8, and 9 have similar tables for the President's Commission's reports. Unlike the Nexis and legal databases, the Medline data base does not contain the full text of articles; the searches reported in Tables 5 and 8 report only mentions of the two commissions in the titles or abstracts of articles, not in the text or footnotes of the articles. Thus, the data provide

TABLE 3 Number of Citations in News Database (Nexis Omni) to the Two Commissions, Through 1992

National Commission: 57
President's Commission: 238

NOTE: The impact of the National Commission is *substantially* undercounted here because this database did not exist until five years after the National Commission began. These data are presented for information only.

TABLE 3A Citations to Both Commissions in National Library of Medicine's BIOETHICSLINE Database, Through 1992

	News and Scholarly Articles and Books	All Citations*
National Commission	177	235
President's Commission	171	214

*Includes such items as commission reports and publications, meeting transcripts, and *Federal Register* notices of proposed and final regulations.

TABLE 4 Citations to the **National Commission** in Court Cases (Lexis—GenFed Mega search) and in the *Federal Register* (Lexis—GenFed Allreg search), 1981–1992

Name of Report	Cites in Court Cases	Cites in *Federal Register* (regulations)	Total
Research on Fetus	3		3
Research Involving Prisoners		6	6
Research Involving Children		1	1
Psychosurgery		1	1
Disclosure of Research Information Under Freedom of Information Act	1		1
Research Involving Institutionalized Mentally Infirm			
Institutional Review Boards		4	4
The Belmont Report		2	2
Ethical Guidelines for Delivery of Health Services by DHEW			
The Special Study on Implications of Advances in Biomedical and Behavioral Research			
*Swine Flu Consent Review**	6		6
Cites to the commission itself	1		1
Total	11	14	25

NOTE: The Lexis data base does not begin until 1981, three years after the last National Commission Report was issued.

*Under the legislation that indemnified manufacturers of swine flu vaccine in 1976, the commission reviewed the consent forms prepared by the Centers for Disease Control for the Swine Flu Program. This activity did not result in a published report.

an indication of the relative frequency of articles about reports of the two commissions, but this approach is far from a full measure of the impact of these reports on the scholarly and scientific literature.

A further caveat about these tables is needed. Except for the Bioethics line (Table 3A), these tables should *not* be interpreted as comparing the two commissions' impact. *The other databases did not come into existence until several years after the National Commission's reports were issued and so do not capture the initial responses to the National Commission's work.* This is important because commission reports generally receive the most intense attention while reports are being prepared and immediately after publication. The value of these tables is in the comparison *across each commission's reports.* The data in the tables are a much more complete indicator of the President's Commission's impact than the National Commission's. Even so,

TABLE 5   Citations to **National Commission** in Medical Journal Databases (Lexis—GenMed—and National Library of Medicine's Medline)*

Name of Report	1975–1989	1990–Present	Total
Research on Fetus	7		7
Research Involving Prisoners	2		2
Research Involving Children	6	1	7
Psychosurgery	3		3
Disclosure of Research Information Under Freedom of Information Act			
Research Involving Institutionalized Mentally Infirm	4		4
Institutional Review Boards	6		6
The Belmont Report	11	3	14
Ethical Guidelines for Delivery of Health Services by DHEW			
The Special Study on Implications of Advances in Biomedical and Behavioral Research			
Cites to the commission itself	12	1	13
Commission cited as identifier of an individual	2		2
Total	53	5	58

*Possible duplicate cites to particular articles have not been eliminated. *Federal Register* cites have been removed. These databases include the *Hastings Center Report*, where many of the cites appear.

the tables do not convey the full impact of even the President's Commission's reports; for example, state legislation is not covered, an omission that particularly understates the influence of the President's Commission's report *Defining Death*, which had a widespread impact on state law.

Cites to National Commission Reports

Table 4 shows cites in the courts and in regulatory activity. Much of the regulatory activity involving National Commission reports was over by the time the Lexis service began coverage of the *Federal Register*. There had already been considerable activity regarding *Research on the Fetus, Research Involving Children, Research Involving Those Institutionalized as Mentally Infirm* (proposed regulations that were never adopted), and *Institutional Review Boards*. Table 4 really shows the end of a substantial period of activity. *Research on the Fetus* was cited in a handful of court cases in the 1980s, but, ironically, the most frequent court reference to the National Commission was on a topic that it did not do a report on at all—the swine flu program.[8]

In medical journals (Table 5), the most frequently cited National Commission reports are *The Belmont Report* (on the ethical principles that should underlie research involving human subjects), *Research on the Fetus, Children, Institutional Review Boards, Those Institutionalized as Mentally Infirm, Psychosurgery,* and *Research Involving Prisoners,* in that order. The other three reports were not cited.

Law review citations (Table 6) were concentrated on *Research on the Fetus* and the *Belmont Report,* with *Children, Prisoners,* and *Psychosurgery* each being cited once or twice. The other five reports were not cited in the law review literature.

In sum, the citation data suggest that the most influential reports of the National Commission were *Research on the Fetus* and *The Belmont Report,* with *Children, Institutional Review Boards,* the *Mentally Infirm, Prisoners,* and *Psychosurgery* following in roughly that order. Three reports appeared to have been completely ignored—they "sank like a rock," in the words of a former staff member. They were *Disclosure of Information under the Freedom of Information Act, Ethical Guidelines for the Delivery of Services by the Department of*

TABLE 6 Law Review Citations to **National Commission** Reports, 1981 to Present (Lexis—Lawrev search)

Name of Report	1981–1989	1990–Present	Total
Research on Fetus	10	4	14
Research Involving Prisoners	2		2
Research Involving Children	1	1	2
Psychosurgery	1		1
Disclosure of Research Information Under Freedom of Information Act			
Research Involving Institutionalized Mentally Infirm	1		
Institutional Review Boards			
The Belmont Report	5	4	9
Ethical Guidelines for Delivery of Health Services by DHEW			
The Special Study on Implications of Advances in Biomedical and Behavioral Research			
Cites to the commission itself	2		2
Commission cited as identifier of an individual	2		2
Total	24	9	33

Health, Education and Welfare, and *The Special Study: Implications of Advances in Biomedical and Behavioral Research.*

Cites to President's Commission Reports

The number of citations to President's Commission reports was much larger in both the mass media (Table 3) and in the courts and scholarly literature (in part because of the dates covered by the database, as discussed above). However, variation across reports appears again, in even more pronounced fashion. *Deciding to Forego Life-Sustaining Treatment* was the most frequently cited report in the courts (Table 7), including three Supreme Court citations[9] and many other prominent cases. *Defining Death* and *Making Health Care Decisions* were also used in several cases. (The main impact of *Defining Death* was on state laws.) The other seven President's Commission reports were cited only once or not at all in a court case.

Cites in the *Federal Register* (Table 7) were concentrated on one report—*Protecting Human Subjects* (1981)—and stemmed from a single commission recommendation: that there be uniform regulations for human subjects' protection across all federal agencies. (Despite this objective measure of impact, it apparently was not a matter about which the commission took much satisfaction, as indicated by their responses—presented

TABLE 7 Citations to the **President's Commission** in Court Cases (Lexis—GenFed Mega search) and in the *Federal Register* (Lexis—Genfed Allreg search), 1981–1993

Name of Report	Cites in Court Cases	Cites in Federal Register (regulations)	Total
Defining Death	7		7
Protecting Human Subjects		37	37
Compensating for Research Injuries	1		1
Making Health Care Decisions	7	3	10
Whistleblowing in Biomedical Research			
Deciding to Forego Life-Sustaining Treatment	36	5	41
Implementing Human Research Regulations			
Screening and Counseling for Genetic Conditions	1		1
Securing Access to Health Care			
Splicing Life		11	11
Total	52	56	108

TABLE 8 Citations to **President's Commission** in Medical Journal Databases (Lexis—GenMed—and National Library of Medicine's MedLine)*

Name of Report	1980–1989	1990–Present	Total
Defining Death	42	8	50
Protecting Human Subjects	2		2
Compensating for Research Injuries	1		1
Making Health Care Decisions	20	14	34
Whistleblowing in Biomedical Research			
Deciding to Forego Life-Sustaining			
Treatment	72	30	105
Implementing Human Research			
Regulations	2		2
Screening and Counseling for			
Genetic Conditions	5	3	8
Securing Access to Health Care	10	11	21
Splicing Life			
Summing Up	2		2
Cites to commission itself	7		7
Commission cited as identifier			
of individual	5		5
Report not identifiable	9	1	10
Total	177	67	247

*Possible duplicate cites to particular articles have not been eliminated. *Federal Register* cites have been removed. These databases include the *Hastings Center Report*, where many of the cites appear.

later—regarding the impact of their work. *Protecting Human Subjects* was hardly mentioned, perhaps because the recommendation in question was reached easily and involved no issues with ethical bite.) *Splicing Life* also appeared several times in the *Federal Register* as NIH established the Human Gene Therapy Subcommittee of the Recombinant DNA Advisory Committee, but most commission reports were in little or no evidence in the federal government's outlet for announcing regulatory activity.

The databases on medical journals (Table 8) showed almost 250 references to President's Commission reports. More than 40 percent were accounted for by one report, *Deciding to Forego Life-Sustaining Treatment.* There were also numerous cites to *Defining Death, Making Health Care Decisions*, and *Securing Access to Health Care,* with other reports cited fewer than ten times.

Deciding to Forego also accounted for 40 percent of the cites in the law review literature (Table 9). Citations thereafter were more broadly dis-

TABLE 9 Citations to **President's Commission** in Law Reviews, 1983 to Present (Lexis—Allrev search)

Name of Report	1983–1989	1990–Present	Total
Defining Death	4	9	13
Protecting Human Subjects			
Compensating for Research Injuries	1		1
Making Health Care Decisions	21	10	31
Whistleblowing in Biomedical Research			
Deciding to Forego Life-Sustaining Treatment	40	31	71
Implementing Human Research Regulations			
Screening and Counseling for Genetic Conditions	6	6	12
Securing Access to Health Care	13	9	22
Splicing Life	5	10	15
Summing Up		1	1
Cites to commission itself	2		2
Commission as identifier to individual	6	1	7
Report not identified		1	1
Testimony at hearings	1		1
Total	99	78	177

persed, with *Making Health Care Decisions, Securing Access, Splicing Life, Defining Death,* and *Genetic Screening* all having at least a dozen cites.

In sum, as with the National Commission's reports, there is striking variability in citations across President's Commission reports. *Deciding to Forego Life-Sustaining Treatment* is in a class by itself as an influential document, but there are also frequent citations to several other reports. *Making Health Care Decisions, Defining Death,* and *Securing Access to Health Care* were in a middle group, with *Genetic Screening* and *Splicing Life* also receiving important attention. The other four reports—*Compensating for Research Injuries, Protecting Human Subjects, Implementing Human Research Regulations,* and *Whistleblowing in Biomedical Research*—received almost no scholarly attention. *Protecting Human Subjects,* however, was a "citation classic" in the *Federal Register.*

Views of Members and Staff

To explore the reasons behind these differences in the impact of the reports of the two commissions, let us turn to the views of former members and staffers of the two bodies. In the Spring of 1993 I sent a questionnaire to former members of both commissions and to professional staff members who had played a major role in drafting commission reports. I received responses from six of nine living members of the National Commission (another wrote to offer to respond orally) and from six of the seven former staff members to which questionnaires had been sent. From the President's Commission, only five of 18 former members to whom the questionnaire was sent returned it, as did nine of 12 former staffers who were surveyed. The minimal response from former members of the President's Commission is consistent with an important difference between the two commissions—the extent to which the commission, rather than the staff, took primary ownership of the process.

Some questions concerned the respondents' own involvement with the various topics addressed by their commission and their assessment of the impact of their commission's reports and the process that produced it. In this regard, they were asked first about which reports had a "critical impact on public policy in the U.S.," which ones had a "significant impact on thought in the field of bioethics," and which ones had gone "on the shelf [to] collect dust." Then they were asked two pages of questions about *each* report. These questions asked them to evaluate their commission's deliberations (how serious and contentious they were and how difficult the intellectual challenge); to evaluate their own investment in each report; to evaluate each report's success, including the ways and reasons that each report succeeded and did not succeed. They were also asked a set of fixed-response questions on factors that affected each report, on different parties' interest in the topics, and on different types of impact.

In this paper, staff and members' responses are presented together; only notable differences will be mentioned. Numbers are small and not all respondents responded to all questions, so responses should be treated accordingly. Some staff did not respond to questions about reports on which they played little or no role; this increased the rate of item non-responses. Nevertheless a reasonably clear picture emerges of how former members and staff defined success and failure of reports and their explanations for both.

Responses are shown in Table 10 (National Commission) and 11 (President's Commission). Broadly speaking, four general types of reports' success were mentioned:

- Characteristics of the report itself—its clarity, the quality of the analysis, the information and data it contained, and so forth;
- Impact on the broader debate and future thinking on the topic, including in the field of bioethics;
- Impact on the behavior of researchers, physicians, or medical institutions;
- Impact on law (judicial decisions or statutes) and regulations.

TABLE 10   Terms in which Respondents Described Various Reports of the **National Commission** as Having Been Successful or Unsuccessful. Open-ended Responses from Survey of Former Members and Staff of the National Commission, Spring 1993

Measures of Success	Measures of Failure
Gathered new and sometimes unexpected data	Lack of intellectual bite; boring; too bland
Exposed facts; provided information; focused debate	Broke no new ground
Provided a model of clear and logical ethical analysis (e.g. *Children*); clear enunciation of issues	A few point left open to multiple interpretations
Clarified issues and key matters (e.g., "therapeutic research"; differences between physicians' and researchers' roles; differentiated scientific and ethical issues)	Recommendations not supported by evidence (e.g., *Prisoners*)
Demythification of some issues (e.g., the nature of fetal research)	Recommendation may have been to restrictive
Provided new concepts/distinctions (e.g., consent/assent in *Children*)	Did not influence professional decisions
Broke new ethical ground	"Sank like a rock"
Shaped subsequent thinking	Not implemented in regulations
Impact on field of bioethics and teaching therein	Did not change public policy
Provided guidance for researchers or IRBS; influenced the affected parties	Failed to permanently resolve a disputed area of policy (e.g., *Fetal Research*)
Buttressed or codified an existing system (e.g., IRBS)	
Report was understood and accepted in the research community	
Changed practices that some commissioners disapproved of (psychosurgery; research on prisoners; nontherapeutic research on children were all cited)	
Provided at least partial or temporary resolution for policy disputes, allowing research to proceed	
Recommendations were implemented in regulations	

TABLE 11 Terms by which Reports of the **President's Commission**
Were Described as a Success and as Having Not Succeeded. Open-ended
Responses from Survey of Members and Staff of President's Commission,
1993

Terms Describing Success	Terms Describing Lack of Success
Raised awareness of significance of a problem (examples mentioned ranged from cites in the literature to Congressional hearings)	Report lacked guts (*Securing Access*); was too timid re medical profession (*Decisions to Forego*); recommendations had little "bite" (*Genetic Screening*)
Good data collection and new empirical information	Recommendations were indecisive (*Compensating Research Injuries*)
Important compilation of data on issue (e.g., *Securing Access*)	Report did not deal well with certain issues
Opened new avenues of discussion; framed future discussions; clarified issues; conceptual impact; provided good overview of problem	Arguments in support of certain conclusions were weak or flawed (e.g., in *Defining Death*)
Achieved consensus, and helped build wider consensus on complex ethical issue and provided basis on which future debate can take place	Report has been largely ignored and has had little impact on practice (*Making Health Care Decisions*)
Resolved some contentious issues; shaped public policy	Recommendations not implemented
Provided authoritative crystallization of work in field; provided groundwork for subsequent policymaking	
Highly influential on professional thinking and public discourse; background effect on medical education	
Demonstrated need for and usefulness of IRB site visits by knowledgeable people	
Became standard citation on issue; frequent and/or continued citation	
Became the model (the "Bible") for decision making in care of terminally ill nationally (*Deciding to Forego*)	
Major impact on institutional policy; influence on consent forms	
Impact on ethics committees	
Major impact on law; provided rationale accepted by legislators, courts, and policy makers; highly influential on court decisions and statutory law (*Deciding to Forego*); accelerated statutory uniformity (*Defining Death*); became standard citation in law and hospital policy	

The terms in which failures were described were by-and-large mirror images of these.

Although the success/failure categories were similar for the two commissions, more examples of characteristics of reports and types of impacts were mentioned by respondents from the President's Commission. This may be due to the President's Commission's broader mandate, but it may also reflect greater diversity within the staff.

The multiple dimensions of success create the possibility, already alluded to, that a report could be a success in some terms and a failure in others. We will return to this point.

WHICH REPORTS SUCCEEDED AND WHICH FAILED?

The National Commission's Reports

Based on the views of former members and staff of the National Commission, its reports can be divided into three categories—successful ones (4), partially successful ones (3), and unsuccessful ones (3). Responses to open-ended questions about which reports had an impact on public policy, which influenced the field of bioethics, and which had gone on to collect dust are shown in Table 12. Responses to questions that asked for success ratings for each individual report are shown in Table 13.

The Successes

Four reports were identified by most respondents as having had a critical impact on public policy and/or a significant impact on the field of bioethics: *The Belmont Report,* which identified the basic ethical principles that should underlie the conduct of research involving human subjects; *Research on the Fetus* and *Research Involving Children,* which defined the boundaries on ethically permissible research involving these two categories; and *Institutional Review Boards,* which examined the primary mechanism for protecting the rights and welfare of human subjects. (Although half of the respondents saw *Research Involving Prisoners* as having had a significant impact on public policy, they did not all agree that this impact was beneficial.) These same reports were also evaluated most favorably on the fixed-response question regarding the success of individual reports.

Interestingly, though these reports all dealt with issues at the core of the Commission's congressional mandate, they are of quite different natures. *Fetus and Children* defined what types of research could be ethically supported by the federal government; to reach its recommendations, commissioners had to find their way through some fundamental ethical conflicts among themselves. *Belmont* did not have direct regulatory applicabil-

TABLE 12 National Commission Reports Identified as: (a) Having Had a Critical Impact on Public Policy, (b) Having Had a Significant Impact on Thought in the Field of Bioethics, and (c) Having Gone on the Shelf to Collect Dust. Open-ended Responses from Survey of Former Members and Staff of the National Commission, Spring 1993

Name of Report	Number of Respondents Offering each Assessment		
	Report Had Critical Impact on Public Policy	Report Had Significant Impact on Bioethics	Reports that Are Collecting Dust
Research on Fetus	11	2	1
Research Involving Prisoners	6	0	0
Research Involving Children	7	3	0
Psychosurgery	4	1	7
Disclosure of Research Information under Freedom of Information Act	2	0	6
Research Involving Institutionalized Mentally Infirm	2	0	4
Institutional Review Boards	10	4	0
The Belmont Report	9	12	0
Ethical Guidelines for Delivery of Health Services by DHEW	0	0	10
The Special Study on Implications of Advances in Biomedical and Behavioral Research	0	0	8

TABLE 13 Respondents' Evaluations of Whether Individual Reports of the **National Commission** Were (a) Very Successful, (b) Partially or Somewhat Successful, or (c) Largely or Wholly Unsuccessful. Fixed-response Items from Survey of Former Members and Staff of the National Commission, 1993

Name of Report	Number of Respondents Offering each Assessment			
	Very Successful	Partially Successful	Largely/Wholly Unsuccessful	No Response
Research on the Fetus	7	5	0	0
Research Involving Prisoners	5	2	0	0
Research Involving Children	9	2	0	1
Psychosurgery	1	4	4	2
Disclosure of Research Information	1	4	2	5
Research Involving Institutionalized Mentally Infirm	2	6	3	1
Institutional Review Boards	9	1	0	2
The Belmont Report	10	1	0	1
Ethical Guidelines for Health Services	1	1	4	4
Special Study	1	3	5	3

Note: One commissioner found all reports successful; one responded only to the first question. Non-responses often meant no recollection.

ity (as did the reports on subject populations); the identification of the ethical principles that should underlie research was primarily an intellectual challenge that commissioners (and their staff and consultants) grappled with together. *Institutional Review Boards* evaluated an existing regulatory mechanism for protecting human subjects and made recommendations for improvements; matters of fundamental disagreements over ethics were not involved.

Descriptions of these reports' impact reflect these differences. Respondents pointed to the impact of *Fetus* in lifting a congressional ban on research, on regulations, and on future debate on the topic. On *Children*, they pointed to the regulatory impact, acceptance by the research community, and the impact on research, as well as the clarity and logic of the report's analysis. On *IRBs*, they cited the regulatory impact and the reinforcement of the existing system. On *Belmont*, they cited the report's importance in providing principles for use by IRBs and in influencing the field of bioethics. (The impact of *Belmont* was so substantial that some respondents were actually troubled that the three basic principles identified in the report—beneficence, respect for persons, and justice—had become an uncritically used "mantra," in the words of one respondent.)

The Mixed Cases

The reports *Research Involving Those Institutionalized as Mentally Infirm, Research Involving Prisoners*, and *Psychosurgery* were viewed in more complicated terms. Most respondents believed that these reports (with the partial exception of *Prisoners*) had been well done—with good evidence and ethical analyses. In addition, several respondents in each case perceived an impact on public policy; in the latter two reports, the perceived impact was primarily negative—the ending of research involving prisoners and a discouraging impact on psychosurgery. (Not all respondents agreed that these had been good policy impacts.) Several respondents saw *Mentally Infirm* and *Psychosurgery* as only gathering dust. At least half of the respondents saw both *Mentally Infirm* and *Prisoners* as at least partially successful, though only three judged *Psychosurgery* so favorably.

Why were these reports viewed as failures by some? The *Mentally Infirm* report was seen as a failure because the recommendations (which respondents still viewed as sound) were never implemented in regulations. Simply put, a report that made recommendations for regulatory change could not be deemed a success if those recommendations had largely been ignored. Some also believed the report had suffered because of the legislative mandate's focus on the *institutionalized* mentally infirm, which gave the report a peculiar emphasis in an era of deinstitutionalization. Moreover, the commission's administrative location in NIH seemed anomalous for this topic since most funding for research on this population came from other federal agencies (particularly the National Institute of Mental Health).

Criticism of *Prisoners* focused largely on its lack of impact and the quality of the report (illogical, excessively paternalistic, unoriginal; a well-intentioned but unrealistic attempt at prison reform). Moreover, this was also a topic of little relevance to NIH and the Public Health Service regulations for protection of human subjects, since most research involving prisoners was being financed and performed by pharmaceutical companies or by other federal agencies and were thus not subject to those regulations.

Psychosurgery was seen as a partial failure because of a lack of impact on either public policy or professional decisions. Although this topic had been included in the commission's mandate, it was nevertheless seen as having been outside the commission's primary expertise (as practice rather than research). Accordingly, some respondents believed that the commission's views were not regarded as authoritative.

The Failures

Former members and staff of the National Commission saw three of its reports as failures. (Indeed, several respondents had difficulty discussing these reports because they were gone from the memory bank.) *Disclosure of Research Information* dealt with whether research proposals submitted to NIH should be available to the public (including competing researchers) under the Freedom of Information Act. In *Ethical Guidelines for the Delivery of Health Services by DHEW* the commission attempted to apply the principles developed in *The Belmont Report* to health services delivery programs. In preparing *The Special Study* of the "*Implications of Advances in Biomedical and Behavioral Research,*" the commission relied heavily on a Delphi study— a method viewed skeptically by the staff director and several commissioners—by a contractor that had little contact with the commission. Although a thick volume was published, the commission's report made up only the first ten pages; the remainder was appendices.

A common characteristic of the failures was their periphery to the commission's core concern about the ethics of research involving human subjects. (In the view of some, this was also true of *Psychosurgery* because the topic was one of medical practice and therefore a matter for clinical research and medical consensus rather than for a commission concerned with research ethics.) Many respondents noted these topics' lack of centrality to the commission's mandate in explaining why these reports had not been successes. Responses to my questions about their personal investment in the various reports showed that these topics did not engage commissioners nearly as much as did the subject populations, *Belmont,* and *IRBs.* They observed that these topics were not seen as major agenda items, that the commission lacked expertise and/or moral authority regarding them, and that these topics had no direct connection with regulations and NIH's responsibilities, as did the core mandates. Even the location of the commission in NIH was seen as inappropriate by some on such topics.[10]

The National Commission's failures point to an important aspect of commissions. An existing study commission—or a legislative vehicle that is going to create one—tends to attract topics, much as certain types of legislation become Christmas trees for different legislators' pet projects. In some cases, topics added to a commission's legislative mandate through such processes have little to do with the rest of the commission's mandate. What happens then may depend on whether influential commissioners or key staff members take a keen interest. Topics need champions, even if assigned to a study commission by Congress or the White House.

As we shall see, some topics addressed in partly successful reports of the President's Commission were added after it was created; in each case, the topic was of great interest to the executive director and key staffers. However, in the case of the National Commission, neither commissioners nor the staff director had much interest in the topics outside of the commission's core concerns with research involving human subjects. Even the appointments to the commission reflected its core duties. Those who were responsible for appointing members of the National Commission seemed to have in mind only its responsibilities in the areas of fetal research, research involving children, and research involving the mentally infirm; none of the appointees had particular expertise or interest in the topics of the reports that became failures.

For a member-driven (as opposed to a staff-driven) commission, the lack of commissioner interest in a topic almost guarantees that any report will be cursory, superficial, and likely to gather dust. Of course, this is not necessarily incompatible with the intentions of those who assigned the topic to the commission, since this is a convenient, painless way for a legislature or agency to deal with a prickly or unwelcome topic.

The President's Commission's Reports

Like the National Commission, the President's Commission issued ten reports which its members and staff view in retrospect as of variable success.[11] Based on responses shown in Tables 14 and 15, only one report can be classified as a clear success; five were partial successes; and four were dust collectors, even if not outright failures.

The Successes

From the perspective of 1993, the commissioners and staff members who completed my survey viewed only one report—*Decisions to Forego Life-Sustaining Treatment*—as an unambiguous success in terms of having both "critical impact on public policy" and "significant impact on bioethics" (Table 14), as well as having been "very successful" (Table 15). All types of success were mentioned. Regarding the report's qualities, respondents pointed to its clarity and depth, its having filled a "tremendous need" in a sensible and thoughtful way, and its having "crystallized the most progressive mainstream thinking." As one respondent put it, "it is still an authoritative text to this day." Respondents also noted the impact on public and professional discussion and on court cases, institutional policies, professional practices, and public policy. Though several respondents criticized the report—for not being sufficiently critical of medical professionals who ignore patients' desires, or for not dealing with all issues adequately—this report seemed to have had the desired impact at all levels.

The Partial Successes

On the basis of the responses of former members and staff, five President's Commission reports could be classified as partial successes with regard to impacts on public policy and bioethics.

Defining Death was unanimously regarded as a success from one standpoint—its influence on state laws. The commission's recommended revision in the definition of death has been adopted in a majority of states. Nevertheless, there are mixed feelings about the quality of the analysis in the report. The criticisms were rooted in a basic disagreement, largely within the staff, over the analysis of alternative brain death definitions; several areas of "incoherence" or "intellectual unsoundness" were perceived. There was a sense that the executive director (and the commission) had been unwilling to deal with some valid issues and that power rather than persuasive argument had carried the day; a decade later those feelings remain strong. One former staff member said: "The executive director had clear and fixed ideas on the topic, which he sought to implement with a minimum of dispute or controversy. Staff dissent was largely suppressed." Another observed that "the commission was determined to uphold the emerging consensus, whether or not it had any theoretical basis." These criticisms of the former staffers are supported by a number of published critiques over the years.

The commission's report on informed consent, *Making Health Care Decisions,* was viewed by almost all respondents as having had an effect on public policy and/or on bioethics, but a majority saw it as, at most, partially

TABLE 14 President's Commission Reports Identified as: (a) Having Had a Critical Impact on Public Policy, (b) Having Had a Significant Impact on Thought in the Field of Bioethics, and (c) Having Gone on the Shelf to Collect Dust. Open-ended Responses to Survey of Former Members and Staff of the President's Commission, Spring 1993

Name of Report	Number of Respondents Offering each Assessment		
	Report Had Critical Impact on Public Policy	Report had Significant Impact on Bioethics	Reports that Are Collecting Dust
Defining Death	13	6	0
Protecting Human Subjects	2	0	5
Compensating for Research Injuries	2	1	7
Making Health Care Decisions	6	8	1
Whistleblowing in Biomedical Research	3	1	6
Deciding to Forego Life-Sustaining Treatment	12	13	0
Implementing Human Research Regulations	3	0	5
Genetic Screening and Counseling	2	5	4
Securing Access to Health Care	4	6	4
Splicing Life	3	5	2

TABLE 15 Respondents' Evaluations of Whether Individual **President's Commission** Reports Were (a) Very Successful, (b) Partially or Somewhat Successful, or (c) Largely or Wholly Unsuccessful. Fixed-response Items from Survey of Former Members and Staff of the President's Commission, 1993

Name of Report	Number of Respondents Offering each Assessment*			
	Very Successful	Partially Successful	Largely/Wholly Unsuccessful	No Response
Defining Death	9	2	0	3
Protecting Human Subjects	1	6	1	6
Compensating for Research Injuries	1	4	7	2
Making Health Care Decisions	4	7	2	1
Whistleblowing in Biomedical Research	1	2	4	7
Deciding to Forego Life-Sustaining Treatment	12	1	0	1
Implementing Human Research Regulations	2	5	1	6
Screening and Counseling for Genetic Conditions	1	7	1	5
Securing Access to Health Care	1	7	3	3
Splicing Life	2	4	2	6

*The number of nonresponses in President's Commission is due in part to commission member and staff turnover and staff specialization. Many non-respondent's had no involvement with some particular reports.

successful. The positive assessments focused on the report's quality—its "lucid, constructive analysis" and the survey research results it included—and its value as an educational document. But the perception of most respondents was that the report had had little or no impact on professional practice ("Doctors don't take informed consent seriously and no amount of writing, however good, makes any difference"), and no one cited any specific public policy impact.

The other three partial successes—*Securing Access to Health Care*, *Splicing Life*, and *Screening and Counseling for Genetic Disorders*—followed a similar pattern. In each case, several respondents saw the report as having had a significant impact on bioethics and, in the case of *Securing Access*, on public discourse. But most respondents perceived little or no public policy impact.

Securing Access was praised for the data it brought together on the uninsured and for articulating what became an influential ethical argument about the access issue (stated in terms of societal obligations rather than individual rights). But some were critical of the report, feeling that it had been watered down at the insistence of the conservative Reagan-appointed commissioners, and several noted the report's lack of impact on public policy.

Splicing Life was also seen as a clear, careful, and thoughtful report that had included good material, been the subject of a Senate hearing, influenced public debate, and helped lead to the establishment of the Human Gene Therapy Subcommittee of the NIH Recombinant DNA Advisory Committee. But some respondents thought that the overall tone was perhaps too "soothing" with regard to the implications of the issues that it addressed. The main impact that most respondents cited was intellectual.

Screening and Counseling was praised for its characterization of the issues, for providing a good overview, for its foresightedness and comprehensiveness, and for having avoided the "abortion quagmire." But there was little sense that the report had had any substantial public policy impact, though the report has been rediscovered to some extent in recent years owing to developments in genetic screening for cystic fibrosis.

The Dust Collectors

Four reports of the President's Commission were seen by most respondents as having had little effect on public policy or on the field of bioethics and as having gone on the shelf to collect dust. These were the three reports on research with human subjects—the two biennial reports that were part of the commission's mandated oversight function, and the report on *Compensating for Research Injuries*—and the report on *Whistle-Blowing*.

The perceived lack of effects of the two biennial reports—*Implementing Human Subjects Regulations* and *Protecting Human Subjects*—may have been partly due to some respondents' inability to distinguish between them in attempting to respond to the questionnaire. Moreover, staff who had been close to these reports were aware of regulatory impacts that were largely invisible to nonspecialists.

These two reports also reveal a further complexity in trying to assess the impact of a commission, because the mandated task that led to these reports was distinctive. The National Commission had already made recommendations for protecting human subjects, and these had been partly incorporated into DHHS regulations. The President's Commission was directed to monitor the situation and to report biennially. The heart of the first report was the recommendation for uniform regulations across all government agencies. As was noted earlier, this recommendation was in fact adopted by the federal government over the course of the next decade. So this report clearly had a regulatory impact, though not of the sort to excite persons who were intellectually engaged with the dilemmas of bioethics. The heart of the second report, issued with little publicity at the end of the commission's existence, was whether (and how) federal agencies could know whether institutions were actually implementing the regulations in ways that would protect human subjects. Whatever impact this report might have had was not visible to the members and staff who responded to my questionnaire.

Compensating for Research Injuries was seen as a failure because its only purpose was a public policy change, and none occurred. The report itself was praised for the thoroughness and ethical sophistication of the analysis (although the final recommendations were seen as "indecisive" by some). But the recommendations were not adopted by the Department of Health and Human Services, in part because the problem was not as serious as had been thought (i.e., few research injuries were identified) and in part because of opposition from the "research establishment."

The final report, *Whistleblowing in Biomedical Research*, was the summary of a conference that was jointly sponsored by the commission, rather than a full-fledged commission report. The case could be made that this report cannot be fairly judged on the same scale as the reports on which commissioners argued, and staffers wrote and revised, over the course of several meetings. The fact that only a few respondents perceived an impact is probably not surprising, although some noted that the report had opened a topic that has become more important in subsequent years.

In sum, respondents agreed that only two reports, *Defining Death* and *Decisions to Forego,* had a critical impact on public policy, and several mentioned *Making Health Care Decisions* in this regard. More reports were given credit for a significant impact on the field of bioethics. At least five respondents saw six reports as having had this effect—*Defining Death, Deciding to Forego, Making Health Care Decisions, Securing Access to Health Care, Genetic Screening and Counseling,* and *Splicing Life.* Most respondents thought the description of sitting on shelves and collecting dust applied to the other four reports—*Compensating for Research Injuries, Protecting Human Subjects, Implementing Human Research Regulations,* and *Whistleblowing in Scientific Research.* (Four respondents also put *Genetic Screening and Counseling* and *Securing Access* into this category.)

Responses to the series of questions asking for evaluations of the success of each report were consistent with these results. Only three reports were classified as "very successful" by more than two respondents—*Deciding to Forego* (12), *Defining Death* (9), and *Making Health Care Decisions* (4). However, in contrast to the National Commission, *all* of the other reports were seen by at least two respondents as at least "partially successful."

So, compared to the members and staff of the National Commission, respondents from the President's Commission saw it has having hit fewer home runs, but also as having struck out less often.

Accounting for Success and Failure

National Commission

National Commission respondents attributed reports' success to several types of factors (Table 16): the quality of the process, the efforts of members and staff in playing their roles, and the commitment to reason and to obtaining needed information. Interestingly, no one mentioned the fact that the law creating the commission required the Secretary of Health, Education, and Welfare to respond in writing to commission recommendations, including an explanation for any decisions not to implement them. (Interestingly, the *absence* of this factor was mentioned by President's Commission staff in explaining the lack of impact of its report, *Compensating for Research Injuries.* The National Commission staff may have come to take this important statutory provision for granted.)

Explanations of the National Commission's failures were more diverse and interesting: the commission's lack of expertise or authority on certain topics; the failure of politicians and bureaucrats to implement good recommendations; flaws in the commission's mandate and bureaucratic location; time constraints; conflicts between multiple goals; and some commissioners' and staff members' unwillingness to free themselves from their preconceptions. The conflict with the original executive director that was resolved by his resignation was recalled as a crucial period in establishing the commission's independence from NIH.

More information on the factors that positively or negatively influ-

TABLE 16 Explanations Offered by Respondents to Account for the
Success or Failure of Reports of the **National Commission.** Open-ended
Responses from Survey of Former Members and Staff of the National
Commission, Spring 1993

Explanations of Success	Explanations of Failure
An open honest process of debate; depth of inquiry; extensive analysis by commissioners	Some topics were outside the commission's expertise
Interest and commitment of commissioners and staff	Impact of some reports on vulnerable populations was reduced once the *Belmont Report* and the principles it identified were released
Commission's commitment to getting the facts and the full range of ethical opinion on topics	Commission had no authority on some topics
Reports were well-argued, based on facts, and reasonable	Subsequent interventions by politicians (e.g., *Fetal research*)
Commission's operating out of academic rather than political values	Subsequent poor regulation writing by DHHS (e.g., *Institutionalized Mentally Infirm*)
Reports were developed in a public process with press coverage; the public nature of the commission's debates	Technology or medical practice changed and left report largely irrelevant (e.g., *Psychosurgery*)
Leadership by the chairman	Commission's mandate was faulty (e.g., the focus on the *institutionalized* mentally infirm)
Was willing to allow publication of dissents rather than reach bland consensus (e.g., *Fetus, Children*)	The commission's location within NIH was seen as inappropriate for certain topics
Excellent staff work	Time constraints and the end of the commission
Assembly or development of pertinent information through commissioned papers, new research, and site visits	Multiple goals (encourage research and protect human subjects)
Public policy and scientific need; public interest in the topic	Commissioners or staff with ax to grind could derail debate

enced the National Commission's reports is shown in Tables 17 and 18. Looking across all reports, four influences stand out as having a positive impact: the composition of the commission, the role of staff, the framing of the commission's charge, and reports and papers written for the commission. The main negatives cited were time constraints, external interest (a complicated factor—there was a lack of interest in certain topics, but the main problem was the excessive external interest in the topic of psychosurgery, in which a group of activists disrupted and ended a public hearing of the commission), congressional politics, and the commission's bureaucratic location. There were also a scattering of complaints about the composition of the commission; these mostly pertained to idiosyncracies of particular commissioners on particular topics.

President's Commission

President's Commission respondents (Table 19) explained its successes (or lack of success) in somewhat similar terms to those of respondents from the National Commission. However, the President's Commission respondents placed much more emphasis on the subject matter as an explanation of success—certain topics being of high public interest, the time being ripe for resolution of the issue, the pressing need for clarification.[12] Characteristics of topics—their not being terribly important or sexy or their having already been dealt with by the National Commission—were also cited as an explanation of the lack of success of some reports.

There were also references to detrimental conflicts. Some involved the Reagan-appointed commissioners who entered the fray as the final group of reports was nearing completion. (The enabling legislation provided for a rotating membership of the commission. Ronald Reagan's election occurred during the Commission's life, and he appointed members with stronger political than substantive qualifications. Moreover, the Reagan appointees mostly had different ideological views on certain issues than did the commissioners and staff that had already done substantial work on a topic, particularly the report on access to health care.) There were also allusions to conflicts between the executive director and staff members assigned to particular topics, perhaps an inevitability when both roles are filled with people with strong credentials and, in some cases, with disciplinary differences.

More information on the factors that positively or negatively influenced the President's Commission's reports is shown in Tables 20 and 21. Looking across all reports, three factors stand out as having a major positive impact: external interest in the topic, the role of staff, and reports and papers written for the commission. What is remarkable, particularly in contrast to the National Commission, is how rarely the commission's mem-

TABLE 17   Factors that Respondents Saw as Having a "Major Positive" Impact on **National Commission** Reports. Fixed-response Items from Survey of Members and Staff, 1993

Name of Report	Factors Cited as *Positively Affecting* each Report by any Respondent (number citing each factor)				
	Time Constraint	Budget Constraint*	External Interest	Congress. Politics	White House Politics
Research on the Fetus	2	1	5	5	1
Research Involving Prisoners		1	1		
Research Involving Children			3		
Psychosurgery		1	1		
Disclosure of Research Information					
Research Involving Institutionalized Mentally Infirm				1	
Institutional Review Boards	1	2	1		
The Belmont Report	1	1	1		
Ethical Guidelines for Health Services					
Special Study					
Total Mentions	4	6	12	6	1

* Those citing budget constraints were referring to the *absence* of budget constraints.

bership was mentioned as a positive factor. Looking across all ten reports it was mentioned only 14 times. (Four respondent commissioners accounted for all of these mentions.)

In terms of the negatives, two factors stand out—time constraints and the composition of the commission. The latter again reflects the political change that came with the eight Reagan appointees in 1982. (This also underlies the characterization of White House politics as a problem.) The other factor that was mentioned more than ten times was the lack of external interest in the topic, a particular problem with regard to the reports on compensating injured research subjects and the implementation of the human research regulations.

LESSONS AND CONCLUSIONS

The National Commission, because of its mandate and the composition of its membership and staff, seems to have produced narrower reports that were tightly focused on regulatory questions. The success or failure of

Composition of Commission	Role of Staff	Framing of Charge	Bureaucratic Location	Papers/ Studies Done for Commission	Public Hearings
6	5	6	1	9	5
1	4	2		4	5
6	7	3	2	7	6
3	3	2	2	5	
			1	1	1
4	4	2	1	3	3
4	9	3	4	9	3
7	9	5	2	8	3
	1	1			
	2	1		1	
31	44	25	13	47	26

such reports is closely tied to success of the recommendation in the policy process. The President's Commission had a more wide-ranging agenda, with several important topics having no specific tie to a particular policy decision. Thus, while a typical National Commission recommendation included specification of regulatory actions a particular agency should take, the President's Commission's conclusions and recommendations (*Defining Death, Protecting Human Subjects,* and *Compensating Injured Research Subjects* excepted) were aimed at a broad audience of policymakers, professionals, and the public at large. Perhaps because so many staff members were oriented toward the fields of bioethics and real-world problems, President's Commission reports had a kind of broad orientation that was found primarily only in *The Belmont Report* of the National Commission.

The performance of the National Commission seems to have been more uneven than the President's Commission's. Four of the National Commission's reports were viewed as successes, but three were seen as failures. None of the President's Commission reports were complete failures, but only one was seen as an unqualified success. It is difficult to know

TABLE 18   Factors that at Least One Respondent Saw as Having a *Negative* Effect on **National Commission** Reports. Fixed-response Items from Survey of Members and Staff, 1993

	Factors Cited as *Negatively Affecting* each Report by any Respondent (number citing each factor)				
Name of Report	Time Constraint	Budget Constraint	External Interest	Congress. Politics	White House Politics
Research on the Fetus	5			4	
Research Involving Prisoners			4	2	1
Research Involving Children	1		1		
Psychosurgery	3		6	4	1
Disclosure of Research Information	3	1	2	2	
Research Involving Institutionalized Mentally Infirm	3		2	2	2
Institutional Review Boards	1				
The Belmont Report					
Ethical Guidelines for Health Services	5	3	3	2	1
Special Study	4	2	2	1	1
Total Mentions	25	6	20	17	6

whether these are objective differences, since different evaluators are involved. Critics of the President's Commission may be tougher, because the experience is fresher, because there was more conflict and disagreement between staff members and the executive director and commission, and because more of the former staff members are academics who may apply scholarly, rather than policy, criteria to reports.

Even so, the commissioner-driven versus staff-driven character of the two commissions, described earlier in this paper, may explain the difference. The National Commission staff tended to take its lead from the commission itself, so a topic might be handled in a cursory way if no commissioners cared much about it. By contrast, the executive director of the President's Commission made staffing provisions for all topics, and the staff's performance reflected both on their professional credibility and on the executive director himself.

The work of a commission is a combination of three broad factors—topics, commissioners, and staff.[13] The experience of these two commissions, each of which issued reports that were of highly variable success, demonstrates the importance of all three factors.[14] Complex relation-

Composition of Commission	Role of Staff	Framing of Charge	Bureaucratic Location	Papers/ Studies Done for Commission	Public Hearings
	1	1	1		
1		1	3		
3	1		1		
2			2		3
1	1	1	1		
		2	1		
			1		
			1		
2	2	1	3	1	1
4	1	3	3	2	1
13	6	9	17	3	5

ships between these three factors have enormous implications for commission success. Many of these implications can be summarized into seven "lessons."

Lesson One

Ethics commissions can play a useful role in helping policymakers, practitioners, and the public at large deal with the value conflicts and ethical dilemmas that accompany new developments in biomedical and behavioral research and technology.

A substantial list can be made of the beneficial consequences of the work of these two commissions. (It must be acknowledged that the methods used in this project were not likely to elicit the most critical of views.) The National Commission made recommendations that enabled important research to proceed within a regulatory framework that both policymakers and the research community found acceptable. There were times when that did not seem possible. President's Commission's reports had an

TABLE 19 Explanations Offered to Account for Success or Failure of Reports of the **President's Commission**. Open-ended Responses from Survey of Former Members and Staff of President's Commission, 1993

Explanations for Successes	Explanations for Lack of Success
The characteristic of the topic—with clear need for clarification and high public interest; time ripe for an authoritative analysis; an eager audience awaited it; issue susceptible to philosophical analysis	The particular problem turned out not to be serious or extensive; not a burning issue; little interest in issue
	No natural audience for a particular report
Existence of substantial scholarly literature on topic	Report difficult to translate into action (*Making Health Care Decisions*)
Good background papers by consultants	Key aspects of issue had been dealt with already (i.e., by National Commission)
Involvement of legal and medical community (*Defining Death*); involvement of agency liaisons (*Implementing Human Research Regulations*)	Topic did not hold attention of commissioners (*Compensating Research Injuries*) because of technical difficulty and seeming lack of importance
Solid work on law, philosophy, sociology, and history of topic	Topic not sexy (*Making Health Care Decisions*)
Investment of time and effort; depth and quality of report; scholarly analysis; new data; strength of underlying philosophical analysis	Some arguments in staff drafts were watered down by commissioners
Hard and excellent staff work	Staff views (and intellectual rigor) suppressed because of commission's or staff director's views and desire for professional support of report and to keep report in line with emerging consensus in field (*Defining Death*)
Critical interaction between commission and intellectual staff; good staff diplomacy re the commission	
Individual commissioners' contributions on certain new topics	Commissioners generally less qualified and involved than staff
Report crystallized "progressive mainstream thinking" and took apart myths and dogmas	Some topics were not priorities; some reports less substantial
Clarity of the analysis and writing in the report	Strong language in one report (*Securing Access*) gutted because of changing commission membership; recommendations not specific enough
The grounding of difficult issues (e.g., *Deciding to Forego Life- Sustaining Treatment*) not only in philosophical, theological, sociological, and legal terms but also in the experiences of health professionals, families, and patients	Report's reasoning too arcane (*Compensating Research Injuries*)
	There are limits to what can be accomplished at once; competing priorities on reports
	Acceptance or implementation was defeated by vested interests, bureaucratic resistance, or Reagan era ideology/ political climate

enormous effect on very difficult issues regarding the terminally ill and the definition of death. While they existed, both commissions played a valuable role in providing a focal point for work in the field of bioethics, and reports from both groups both lowered the temperature on some heated issues (research involving children, genetic screening) and became important points of reference for much subsequent scholarly work and policy debate.

Lesson Two

Design details can make an enormous difference in the performance of commissions.

Although it is difficult to draw sweeping conclusions based on two case studies, a number of aspects of the ways these commissions were designed seemed to have important consequences. These include:

(a) The creation of these bodies as governmental, rather than private entities. Governmental bodies are required to operate under sunshine laws. This was still new when the National Commission was in operation; despite initial concerns, broad agreement eventually developed that the attendance of the press and interested members of the public had a beneficial effect on the process.

(b) Appointment versus election of the chair. The National Research Act's unusual requirement that the chair of the National Commission be elected from within its membership had important, positive consequences for the leadership of the commission.

(c) Establishing rotating, overlapping terms for commissioners. These create difficult problems for a study commission that is striving to reach agreement on difficult value questions. Time-consuming conflicts on reports-in-progress can result from membership changes. The rotation of membership will also tend to increase the power of staff. It seems wiser to give a commission a life span and a mandate and to appoint a new commission (with a new mandate) at the end of that life span.

(d) Administrative location of the commission. Independence has both perceptual and substantive importance for ethics commissions. The President's Commission's existence as an independent agency had significant advantages over the National Commission's NIH location.

(e) Where ideological divisions exist, the appointment process is fraught with potential problems. This is particularly true when political control of the appointing authority changes, as with the Reagan election of 1980. That experience proved that legislative language about "distinguished" appointees or categories of expertise are subject to widely differing interpretations.

TABLE 20 Factors that Respondents Saw as Having a "Major Positive" Impact on **President's Commission** reports. Fixed-response Items from Survey of Members and Staff, Spring 1993

	Factors Cited as Positively Affecting each Report by any Respondent (number citing each factor)				
Name of Report	Time Constraint	Budget Constraint	External Interest	Congress. Politics	White House Politics
Defining Death	1	1	4		
Protecting Human Subjects			1		
Compensating for Research Injuries			2		
Making Health Care Decisions			3		
Whistleblowing in Biomedical Research			1	1	
Deciding to Forego Life-Sustaining Treatment	1	1	12		
Implementing Human Research Regulations			1		
Screening and Counseling for Genetic Conditions			1	1	1
Securing Access to Health Care	2	2	3	1	1
Splicing Life			1	1	1
Total Mentions	4	4	29	4	3

Lesson Three

The appointment of commissions is a very complicated matter, full of trade-offs and dangers.

Clearly, trade-offs and competing considerations exist in many aspects of creating a commission and carrying out its work. Will members be appointed for their expertise or because membership is a plum to be given to acknowledge past political favors? How much does the official who is making the appointments care about the commission and its mandate? Might the official care too much about one or another possible outcome? The experience of the President's Commission shows how the process can be politicized. The combination of a rotating membership and a presidential election can be volatile. And it was not only the Reagan appointees that are the issue here; some observers looking at the commission and staff assembled under the Carter administration found the staff to be better

Composition of Commission	Role of Staff	Framing of Charge	Bureaucratic Location	Papers/ Studies Done for Commission	Public Hearings
	6	2	2	4	2
1	3	3	2	1	
	2			1	
4	11	3	1	9	2
	3			4	2
3	10	4	2	7	6
1	4	3	2	3	1
3	5	1	1	3	1
1	9	2	2	7	7
1	3	1		2	1
14	56	19	12	41	22

qualified than the commission. Such a perception on the part of a staff makes for complicated dealings with the commission, but no one would suggest that the answer is to appoint a weaker staff. But how does one guarantee that a highly qualified commission will be appointed?

Many other trade-offs could be noted: between commissioners who bring visibility to the activity (e.g., Magic Johnson on the AIDS Commission) and those who bring substantive expertise; between recommendations designed to be adopted by policymakers and recommendations that are intellectually satisfying to rigorous thinkers; between recommendations that will solve an immediate problem and recommendations that will not be accepted but may be admired and even adopted some years later; between consensus achieved by making language general or fuzzy and a strong, clear recommendation accompanied by a strong, clear dissent. There is no one right answer for any of these matters, but the itemization shows how many balances must be stuck in the course of designing and executing the work of a commission.

TABLE 21   Factors that at Least One Respondent Saw as Having a
Negative Effect on **President's Commission** Reports. Fixed-response Items
from Survey of Members and Staff, 1993

	Factors Cited as Negatively Affecting each Report by any Respondent (number citing each factor)				
Name of Report	Time Constraint	Budget Constraint	External Interest	Congress. Politics	White House Politics
Defining Death	1				1
Protecting Human Subjects		2	1	1	
Compensating for Research Injuries	2	1	5	2	2
Making Health Care Decisions	5				
Whistleblowing in Biomedical Research	1		1		
Deciding to Forego Life-Sustaining Treatment	5	1		1	1
Implementing Human Research Regulations	3	1	3	1	1
Screening and Counseling for Genetic Conditions	4	1	1		
Securing Access to Health Care	3		2	4	8
Splicing Life	3	1	2	1	1
Total Mentions	27	7	15	10	14

Lesson Four

**A strong staff can overcome serious shortcomings of a commission
itself. Conversely, a strong commission can overcome serious staff
problems.**

Both of these commissions are widely viewed as successful. But, as was
described earlier, the relative strengths of the membership and staff of the
two commissions were quite different. The strength of the National Commission lay in its membership and chair, and to a lesser extent its staff. The
President's Commission's strength lay in its staff.

Accordingly, the two commissions were characterized by different staff/
commissioner relations. Members of the National Commission debated
among themselves down to the smallest details of reports, in many cases
going line by line over staff drafts to make sure that the staff had captured
exactly what commission members had agreed to among themselves. By
contrast, staff members of the President's Commission were much more

Composition of Commission	Role of Staff	Framing of Charge	Bureaucratic Location	Papers/ Studies Done for Commission	Public Hearings
	1	1			
2					
5		3	2	1	3
1					
	1	1			
6					
1		1			
1					
9	1	1	1		
2	2	2	2	2	1
27	5	9	5	3	4

engaged in trying to work through their own ideas and solutions to the problems assigned to the commission, and meetings had more of a flavor of commissioners providing oversight over what staff had done and of staff trying to sell the ideas that had been developed.

Lesson Five

Topics need champions—an influential member or staffer who cares about it and insists that the commission care.

If a commission is asked to study and make recommendations on several topics, a particular topic can become an orphan. If this happens, a perfunctory report may result (as with the National Commission's *Special Study* or its report on ethical issues in the delivery of services by the Department of Health, Education, and Welfare). Or the commission may decide not to even issue a separate report (as with the President's Commission's statutory mandate regarding privacy and confidentiality issues in research and medical care).

Because the personal interest of influential commissioners or staff members is so important, the experience of the President's Commission demonstrates that topics that are self-assigned by the commission itself can be handled with enormous distinction. The report *Deciding to Forego Life-Sustaining Treatment* was not part of the commission's legislative mandate; it was a topic that was undertaken in response to issues that came to the fore during the work that led to the report *Defining Death.*

Lesson Six

Although several definitions of success can be applied to commissions, nothing substitutes for having a perceptible impact on either policy or practice.

Although the success of a commission is multidimensional and may be difficult to assess objectively, people who are engaged in the enterprise as commissioners or staffers clearly believe a report must make a difference if it is to be considered a success. No matter how well reasoned and carefully documented a report may be, if it does not change something in the world it will be viewed as a failure.

Even very high quality reports can fail to have a significant impact on policy or practice. A commission report can contribute to the ripening of a topic by bringing attention to it, but it is also true that carefully documented reports with clear recommendations can be ignored. This is particularly likely under two circumstances.

The first is when the policy changes that implementation would require are tightly controlled by vested interests and there is no significant constituency behind the recommendation. (The President's Commission's report *Compensating for Research Injuries* is a case in point, requiring action by the Department of Health and Human Services with virtually no outside prodding, except from the commission; bureaucratic inertia easily killed the recommended ideas. The same was true of the National Commission's report on *Those Institutionalized as Mentally Infirm.*)

Second, reports can fail to have an impact when there is no particular target for the recommendations, as was the case with the President's Commission's report *Making Health Care Decisions.* The most that staffers could realistically expect of the report's call for more shared decision making between doctors and patients was to have an influence on medical education; this is a very diffuse kind of impact and no one had much confidence that the issuance of a commission report—even one that based a satisfying ethical argument on solid empirical grounds (including survey data on people's desire for information and data linking good communication to positive health outcomes)—was likely to have a substantial impact on entrenched patterns.

Lesson Seven

Recommendations are not self-implementing.

Commissions that want to see their recommendations enacted in law or policy need to keep an eye on how agencies or legislative bodies deal with their recommendations. Recommendations issued near the time that a commission disbands and with little publicity and no follow-up are easily ignored by policymakers who have other agendas. The early reports by both commissions tended to have the best chance of being adopted in policy.

Requirements that agencies respond publicly to commission recommendations can play a valuable role in this regard—it was particularly important for the National Commission's regulatory recommendations—but other mechanisms (e.g., congressional hearings) can play a role. The importance of the public information function and the dissemination of findings in forms in addition to formal reports should be recognized.

ACKNOWLEDGMENTS

The author acknowledges with gratitude the assistance of Andrea Adams, Mary Anastasio, Jennifer Morgan, and Annie Elizabeth VanDusen.

NOTES

1. Other bodies have had less success. The congressionally created Biomedical Ethics Advisory Committee foundered over issues of mandate and appropriations and disbanded without ever issuing a report. Earlier, the Ethics Advisory Board, which was created by the Department of Health, Education and Welfare in 1978, demonstrated its ability to respond in a timely fashion to issues of biomedical ethics, but was eliminated with the stroke of a bureaucrat's pen when funds were needed elsewhere.

2. A substantial literature exists on presidential commissions. Examples include David Flictner, 1986, *The Politics of Presidential Commissions: A Public Policy Perspective (Dobbs Ferry, NY: Transnational);* Terrence R. Tuchings, 1979, *Rhetoric and Reality: Presidential Commissions and the Making of Public Policy (Boulder: Westview),* and Thomas R. Wolanin, 1975, *Presidential Advisory Commissions: Truman to Nixon (Madison: University of Wisconsin Press).*

3. Prestige is to some extent a function of the prominence of the individual members, but the designation, "President's Commission," itself carries weight and commands attention from the press and the public. This is one reason why the politically powerful sometimes like to create commissions and the politically vulnerable worry about the attention and legitimacy that may be given to a cause or point of view to which they are opposed, and why people from many camps will seek to influence the membership of the commission.

4. For example, both Senator Kennedy and Senator Buckley, who had reached a key legislative compromise involving fetal research—creating a moratorium pending recommendations from the Commission—had visible hands in the selection of commission members, and the chair of the President's Commission was owed a large political debt by President Carter. Political connections undoubtedly had a role in other members' appointments; the least subtle instances occurred when President Reagan made several appointments to the President's Commission after the terms of several Carter-appointed commissioners expired.

5. The major examples were the National Commission's study of the Institutional Review Board system and the President's Commission's extensive survey research project of the public and physicians to provide documentation for its report *Making Health Care Decisions*.

6. This statement requires some qualification, since there was some turnover of commissioners and staff, especially in the instance of the President's Commission. Moreover, since staff members tended to concentrate on certain reports and since the interest and commitment of individual commissioners varied across topics, it could be argued that in a sense the commission and staff both varied from topic to topic or report to report. Yet, for both commissions, there was one staff director and one chairman and substantially the same set of commissioners and staffers throughout the commission's life.

7. *Federal Register* citations should be interpreted with caution because the same action may appear numerous times. Moreover, a report may be cited more than once without final regulatory action ever taking place.

8. In legislation to indemnify vaccine manufacturers so that they would produce the swine flu vaccine, Congress required the Centers for Disease Control to consult with the National Commission regarding the issue of informed consent; the commission met with CDC officials and sent them a letter with recommendations. The consultation (though not the commission's letter) was cited in several lawsuits alleging injuries from the swine flu vaccine.

9. *Rust v. Sullivan; Cruzan v. Missouri Department of Health; Bowen v. American Hospital Association.*

10. In the view of some, this was also a problem with the report on the institutionalized mentally infirm.

11. A methodological point arose with regard to responses of staffers of the President's Commission, many of whom devoted much or all of their effort to particular topics and who had little or no involvement with other topics. Unlike staffers of the National Commission, who generally attended all parts of all meetings, many President's Commission staffers went to commission meetings (or parts of meetings) only when their particular topic was on the agenda. As a result, President's Commission staffers had more difficulty assessing the process and outcome of the whole group of reports than did National Commission staffers.

12. Perhaps the best example of timing was the coincidental release of the report on *Definition of Death* on the same day that an anti-abortion Constitutional amendment that would define the beginning of human life was introduced on Capitol Hill. The juxtaposition was too delicious to be ignored by the media and led to a Nightline appearance that night by the executive director and a member of the Commission, as well as other news coverage.

13. I first heard a similar formulation from David Goslin regarding projects at the National Research Council.

14. Adequate resources are also a requisite, but this was not an issue in either of these cases.

Limiting Life-Prolonging Medical Treatment: A Comparative Analysis of the President's Commission and the New York State Task Force

BARUCH A. BRODY, Ph.D.

Professor of Medicine, Baylor College of Medicine

In 1983, the President's Commission for the study of Ethical Problems in Medicine and Biomedical and Behavioral Research produced a report on the topic of limiting life-prolonging therapy entitled *Deciding to Forego Life-Sustaining Treatment.*[1] Three years later, in 1986, the New York State Task Force on Life and the Law produced a report on some aspects of this topic entitled *Do Not Resuscitate Orders.* It produced in 1987 a second report on other aspects entitled *Life-Sustaining Treatment: Making Decisions and Appointing a Health Care Agent.* In 1992, it produced still a third report entitled *When Others Must Choose.*[2]

The report of the President's Commission has been widely acclaimed. It is often felt that its report shaped a social consensus on this difficult topic. On the other hand, the work of the Task Force has attracted considerable criticism and controversy. It seems to have been much less of a success.

If one accepts these perceptions, then it seems natural to raise a series of questions in the hope of learning what makes some commissions work better than others. Was it a function of the membership? Did the President's Commission benefit, for example, from not attempting to include representatives of many diverse religious groups, all of whose concerns needed to be addressed? Was it a function of how the work was done? Did the President's Commission benefit from holding many public hearings before it began shaping its report? Was it a function of the duration of the commission? Did the President's Commission benefit from knowing that it was working under a strict time limit and that it would have to accomplish its goals in that confined period? Such procedural questions are inevitable if the above-mentioned perceptions are accepted.

The main thesis of this paper, to which the bulk of it is devoted, is that these perceptions are incorrect, both about the President's Commission and about the New York State Task Force. The report of the President's Commission was a success in summarizing a consensus that had emerged, and in beginning the process of moving beyond it, not in shaping that consensus. The reports of the New York State Task Force were a success in producing legislation that incorporated this consensus, and the controversy was nothing more than the expected accompaniment of any important legislative initiative. The nature of their successes differed because they were operating in different contexts and had different roles. A second thesis, to which we shall return briefly in the conclusion, is that the structural and procedural differences mentioned above are reflections of these different contexts and roles, and that the proper conclusion to be drawn is that structure and process should be a function of context and roles.

The strategy for my analysis is as follows: In the rest of this introduction, I will present a statement of the current consensus about limiting life-prolonging treatment. For the sake of this analysis, I will take its validity for granted. In the next two sections, I will discuss the relation of the work of the two groups to the current consensus, to the context in which they operated, and to their roles. It is in those two sections that I will defend my claims about the nature of their successes. Finally, in the conclusion, I will briefly return to some of the structural and procedural issues.

I offer the following, which is a modification of an analysis recently presented by Meisel,[3] as my statement of the current consensus:

(a) The mere fact that some treatment exists that would prolong the life of some patient does not by itself suffice to justify providing that therapy to that patient, because extending life by providing the treatment in question may not be beneficial to the patient in light of the patient's values and patients have a right to refuse therapy whose provision they judge to be against their interests.

(b) Both competent and incompetent patients have that right to refuse life-prolonging therapy; of necessity, the way in which that right is exercised is different in the two cases.

(c) Despite the differences, decision making for both types of patients should usually occur in the clinical setting without recourse to the courts.

(d) The main role of legislatures is to see that these rights are adequately recognized in law, and the main role of health care institutions is to insure that there are proper policies and mechanisms in their institutions for facilitating proper processes for such decision making and for insuring that they are appropriately documented.

(e) These refusals may be of all forms of therapy, including artificial nutrition and hydration, and they may involve both the withholding of life-preserving therapy and the withdrawing of such therapy.

(f) Such refusals of life-prolonging therapy must be distinguished both from active euthanasia and from assisted suicide.

(g) When the patient is not competent, the attending physician, who normally makes that decision of incompetency, may rely upon a patient's advance directive to refuse treatment incorporated in such documents as living wills.

(h) If there is no living will or its equivalent, the patient's right to refuse treatment may be exercised on behalf of the patient by a surrogate decision maker appointed by the patient in advance (by use of such mechanisms as the durable power of attorney) or specified by some statutory scheme (usually, family members in some ordering of priority). The surrogates should apply a substituted judgment standard, or, if they cannot, a best interests standard.

(i) The same principles should apply to parental decision making about life-prolonging therapy for their children, especially severely ill newborns, but the emphasis must be on the child's best interests since the substituted judgment standard cannot apply.

With this statement of the current consensus in mind, I turn to an analysis of the work of the President's Commission and of the New York State Task Force on limiting life-prolonging treatment.

ACCOMPLISHMENTS OF THE PRESIDENT'S COMMISSION

As indicated above, the received view is that the report of the President's Commission, *Deciding to Forego Life-Sustaining Treatment*, was very successful in shaping the current consensus about decisions to limit life-prolonging treatment. My argument will be that this claim is much too simplistic, and that once the factors of context and role are taken into account, a much more complex picture emerges. In particular, we shall see (a) that most of the elements of the consensus were prominently present in the public debate before the appearance of that report; (b) that the report organized and added one crucial element to, offered a sound foundation for, and placed an official imprimatur on, a very new consensus that had just emerged; (c) that the report raised many crucial issues that were to become central to the later debate, and adopted positions, often quite ambiguous, on these issues. This ambiguity was possible because the report was not designed to lead to any specific legislation or hospital policy. None of this is to say that the report was unsuccessful. It is rather to say that its success needs to be understood in terms of its context and its role.

The report contains a detailed account (pp. 9–11 and pp. 259–74) of its own genesis and it is worthwhile noting a number of major points made by the Commission to which we shall return. The first is that the whole topic of limiting life-prolonging treatment was not part of the statutory mandate for the President's Commission. The definition of death was however part of that mandate and the Commission began work on that topic in January of 1980. But in the course of hearings on that topic, it was led to realize that a report was also needed on limiting care to certain patients, especially vegetative patients. Secondly, the report was seen by the Commission as an outgrowth of what it had to say in two other reports which dealt with mandated topics, its report on decision making, *Making Health Care Decisions*,[4] and its report on the allocation of health care resources, *Securing Access to Health Care*.[5] Finally, as in the case of all of its other activities, the Commission began with public hearings on the topic and then moved on to extensive internal deliberations aided by external reports and additional public comments. Throughout the work on its report, the Commission's process was a very open process.

With this understanding of the Commission's process, let us turn to the substance of its report. A comparison of the principles of the current consensus with the summary of the 24 conclusions contained in the introduction to *Deciding to Forego Life-Sustaining Treatment* reveals both considerable overlap and some differences. We will first examine the extent to which our consensus principles are incorporated in its summary conclusions and we will then examine those of its summary conclusions which are not included in our consensus principles.

Our principle (a) is incorporated in its summary conclusions (1), (2), and (21b). Our principle (b) is incorporated in its summary conclusions (9), (11), (17c), and (20), although the reference to limitations on surrogate authority in (9a) and (21c) is not fully in accord with principle (b), and will be analyzed below when we discuss ambiguities in the report. Our principle (c) is incorporated in its summary conclusions (6), (9e), and (18), with some useful comments about when recourse to the courts would be appropriate. Our principle (d) is incorporated in its summary conclusions (7), (9b), (9d), (17a), (22), and (23). Our principle (e) is incorporated in its summary conclusions (5) and (11). Our principle (g) is incorporated in its summary conclusion (8) about the assessment of incompetency and (9c) about living wills, although (9c) offers only lukewarm support for living wills, preferring the use of durable powers of attorney. Our principle (h) is incorporated in its summary conclusions (9a) and (9c). Finally, our principle (i) is incorporated in its summary conclusions (13), (15), and (17). There is no doubt then that the President's Commission advocated nearly all of the elements of the current consensus. The only exception is principle (f), which is not clearly articulated in the summary of the conclusions but is discussed in the text of the report. We shall return to it below when we discuss ambiguities in the report.

What other conclusions are presented in the report which are not part of our list of consensus principles? A few are unproblematic. These include summary conclusion (4) calling for better options for those who refuse life-prolonging therapy, summary conclusion (16) calling for decision makers to have access to the best up-to-date information, and summary conclusion (24) calling for better education of health care professionals about these issues. Much more important are summary conclusions (3b), (3c), and (12) on the impact of resource allocation on this type of decision making, summary conclusion (10) on the special status of PVS patients, and summary conclusion (14) on the lack of any need to provide futile care to severely ill newborns. We shall return to these issues below when we discuss ambiguities in the report.

Although there are differences then between the principles of the current consensus and the summary conclusions of the President's Commission, differences which we shall discuss below, they should not blind us to the obvious tremendous overlap between the current consensus and the views of the President's Commission. All of this leads us to ask about the role of the Commission in forging that consensus. To what extent was the consensus present before the appearance of *Deciding to Forego Life-Sustaining Treatment?* What were its contributions to the emergence of that consensus? In order to answer these questions, we need to examine the report in the context of the discussions about limiting life-prolonging therapy in the period 1975–1983. Our goal will not be to identify who said what first; it will be, instead, to identify major trends in prominent discussions during that crucial period.

I want to begin with several prominent discussions in the professional literature. The first is a well-known and very influential article in the *New England Journal of Medicine* in 1976 authored by the Clinical Care Committee of the Massachusetts General Hospital.[6] The article describes a newly introduced system for classifying patients according to the level of therapeutic effort they would receive. Patients in Class C had selective limitations placed on the therapeutic measures provided while patients in Class D had all therapeutic measures, except those indicated for comfort, discontinued. Many of the elements of the current consensus are clearly present in that policy. It is recognized that life-prolonging treatments may be inappropriate in some cases. That decision is to be made in the hospital without recourse to the courts. The role of the institution is to insure that there are policies and procedures in place (including a consultation committee) to facilitate such decision making and its documentation. All forms of therapy may be withheld or withdrawn. Other elements of the current consensus are missing from that document. It places the locus of decision making in the attending physician rather than in the patient or those who speak for the patient. The only exception is for Class D patients, where consultation with, and concurrence of, the family is required. As a result of this emphasis on physician decision making, there is no mention of certain crucial patient-centered elements of the consensus such as the rights of patients to refuse treatment, the use of advance directives, and the family as surrogate decision makers attempting to apply the substituted judgment rule.

Another important discussion was published in *Critical Care Medicine* in 1978 by members of the Critical Care faculty at Presbyterian University Hospital in Pittsburgh.[7] It also described a system introduced in 1975 for classifying patients according to the level of therapeutic effort they would receive. This system is closer to the system currently used in many institutions, as it divides patients into four categories: total support, all but CPR, no extraordinary measures (ranging all the way from ICU admission to parenteral nutrition), and dead. The system described contains all of the elements of the current consensus contained in the Massachusetts General Hospital system. Most crucially for our purposes, the policy required that orders about the level of care to be provided be accompanied by a progress note indicating that a discussion had taken place with the patient or the family and that they agreed with the order. As a result of that change from physician-centered decision making, the document also referred in its discussion of the policy to the patient's right to refuse treatment and to advance directives such as living wills. So the Pittsburgh publication contains many of the patient-centered elements of the current consensus. The only ones to which I see no allusion are the emphasis on substituted judgment by surrogate decision makers and the question of parental decision making for newborns. I am not claiming that the Pittsburgh policy is a fully articulated statement of nearly all of the elements of the current consensus; the patient-centered elements are not given the emphasis they are given either in the report of the President's Commission or in the current consensus. What I am saying is that the Pittsburgh policy moves us much closer to most of the elements of that consensus.

Many elements of that consensus were also present in two statements by the Judicial Council of the American Medical Association, published in 1982.[8] One discussed issues related to quality of life in both newborns and adult patients and the other discussed issues related to terminal illness. Both statements affirmed that life-prolonging therapy can sometimes be withheld or withdrawn. Both statements assigned a significant role to those who speak for the patient, although parents of newborns are identified as the decision makers for them while the wishes of the family speaking on behalf of the adult patient are only factors to be considered by the physician who makes the decision. Both statements dealt with all forms of life-prolonging therapy.

There are many more statements in the professional medical literature in the period 1975–1982 related to limiting life-prolonging medical treatment; we have only presented a small selection from that much more extensive literature, a literature whose history deserves a much fuller analysis. But we have seen that *Deciding to Forego Life-Sustaining Treatment* goes beyond what was already in the professional literature primarily by emphasizing the point that the organizing theme for all policies and decisions to limit care should be the decisions of the patient or those who speak on behalf of the patient, because the patient has the right to refuse life-prolonging therapy. Even that theme was present in some of the professional literature, but none of that literature made it the organizing theme. In this way, *Deciding to Forego Life-Sustaining Treatment* is an application of the general principles about decision making enunciated in *Making Health Care Decisions.*

We turn from the medical literature to legal developments. I want to emphasize at least two developments, the development of natural death statutes and the development of right-to-die decisions in the courts. We shall see in that material ample evidence of the acceptance of most of the elements of the current consensus.

California passed the first natural death statute in 1976. It was followed in 1977 by Arkansas, Idaho, Nevada, North Carolina, Oregon, and Texas.[9] By the time the Commission report came out, 14 states and the District of Columbia had passed such statutes. This is not the place to offer a full analysis of all of them. We shall only focus on the extent to which the first seven, which antedated by several years the work of the President's Commission, incorporated the elements of the current consensus.

The full force of principle (a) of the current consensus, that life-prolonging care can be withheld because the patient has a right to refuse it, is the whole point of all of these natural death statutes. But it is worth noting that several of them (Arkansas, California, Idaho, and North Carolina) begin with an explicit statement of that right. I note, parenthetically, that Arkansas defines it as both the right to refuse such therapy and the right to request it and that North Carolina defines it as the right to a peaceful and natural death. It is also worth noting that while most of them (California, Idaho, Nevada, Oregon, and Texas) confine their provisions to patient refusals in certain cases, thereby seeming to limit the recognition of patient rights, all who do so make it clear that the statute does not limit any more general right to refuse treatment. Principle (b), that the right extends to incompetent as well as competent patients, is once more the whole point of these statutes, but it is worth noting that two of the statutes (Arkansas and North Carolina) add more provisions which provide for surrogate decision making on behalf of incompetent patients. As all of the statutes allow attending physicians to rely upon directives without the authorization of a court, they all incorporate principle (c) of the current consensus. None of them talk about the role of health care institutions mentioned in principle (d), but they all exemplify the role for legislatures mentioned in principle (d), viz., seeing that the right to refuse treatment is recognized in the law. Five of the seven (California, Idaho, Nevada, Oregon, and Texas) both offer very broad definitions of the forms of therapy that are covered and explicitly cover both withdrawings and withholdings of these therapies; the other two offer somewhat more limited definitions of the forms of therapy covered, but North Carolina does explicitly cover both withdrawings and withholdings of the covered therapies. So while none explicitly mention artificial nutrition and hydration (perhaps because that issue was not very prominent in 1976–1977), principle (e)'s spirit is found in all seven statutes. Principle (f), the distinction between authorizing the limiting of life-prolonging therapy and authorizing suicide or euthanasia, is articulated in six of the seven statutes (all but the Arkansas statute). Principle (g), the recognition of living wills, is, of course, the whole point of these statutes. Elements of principles (h) and (i), about other aspects of surrogate decision making, are found in several of the statutes, although that is obviously not their main point. Of particular importance is the fact that Arkansas addressed the issue of pediatric patients.

The conclusion that emerges from this analysis is that by 1977, seven states had passed statutes that incorporated most of the elements of the current consensus. And, of course, eight more jurisdictions passed such statutes by the time that the report of the Commission came out. Of particular importance is that these statutes, unlike the professional medical policies analyzed above, were firmly grounded in an emphasis on the right of individuals to refuse therapy. However, some elements of the current consensus (the role of institutional policies, the standards for surrogate decision making, and the use of durable powers of attorney) were not present, usually because they were not relevant to the purposes of the statutes.

The period in question also saw the appearance of many fundamental court decisions about limiting life-prolonging therapy. We will focus on decisions that predated the work of the President's Commission. The most important are the New Jersey case of *In re Quinlan* (1976),[10] the Florida case of *Satz v. Perlmutter* (1978)[11], the New York cases of *In re Eichner* (1981),[12] and *In re Storar* (1981),[13] and the Massachusetts cases of *Superintendent of Belchertown State Hospital v. Saikewicz* (1977),[14] *In re Dinnerstein* (1978),[15] and *In re Spring* (1980).[16]

Nearly all of the principles of the current consensus that were relevant were adopted in 1976 by the Supreme Court of New Jersey in the case of Karen Quinlan, where the father of a PVS (persistent vegetative state) patient was appointed as her guardian with the authority to authorize the discontinuation of all extraordinary life-prolonging therapy. This decision overruled the opinion of a lower court that thought that the decision should be left in the hands of the medical profession. Treatment could be withdrawn because the patient's right to refuse treatment was to be exercised on her behalf by her father. So the opinion incorporated principles (a) and (b) of the current consensus as they apply to that case. The opinion also ruled that recourse to a court would be inappropriate, so it adopted principle (c) of the current consensus. In calling for hospital processes including consultation with an ethics committee (not necessarily what is currently meant by that term), it incorporated much of principle (d). In authorizing the withdrawal of a respirator, it incorporated much of principle (e). It adopted principle (f) by explicitly distinguishing the refusal of life-prolonging therapy from suicide. Finally, since the court authorized a parent to make the decision for his child, it incorporated some components of principle (i). Moreover, it explicitly indicated that he was to do so on the basis of his best judgment as to whether she would refuse the therapy; this emphasis on substituted judgment incorporates some of principle (h). None of the other principles were relevant in that case. So the opinion in the Quinlan case was a major statement of the current consensus. Perhaps the one exception was its somewhat confusing discussion of ordinary and extraordinary measures. In fact, when the respirator was removed from Karen Quinlan, she lived for nine years sustained by antibiotics and nasogastric feedings. It is hard to be sure, however, whether this represented the wishes of her father or the court's unwillingness to accept the full force of principle (e).

In 1978, a Florida District Court of Appeal authorized a 73-year-old competent ALS patient, Abe Perlmutter, to remove his respirator. It based its decision on a broad appeal to the patient's rights of self-determination and privacy, thereby incorporating principle (a). Because the case involved a withdrawal of life-prolonging therapy, the decision incorporated components of principle (e). It explicitly incorporated principle (f) by distinguishing the removal of the respirator from suicide. When the Supreme Court of Florida affirmed the decision in 1980, it called upon the legislature to legislate in this area, thereby incorporating an element of (d).

The Saikewicz case, the first of our Massachusetts cases, represents the first of our cases that challenged a component of the current consensus, principle (c). In its decision, the Supreme Judicial Council of Massachusetts ruled in 1987 that decisions involving incompetent patients must be brought to a court. Nevertheless, even that decision incorporated many components of the current consensus. It incorporated principle (a) by grounding withholdings of therapy in the right of patients to privacy and self-determination. It incorporated principle (b) by insisting that incompetent patients have the same right to refuse treatment as competent patients, although the process would have to be different. It explicitly adopted the substituted judgment principle, thereby incorporating elements of (h). This emphasis on judicial intervention was limited in the subsequent cases of *In re Dinnerstein* (1978) and *In re Spring* (1980). So while it is true that one element of the current consensus was rejected by the Massachusetts courts in the period before the appearance of the Commission's report, it is also true that many more elements of that consensus were affirmed by those courts and by the subsequent professional literature reflecting on its decisions.

The court that was the furthest from adopting what was to become the consensus was the New York Court of Appeals in two companion cases, *In re Eichner* and *In re Storar* (1981). In the former case, the New York Court of Appeals upheld a decision that a respirator could be removed from a PVS patient who had clearly expressed his wishes that he not receive such life-prolonging therapy in such a case. In the latter case, the court rejected a decision authorizing a denial of life-prolonging blood transfusions to a never competent, retarded patient. Several observations need to be made here: (1) the elements of the current consensus most clearly rejected were the insistence in *Eichner* on clear and convincing evidence of the patient's previously expressed wishes rather than substituted judgments by others about what the patient would have wished, thereby rejecting a portion of (h), and the unwillingness in *Storar* to rely upon any surrogate's judgment about the patient's best interests, thereby rejecting another portion of (h); (2) nevertheless, the Court of Appeals still accepted limitations on life-prolonging therapy based upon the right to refuse treatment, thereby accepting principle (a), and extended that to incompetent patients, thereby accepting principle (b). As *Eichner* involved the withdrawing of a respirator, the Court of Appeals accepted an important element of (e). Since living wills are excellent examples of clear and convincing evidence of the patient's previously expressed wishes, the *Eichner* decision laid the foundation for their recognition, thereby laying the foundation for the acceptance of (g).

In short, an analysis of court decisions which preceded the work of the Commission reveals that major elements of the consensus were accepted in the most important judicial rulings on these issues. While it is true that there were some elements rejected by some courts, this cannot take away from the extent to which the judicial rulings were in consonance with both the legislation and the professional medical literature analyzed above.

Our first conclusion must therefore be that most of the elements of the current consensus were prominently present and widely accepted before the appearance of *Deciding to Forego Life-Sustaining Treatment.* If it were needed, one could provide further evidence from both the secular and religious bioethics literature, but I believe that the evidence already presented is sufficient. What then was the role of that report in the development of the current consensus?

I believe that the report of the Commission played four roles in the development of the current consensus: (1) It summarized in one well-organized and authoritative statement the consensus whose elements had emerged in the years just before its work. It needs to be remembered that all of the material we analyzed was from the last ten years before the publication of its report. There is some even earlier material, but it is neither very extensive nor very authoritative. Moreover, no one other document contained all of the elements of the consensus. The report of the Commission was needed to give very authoritative approval to, and advocacy of, the full consensus that had just emerged. (2) It offered valuable criticisms (pp. 159–60) explicitly directed at the Massachusetts view about the need for judicial approval, suggesting ethics committees as an alternative, and it offered a valuable defense (pp. 132–6) of the substituted judgment/ best interests approach, thereby implicitly criticizing the New York decision in *In re Storar.* In these ways, it defended the new consensus against some alternatives. (3) It also placed great emphasis on durable powers of attorney for health care decision making, a tool that had not received enough attention before the report of the Commission. (4) Finally, the report made it very clear that the organizing theme for the new consensus was the patient's right to refuse treatment based upon the patient's perception of what was in the patient's best interest. Although much of the legal material we examined contained that theme, this was not as true of the professional material. There was a real need then for this emphasis. In all four of these ways, then, the report of the President's Commission made a valuable contribution to the emergence of the current consensus, even if its outline and most of its elements were widely accepted before the appearance of the report.

I believe that there was another contribution made by the report, a contribution that has not been adequately noticed. On a considerable number of issues, the President's Commission took positions that went beyond the consensus then and even the consensus now. Some of the positions were not clearly articulated, but this ambiguity was possible because the report was not advocating some specific legislation or some specific hospital policy. Despite these ambiguities, the report was often the starting point for further discussions about limiting life-prolonging therapy, discussions that still continue today. The issues were: (1) What is the best form of advance directives, living wills or durable powers of attorney? (2) What are the limits of surrogate decision making, both in the case of newborns and in the case of incapacitated adults? (3) Can society legitimately prohibit active euthanasia and/or assisted suicide when requested by competent adults? (4) Do the special features of PVS patients mean that decision making to limit life-prolonging therapy for them is different from decision making to limit such therapy for other patients? (5) Can physicians unilaterally limit futile care? (6) To what extent, and by what process, can life-prolonging therapy be limited because of economic considerations? Let us briefly analyze the contribution of the Commission's report on each of these issues.

In the last ten years, there has been a considerable debate about the respective merits of two major forms of advance directives, living wills and durable powers of attorney.[17] No consensus has emerged on this question. The concern today about living wills is their lack of specificity. The concern today about the durable power of attorney is whether the surrogate decision maker really knows what the patient would have wanted. At the time of the Commission's report, the concerns about the living will statutes then in existence were that they were too narrowly drawn and lacking in assurances that they would be honored, while the concern about the durable power of attorney statutes then in existence was that they had not been drafted for use in a medical setting and did not have appropriate safeguards for that setting. As far as I can see, the report was the first to raise the issue of the merits and demerits of these two approaches. Moreover, while summary conclusion (9c) states that durable powers of attorney are preferable, the text of the report (pp. 136–53) offers a much more balanced account, emphasizing the problems as well as the strengths of both, and the need for legislation to deal with potential problems with both. But since no specific legislation is proposed as a model statute, akin to the model statute for brain death proposed in another report by the Commission, the issue of preferability and of emphasis in legislation is never really resolved in the text of the report.

Are there any limitations on the right of surrogate decision makers to refuse life-prolonging therapy for those for whom they make decisions which extend beyond the limitations on the right of competent adults to refuse life-prolonging therapy for themselves? While the report discusses that issue at two points, once (p. 133) in connection with surrogate decision making for incompetent adults and once (pp. 217–23) in connection with surrogate decision making for severely ill newborns, the more substantial discussion is in the second context. The continuing controversy on this issue, both before and after the passage of the current Baby Doe law,[18] testifies to the fact that there is no consensus on this issue. The report of the Commission clearly limits the right of parents, acting as surrogates for their severely ill newborn child, to refuse life-prolonging therapy which is in the best interests of the infant; such therapy can be refused only when the child's handicaps "are so severe that continued existence would not be a net benefit to the infant" (p. 218). An important footnote (footnote 79 on page 219) even cautions that such assessments must be made from the perspective of the infant, who will grow up with these handicaps and who will often be able to make adjustments for them, and not from the perspective of the normal adult surrogate decision maker who may find life with those handicaps excessively burdensome. But the only example of treatment refusals explicitly criticized (p. 219) is the refusal of needed surgery on Down's Syndrome children with intestinal abnormalities. Nothing clear is said about the harder cases ranging all the way from spina bifida to bilateral severe intraventricular hemorrhages. After reviewing the discussion (on pp. 221–3) of the Lorber criteria for withholding life-prolonging therapy from children with spina bifida, I cannot tell whether the Commission thought that prolonging life for some of these infants, the better cases according to Lorber's criteria, was clearly beneficial and mandatory or whether they thought that such care is always of ambiguous benefit and therefore optional in such cases. When do treatments stop being clearly beneficial, and mandatory regardless of parental wishes, and become of ambiguous benefit, and therefore open to parental refusal? The report is unclear on this crucial issue, offering a process of review without a clear standard for that review. This is in clear contrast with the current Baby Doe law, which says, for better or worse, that this point is reached only when the child is irreversibly comatose or clearly dying. Once more, the Commission raised an important question that takes us beyond the consensus, but offered an ambiguous answer, the type of answer that could not ground an operating policy or law. The substantive standard that a hospital committee might enforce by policy or by law need not be the Baby Doe standard, but it does need to be something more concrete than a reference to the best interest of the child, even if we agree with the Commission that any standards will leave some ambiguities.

Do the arguments justifying honoring refusals of life-prolonging therapy also justify honoring requests for active euthanasia and/or assistance in suicide? That issue is today a matter of great controversy; there is certainly no consensus about it.[19] The treatment of that issue in the report is very interesting. The report (pp. 60–89) challenges the conceptual and moral significance of those distinctions (e.g., causing death vs. allowing to die) which are usually used to differentiate active euthanasia from refusing life-prolonging therapy, and its rationales for honoring the refusals, especially the appeal to patient rights, seem to apply to honoring requests for active euthanasia as well. Nevertheless, the report supports (on pp. 71–3) the prohibition against mercy killing as a way of continuing a public affirmation of the high value of human life. However, that support is conditioned on the prohibition's not causing too much suffering to patients because of a broad understanding of the legitimacy of limiting care and of supplying adequate pain relief. Those who support the current ban on honoring such requests can appeal to the report's explicit conclusion, while those who oppose the current ban can argue that the report's analysis, supplemented by a fuller understanding of the extent to which patient suffering cannot otherwise be alleviated, really supports lifting the ban. It seems to me best to describe the report's position on this issue as ambiguous. It raised the right questions, and it indicated the factors to be considered on both sides, but its conclusions were far from unambiguous.

The question of whether or not decision making about life-prolonging therapy is different in the case of PVS patients is currently a matter of great controversy. Those[20] who support the concept of qualitative futility as a source for legitimate physician limiting of care independent of patient or family wishes usually treat PVS patients as their clearest example of when care can be limited on grounds of qualitative futility; PVS patients are so different that decision making in their case must also be different. Those who support the usual processes of decision making in these cases insist that there is a value judgment being made that should be made in light of the patient's values as assessed by their surrogates.[21] The controversy surrounding the Wanglie case[22] typified this continuing controversy. The report clearly treats PVS patients as different, emphasizing (p. 186) the very limited interests such patients have in their continued existence given that they have permanently lost consciousness. I have elsewhere[23] criticized this claim, arguing that it presupposes the wrong conception of interests. I have also suggested that the report should instead have relied on the nonpersonhood of PVS patients. But that is not the point that I want to make here. What I want to note for now is the ambiguity of what is supposed to follow from either the limited interests PVS patients have in continued existence or the nonpersonhood of PVS patients. Does this mean that life-prolonging therapy can be limited independently of family concurrence? Support is clearly expressed in the report for the family which agrees to limit such therapy, but, according to the report, even advance patient requests for continuing life-prolonging therapy in such circumstances need not but may be honored (p. 193). No clear-cut answer is provided to our question; even the recommendation to appoint a guardian in such cases (p. 194) is unclear on the crucial issue of how the guardian should respond to patient requests made in advance, or family requests made at the time of decision making, for continued life-prolonging therapy. The report raises the right questions, but remains ambiguous in ways that policies or legislation could not be ambiguous.

The report's discussion of the issue of limiting life-prolonging care to patients who will soon die no matter what is done is in some ways less ambiguous. Those[24] who advocate limiting this type of futile care insist that the normal processes of decision making need not be applied in such cases; physicians need not offer, they insist, to provide life-prolonging therapy in such cases, and the concurrence of the patient or the surrogates to not provide it is not needed in such cases. Those[25] who oppose the concept of futility insist that there is a judgment to be made about the value of the remaining period of life. The patient or the surrogates must decide whether or not it is worth the burden of the life-prolonging therapy. Naturally, there is also much controversy about how quick must the inevitable death be before the case is described as futile. The report discusses these issues most fully in the case of severely ill newborns. It seems to come down clearly on the second side (p. 220), insisting that parental wishes for continued life-prolonging therapy should be honored. But this is quickly limited to those cases where the life-prolonging therapy does not cause substantial suffering. How much suffering is substantial enough? Who makes this decision and by what standard will this decision be made? Also, the report says that health care providers who disagree may withdraw from the case. What happens when all the neonatologists want to withdraw? While the report raises crucial questions and offers some answers, it leaves many ambiguities that would undercut any actual policy or legislation based on it.

No question is more controversial today than the question of whether life-prolonging therapy may be limited on economic grounds. Those who oppose such limitations[26] see them as a failure to be faithful to the needs of, and the commitments to, patients. Those who support such limitations[27] see them as crucial to controlling rapidly escalating health care costs. While supporting such limitations in principle, the report emphasizes (pp. 95–100) that this is not a wise place to focus discussions of cost containment and that it would be better to first develop acceptable policies on equitable limits on health care in general and then apply them to limiting life-prolonging therapy. The report is appealing here to the more general policies developed in *Securing Access to Health Care.* In light of the fact that we as a society are far from having such general policies, and that what we have by way of intuitions and particular limitations is very ambiguous, the report's conclusions leave the whole question of economic limitations on life-prolonging therapy totally unresolved for now.

What are we to conclude about the role of the President's Commission in taking us beyond the consensus about limiting life-prolonging therapy? Its report certainly raised many of the issues that have been heatedly debated since its appearance ten years ago. It often identified the main arguments on both sides. But its conclusions were often very ambiguous. As a starting point for discussion on these matters, the report was a great success. As the foundation for concrete policies and/or legislation on these matters, it was far less successful. An assessment of its success in these areas depends therefore upon one's conception of the role of the report. When one adds this conclusion to our earlier contextual conclusions about how the report did and did not contribute to the development of the consensus, it becomes clear then that a proper assessment of the success of the President's Commission must be very dependent both upon one's understanding of the context in which it operated and upon one's understanding of its role.

ACCOMPLISHMENTS OF THE NEW YORK STATE TASK FORCE

Having seen the importance of context and of role in assessing the accomplishments of the report of the President's Commission, we will begin our assessment of the reports of the New York State Task Force on limiting life-prolonging therapy by looking at the context in which the Task Force was created and in which it issued its reports.

The New York State Task Force was created by Governor Cuomo in 1985 and issued its three major reports in 1986, 1987, and 1992. Two of the six issues it was asked to look at, decision making for those without decisional capacity and discontinuing life-sustaining therapies, relate to our topic.

What was the status of New York law and of thinking in New York on these issues before the Task Force began its work and in the early years of its work? I think that there are a number of points that need to be kept in mind:

(1) New York State had no statutes on the definition of death, on limiting life-prolonging therapy, and on advance directives.

(2) As noted above, the New York courts in 1981 had rejected part of the current consensus. In particular, a decision to limit life-prolonging therapy for an incompetent patient required in New York clear and convincing evidence that the patient would have requested those limitations in the circumstances at hand, rather than surrogate substituted judgments or surrogate judgments of the patient's best interests. In 1988, the New York Court of Appeals, in an opinion[28] written by Judge Wachtler (influenced, it has been suggested,[29] by a case involving his own mother), reaffirmed that position and allowed for limiting such therapy only when the evidence of the patient's expressed advance wishes applied very specifically to the patient's actual condition.

(3) At least two very well organized groups in New York, the New York State Catholic Conference and the Agudath Israel (an Orthodox Jewish organization), expressed strong and politically influential concerns about components of the consensus on limiting life-prolonging therapy, concerns growing out of their reverence for human life. Some of those concerns will be discussed below. For now, it is sufficient to say that the New York State Task Force operated in a context in which important ethical/

religious voices were not supportive of elements of the consensus that had emerged elsewhere.

(4) From 1981 to 1984, a grand jury in Queens investigated a hospital DNR (do not rescuscitate) policy that eschewed the use of explicit DNR orders, relying instead on a covert system in which purple dots were placed on the charts of patients, indicating that the patients were not to be resuscitated. The grand jury's report in 1984[30] supported the use of DNR orders with proper procedural safeguards and called for regulations governing the use of explicit DNR orders.

(5) In response to this confusing situation, the Medical Society of the State of New York issued in 1982 a set of guidelines on DNR orders.[31] The guidelines called for the decision on a DNR order to be made by the physician and the patient (or appropriate family members, if the patient was not capable of making a decision). Unfortunately, the guidelines did not address limitations on the use of other forms of life-prolonging therapy, did not discuss the use of advance directives, and did not discuss the crucial question of the nature and evidentiary backing for surrogate decision making.

In short, when the New York State Task Force began its work in 1985, it confronted anything but a consensus on limiting life-prolonging treatment. How did it define its role in that situation? That leads us to our second question, the question of role.

An examination of the governor's executive order[32] establishing the Task Force makes it clear that it was given many roles:

> The Task Force studies shall include: a review of current law and practice pertaining to these issues; an analysis of the proper roles of patients, family members, health care professionals and the courts in making health care decisions; the advisability of adopting legislative or administrative policies affecting these issues, where appropriate; and recommendations to enhance public consideration for those issues not susceptible to immediate legal or administrative resolution.

From the very beginning, however, the Task Force focussed on the development of reports which proposed legislation. In light of the context in which it operated, particularly the limits on surrogate decision making articulated by the New York Court of Appeals, this was a very reasonable choice of role. It was, moreover, a role that was supported by the New York legislature, which adopted in 1987 a DNR law based upon the Task Force's 1986 report,[33] adopted in 1990 a health care proxy law based upon the Task Force's 1987 report,[34] and is currently considering legislation on surrogate decision making based on the Task Force's 1992 report. It is also a role that we need to keep in mind as we assess the accomplishments of the three reports.

What was the content of the reports? Do they incorporate the current consensus outlined above? Do they go beyond that consensus in valuable ways? The answer to these three crucial questions requires a careful analysis of the three reports.

The initial report on DNR orders provided for a presumption for the use of cardiopulmonary resuscitation (CPR) unless the patient or the surrogate consents to the issuance of a DNR order. The report made it clear (pp. 9–12) that this approach is grounded in the value of self-determination and that refusals of CPR should therefore be honored even when the patient does not have a terminal illness (this was one of the items that was dissented from by Rabbi Bleich, a member of the Task Force associated with the Orthodox Jewish community). In these ways, the report accepted principle (a) of the current consensus. By providing for DNR orders for both competent and incompetent patients, the report accepted principle (b) of the current consensus. Although it did provide for judicial review under certain circumstances (pp. 87–8), the report's main emphasis was on decision making outside the judicial system, so it accepted principle (c) of the current consensus. By calling for legislation and for institutional policies and dispute mediation systems (pp. 49–51), the report accepted principle (d) of the current consensus. Principles (e) and (f) were irrelevant to the report's discussion, which was confined to DNR orders because of the immediate needs in New York in light of the factors noted above. The report allowed both for patients indicating in advance that they do not want CPR and for their appointing surrogates to make that decision for them. It also rejected the opinion of the Court of Appeals, at least for the case of CPR (the only therapy it covered), in that it allowed (pp. 43–4) surrogates to use the substituted judgment and/or the best interests standard. Therefore, the report accepted principles (g) and (h) of the current consensus. Finally, the report accepted (pp. 46–9) parental decision making for minor children, thereby incorporating principle (i) of the current consensus.

There were some additional components of the report that went beyond the current consensus and should be noted. To begin with, it dealt with the problem of patients who have no surrogate decision maker, allowing for the writing of a DNR order when resuscitation would be futile (defined by the legislature[35] as "CPR will be unsuccessful in restoring cardiac and respiratory function or that the patient will experience repeated arrest in a short time period before death occurs") or when a court directed that such an order be written (the legislature made it clear that the court could do so using either a substituted judgment or a best interest standard). Secondly, it addressed the issue, raised by the President's Commission, of limitations on surrogate decision making to refuse CPR. The Task Force (pp. 41–3) limited this authority to cases where the patient has a terminal illness, is permanently unconscious, or is so sick that resuscitative measures would probably be unsuccessful and only prolong the dying process. The legislature[36] modified those standards by changing the third to refer to cases in which resuscitation would be futile and by adding the fourth possibility that resuscitation would be extraordinarily burdensome in light of the patient's condition and expected outcome. Both of these standards are quite close to the Baby Doe standards for parental surrogate decision making; more crucially, both provide far more guidance than the standard provided by the President's Commission. Thirdly, it allowed for the unilateral withholding of futile CPR at least in some cases; the precise extent of this became, as we shall see below, a matter of considerable controversy. Fourthly, it began the very difficult process of defining the role of hospital ethics committees (although it used the name of dispute mediation system), addressing such issues as who may call for their use, what happens while their work is going on, and what happens if they fail to bring about agreement (pp. 49–51). Finally, it dealt with a great many questions of concrete details, including the written documentation required for a DNR order, the conditions under which a physician can invoke the therapeutic exception to consult surrogates rather than the patient, the process for determining patient incompetency, the role of friends as surrogates, the special procedural protections needed by institutionalized patients, the need for review of DNR orders, and the validity of DNR orders after interinstitutional transfers.

To summarize, when the legislature adopted with some changes the Task Force's proposed legislation, it incorporated into New York law, at least in connection with CPR, all of the relevant elements of the current consensus. Moreover, it also incorporated, and even added to, some of the crucial ideas of the Task Force that went beyond the current consensus. In light of the context in which the Task Force operated, and given its chosen role, that was a significant accomplishment. No doubt, there was considerable controversy generated both by the report and by the legislation; we shall discuss that controversy below. But none of that takes away from its accomplishments in its initial report.

We turn now to the second of its reports, the 1987 report on appointing a health care agent to make decisions. Once more, context is crucial for understanding the significance of that report. In light of the New York court decisions about surrogate decision making which required surrogates to meet the very high standard of clear and convincing evidence of previous patient wishes, surrogate refusals of life-prolonging therapy were severely limited in New York. The essential point of the report was to propose legislation that would partially remedy this problem. At least in those cases in which the patient, before he or she became incompetent, appointed a health care agent (the name they proposed for the person awarded a durable power of attorney for health care), the report recommended that the agent be authorized to make decisions on all health care matters, including but not limited to decisions about life-prolonging therapy, using either the substituted judgment or the best interest standard (pp. 91–2). The legislature[37] limited this provision in decisions to forego the provision of nutrition and hydration to surrogates who have reasonable knowledge, but not necessarily clear and convincing evidence, of the patient's wishes. Leaving this aside for the moment, we can certainly conclude that one of the accomplishments of the report was to lead to the passage of legislation that moved New York closer to the current consensus, at least for patients who had appointed a health care agent.

The second report, like the first report, did more than that. It moved beyond the current consensus in the following ways: (1) Following the lead of the President's Commission, it emphasized durable powers of attorney over living wills. In addition to noting the traditional problem of the uncertainty of the meaning of living wills, it pointed out (pp. 75–83) that durable powers of attorney cover all health care decisions, not just decisions to forego life-prolonging therapy, and also serve as a vehicle for those who want to direct that life-prolonging therapy be continued even when their condition was grave, and not just as a vehicle for those who want to direct that it be limited. (2) It provided a mechanism for the informal determination that the patient was incompetent and that the agent therefore had authority, it dealt with the patient's right to be notified of that determination, and it structured an appeals process for that determination (pp. 152–3). All of these are crucial details for policies and laws that are to be implemented in the real world; (3) it raised and addressed (pp. 93–4) the question of liability for costs of the health care chosen by the agent.

There was some controversy about this second report, although it was on the whole much less controversial than the first report. We shall discuss this controversy, and the modifications made by the legislature to deal with the freedom of conscience issues that were central to it, below. None of this takes away, however, from its accomplishments in bringing New York closer to the current consensus and in moving beyond it in important ways.

The last of the reports, the 1992 report on deciding for incapacitated patients (together with its April 1993 supplement), attempted to complete the process of incorporating the current consensus into New York law. It called attention (p. ix) to the fact that the major gap in that incorporation is a failure to deal with surrogate decision making that limits life-prolonging treatments other than CPR when the patient has not appointed a health care agent and there is no living will to supply clear and convincing evidence of the patient's wishes, and it attempted to fill that gap. It also attempted to provide for surrogate decision making about health care in general when the patient has not appointed a health care agent. As one

would expect, its major recommendations (pp. x–xi) were that such decision making should be allowed using the substituted judgment and/or the
best interests standards.

As with the other reports, this last most comprehensive report moved
beyond the current consensus to deal with a large number of issues which
need to be resolved if such laws are to be implemented in actual cases.
Many of these issues were already treated by the Task Force in its work on
DNR orders. The following seem to be the most important issues addressed: (1) Incompetent patients without surrogates: the Task Force had
already addressed this issue in its DNR report, but it returned to it in this
latest report. Its recommendations (pp. 157–71) were to allow the physician to provide routine care using his/her own judgment, to provide major
medical treatment after approval by another physician designated by the
hospital, and to forego life sustaining treatment only after additional approval by a hospital bioethics review committee; (2) Limitations on surrogate decision making to limit life-prolonging therapy: the Task Force, following in the path of the President's Commission, had already addressed
this issue as well in its DNR report, but it returned to it both in the third
report and in its 1993 supplement to that report. In the report itself (pp.
109–15), it limited that authority to cases (i) where the surrogate judged,
using the substituted judgment and/or best interests standards, that the
therapy was too burdensome *and* (ii) where the patient would die within
six months, or where the patient was permanently unconscious, or where
an attending physician and a bioethics review committee or a court concurred with the decision. In the supplement (p. 2), the last two conditions
were replaced with the conditions either that two physicians concurred
that the provision of treatment would be inhumane or extraordinary under
the circumstances or that the decision was in accord with the reasonably
known wishes of the patient (3) Issues of futility: as in the CPR report, the
new report allowed for the unilateral withholding of futile therapies (now
called therapies without medical benefit) in some cases. The clearest case
(pp. 259–60) is where life-prolonging treatment can be limited for incompetent patients with no surrogates if the attending physician, with the concurrence of a second physician designated by the hospital, judges that the
patient will die imminently even if the treatment is provided. Restrictions
on that provision, together with a fuller discussion of the Task Force's views
on futility, will be discussed below when we discuss the controversies surrounding its work (4) The role of bioethics review committees: The Task
Force had already begun working on the role of bioethics committees in
hospitals in its DNR report, but it saw them in that report serving only in an
advisory capacity. This may explain the name given to them in that report,
where they were seen as one of several alternative "dispute mediation systems." The new report goes way beyond that. Such committees are now

mandatory, and there are certain cases of limiting life-prolonging therapy (e.g., from incompetent patients without surrogates) in which their prospective approval is now required. As a result, the report (pp. 137–55) now contains extensive provisions about composition, procedure, documentation, etc. (5) Finally, as a continuation of modifications made by the legislature in response to criticisms of the Task Force's second report, the third report contains (pp. 187–93) extensive provisions protecting the right of conscientious objection by institutions and providers. We will return to these provisions below when we talk about the controversies surrounding the Task Force's work.

Having reviewed the content of all three reports, and some aspects of the legislation adopting, in a modified fashion, the first two reports, what can we say in response to our initial questions about the content of the Task Force's reports? I think that we can say that the reports were based primarily on the current consensus. I think we can say that the legislation based upon them incorporated into New York law much of the current consensus, and that what is missing will be incorporated if and when the proposed legislation in the third report is enacted into law. I think that we can say that the reports and the legislation based upon them also attempted to deal with many crucial issues left unresolved by the current consensus. In light of the context in which the Task Force operated, and given its legislative role, these are very considerable accomplishments.

But what about the controversies surrounding the work of the Task Force? Don't they reveal some very fundamental problems and shortcomings either in the content of the reports or in the operating methods of the Task Force? In order to answer these questions, we need to look more carefully at those controversies.

There is one that I want to note and to then put aside. This is the internal controversy within the Task Force represented by the dissenting opinions of one of its members, Rabbi J. David Bleich. In each of the reports on life-prolonging therapy, Rabbi Bleich dissented because of his strong moral/religious convictions, based on his reading[38] of the Orthodox Jewish sources, that the goal of decision making should be ". . . cure or, *de minimis*, maximum prolongation of life."[39] This led him to want to confine the writing of DNR orders to cases in which little or nothing can be gained by resuscitation and to want to limit the authority of surrogates, appointed by the patient or by the law, to refuse life-prolonging therapy. These dissents have not, as far as I can tell, attracted that much of a following outside of his own particular community, so I will not focus on them here.

Most of the controversy centered around the initial DNR report and the legislation based on it. Fortunately, a great deal of the material associated with that controversy was presented and analyzed in a 1990 conference at Union College, the proceedings of which were to shortly appear.[40] I think that there are really several different issues at stake in that controversy, and I want to analyze each of them separately.

Two of the controversies dealt with items of detail that were readily correctable and were corrected in the 1991 amendments to the DNR statute.[41] The first had to do with whether or not patient and/or surrogate agreements to DNR orders had to be in writing. The original statute required written agreements from surrogates, although oral agreements from patients were acceptable. Despite this clear difference, it was widely reported that many hospitals required written agreements both from patients and from surrogates. It was also widely believed that this requirement was burdensome on staff and difficult for patients and/or surrogates. All of this led to the claim that increased paperwork and inhumane demands on patients and/or families, rather than improved discussion and communication, were the main outcomes of the statute.[42] The 1991 amendments resolved this problem by allowing both surrogates and patients to agree orally to a DNR order, requiring only that physicians record that agreement in the medical record. The second had to do with DNR orders on nonhospitalized patients who were anticipated to suffer an arrest at home. Would the emergency medical technicians have to resuscitate them? Several clinicians and family members had highlighted the difficulties posed by inadequate attention to that issue.[43] The 1991 amendments clarified the procedures for such orders being written and honored, addressing even the very difficult question of what to do when family members insist to the emergency medical personnel that resuscitative efforts be attempted despite such orders. These controversies are reflective of what you would expect when broad philosophies are operationalized in specific legislation; important problems about details that were not anticipated emerge. The occurrence of these controversies is a sign of a problem only if they persist because of legislative inaction. In fact, however, the legislature did correct these problems. If there were controversies that reflected problems with the work of the Task Force, they had to be more fundamental controversies. Two possibilities exist.

The first was the controversy over whether or not it was appropriate to discuss DNR orders with patients who were competent rather than with their family members. There was a feeling on the part of some that this was inhumane and inappropriate. This claim is, of course, a challenge to the fundamental presuppositions of the current consensus (a) that the foundation of limiting life-prolonging therapy is the decision of the competent patient that the benefits of such therapy are not sufficient and (b) that all surrogate decision making is an attempt to deal with cases in which the patient is no longer competent. Both the Task Force's initial report and the DNR legislation based on it allowed for a carefully defined exception to consulting patients when that would pose a serious threat of an immediate and severe injury to the patient, but both continued to insist upon the fundamental validity of the current consensus. I find it hard to fault the Task Force for doing so.

The second was the controversy over futile DNR orders. The claim was made that the Task Force's report, and the legislation based upon it, required the provision of CPR even when it was futile as long as the competent patient or the incompetent patient's surrogate insisted on it. The only case where the report and the legislation explicitly and unambiguously allowed physicians to write DNR orders on the grounds of futility was when there was no surrogate available. Many felt that this led to inappropriate resuscitative efforts. This controversy is not about details, but about a fundamental issue of principle. It is not about a challenge to the current consensus, but about what the Task Force did when it went beyond the current consensus. Does this controversy, which was probably the most contentious controversy surrounding the Task Force's work in this area, reveal a fundamental shortcoming in its approach?

Before answering this question, I want to note the Task Force's own response to this issue. Although Commissioner Axelrod[44] attempted to defend the above understanding of the law at the Union College conference, arguing to an unsympathetic audience that futile resuscitation was not that common, the Task Force has adopted a different approach: (a) Since 1988, the Department of Health, with the support of the Task Force, has maintained the view that despite the lack of an explicit provision saying so, the law creates no requirement to provide futile CPR so long as physicians don't use the invocation of futility so commonly as to create a new system of unwritten DNR orders.[45] In the current proposed legislation, that view is incorporated in the provision that physicians are not required to provide at the request of a surrogate any form of care they "would have no duty to provide at the request of a patient with decision-making capacity."[46] Unfortunately, that concept is left undefined both in the report and in the legislation (b) At the same time, the final version of the current proposed legislation[47] actually makes it harder to invoke futility even in decision making for incompetent patients without surrogates since it imposes the additional requirement that the provision of the life-prolonging treatment "would violate acceptable medical standards."

It seems clear to me that the Task Force has not yet found an acceptable solution to this most vexing problem, one that has produced tremendous controversy. In a crucial footnote in the third report (p. 203), it admits that its own members are split on this issue. But this failure is hardly a criticism of the Task Force. The uncertainties it feels about this issue are reflective of a lack of a social consensus rather than of a Task Force failing. When the President's Commission raised this issue but failed to resolve it, this gave rise to continued discussion but not to criticism of the President's Commission. When the New York Task Force failed to resolve it, there was controversy and criticism. Why the difference? I think that it was due to the fact that the ambiguity was left in legislation that people had to live with on a day-to-day basis, rather than in a general policy statement. Once more, we see the importance of understanding context and role when we assess accomplishments and failures.

Let me conclude with a brief analysis of the controversies surrounding the health care agent report and the resulting legislation. The two major issues, raised primarily by the Catholic Conference, related to surrogate decision making to limit the provision of nutrition and hydration and to protecting the rights of conscience of individuals and institutions. Resolving the first issue in the legislative process did require a modest withdrawal from the current consensus, since surrogate decisions to limit such therapies must by statute be based upon more substantial evidence of patient wishes than decisions to limit other therapies. Resolving the second issue in the legislative process actually moved New York beyond the current consensus in very sensitive and informative ways. New York now has separate and very thoughtful rules on these matters. If we see the Task Force's efforts as part of a larger legislative process, then a quick analysis suggests that this larger process worked very well to insure that the resulting legislation was sensitive to the context of a state in which there is tremendous religious/ethical pluralism on the difficult questions raised by the limiting of life-prolonging therapy.

What are we to conclude then about the accomplishments of the New York State Task Force in its work on limiting life-prolonging therapy? I would conclude that if its third report is incorporated into legislation, it will have succeeded, in a context in which these issues were very controversial, in incorporating the current consensus into law, in making that consensus operational by filling in many of the details, and in moving beyond that consensus in important ways. Some controversy surrounding its work was inevitable as broad policy was incorporated into legislation and followed on a daily basis, but the New York legislative process has successfully handled much of that controversy. The remaining controversy about futility is a very different matter, but its continuation is more of a reflection on a current social uncertainty about that issue than a reflection on the work of the Task Force.

CONCLUSION

The analysis we have offered of the President's Commission and of the New York State Task Force has shown the centrality of the understanding of context and of role in the assessment of these two commissions. This is, of course, the main thesis of the paper. But I want in this conclusion to add a speculative suggestion relating to the structure of, and the processes used by, these two commissions. In particular, I want to suggest that their different contexts and roles made different structures and processes appropriate for these two groups.

If your role is to develop, and to serve as advocates for, legislation in a context in which there is much disagreement on the topic of the proposed legislation, it is probably very important that the many groups (including the religious groups) with the diverse views on the topic be represented in the process of developing the legislation so that as few as possible feel that the legislation is being imposed on them. It may well be a good idea to first try to work out a common legislative proposal in informal private discussions, allowing for less posturing and for more attempting to find a common consensus, and to present it for public discussion only after a common plan has emerged. Given the vagaries of legislative timetables and given the need to fashion further compromises in a legislative process, it is probably a mistake to set a firm date for the conclusion of activities.

The situation is very different if your role is to articulate and systematize a recently emerged consensus and to begin discussions of moving beyond the consensus. Here, what may be needed is a very public process, where the diverse groups appear and present their positions before a group of well-respected individuals (with a strong staff) who are good at listening and synthesizing. It is, moreover, easier to talk of a limited time frame for these activities.

These are, of course, very speculative claims, but I find them quite plausible. Moreover, they help complete the explanation of the successes of the two commissions. I do think therefore that they are deserving of serious consideration.

NOTES

1. President's Commission for the Study of Ethical Problems in Medicine and Biomedical and Behavioral Research, *Deciding to Forego Life-Sustaining Treatment* (Washington, D.C.: U.S. Government Printing Office, 1983).

2. The New York State Task Force on Life and the Law, *Do Not Resuscitate Orders* (New York: Task Force, 1986), *Life-Sustaining Treatment: Making Decisions and Appointing a Health Care Agent* (New York: Task Force, 1987), and *When Others Must Choose* (New York: Task Force, 1992). That last publication is supplemented by *Supplement to Report and Proposed Legislation* (New York: Task Force, 1993).

3. Meisel, A. "The Legal Consensus about Forgoing Life-Sustaining Treatment: Its Status and its Prospects" *Kennedy Institute of Ethics Journal* vol. 2 (1993) pp. 309–45.

4. President's Commission for the Study of Ethical Problems in Medicine and Biomedical and Behavioral Research, *Making Health Care Decisions* (Washington, D.C.: U.S. Government Printing Office, 1982).

5. President's Commission for the Study of Ethical Problems in Medicine and Biomedi-

cal and Behavioral Research, *Securing Access to Health Care* (Washington, D.C.: U.S. Government Printing Office, 1983).

6. Clinical Care Committee of the Massachusetts General Hospital, "Optimum Care for the Hopelessly Ill" *New England Journal of Medicine* vol. 295 (1976) pp. 362–4.

7. Grenvik, A. *et al.* "Cessation of Therapy in Terminal Illness and Brain Death" *Critical Care Medicine* vol. 6 (1978) pp. 284–91.

8. Judicial Council, *Current Opinions of the Judicial Council of the American Medical Association* (Chicago: American Medical Association, 1982). The opinions in question are numbered 2.10 ("Quality of Life") and 2.11 ("Terminal Illness").

9. The statutes in question are *Ark. Stat. Ann.* 82-3801–3804 (March 30, 1977), 1976 *Cal Stat* Chapter 1439, Health and Safety Code, 7185–7195 (Sept. 30, 1976), *Idaho Code* 39-4501–4508 (March, 1977), *Nev. Rev. Stat.* 449.550–590 (May 6, 1977), *N.C. Gen. Stat.* 90-320–322 (July 1, 1977), *Or. Rev. Stat.* 97.050–090 (June 9, 1977), and *Tex. Rev. Civ. Stat. Ann.* 4590h (August 29, 1977).

10. *In re Quinlan* 70 N.J. 10, 355 A. 2d 647

11. *Satz v. Perlmutter* 362 So. 2d 160.

12. *In re Eichner* 52 N.Y. 2d 363, 420 N.E. 2d 64

13. *In re Storar* 52 N.Y. 2d 363, 420 N.E. 2d 64

14. *Superintendent of Belchertown State Hospital v. Saikewicz* 373 Mass. 728, 370 N.E. 2d 417.

15. *In re Dinnerstein* 6 Mass. App. 466, 380 N.E. 2d 134

16. *In re Spring* 380 Mass. 629, 405 N.E. 2d 115

17. For an introduction to some of these issues, see Emanuel, E.J. and Emanuel, L.L. "Proxy Decision Making for Incompetent Patients" *JAMA* vol. 267 (1992) pp. 2067–71.

18. P.L. 98-457 (Oct. 9, 1984). A good introduction to the continuing controversy is Kopelman, L.M. *et al.* "Neonatologists Judge the 'Baby Doe' Regulations" *New England Journal of Medicine* vol. 318 (1988) pp. 677–83.

19. As a good example of that controversy, consider the discussion prompted by publication of Quill, T.E. "Death and Dignity: A Case of Individualized Decision Making" *New England Journal of Medicine* vol. 324 (1991) pp. 691–4.

20. Schneiderman, L.J. *et. al.* "Medical Futility: Its Meaning and Ethical Implications" *Annals of Internal Medicine* vol. 112 (1990) 949–54.

21. Truog, R.D. *et al.* "The Problem with Futility" *New England Journal of Medicine* vol. 326 (1992) 1560–4.

22. Angell, M. "The Case of Helen Wanglie" *New England Journal of Medicine* vol. 325 (1991) pp. 511–2.

23. Brody, B.A. "Special Ethical Issues in the Management of PVS Patients" *Law Medicine and Health Care* vol. 20 (1992) pp. 104–15.

24. Blackhall, L.J. "Must we Always Use CPR" *New England Journal of Medicine* vol. 317 (1987) pp. 1281–4.

25. Youngner, S.J. "Who Defines Futility" *JAMA* vol. 260 (1988) 620–1.

26. A classical statement, which still recognizes some physician roles in cost-containment, is Angell, M. "Cost Containment and the Physician" *JAMA* vol. 254 (1985) 1203–7.

27. Menzel, P. *Strong Medicine* (New York: Oxford University Press, 1990) and Morreim, E.H. *Balancing Act: The New Medical Ethics of Medicine's New Economics* (Dordrecht: Kluwer, 1991).

28. In re Westchester County Medical Center (O'Connor) 72 N.Y. 2d 517, 531 N.E. 2d 607. Judge Wachtler has defended his position in Wachtler, S. "A Judge's Perspective: The New York Rulings" *Law Medicine and Health Care* vol. 19 (1991) pp. 60–2.

29. Belkin, L. "New York Rule Compounds Dilemma over Life Support" *New York Times* May 11, 1992, p. 1

30. McClung, J.A., and Kamer, R.S. "Legislating Ethics: Implications of New York's Do-Not-Resuscitate Law" *New England Journal of Medicine* vol. 323 (1990) pp. 270–2.

31. *ibid.*

32. Reprinted in *Annual Report of New York State Task Force on Life and the Law for 1988* pp. 10–11.

33. N.Y. Public Health Law Article 29-B.

34. N.Y. Public Health Law Article 29-C.

35. Article 29-B, Section 2961.

36. Article 29-B, Section 2965.

37. This special provision is discussed in New York State Department of Health, *The Health Care Proxy Law: A Guidebook for Health Care Professionals* (Albany: Department of Health, 1991) pp. 16–7.

38. For an alternative reading, see Brody, B. "A Historical Introduction to Jewish Casuistry on Suicide and Euthanasia" in Brody, B. *Suicide and Euthanasia* (Dordrecht: Kluwer, 1989) pp. 39–75.

39. *Life Sustaining Treatment, supra* note 2. pp. 147–8.

40. Baker, R. and Strosberg, M.A. *Legislating Medical Ethics* (Dordrecht: Kluwer, 1994).

41. Amendments to New York Public Health Law 29-B (July 15, 1991).

42. Letter of Baker and Strosberg (April 23, 1991), reprinted in Baker and Strosberg, *supra* note 40.

43. O'Brien, D.D. "One Family's Experience with the New York DNR Law" and Quill, T.E. "When the Ambulance Goes Home", both to appear in Baker and Strosberg, *supra* note 40.

44. Rosenthal, E. "Rules on Reviving the Dying Bring Undue Suffering, Doctors Contend" *New York Times* (October 4, 1990) p. 1.

45. Swidler, R.N. "The Presumption of Consent in New York State's Do-Not-Resuscitate Law" *New York State Journal of Medicine* (Feb. 1989) pp. 69–72.

46. Found in the 1993 supplement, p. 16.

47. *Ibid* p. 23.

48. See Gutis, P.S. "Accord Near on Proxy Plan for Life-Support Decisions" *New York Times* (May 30, 1989) p. B3 and Miler, T. "New York State's Health Proxy Law" *New York Law Journal* (August 16, 1990) p. 1.

The Formulation of Health Policy by the Three Branches of Government

LAWRENCE GOSTIN, J.D., L.L.D. (Hon.)

Professor and Co-Director, Georgetown University Law Center/
Johns Hopkins School of Hygiene and Public Health
Program on Law and Public Health

Modern health policy poses complex legal, ethical, and social questions. The goal of health policy is to protect and promote the health of individuals and the community. Government officials can accomplish this objective in ways that respect human rights, including the right to self-determination, privacy, and nondiscrimination. Numerous papers have addressed the question, What is sound health policy?[1] However, assessments rarely address the following important questions: Which bodies are best equipped to solve which health policy problems and why? What data do policymaking bodies need? How can that data best be made available to decision makers?

The United States is a highly diverse and complicated society. Many groups "weigh in" on significant health policy issues. America's expansive range of policymaking bodies and groups seeking to influence policy render it impossible to offer a systematic and comprehensive analysis of health policy formulation. To make an examination of policy development manageable, I will work from the following assumption, which is partly, but not wholly, valid. I will assume that formal development of health policy is the primary preserve of the three branches of government—the executive, legislature, and judiciary—at the state and federal levels. In practice, many other bodies make policy (such as professional associations or ethics groups through guidelines.)[2] This essay focuses on official government policymaking that is legally binding or at least has persuasive force in law. It evaluates the relative strengths and weaknesses of each branch of government with respect to health policy formulation. It also examines sources of information and influence that help drive policymaking. These include presidential and congressional commissions, task forces and advisory bodies, professional and trade associations, and public interest, consumer, and community-based groups.

Although I argue below that health policy is best formulated through rigorous and objective assessment of data, I do not support any restriction on the right of interest groups to publish their views and to appropriately lobby policy makers. A robust constitutional society that values freedom of expression and unrestricted participation in the political process should support a role for interest groups in health policy formulation. It should not censor or fetter the views of those who seek to participate in the process. Yet, the various branches of government should be able to rely on full, objective information and advice based upon sound scientific evidence. This essay will explore some mechanisms for achieving these aims.

Health policy encompasses a vast range of issues in health care, public health, and biotechnology. This essay selects illustrations from several areas that, over a period of time, have generated a great deal of policy formulated by each branch of government. These include reproductive rights, the right to die, and mental health. I will also use examples in the fields of health care reform, AIDS, and civil rights of persons with disabilities.

CHARACTERISTICS OF SOUND POLICY DEVELOPMENT

What factors are important in developing sound health policies? The policies themselves are rarely subjected to scientific scrutiny. Whether society seeks to reform the health care system, to restrict or to expand women's choices to receive an abortion, or to authorize or to criminalize physician-assisted dying, it has no precise means by which to test for the "correct" approach. Health policy decisions often reflect choices between competing values, as well as assessments of available data. Interest groups, including organizations representing various health care professionals, select their values and evaluate data through their own lenses. Clearly, groups comprised of highly expert and well-intentioned professionals often make markedly different decisions about health policy.

The New York case of *New York State Society of Surgeons v. Axelrod*[3] exemplifies the difficulty of deciding on one "correct" policy solution to complex health problems. The highest state court considered whether the state health commissioner had correctly categorized HIV infection as a communicable disease. This policy, on its face, appears noncontroversial and subject to neutral assessment. Yet, health professionals strongly split on this issue. Many public health organizations (e.g., the American Public Health Association) supported the commissioner, because the communicable disease classification under New York law adopted a voluntary approach to controlling the HIV epidemic. However, many medical and surgical organizations (e.g., the American Medical Association) favored the classification of HIV infection as a sexually transmitted disease. This would authorize greater use of compulsory testing, reporting, and contact tracing. What factors should have guided the court's decision between these two sets of respected professionals, who each used reasoned argument and data to argue that their preferred health policy was more effective?

Governmental officials need a framework for the development of sound health policy. Adopting the model I set out below does not guarantee that policies will be "effective"; but it does provide a way to filter out obvious biases and to focus attention on scientific data and reasonably objective assessments of arguments. Applying this framework allows interest groups to continue making their voices heard, while it encourages decision makers to obtain information from more neutral sources as well.

Several factors are important for developing sound health policies. First, to the extent possible, the policymaker should be objective and dispassionate. This means that decision makers should have no conflict of interest or improper financial or professional incentive. Policymakers should be able to understand the data and arguments presented, to assess them reasonably objectively, and to balance competing values fairly. In many areas of health policy, it is not necessary or even desirable for policymakers to be "experts" themselves, as long as they have access to expert advice.

Second, policymaking bodies should be publicly accountable for their decisions. If science or existing societal values do not support a decision, a democratic means for altering the decision is often desirable. Democratic societies thrive on the principle that government action that affects individuals and communities is subject to public review. Periodic elections provide an opportunity for the public to demand explanations and for public officials to articulate and justify their decisions.

At least one kind of health policy is not always best made through fully accountable decision makers: the kind that fundamentally affects the human rights of individuals and minority communities. Health policies that seriously burden individual rights to liberty, privacy, and nondiscrimination may require judicial, rather than majoritarian, determinations. For example, a fetal protection policy that excludes all women from unsafe work places to promote the health of infants may violate fundamental rights of nondiscrimination. In *Johnson Controls,* the U.S. Supreme Court unanimously ruled that a fetal protection policy was discriminatory even though the company presented some scientific evidence that the fetus of a pregnant worker could be at risk.[4]

Third, the decision making body should be positioned to receive and to evaluate full and objective information on all aspects of a health policy. Government entities often have access to a great deal of information, but assessing the reliability of that information may be difficult. Judges receive information from legal advocates as well as "experts" selected by each side of a case; likewise, legislators and executive officials receive information from a wide array of lobbyists and professional groups. Policymakers may recognize that information is coming from a potentially biased source, but may have difficulty weighing the relative value of the information they receive.

In addition to receiving information from the wide variety of traditional sources, policymakers need access to objective and complete information from reasonably neutral sources. This includes data and argument on the scientific, ethical, social, and legal aspects of the issue. Decision makers may seek information from one or several different objective sources in order to develop sound health policy.

Fourth, policymakers must have well-considered criteria for making the decision. Objective criteria help to guide decision makers in formulating goals, selecting means, and establishing the scientific, social, and ethical parameters for decision making. They also reduce the arbitrariness or biases that often are inherent in decision making processes. I suggest the following steps to guide policymakers:[5]

(a) *Examine the public health interest.* Does the proposed policy seek to achieve a compelling health objective? The policymaker should clearly and narrowly define the health purpose(s) of the policy. This protects against biases in decision making, helps communities to understand the policy rationale, and facilitates public debate.

(b) *Examine the overall effectiveness of the policy.* Is the proposed policy likely to be effective in achieving the stated goal(s)? This step requires an assessment of whether the policy is an appropriate intervention to achieve the stated objectives and whether it is reasonably likely to lead to effective action. The policymaker should gather scientific data and apply logic to analyze whether a policy will be effective.

(c) *Evaluate whether the policy is well-targeted.* Is the proposed policy narrowly focused on the health problem? A decision maker should determine whether a policy is narrowly tailored to address the specific health problem, or whether it is over- or underinclusive. Overbroad policies target a population that is much larger than necessary to achieve the health objective. For example, the Bush and Clinton policy that interned or repatriated all Haitian refugees with HIV infection was overbroad, because it affected all of the group, regardless of whether individuals engaged in safe sex or other practices. It adversely affected individuals who did not pose a significant risk of transmission of HIV.[6]

(d) *Identify the human rights burdens.* This step requires an inquiry into the nature, invasiveness, scope, and duration of human rights violations. Does the policy interfere with the right to liberty, autonomy, privacy, or nondiscrimination? For example, a policy that requires women to use contraceptives as a condition of receiving welfare benefits might interfere with the right to reproductive privacy and discriminate against women (because the policy does not apply to men) and the poor (because the policy does not affect higher-income women). It may also burden the social and economic rights of dependent children if benefits were withdrawn.

(e) *Examine whether the policy is the least restrictive alternative.* A policymaker should assess whether the health objective could be achieved as well, or better, with fewer restrictions on human rights. This step helps to ensure that a policymaker considers alternatives that may better accommodate societal and individual interests.

Fifth, the policymaker should pursue a fair process to arrive at the decision. This requires a careful examination of all relevant facts and arguments. Procedures may include inquisitorial or adversarial hearings, investigations, or other rigorous methods for finding facts and examining arguments. A fair process requires that all persons or organizations that have a legitimate interest in the outcome should have a reasonable means of presenting evidence or arguments. Careful attention to decision making processes achieves both more accurate fact finding and greater equality and fairness to interested individuals and groups.

These five elements of policymaking (impartial decision making, accountability, collecting full and objective information, applying well-considered criteria, and following a rigorous and fair process) are often helpful in developing sound health policies. In the following section, I apply these criteria to decision making by each of the three branches of government and assess which bodies are most capable of resolving which health policy problems and why.

GOVERNMENT BODIES AND THE CAPACITY TO ADDRESS HEALTH ISSUES EFFECTIVELY

The Judiciary

In theory, the judiciary provides the least ideal forum for the development of many health policies. Certainly, judges are thought to be impartial and able to assess evidence and arguments from a variety of sources objectively. However, many judges are insulated from public accountability. They are appointed by political figures, often for their political ideologies;

they may have long-term or life appointments; and many are not subject to election or reappointment. Judges usually bring legal skills to the bench; they may lack experience with scientific or ethical thinking. They rarely receive education or training in health issues.[7]

More importantly, the adversarial nature of judicial proceedings militates against a prominent role for judges in health care policy formulation. The information that judges receive is often partial and incomplete; also, attorneys usually present narrow legal arguments that may not endorse the most desirable policy position. The legal system frequently assumes judges can produce a balanced, accurate decision after hearing two extremist versions of an issue. Yet, each version may be biased or unreliable. Courts lack the tools for assessing the validity of complex scientific or technological evidence and arguments. Courts rely on "expert" witnesses. However, expert witnesses are usually paid for their testimony; this presents a conflict of interest. Also, they may not be the most qualified in their fields, and they may offer opinions that the majority of their peers do not accept and/or that may not have been subjected to adequate scientific inquiry.

In *Daubert v. Merrell Dow Pharmaceuticals,* the U.S. Supreme Court ruled for the first time on the place of scientific evidence in federal proceedings.[8] The decision involved an appeal about whether the drug Bendectin caused birth defects. The federal district court and the court of appeals had dismissed the lawsuit, ruling that data concerning birth defects were inadmissible because they were not "generally accepted" in the scientific community.

The Supreme Court rejected the "general acceptance" standard that looked to the conclusions of the expert witness, and it took a broader view of the scientific process, with an emphasis on "methods and procedures." The Court established judges as active gatekeepers charged with insuring that "any and all scientific testimony or evidence admitted is not only relevant, but reliable." It asked judges to screen out ill-founded or speculative scientific theories. The Court held that judges should focus on the reasoning or methodology behind scientific testimony, rather than on whether the conclusions of an expert witness have won general acceptance in the scientific community. Speaking for the Court, Justice Blackmun said, "In order to qualify as scientific knowledge, an inference or assertion must be derived by the scientific method" and must have been tested or at least subject to testing. While publication in a peer reviewed journal was not essential, it was relevant."[9] In dissent, Chief Justice Rehnquist, joined by Justice Stevens, warned that the decision would require judges to become "amateur scientists."

The *Daubert* case may well enable judges to assess expert testimony with somewhat greater reliability by reference to the scientific method. But, as Justice Blackmun stated, "There are important differences between the quest for truth in the courtroom and the quest for truth in the laboratory." These differences still place courts in a uniquely difficult position to assess health policy. Courts must frame their questions under the terms of a case or controversy and the applicable law. Courts do not adopt criteria to help them assess the benefits and harms of a health policy; they only resolve whether a policy is lawful. Also, courts rarely appoint neutral experts. Accordingly, even if they are able to filter out confounded scientific theories, they lack access to the objective expertise necessary for developing health policy. Courts could considerably enhance their ability to assess scientific questions if they systematically appointed neutral experts paid only by the state. Appointed experts could help the court perform a thorough, objective examination of the state of the science, which is essential for sound decision making.

Despite these numerous disadvantages courts have been instrumental in developing several important health policies. I will discuss three areas where courts have made major contributions to health policy—reproductive rights, the right to die, and mental health. The important role of the judiciary in the field of reproductive rights has been well discussed.[10] Beginning with the seminal cases of *Griswold v. Connecticut*[11] and, later, *Roe v. Wade*,[12] the courts for nearly two decades defended the reproductive rights of women. The Supreme Court found a constitutional right to "privacy" even though no mention of the concept appears in the Bill of Rights. The courts used the newly construed right to privacy to prevent the state from interfering with the sale and distribution of contraception.[13] The Supreme Court explained that contraception concerns "the most intimate of human activities and relationships."[14]

The Supreme Court stated that the constitutional promise of privacy protects not only the right to use contraception, but also the right to decide whether to carry a fetus to term.[15] It defended a woman's right to choose, and the privacy of her relationship with her physician, through the mid-1980s.[16]

In recent years, the changing composition of the Supreme Court has led to a significant erosion of reproductive rights and medical privacy. The Court upheld the authority of the state to restrict the use of public employees and facilities for the performance of nontherapeutic abortions.[17] The Court also upheld a Department of Health and Human Services regulation prohibiting federally funded family planning clinics from counseling or referring women for abortions.[18] The DHHS regulation became known as the "gag rule" because it prohibited funded programs from providing women with objective clinical information about reproductive choices. In *Planned Parenthood of Southeastern Pennsylvania v. Casey*,[19] the Supreme Court changed the legal standard by which to evaluate restrictions on abortion. This decision will have a profound effect on access to reproductive health care.[20] It will allow states to place restrictions on access, such as requirements that abortions be performed in hospitals that are not publicly funded; restrictions on the timing, such as waiting periods for abortions; and mandatory justification and information requirements, such as limiting the reasons women can use for an abortion and requiring the doctor to present state-approved information.[21] This shift in the composition and decision of the Supreme Court vividly shows how changeable the courts can be in assessing health policy and defending human rights.[22]

Many argue that the development of the right to privacy from 1965 through the early to mid-1980s had profound, positive effects on reproductive policy. Neither the legislative nor the executive branch produced similarly clear and consistent policies on contraception and abortion. Current efforts in Congress (e.g., the Freedom of Choice Act) and in state legislatures to protect reproductive privacy use the same "fundamental rights" analysis that the Supreme Court employed in *Roe*.[23] Courts also developed thoughtful rulings on surrogate motherhood[24] and artificial reproduction that some state legislatures are emulating.[25]

The judiciary has also displayed leadership in formulating policy around the right to withdraw life-sustaining treatment, beginning with the Karen Ann Quinlan decision of the New Jersey Supreme Court in 1976.[26] While the U.S. Supreme Court has rarely extended the right to privacy beyond reproductive decisions,[27] many state courts have interpreted the federal and state constitutions as conferring a right to refuse life-sustaining medical treatment.[28] The court in *Bouvia* held that a patient's decision to forego medical treatment "is a moral and philosophical decision that, being a competent adult, is hers alone."[29] The right to refuse medical intervention has been extended to persons who have become incapable of making a decision[30] and those who have always been incapable.[31] The courts have almost uniformly respected the decisions of surrogates, particularly family members, in making choices for persons who could not decide for themselves.[32]

The courts have defined the circumstances under which treatment could be terminated with greater specificity over the years. Most courts have rejected the distinction between withholding and withdrawing treatment, between ordinary and extraordinary treatments, and between terminally ill and nonterminal cases. The courts have protected the right to refuse treatment in cases involving ventilators and blood transfusions, as well as those involving nutrition and hydration.[33] Many courts have set out procedures and criteria for decision making ranging from second opinions, prognosis, and ethics committees[34] to ombudsmen.[35]

Despite the courts' own insistence that legislatures would make these decisions better, the judiciary has formulated much of the policy surrounding termination of life-sustaining treatment. Only recently has the locus of policy begun to shift to federal and state legislatures. The Supreme Court's decision in *Cruzan* provided an impetus for the move to legislative policymaking on the right to die.[36] In *Cruzan*, the U.S. Supreme Court upheld the decision of the Missouri Supreme Court to adopt a clear and convincing evidence standard for the termination of life-sustaining treatment. The Supreme Court never mentioned the word "privacy" in its decision. Instead, it found that competent patients had a "liberty interest" to refuse treatments. The Court did not view the individual's liberty interest as "fundamental"; this suggested that the state interest in preserving life could prevail.

Legislatures began to conceive of ways in which the decisions of persons to refuse life-sustaining treatments could be more routinely respected. In her concurrence in *Cruzan*, Justice O'Connor gave some guidance by suggesting that the Court might in the future constitutionally protect the advance directives of patients. In 1990, Congress enacted the federal Patient Self-Determination Act, with an implementation date of December 1, 1991. The Act conditions health care providers' receipt of Medicare or Medicaid dollars on their provision of written information at the time of admission about patients' rights under state law to accept or refuse medical treatment and to formulate advance directives. Since *Cruzan*, state law on advance directives has increasingly been crafted by legislatures.

The field of mental health policy shows a similar pattern of judicial leadership followed by legislative enactment. During the 1970s, the courts began a process that would transform mental health policy in America. The courts struck down mental health statutes as unconstitutionally vague and insufficiently related to the states' valid interests in protecting the public from harm.[37] The courts refused to allow broad discretionary language in civil commitment statutes if it described psychiatric decision making purely in medical terms, such as "mentally ill," "in need of treatment," personal "welfare," or "best interests." Nor would the courts allow civil commitment in the absence of rigorous due process including the right to notice, counsel, and a hearing.[38] The courts constitutionally required the standard of proof at civil commitment hearings to be more than a preponderance of evidence; typically, commitment demands "clear and convincing evidence."[39] More recently, the courts also developed standards for refusal of treatment by persons with mental illness.[40] Mental health legislation in America has been fundamentally reformed to comply with the constitutional requirements set by the judiciary.

I do not argue here about whether judicial policies in these three areas have been effective. Some have claimed that abortion cases too rigidly adhered to the scientifically and socially questionable trimester framework; that the right to die cases gave insufficient weight to the need to preserve life; and that the mental health cases led to a decade of deinstitutionalization that increased human suffering, homelessness, and violence in America. I do observe that the judiciary has had a profound, lasting effect in these and other areas of health policy, which other branches of government have emulated.

What factors made these issues particularly suited for judicial decision making? At least one of three factors was common to each of these areas of health policy. First, each issue involved emotionally charged social questions that divided the public. The right to life is perhaps the single most controversial and enduring problem in health policy formulation. The issue of preservation of life is central to both abortion and termination of life-sustaining treatment. While the mental health cases do not engender the same emotion, they still involve sharp differences between professionals and civil libertarians about the right of society to confine and to treat persons with mental illness. Indeed, the culture of the time influenced much of the discourse, and ultimately, litigation. Rosenhan's " On Being Sane in Insane Places,"[41] Szasz's "*Myth of Mental Illness,*"[42] and Goffman's "*Asylums*"[43] each symbolized the antipsychiatry movement of the day. Courts in some ways are uniquely suited for dealing with such areas of social divisiveness. They can often remain aloof from the controversy and rely on "neutral" legal doctrine. The legislative and executive branches of government are more vulnerable to interest groups, lobbyists, and financial pressures.

The second factor common to at least one of these health issues is the absence of formal policy existing at the time of the litigation. When the New Jersey Supreme Court was deciding Karen Quinlan's case, there was little legislative or executive guidance on the termination of life-sustaining treatment. The court was simply deciding the case with which it was presented. It had to craft a reasoned decision based upon traditional legal and ethical principles: respect for persons, autonomy, and privacy. The courts that followed *Quinlan* had to look to prior judicial decisions in other jurisdictions because the legislatures, for the most part, still had not acted.[44] The courts in the right-to-die cases appeared to be filling a vacuum in policy. This second factor suggests that the courts are more likely to intervene in areas where there was lack of consensus or established policy.

Prior to 1973, some liberalization in the scope of lawful abortions was evident in several legislatures, but few statutes approached the breadth of the privacy right decreed by the court in *Roe*. Most of the existing legislation was haphazard and inconsistent. It often did not balance individual interests with those of the state.[45] It is an open question as to whether the Supreme Court would have intervened in quite so decisive a manner if more settled policy on abortion rights had existed. The Court moved, at least in part, because of the absence of a national consensus on the issue.

Judicial decisions in mental health cases, unlike abortion or right-to-die cases, did not simply fill a policy vacuum. At the time of this litigation, all 50 states had civil commitment statutes that were fairly uniform in content. The courts appeared to usurp the field by requiring the legislatures to enact new statutes to comply with constitutional guarantees.

The judiciary, then, has sometimes acted as a pathfinder when there was a paucity of established policy. In an atmosphere of uncertainty in health policy, the courts can answer questions on a case-by-case basis. It is only after years of case law that a consistent policy emerges and gains public acceptance. At that time, the legislature can begin its work in clarifying and codifying policy choices.

A third characteristic shared by all three health issues is the presence of a fundamental claim to human rights by individuals and groups. These human rights claims weighed heavily in the balance of scientific, social, and ethical issues. In the fields of reproductive rights and the right to die, the courts repeatedly echoed the theme of individual choice, self-determination, and privacy. In the mental health cases, the courts emphasized fundamental claims to due process and liberty. This third factor (i.e., the central importance of human rights) is likely to be the most important in deciding whether the courts will, or should, intervene in significant cases of health policy. Unlike the executive and legislative branches of government, the courts are suited to protect the rights of individuals or groups. They are less concerned with pleasing the majority and less likely to give in to majoritarian pressures that may oppress vulnerable individuals or groups or restrict their rights. The judiciary also has appropriate criteria and procedures for ensuring the protection of individual rights. Courts can invalidate oppressive state action through constitutional review, and can protect minorities through civil rights decisions.[46] While the legislature or executive may focus more strongly on using science to promote the health of the community, these two branches sometimes overlook or insufficiently weigh human rights concerns. Where human rights become a defining value in health policy, courts may be the most appropriate body to make decisions.

The Legislature

If the judiciary is the least suited branch of government to develop health policy in many areas, the legislature may be the most suited. The legislature is thought to be impartial and publicly accountable; it has the capacity to collect full information from a wide range of objective sources; part of its mandate is to protect and promote the health of the public; and it has the power to engage in a lengthy and deliberative process in enacting legislation.

Classic American federalism suggests that the legislature possesses special authority to develop policy.[47] In essence, the power to make law reposes exclusively in the legislature, though it may delegate rule-making and regulatory powers to departments in the executive branch. The judiciary and the executive (apart from the veto power) are not permitted to intrude into its legislative powers. Article I, Clause 8, of the U.S. Constitution empowers Congress to "make all Laws which shall be necessary and proper for carrying into Execution. . . . the powers vested by this Constitution in the Government of the United States, or in any Department or Offices thereof." The state legislatures have police powers to protect and promote the health, safety, and morals of the community.[48] This power may establish the legislature as the appropriate policymaking body in most circumstances.

In theory, neither the executive nor the judiciary has a mandate to create health policy. The court system, apart from its historic role of constitutional or judicial review,[49] principally interprets, construes, and applies the law. Moreover, the federal courts exercise their powers only to resolve "cases" or "controversies" (Article III). The principal power of the executive in domestic affairs is to carry the laws into effect and secure their observance.[50] The scope of executive rule making cannot constitutionally reach beyond the bounds of the applicable legislation.[51] Thus, while the various agencies of the federal and state governments that deal with health can powerfully affect policy through rule making, the direction and limits are placed by the legislature.

Democracies usually pride themselves on having elected legislatures that are independent and fully accountable to the public. It is for this reason that so much concern is focused on tightening legal and ethical rules for financing campaigns, controlling lobbyists and pressure groups, and prohibiting conflicts of interest. To be sure, questions remain about whether legislators have financial conflicts of interest or have been unduly influenced. Nevertheless, legislators must meet increasingly strong legal and ethical standards and are subject to periodic elections.

Legislatures are also appropriate policymakers because they draw on the experience of a diverse membership and staff. Importantly, they can collect information from a wide variety of sources. Legislative committees receive written and verbal suggestions from interested groups, and often request information from more objective sources.

Legislatures, if provided with adequate resources, can establish standing bodies designed to help gather and analyze the scientific data necessary for sound policy development. They can also create commissions to advise on particular health policy issues such as AIDS[52] or bioethics. Congress's Office of Technology Assessment (OTA)[53] provides an apt model of a standing advisory body. The OTA is an analytical support agency of the U.S. Congress. It helps congressional committees understand policy that often involves highly complex technological issues. Congress can frame health policy questions that are most useful to its legislative agenda and receive timely assistance. The OTA can issue contracts and assemble interdisciplinary working groups to obtain specialized information. The OTA has provided extensive data and analysis to Congress in numerous areas of health policy ranging from the human genome to HIV disease[54] and tuberculosis.[55]

Congress can also request studies from the U.S. General Accounting Office on health policy issues. Recent reports of the General Accounting Office include studies of organ transplantation,[56] needle exchange programs,[57] and Medicaid.[58]

While legislatures rarely operate according to clear, written criteria, their constitutional mission to preserve the health, safety, and morals of the community sets the parameters for their activities. Moreover, legislatures can require committees to observe the criteria for sound decision making that have already been suggested—i.e., to establish policies that are effective, well-targeted, and minimally burdensome of human rights.

Legislatures have the capacity to follow a rigorous, fair decision making process. Legislative hearings can be thorough and expansive in ways that are simply not feasible in other branches of government. While judicial hearings are adversarial in nature, legislative committees may use many methods to gather information and hear from interested parties. Legislatures may provide forums to review societal perspectives, as Congress did in the hearings involving Justice Clarence Thomas; they also can invite interest groups, consumers, professionals, and academics to present testimony. In sum, legislatures can garner a massive amount of information in open, impartial ways that make them strong candidates for sound policymakers.

There are, of course, major detriments to legislative policymaking. First, most legislators belong to political parties whose partisan character may lead them to view policy issues through a narrow lens. Rather than independently seeking the most effective health policy, leaders of a political party may powerfully influence legislators. For example, the 1992 presidential candidates spent a great deal of time discussing the "gridlock" in Congress. On almost every policy issue of consequence, political parties found little common ground. Indeed, when particularly divisive issues such as abortion policy or fetal tissue research are at stake, entire pieces of legislation can be thwarted through noncooperation, filibusters, and threats of a presidential veto from the opposing political party.

Second, legislators may be indebted to particular individuals and groups that helped them to get elected. Financing modern political campaigns is extraordinarily expensive. Legislators may have to think long and hard before making decisions against the interests of large contributors. For example, substantial contributions from the pharmaceutical, tobacco, agricultural, or automobile industries can strongly influence legislators' judgments on policies affecting the public health and safety.

Third, legislators are highly sensitive to well-organized interest groups. These include professional associations such as the American Medical Association (AMA) or American Bar Association (ABA). These organizations are perceived to be able to influence a large number of voters. A legislator may be concerned as much with the way he or she will be viewed by powerful interest groups as with the impact of the health policy under consideration. Many health policy analysts, for example, believe that Medicare benefits should be modified to provide more cost effective coverage for persons who can least afford health insurance. Yet, this is a politically difficult area to tackle because of the influence of organizations representing older populations. Similarly, legislators often give deference to the plaintiff's bar on medical malpractice or the AMA or health insurers on health care reform.

Fourth, legislators frequently operate on a limited horizon. Legislators are elected for a short term, and may not be interested in the longer term benefits of a policy. They may, for example, be concerned more with the immediate electoral problems caused by increased taxes necessary to provide universal health care coverage, than with the long-term health and financial benefits of reforming the health care system.

The Americans with Disabilities Act (ADA) provides an illustration of a statute that fulfills all of the promise of the legislature as an effective policymaker. While the ADA provides a strong weapon against discrimination against persons with disabilities, its impact on the health care system is less well understood. Several areas of impact on the health care system have been observed by courts and commentators: the duty of health care professionals to treat patients with disfavored health conditions such as AIDS, the duty not to discriminate in health care benefits coverage, and the duty to exercise compulsory public health powers fairly.[59]

The ADA was born of a remarkable coalescence of the interests of a large and diverse group of people. The act was supported by groups representing persons with disabilities, civil liberties groups, AIDS advocacy organizations, and mental health associations. It was supported on a broad bipartisan basis with leadership from Republicans (e.g., Senators Dole and Weicker) as well as Democrats (e.g., Senator Kennedy and Congressman Waxman). Notably, it had the support of President Bush, who signed legislation passed by a Democratic Congress.[60,61]

The ADA is the latest in a series of statutes enacted by Congress that proscribe discrimination on the basis of race, sex, age, and disability. These accomplishments in the field of civil rights are widely perceived as critically important policies that have been the preserve of the legislative branch of government. More recently, many state legislatures have enacted antidiscrimination statutes to protect persons with HIV infection or disease[62] or persons with genetic traits or conditions.[63]

What are the qualities of the legislative process that made it possible to achieve the social good that has emerged from civil rights legislation? And why has the legislature had such difficulty replicating this success in other areas where social change is equally imperative, such as health care reform?

The success of legislatures in the field of civil rights is largely attributable to the growing consensus in society about the evils of discrimination based upon personal characteristics such as race, sex, disability, or health status. Historians may well observe one striking feature in the passage of the ADA. There was widespread consensus around the antidiscrimination principles inherent in the legislation. The legislative debates literally rang with the virtues of equal opportunity and human rights for persons with disabilities in society;[64] diverse interest groups came together and worked in a coordinated fashion in their lobbying efforts; and there was an absence of a vocal and organized opposition.

Even the individuals and groups that would have been expected to stand in the way of these changes refrained from doing so. Conservative persons in Congress never actively opposed the legislation, but narrowed their objections to certain "undeserving" groups such as drug users, homosexuals, and persons with psychiatric disorders involving antisocial behavior or gender identity.[65] They also objected to parts of the ADA that fed directly into the fears of the public, even though those fears were not supported by the epidemiologic evidence. Considerable congressional debate was engendered concerning food handlers with HIV infection. A compromise was ultimately reached to direct the Secretary of Health and Human Services to prepare a list of food-borne diseases where persons could be restricted from working in the food service industry.[66] Predictably, when the list was published a year after the passage of the ADA, HIV disease was not mentioned by the Secretary.*

The absence of significant opposition to the ADA was due, in part, to the fact that in wider society it was becoming culturally and socially inappropriate to vocally oppose civil rights for persons with disabilities.

---

*The desire to override antidiscrimination principles for persons infected with HIV continued in Congress after the enactment of the ADA. The Kimberly Bergalis Act required states to determine whether HIV-infected health care professionals could safely practice invasive, exposure-prone procedures. The statute was passed despite the opposition of virtually all of the national medical and public health associations. Similarly, Congress added HIV infection to the list of dangerous contagious diseases that would allow compulsory screening and exclusion of travelers and immigrants. The statute was passed against the advice of the Department of Health and Human Services.

The experience of the passage of the ADA suggests that the legislature can most effectively act in situations where it is implementing the will of society, where pressure groups act in unity, and the opposition is muted. This is true majoritarian politics. When it works, it can provide powerful and lasting benefits to society. The problem, however, is that legislative processes rarely work in an atmosphere of consensus, especially in the highly controversial health policy arena.

In health policy, the issues are often bitterly contested and divisive. One disease may be pitted against another. For example, legislators may be lobbied to divide scarce resources between competing diseases such as AIDS, tuberculosis, cancer, heart disease, and mental illness[67] or between competing segments of the health care industry such as prevention, acute care, long-term care, and research. The interests of patients may be pitted against those of health care professionals. A pertinent case is the ongoing struggle between doctors and patients for the "right to know" the HIV status of the other. Struggles between generations are even apparent as debates ensue about who should bear the financial burden of paying for health care and who should receive the benefits—the young versus the old, the poor versus the rich, the healthy versus the sick.

A classic example of legislative failure to produce a badly needed public benefit is in health care reform.[68] Health care reform, on its face, ought not to be inordinately difficult for legislatures. A substantial majority of Americans express dissatisfaction with the health care system.[69] Indeed, both candidates in the 1992 presidential campaign supported health care reform.[70,71]

The current system has failed to provide universal access to health care with an equitable sharing of benefits and burdens. An estimated 37 million people do not have health care coverage, with many more people inadequately covered.[72] Disparities in access to health care and poor health outcomes have been shown on grounds of socioeconomic status,[73,74] race and ethnicity,[75] and gender.[76]

The current system has also failed to control escalating health care costs relative to health care expenditures in other countries. The United States spent more than $666 billion on health care in 1990, approximately 12 percent of the nation's gross national product.[77] Health care expenditures are projected to reach $1.6 trillion, between 16 and 18 perent of the gross domestic product by the end of the decade if effective controls are not instituted.[78]

Given the fact that the current system appears not to serve the interests of large numbers of individuals, as well as the fiscal interests of American society, one would have expected Congress to act. Prominent members of Congress have worked on commissions and other initiatives to accomplish that objective,[79] and congressional committees have conducted many hearings. The gridlock can probably be attributed to the powerful interest groups whose vision of reform differs substantially. Organized medicine is concerned with limits on the doctor's income and freedom to practice; the organized bar is concerned about malpractice reform; the health insurance industry is concerned about its survival and the ability to continue traditional underwriting practices; consumers worry about loss of the absolute right to choose their doctor; and the business community and taxpayers are concerned about the cost. The ability of Congress to rise above the strong competing interests and influences to provide a fair and effective health care system remains in doubt.

The Executive

The executive branch of government brings to health policy formation many of the same benefits as the legislature. The executive branch can be both objective and accountable. Certainly, the chief executive is a political party figure subject to many of the ingrained ideologies that many politicians bring to their decision making. Yet, as the head of his or her party, the chief executive may be free to divert from party political positions or to change those positions. The executive branch, moreover, usually has many agencies concerned with health and social policy. Individuals who work in those agencies often are not connected to political parties and bring a wide body of knowledge and expertise to their fields. This creates enormous possibilities for impartial, accountable, and comprehensive assessments of health policy.

In many ways, the executive branch of government is in the best position to marshall all of the evidence, data, and reasoning necessary for the formulation of sound health policies. The U.S. Department of Health and Human Services, for example, has an unequaled capacity to obtain data in areas of clinical and policy research (e.g., the National Institutes of Health and the Agency for Health Care Policy and Research), prevention and public health strategies (e.g. the Centers for Disease Control and Prevention), and financial impacts (e.g., the Health Care Financing Administration). While the executive branch does not hold hearings like the judiciary or the legislature, it can solicit written and oral comment from organizations and experts. It frequently holds open meetings to discuss public health strategies.[80] It can, moreover, receive rigorous assessments of difficult health science and policy questions through contracts and grants with research institutions.

Presidents and governors can use their agencies wisely to achieve substantial health benefits for the public. The Human Genome Initiative, for example, was designed not only to answer many of the essential scientific questions about the detection, prevention, and treatment of genetic conditions, but also the ethical, social, and legal questions.[81]

The executive branch of government has considerable power to develop, shape, and expand health policy through executive orders, rule making, and interpretive guidance. The Equal Employment Opportunity Commission (EEOC), for example, has been active in pursuing claims under federal disability law. The EEOC has recently issued interpretive guidance suggesting that the ADA prohibits discrimination in health insurance coverage against particular individuals or groups with specific diseases.[82]

Despite the significant potential for the executive branch to develop health policy with all the benefits of the best research and rigorous assessments, it has frequently failed to follow sound scientific recommendations. This has resulted in administrations ignoring or rejecting the advice of scientific and policy commissions. It has also resulted in substantial swings in health policy from one administration to the next. The probable reason for discounting the objective advice of its agencies and commissions is that the executive, perhaps more than any other branch of government, is ideologically driven.

Many illustrations can be found to demonstrate the fragility of the commitment of administrations to neutral scientific assessments of health policy. The Reagan and Bush administrations both refused to allow federal funding for fetal tissue research in spite of the recommendation of an NIH advisory panel. President Reagan barely acknowledged the work of the President's Commission on AIDS. The Commission reported after extensive investigation, and made hundreds of recommendations. The only recognition the Administration gave to the 200-plus-page Commission report was a short press release. The Commission's central recommendations were never implemented.[83] Later, the National Commission on AIDS complained vehemently about being ignored by President Bush.[84] Very few of the recommendations made in several reports were ever seriously considered in the White House.[85]

Administrations sometimes act in ideological ways that anger virtually all of the health policy community. In *McGann*, a federal court of appeals held that an employer who reduced an employee's health coverage from $1 million to $5,000 after he made claims for HIV disease had not unlawfully discriminated under ERISA.[86] Many public health and medical organizations filed amicus curiae briefs asking the Supreme Court to overturn the decision. Yet, the court decided not to hear the case largely because the Bush Administration opposed the appeal.[87]

The disrespect administrations sometimes show for scientific advice is also illustrated by substantial swings in health policy on controversial issues. The behavior of successive administrations on reproductive health policy provides a vivid illustration. For a dozen years Republican administrations developed and maintained highly restrictive policies on abortion rights: (i) in a 1984 order known as the "Mexico City Policy," President Reagan prohibited the United States from providing foreign aid to family planning programs that were involved in abortion-related activities; (ii) in memoranda in 1987 and 1988, the National Institutes of Health placed a moratorium on federal funding of research involving the implantation of fetal tissue from induced abortions; (iii) by memoranda of 1987–1988, the Department of Defense banned all abortions at U.S. military facilities, even where the procedure was privately funded; (iv) in a 1988 regulation known as the "gag rule," the Department of Health and Human Services prohibited family planning clinics funded under Title X of the Public Health Service Act from counseling or referring women for abortion; and (v) in two Import Alerts issued in 1988–1989, the Food and Drug Administration excluded Mifepristone (RU-486) from the list of drugs that individuals can import into the United States.

On the twentieth anniversary of *Roe v. Wade,* January 23, 1993, President Clinton signed five memoranda that repealed all five of these policies—reversing a dozen years of policy on reproductive rights and medical privacy. The result of these sharp changes in policy by the executive is that America never seems to attain a settled policy on the issue of reproductive rights. The strongly ideological positions of the executive branch often allows it to lose sight of the questions that are central to the development of sound health policy—will the policy be effective in protecting and promoting the health of the public and will it adequately safeguard human rights?

CONCLUSION

As this paper is being written, the President's Task Force on National Health Care Reform, chaired by the First Lady, has completed its work, and the President has sent a bill to Congress for systematic reform of the health care system.[88] The President and the First Lady have compared this initiative of the executive to the Manhattan Project and the New Deal. The President was able to marshall the resources of several hundred experts within and outside of government to fundamentally reform the financing, organization, and delivery of health care in the United States.

This will provide a unique opportunity to observe the workings of two powerful branches of government on a health policy issue that can produce enormous social good for millions of Americans by enhancing their access to care, reducing inequalities, and allocating benefits and burdens more equitably. Will the President and Congress jointly develop a new health care system that is beneficial and just? Or will they become stalled in conflict and paralyzed by competing interest groups and ideologies? As years of careful thinking and writing on health care reform turns into a season of political debate and decision, the strengths or inadequacies of the two branches of government may become painfully obvious.

NOTES

1. E.g., National Research Council. *AIDS: The Second Decade*. Washington, D.C.: National Academy Press, 1990.

2. E.g., Hastings Center. *Guidelines on the Termination of Life-Sustaining Treatment and the Care of the Dying*. Briar Cliff Manor, N.Y., 1987.

3. *New York State Society of Surgeons v. Axelrod*, 77 N.Y.2d 677 (1991).

4. *International Union, UAW v. Johnson Controls, Inc.*, 499 U.S. 187 (1991).

5. A considerably more detailed "human rights impact assessment" is contained in Gostin L., Lazzarini, Z., *Public Health and Human Rights in the AIDS Pandemic*. Geneva, Switzerland: World Health Organization, in press.

6. *Haitian Centers Council, Inc., v. Sale*, 823 F. Supp. 1028 (E.D.N.Y. 1993).

7. In 1993, the U.S. Public Health Service conducted the first PHS workshop for state judges on tuberculosis and AIDS. See Gostin, L., Lazzarini, Z., *Tuberculosis, the Law, and Public Health*. Agency for Health Care Policy and Research, in press.

8. *Daubert v. Merrell Dow Pharmaceuticals*, 113 S.Ct. 2786 (1993).

9. Greenhouse L. Justices put judges in charge of deciding reliability of scientific testimony. *New York Times*, June 29, 1993: A13.

10. Butler, J.D., Walbert D.F., eds. 1992. *Abortion, Medicine, and the Law*, 4th ed. New York: Facts on File.

11. *Griswold v. Connecticut*, 85 S.Ct. 1678 (1965). See also *Loving v. Virginia*, 388 U.S. 1(1967); *Eisenstadt v. Baird*, 405 U.S. 438 (1972).

12. *Roe v. Wade*, 410 U.S. 113 (1973).

13. *Griswold v. Connecticut*, 85 S.Ct. 1678 (1965).

14. *Carey v. Population Services International*, 97 S.Ct. 2010 at 2016 (1977). See *Eisenstadt v. Baird*, 405 U.S. 438 (1972).

15. *Roe v. Wade*, 410 U.S. 113 (1973).

16. See, e.g., *City of Akron v. Akron Center for Reproductive Health*, 462 U.S. 416 (1983); *Thornburgh v. American College of Obstetrics and Gynecologists*, 476 U.S. 747 (1986).

17. *Webster v. Reproductive Health Services*, 492 U.S. 490 (1989).

18. *Rust v. Sullivan*, 111 S.Ct. 1759 (1991).

19. 112 S.Ct. 2791 (1992).

20. Benshoof, J. *Planned Parenthood v. Casey*: The impact of the new undue burden standard on reproductive health care. *JAMA* 1993: 269:2249–2257.

21. Dellinger, W. Abortion: The case against compromise. In: Butler, J.D., Walbert, D.F., eds. *Abortion, Medicine, and the Law*, 4th ed. New York: Facts on File, 1992: 90–98.

22. Van Alstyne, W.W. The cycle of constitutional uncertainty in American abortion law. In: Butler, J.D., Walbert, D.F., eds. *Abortion, Medicine, and the Law*, 4th ed. New York: Facts on File, 1992:79–89.

23. Benshoof, op. cit.

24. In re *Baby M.*, 217 N.J. Super. 313 (1987), *rev'd in part*, 525 A.2d 1128 (1988).

25. Yoon, M. The Uniform Status of Children of Assisted Contraception Act: Does it protect the best interests of the child in a surrogate arrangement? *American Journal of Law and Medicine* 1990, 16:525-553.

26. In re *Quinlan*, 70 N.J. 10, 355 A.2d 647, cert. denied sub. nom., *Garger v. New Jersey*, 429 U.S. 922 (1976).

27. See *Bowers v. Hardwick,* 106 S.Ct. 2841 (1986).

28. See, e.g., *John F. Kennedy Memorial Hospital, Inc. v. Bludworth,* 452 So.2d 921 (Fla. Sup. Ct. 1984); In re *Guardianship of Grant,* 109 Wash. 2d 545, 747 P.2d 445 (1987), modified 757 P.2d 534 (Wash. July 15, 1988); *Rasmussen v. Fleming,* 154 Ariz. 207, 741 P.2d 674 (1987); *Brophy v. New England Sinai Hospital, Inc.,* 398 Mass. 417, 497 N.E.2d 626 (1986). See Gostin, L. and Weir, R., Life and death decisions after *Cruzan:* Caselaw and standards of professional care. *Milbank Quarterly* 1991, 69:143–173.

29. *Bouvia v. Supreme Court* (Glenchur), 225 Cal. Rptr. 297 (Ct. App. 1986).

30. E.g., In re *Guardianship of Browning,* 568 So.2d 4 (Fla. Sup. Ct. 1990); In re *Severns,* 425 A.2d 156 (Del. Ch 1980); In re *Torres,* 357 N.W.2d 332 (Minn. 1984).

31. E.g., In re *Guardianship of Grant,* 747 P.2d 445 (1985), modified, 757 P.2d 534 (Wash. July 15, 1988); *Superintendent of Belchertown State School v. Saikewicz,* 370 N.E.2d 417 (Mass. 1977); In re *Eichner* (In re *Storar)* 438 N.Y.S.2d 266 (1981).

32. E.g., In re *Guardianship of Ingram,* 689 P.2d 1363 (Wash. 1984); In re *Guardianship of Hamlin,* 689 P.2d 1372 (Wash. 1984).

33. See Rhoden, N.K. Litigating life and death. *Harvard Law Review* 1988, 102:375–446.

34. See, e.g., In re *Jobes,* 529 A.2d 434 (N.J. 1987); *In re Guardianship of Hamlin,* 102 Wash.2d 810 (1984).

35. In re *Conroy,* 486 A.2d 1209 (N.J. 1985); In re *Peter,* 529 A.2d 419 (N.J. 1987).

36. *Cruzan v. Director, Missouri Department of Health,* 110 S.Ct. 2841 (1990).

37. E.g., *Lessard v. Schmidt,* 349 F. Supp.1078 (E.D. Wis. 1972); *Johnson v. Solomon,* 484 F. Supp. 278 (D. Md. 1979).

38. E.g., *Vitek v. Jones,* 445 U.S. 480 (1980); *Colyar v. Third Judicial Dist. Court,* 469 F. Supp. 424 (D. Utah 1979); *Suzuki v. Yuen,* 617 F.2d 173 (9th Cir. 1980).

39. *Addington v. Texas,* 441 U.S. 418 (1979).

40. E.g., *Washington v. Harper,* 110 S.Ct. 1028 (1990); *Mills v. Rodgers,* 457 U.S. 291 (1982).

41. Rosenhan, D.L. On being sane in insane places. *Santa Clara L. Rev.* 1973; 13:379.

42. Szasz, T.S. *The Myth of Mental Illness: Foundations of a Theory of Personal Conduct.* 1961, rev. ed. 1974.

43. Goffman, E. *Asylums: Essays on the Social Situation of Mental Patients and Other Inmates.* Garden City, N.Y.: Anchor Books Doubleday, 1961.

44. The courts did have a growing body of ethics literature in this area to guide its decisions, notably the President's Commission report.

45. George, B.J. State legislatures versus the Supreme Court: Abortion legislation into the 1990s. In: Butler, J.D., Walbert, D.F., eds. *Abortion, Medicine, and the Law,* 4th ed. New York: Facts on File; 1992:3–77.

46. See Gostin, L. The AIDS Litigation Project: A national review of court and human rights commission decisions, Part II: Discrimination. *JAMA* 1990; 263:2086–2093.

47. For a comprehensive examination of the constitutional role of federal judicial, legislative and executive power, see Tribe, L. *American Constitutional Law,* 2d ed., Mineola, N.Y.: Foundation Press, 1988.

48. *Jacobson v. Massachusetts,* 197 U.S. 11 (1905).

49. *Marbury v. Madison,* 5 U.S. (1 Cranch) 137 (1803).

50. *Tucker v. State,* 35 N.E. 2d 270, 291 (Ind. 1941).

51. *American Medical Assn. v. Heckler,* 606 F. Supp. 1422, 1439 (S.D. Ind. 1985).

52. National Commission on AIDS. *AIDS: An Expanding Tragedy, Final Report.* Washington, D.C.: 1993.

53. U.S. Congress, Office of Technology Assessment. *Genetic Monitoring and Screening in the Workplace.* Washington, D.C.: OTA, 1990. *The Role of Genetic Testing in the Prevention of Occupational Disease.* Washington, D.C.: 1983.

54. U.S. Congress, Office of Technology Assessment. *The CDC's Case Definition of AIDS:*

Implications of the Proposed Revisions—Background Paper. OTA-BP-H-89 Washington, D.C.: U.S. Government Printing Office, August 1992 (listing a dozen other OTA reports on HIV disease).

55. U.S. Congress, Office of Technology Assessment, *The Continuing Challenge of Tuberculosis,* OTA-H-574 (Washington, D.C.: U.S. Government Printing Office, Sept. 1993).

56. U.S. General Accounting Office. *Organ Transplants: Increased Effort Needed to Boost Supply and Ensure Equitable Distribution.* GAO/HRD-93-56, Washington, D.C., April 1993.

57. U.S. General Accounting Office. *Needle Exchange Programs: Research Suggests Promise as an AIDS Prevention Strategy.* GAO/HRD-93-60, Washington, D.C.: March 1993.

58. U.S. General Accounting Office. *Medicaid: States Turn to Managed Care to Improve Access and Control Costs.* GAO/HRD-93-46, Washington, D.C.: March 1993.

59. Goston, L. The Americans with Disability Act and the U.S. Health care system, *Health Affairs* 1992; 11:248–257.

60. West, J. The social and policy context of the Act. *Milbank Quarterly* 1991; 69 (Supp. 1/2):3-24.

61. Gostin, L., Beyer, H., eds. *Implementing the Americans with Disabilities Act: Rights and Responsibilities of All Americans.* Baltimore: Brookes Publishing Co., 1993.

62. Gostin, L. Public health strategies for confronting AIDS: legislative and regulatory policy in the United States. *JAMA* 1989; 261:1621–1630.

63. Gostin, L. Genetic discrimination: the use of genetically based diagnostic tests by employers and insurers. *American Journal of Law and Medicine* 1991; 17:109–144.

64. See volume 136 of the Congressional Record, July 1990 for legislative history.

65. The ADA does not protect persons currently using illegal drugs (s.510) or a range of socially disapproved behaviors such as gender identity disorders, pedophilia, exhibitionism, compulsive gambling, kleptomania and pyromania (s.511).

66. Report of the Judiciary Committee, no. 101–485, part 3 (to accompany H.R. 2273 at 146–147. See Gostin, L., Public health powers: the imminence of radical change. *Milbank Quarterly* 1991; 69 (supp. 1/2):268–290.

67. Bayer, R. Public health policy and the AIDS epidemic. An end to HIV exceptionalism? *New England Journal of Medicine* 1991; 324:1500–1504.

68. But see the successful reform efforts in several states such as Hawaii and Maryland. General Accounting Office. *Access to Health Care: States Respond to the Growing Crisis.* Washington, D.C.: Government Printing Office; 1992.

69. Blendon, R. Bridging the gap between expert and public views on health care reform. *JAMA* 1993; 263:2573–2578.

70. Clinton, B. The Clinton health care plan. *New England Journal of Medicine* 1992; 327–804.

71. Sullivan, L. The Bush Administration's health care plan. *New England Journal of Medicine* 1992; 327:801.

72. Bureau of National Affairs. Number of uninsured persons increases to 36.6 million in 1991. *Daily Labor Report* Jan. 12, 1993.

73. Wise, P.H., et al. Racial and socioeconomic disparities in childhood mortality in Boston. *New England Journal of Medicine* 1985; 313:360.

74. Pear, R. Big health gap tied to income is found in U.S. *New York Times.* July 8, 1993:A1, B10.

75. Council of Ethical and Judicial Affairs. Black-white disparities in health care. *JAMA* 1990; 263:2344.

76. Ayanian, J.Z., Epstein, A.M. Difference in the use of procedures between women and men hospitalized for coronary heart disease. *New England Journal of Medicine* 1991; 325:221.

77. Sullivan, L. The Bush Administration's health care plan. Op cit.

78. Congressional Budget Office. Projections of National Health Expenditures. Washington, D.C.: U.S. Government Printing Office; 1992.

79. Rockefeller, IV, J.D. A call for action: the Pepper Commission's blueprint for health care reform. *JAMA* 1991; 265:2507.

80. See, e.g., National Institutes of Health Workshop on Breastfeeding Research, July 1993.

81. U.S. Department of Health and Human Services and U.S. Dept. of Energy. *Understanding Our Genetic Inheritance: The U.S. Human Genome Project: The First Five Years (FY1991– 1995).* Washington, D.C., 1990.

82. Equal Employment Opportunity Commission. *Interim Enforcement Guidance on the Application of the ADA to Disability-Based Provisions of Employer-Provided Health Insurance.* June 8, 1993. See Freudenheim, M. Insurers accused of discrimination in AIDS coverage: Disability law is cited. *New York Times.* June 1, 1993: A1, D2.

83. The White House. *Implementing Recommendations of the Presidential Commission on Human Immunodeficiency Virus: The 10-Part Plan.* August 2, 1988.

84. National Commission on Acquired Immunodeficiency Syndrome. Report Number One, at p. 2, 6, December 5, 1989. See Rudavsky, S., AIDS Panel Faults Bush Administration Leadership. *Washington Post,* June 25, 1992:A3.

85. Gostin, L. Preface to the Harvard Model AIDS Legislation Project: A decade of a maturing epidemic: an assessment and directions for future public policy. *American Journal of Law and Medicine* 1990; 16:1–32.

86. *McGann v. H&H Music Company,* 946 F.2d 401 (5th Cir. 1991), cert. denied sub. nom., *Greenberg v. H&H Music Company,* 113 S.Ct. 482 (1992).

87. Freudenheim, M. Patients cite bias in AIDS coverage by health plans. *New York Times,* June 1, 1993:A1.

88. Gostin, L. Foreword: Health care reform in the United States—The Presidential Task Force. *American Journal of Law and Medicine* 1993; XIX:1–20.

The Role of Religious Participation and Religious Belief in Biomedical Decision Making

CHARLES M. SWEZEY, Ph.D.

Dean of the Faculty, Union Theological Seminary in Virginia

Biomedical decisions usually focus on specific problems or cases, and particular decisions gain standing and legitimacy when they become part of a practice. By practice, I mean standard ways to deal with typical cases that emerge over time and are accepted by medical practitioners and society. Practices are justified by explicitly stated moral values and characteristic ways of understanding and so interpreting illness. Also important are a long history of care, professional training and socialization, and accepted ways of assimilating new knowledge. These and other factors, however, require an ethos of support.

The explosion of knowledge in biology and other fields of inquiry, combined with recent innovations in medical technology, dramatically increase the human capacity to intervene in the natural life process. They also call into question some of the standard ways of dealing with typical cases. Well-known examples are subject to public debate. May physicians assist in actively terminating human lives? Is it permissible to use human fetal tissue in medical research? Under what conditions, if any, should patients receive organ transplants from nonhuman animals? The central issue in these and other questions is whether what *can* be done technically *ought* to be done morally. The issue has attitudinal dimensions. We respond to innovations in medical technology with wonder and awe. We are grateful for benefits, yet we fear deleterious consequences, so we search for guidance by exploring possibilities and seeking limits, understanding that limits have their own consequences. To set limits and attain possibilities, of course, are ways of specifying what may be done in particular cases, that is, of redefining medical practice.

The search for guidance does not take place in a vacuum, but in the context of a perceived erosion of confidence. The costs of health care rise amid serious debates about access to care and the adequacy of health insurance. Litigation increases amid important questions about the relation of causal accountability to moral and legal responsibility. Questions about the rationing of care appear just when physicians are charged with overtreating patients. Though all of medical practice is not disputed, the number of significant problems and the lack of consensus in dealing with them set a context for scrutiny by an increasingly broad public. The interacting roles of patient and physician are reexamined; the numbers of ethics committees and review boards grow; pressure groups and lobbies emerge. Medical practice seems to have become everybody's business. Along with other aspects of life, it becomes increasingly specialized and at the same time seeks legitimation in a democratic forum.

At the heart of these discussions are disagreements about proper modes of treatment. These disagreements are the source of fears that are larger than disputes about individual cases. One fear concerns the possible effects of a lack of uniformity in practices. The desire for uniformity is rooted in part in an understanding of fairness, the principle that similar cases should be treated similarly. When similar cases are not treated similarly, something seems askew morally. Judgments are difficult here, for there is room for diversity. Adult Jehovah's Witnesses, for example, undoubtedly will continue to refuse blood transfusions, a refusal generally accepted as an exception to standard practice. At issue is the amount of diversity a practice will tolerate. The specter which haunts is that the ethos that sustains standard practices will falter. Thus the second fear is that the very practice of medicine will erode, a practice inherited from the past which has served society well. These fears are strong enough to set a context for addressing the issue of the role of religious belief and participation in biomedical decision making. Clearly religion has the potential to erode, sustain, or enrich at least the ethos that nourishes standard medical practice.

FACTORS IN RELIGIOUS BELIEF

The topic this paper addresses is part of the more general problem of the relation of religion to modern society. The pioneering studies of Max Weber and Ernst Troeltsch have been followed by an enormous literature from several fields.[1] Though not unmindful of these studies, the primary intention of this paper is to provide a framework for understanding the relation between religion and biomedical decision making, and it undoubtedly reflects the viewpoint of a mainline Protestant ethicist. I first provide a scheme which points to important dimensions of religious belief. Although this scheme oversimplifies in ways that offend even my own scholarly sensibilities, it draws attention to several important factors. I next sketch the elements of decision making. Interactions are then traced, and a concluding section follows.

The Vision of God

In the traditions of the West, religious beliefs are intellectual constructs grounded in an experience of the reality of God. Piety, faith, and ecstasy, as well as other terms, refer to this experience. A religious object, God, is disclosed, and this object is characterized in different ways, e.g., king, lord, father, steadfast love, shepherd, judge, deliverer. This experience and its corresponding object is a vision of God, and its effects vary. Different sensibilities are evoked, e.g., reverence, wonder, and gratitude. Liturgical performance is elicited, e.g., praise, confession, and supplication. Certain deeds or acts are enjoined or prohibited, e.g., honoring parents or not bearing false witness.

Believers also articulate the character of the religious object in the form of beliefs. This response has multiple roots, e.g., attempts to clarify liturgical practice, efforts to persuade others of the authenticity of a vision, or simply the struggle to better comprehend and explain the deity. Many who formulate these beliefs are aware of the inadequacy and shortcomings of propositional statements. Indeed, a certain poignancy accompanies the work of theologians who are aware of the agonies of excess or defect, or of claiming either too much or too little for knowledge of God. Still the attempt is as important as it is inevitable, for what is believed about God is decisive in specifying God's relation to the world.

One difficulty is that religion is located in an institution, whereas, presumably, God is not so confined. This difficulty is compounded by the complexity of the world. James M. Gustafson, for example, writes about different "arenas" in which God's presence may be discerned—nature, history, culture, and society.[2] To claim that God is present to society and culture, for example, requires that something be said about God's relation to family life, economic institutions, government, technology, the arts, and the sciences. In the face of these difficulties, some theologians affirm that God is absent from the world, or perhaps present as a condemning judge who calls the faithful away to a better life. Others argue that God's governance includes sustaining and ordering powers that may be discerned in each of these arenas. Still others suggest that God as creator provides the occasions for new possibilities and so enables human innovation. Each of these beliefs, and many others, are thematizations. It is a mistake to reduce them to the status of intellectual propositions to which believers give cognitive assent. This move abstracts from important dimensions of religious belief and fails to see them as construals which, by specifying God's relation to the world, interpret all of life in theological dimension. Theological beliefs seek a coherence and consistency which, faithful to the divine reality, make sense in relation to the world.

If the task of theology in a strict sense is to articulate the vision of God in the form of stated beliefs so that the relation of God to the world gains specificity,[3] its larger task is to elaborate this vision by addressing four issues that recur perennially.[4] The four issues are the relation of good and evil, the nature of religious participation, estimates of reliable sources of knowledge, and the character of moral guidance. Each is part of religious belief, and the vision of God becomes clearer as they are answered. If these questions are not always answered explicitly, they are nonetheless present in the lives of believers as implicit, unstated assumptions. Those who do not share a religious vision offer nonreligious counterparts to explicitly religious answers to these questions.

Good and Evil

The first issue is the relation of good and evil. More precisely, the question concerns their *location* and *extent* as well as their relation. This problem emerges in everyday life when judgments are made about relative goods. One television program rather than another is watched, an adolescent selects a college to attend, a second career is chosen, and so forth.

A key for understanding the interaction of good and evil is found in human responses to certain events. When college students receive midterm grades, for example, responses range from indifference to overly enthusiastic optimism. These and other moods may occur fleetingly in response to particular events. Over time, however, moods may persist and become attitudes adopted toward the world. With apathy, what one does makes little difference; with cynicism, what others say or do makes no difference; with despair, the exercise of intentions is useless. These and other attitudes develop into patterns of being human, so that life is "staged," for example, with deep resignation or with quiet conscientiousness. Attitudes have roots in human nature, but it is human nature patterned in response to a discernment of good and evil forces in the world.

The interaction of good and evil requires an interpretation which sets particular events in a larger frame. Theology provides an interpretation by construing the world in a particular way, and this construal is part of the vision of God. One result may be a thoroughgoing dualism which assigns definite locations to good and evil forces. For example, the dominant culture or mere physical existence becomes the locus of evil, and the pure religious community or spiritual existence is the locus of good. God is envisioned as judge of the dominant culture or as not blessing physical life, and also as the savior who delivers the faithful into true community or spiritual bliss. Certain patterns of life follow. The perception of evil in thoroughgoing dualisms is neither universal nor radical. Since evil is assigned a rather definite *location,* it is not all-pervasive or universal. Since forces for good seem relatively exempt from evil, the *extent* of evil is limited; it is not truly virulent or radical.

Other theological interpretations locate evil more universally and view its extent more radically; they also provide an account of forces for good. The quest genre of literature provides an example. Grasped by a vision of God, a band of pilgrims ventures a journey and sets forth in the world only to encounter pitfalls, dangers, and temptations. Their challenge is to respond to these encounters in ways which faithfully honor the original vision. Those on the journey eventually learn that evil is found not only in the world, but lurks in the heart of each venturer. Moreover, those on the journey inevitably experience moments of grace when, surprisingly, they encounter forces of good outside their own company. The world is thus experienced as an arena of interacting good and evil forces, but without a thoroughgoing dualism. These encounters are means of clarifying the original vision of God who now is perceived as an ordering power who sustains and nurtures human existence as well as the rest of life, and who, as the creator of new possibilities, enables the journey to continue.

To remain with the image of the quest, patterns of life develop which train and equip venturers to deal with the experience of evil. Established ways of living, like the "inner-worldly asceticism" Max Weber attributed to the Puritans, are perduring attitudes adopted toward the world. Because the common experience of believers is that present reality does not exhaust the goodness of God, a way of life can be sustained in the face of truly tragic encounters with evil. What Weber called "the ethical irrationality of the world" is faced, namely, the realization that good results do not always flow from good intentions and that evil persons, despite themselves, may bring benefits.[5] Eschatologies, or beliefs about the way interacting good and evil forces finally play out, are born in these experiences and so expand the vision. Some eschatologies are radically dualistic; others are not. The result, in any case, is a vision of God which interprets human existence in the world.

Perceptions of good and evil, including eschatologies, are not confined to theology. For example, discussions of the consequences of genetic interventions in humans often include estimates of the future which strikingly resemble strands of religious beliefs about the interactions of good and evil, and well-known scientists who are not self-consciously religious spin out their own versions of the human prospect.[6] One cannot but wonder about the possibilities of mutual discourse. At issue is what is known scientifically about the natural world and humanity's place in it, and the role this knowledge plays in interpreting the present and conjuring the future. Also at issue are patterns of existence in the world and the sources of knowledge deemed reliable. In any event, religious belief is clearly a source for understanding the relation of good and evil, though it does this in different ways.

Religious Participation

A second factor in religious belief is the relation of those who share a religious vision to those who do not explicitly acknowledge it. This question is part of everyday life for believers and, in larger form, is present to all. How relate to those who differ in some significant respect? Resolutions of the explicitly religious issue are deeply conditioned by the distinctive form of religious association that first emerged in the West. This form of association is called "congregational religion."

According to Max Weber, congregational religion is an association of persons who embody, though imperfectly, belief in a transcendent God.[7] Transcendent here means the conception of a deity who brings the world into existence, stands over against it, and wills a way of life which differs from that customarily practiced. The embodiment of this belief takes place through three interacting provisions, each of which, again, stabilizes and secures belief in communal form. First, standard ways of venerating and so recalling the nature of the deity in a properly religious way are enacted regularly. Thus a cult is created, including sacraments and other forms of worship. Second, belief in God is fixed in a message that serves as court of appeal and authoritative source of knowledge. This takes place by demarcating canonical writings and by enunciating doctrines which state the meaning of these texts. Third, a means is found to recognize and order religious leaders in the association.

The clergy so ordered take up the task of being true to the transcendent God by leading worship and by interpreting scripture and doctrine. They also bear special responsibility for attracting and maintaining followers in the religious association, and they are successful in this calling to the extent that laity participate in the community, share the religious vision, and comprehend the rest of life in its light. Congregational religion emphasizes two primary methods for interacting with the laity who, notoriously, are unwilling to give up customary ways of living and know better than the clergy the meaning of belief. One is preaching and the other is pastoral care. The two are related, and each is suited to clerical tasks. Pastoral care, or attention to the needs of the laity with a distinctively religious focus, requires clergy to attend to matters which concern the everyday life of parishioners. Preaching affords the regular and formal opportunity to respond to these concerns by interpreting the religious message in the context of worship.

The beginnings of a voluntary principle for human associations are properly found in the emergence of congregational religion.[8] In ways just enumerated, religion differentiates from other forms of human association, including the family, the market, and the state. Being located in one realm raises the question of God's relation to these other realms. This issue is compounded in the modern world which, with its growing segmentation, is increasingly aware of autonomous rationales for differing institutions. Different forms of associations serve independent purposes. The dominant purpose of the economic realm, for example, is to produce and distribute goods and services. The political arena provides a system of governance charged with ensuring order in society. The family fosters mutuality and provides nurture for infants. One purpose of medicine is to provide health care. Religion serves none of these purposes, at least not directly. The irony is that one of the largest challenges faced by religion is posed by its own principle of organization. An enduring task of religion is to comprehend and interpret theologically all of life; but by gaining independence as an organization, its relation to other areas of life is called into question, and so the challenge is set.

Weber's colleague, Ernst Troeltsch, argued that congregational religion exhibits three tendencies in relating to the world.[9] The religious association may *dissociate* from the dominant society by withdrawing in more active or passive ways; it tends more exclusively to its own nurture. The religious community may *oppose* the dominant society by protest, or by seeking to change or overthrow it. Or the dominant society may be *affirmed*, as an inevitable necessity, by critical acceptance, or more wholehearted embrace. These tendencies, then, represent three typical patterns of participation.

A new expression of congregational religion the denomination, appeared with the disestablishment of state-sanctioned religion. For the denomination, the voluntary principle is the organizing feature of congregational life. Persons join, presumably, only when they consent to its norms, that is, to the implicit or explicit consensus that exists in the group. The need to gain the consent of laity introduces a democratic impulse into congregational life and presents a political task to religious leaders who want to attract and retain members. Once the element of democracy is acknowledged and the active consent of laity is present, congregations can become seedbeds of activism.[10] Congregational activities proliferate; new institutions like the Sunday school are formed; alliances with other associations develop. Recent American religious history illustrates that these conditions are an environment for change as in, for example, the emergence of politically conscious evangelicals, the decline of the Protestant mainline, and the growing influence of the Roman Catholic Church.[11]

Denominational life is subject to numerous factors, many outside its control. One thinks of the increase in global interdependence; one thinks of the emergence of pluralism and the recognition of different viewpoints and communities; one even thinks of demographic factors. All of these, and more, are conditions to which congregations must respond. H. Richard Niebuhr once commented, "We are more acted upon than acting," and that may be true of denominations.[12] Still, within whatever limits, denominations retain the capacity to exercise intentions in their many activities. There are different units and levels of participation, including individuals, small groups, congregations, regional bodies, national bureaucracies, etc., and all of these in relation to other organizations and other arenas of existence. Religious participation, then, has many meanings and dimensions.[13]

The basic tendencies noted by Troeltsch illustrate ways in which religious participation takes place in relation to society. Recall that the religious vision grows clearer and God's relation to the world gains specificity with each factor in religious belief. With the factor of religious participation, the relation of God to the community which shares the religious vision is spelled out, and God's relation to the world thereby becomes clearer, that is, God's relation to those who do not explicitly or organizationally acknowledge the religious vision. At least two basic patterns emerge. One pattern identifies God's presence or emphasizes God's relation to the religious association in ways which are not true of God's relation with the larger world. For this pattern, the tendency of the religious association is to oppose the dominant society. On the other hand, the religious community may be viewed as the realm of the conscious acknowledgment of God's more universal presence or relation to the world. The tendency of the religious association in this pattern is to affirm the dominant society.

These patterns have consequences for the vision of God and for the interaction of good and evil. When God is uniquely related to the religious community, it is less likely that the presence of God as an ordering, sustaining, nurturing, and redeeming power will be discerned in the world, which is viewed as the locus of evil. Thus believers tend to oppose the world. If opposition to the dominant society takes the path of changing the world, it is likely that God's positive presence will be selectively identified with certain elements in society, thus modifying the interaction of good and evil. When God's presence is more affirmatively related to the dominant society, discerning the presence of God in the world as an ordering, sustaining, nurturing, and redeeming power is more likely. The location of evil is apt to be viewed as more universal and radical, but enough good is discerned in the world to encourage affirmation, as an inevitable necessity, by critical acceptance, or more wholehearted embrace.

These generalizations are regrettably abstract, and, no doubt, particular historical instances will not conform. They nonetheless draw attention to major patterns of religious participation. In sum, religious participation is multifaceted in depth and breadth.

Sources of Knowledge

The issue for the third factor in religious belief may be posed as a question. What sources of knowledge are reliable, and how are they related? Since answers to any question depend on one or more sources of knowledge, this issue emerges in everyday life. Even the fabled Cynics who rigorously rejected the reliability of all knowledge adopted a stance on this issue, albeit a flatly negative one. Answers in everyday life range from reliance on common sense to disciplined appeals to specialized fields of learning. I concentrate here on sources deemed reliable for morality.

Appeals to sources of knowledge in religion are sometimes more narrow and exclusive, sometimes broader and more inclusive. Sole reliance on an authoritative text illustrates a narrower, more exclusive, answer, which often joins with an appeal to the religious community as the only authentic interpreter of the canonical witness. By contrast, various theories of "natural law" illustrate broader, more inclusive, appeals. They assume that believers and nonbelievers share a common source of reliable knowledge, like perceptions of human nature or a common moral sense. A dominant strand in the Roman Catholic tradition affirms that what is known morally by reason is given by God and universally shared; this knowledge, moreover, is not contradicted by scripture though the latter provides certain commands that go beyond the duties of ordinary living. The so-called quadrilateral of the Methodist Church appeals to four interacting sources of knowledge, namely, scripture, tradition, reason, and experience. It thereby combines more distinctively religious sources with those which presumably are more widely shared. Of course, the exact meaning of each term in the quadrilateral and their relation to each other continue to be debated.

Religious answers to the question about sources of knowledge appeal in some normative fashion to canonical writings. Since the *uses* of authoritative texts vary, the ways scripture actually functions as a normative source also vary. For example, scripture may be viewed as disclosing knowledge of the reality of God, revealing the relation of good and evil, providing guidance in the form of moral values, engendering attitudes, exhibiting virtues, providing direct answers to moral questions, and so forth. It is important to draw fairly precise distinctions in order to understand particular claims.

Some theologians claim on descriptive grounds that multiple sources of knowledge are inevitably present in decision making. Lisa Sowle Cahill argues that four interacting sources of knowledge are invariably present in religious ethics: canonical writings, the religious tradition, normative accounts of the human, and descriptive accounts of the human.[14] Her argument suggests that the normativity of scripture cannot be upheld in actual use unless brought into conscious relation with other sources of knowledge. Judgments, of course, must be rendered about the number of sources and also about their relation. The point here is that some theologians self-consciously use multiple sources, and arguments for their use are not only descriptive but have theological flavor. It is obvious that recourse to "descriptive accounts of the human" places believers on at least some common ground with biomedical decision makers who may not share the religious vision.

These few examples illustrate the plurality of answers to the question about sources. This factor interacts with others. Recall again that the religious vision becomes clearer when each factor of religious belief is taken into account. When the factor is sources of knowledge, God's relation to the world is specified in reference to the availability of reliable moral knowledge to the religious community and to those who do not share the religious vision. In other words, sources of knowledge clearly interact with the factor of religious participation. I delineate two general patterns.

First, to the degree that God's positive presence is identified more exclusively with the religious community in contrast to the rest of humanity, emphasis is placed on the need of the community to rely on more distinctively religious sources of knowledge like canonical writings. For example, if God is more exclusively present to the religious community as lawgiver or commander, a belief grounded in scripture, believers will be enjoined to obey these laws or commands, e.g., do not resist evil or enter the land of Canaan to conquer and occupy. Again, if a religious community gathers around the personality of a leader and does not yet have an authoritative text, the belief that God is present to the world exclusively through those who follow the leader is grounded in a personality; believers are enjoined to follow the leader's directives. A more comprehensive account requires an estimate of the type of knowledge available to nonbelievers; when such accounts are given, they correlate with perceptions of the location and extent of good and evil in the world. For example, the world may be seen as a locus of evil to the extent that it does not follow the teaching of nonviolence or to the extent that it does not follow the teachings which flow from the leader's personality.

Second, to the degree that God's positive presence is related to the world, some emphasis is placed on sources of knowledge which are shared by believers and nonbelievers, at least in moral matters. If God's ordering power is present to the world in sustaining life through the structure of the family, for example, reliable knowledge about being a spouse or a parent may be given through an "order of creation" ordained by the deity and perceived by reason and experience, that is, sources of knowledge universally shared. A more comprehensive account requires an estimate of the role of scripture as a distinctively religious source of knowledge. This estimate may be that reason and scripture do not conflict in moral matters, but that scripture moves beyond reason in certain ways. A more paradoxical claim is that reason and scripture are both required but serve different functions; reason informs us how to restrain evil in the world and scripture gives us reborn hearts. These and other claims also depend upon perceptions of the interaction of good and evil.

These patterns are again regrettably abstract and, of course, particular historical instances may not exactly conform. Although more detailed analysis would require greater nuance, the generalizations indicate two major patterns. They also show that factors in religious belief interact dynamically. If one is persuaded that multiple sources of knowledge are required and also of the reality of God, for example, then one is forced to give a theological account of how God makes reliable knowledge available to the world, say, in the sciences. In sum, the factors of religious belief interact dynamically and are complex.

Moral Guidance

A fourth and final factor in religious belief also takes the form of a question raised in everyday life. What types of guidance, if any, aid in facing the demands of life? By demands of life I refer to a broad array of matters, like choosing a vocation, raising children, electing surgery, or donating money. Possible forms of guidance are also far-ranging, for example, principles and rules, symbols by which to comprehend circumstances, training in character, and distinctions between relative goods. The religious form of this issue is the type of guidance which flows from or is consistent with a vision of God. Religion offers rich resources with respect to these possibilities, but I concentrate here on guidance in the form of moral principles.

Whether the first requirement of a religious vision is a reborn heart or obedient conduct is a perennial debate, often couched in terms of the priority given to inner or outer dimensions of life. The inner dimension emphasizes a new disposition, the outer stresses good deeds. Though exceptions exist, these options are usually viewed as complementary, not as alternatives. Recurring discussions draw boundaries by identifying "legalism" and "antinomianism" as extremes to avoid. An emphasis on inner freedom to the neglect of good conduct is antinomian or "against the law." Legalism emphasizes proper conduct to the neglect of matters of the heart. These distinctions are more successful in indicating extremes to avoid than in stating a middle ground. An agricultural metaphor poses the issue of relating inner and outer dimensions of life in a pattern responsive to the religious vision. How are the "roots" of a plant related to its "fruits," that is, how are the inner dispositions of a way of life related to conduct? The image assumes that both roots and fruits are required and related.

Moral principles are a means to guide conduct. Their *form and content,* as well as their *use and purpose,* stem from a relation between roots and fruits. They are also conditioned by the religious factors of belief which specify God's relation to the world. The relation of good and evil, we have seen, may lead to a thoroughgoing dualism. When the location and extent of evil are more universal and radical, however, this dualism moderates. With the factor of religious participation, tendencies to dissociate or oppose the world stand in contrast with more affirmative stances. With the issue of sources, reliable moral knowledge may be more exclusively available to the religious community or more universally distributed. The religious vision clearly directs these possibilities, but the vision is also shaped by these other factors in belief.

Many combinations of these factors are possible, and I shall indicate two major patterns. In the first, a vision of God with a thoroughgoing dualism which lacks a radical and universal sense of evil links with a tendency to oppose the world. These factors, in turn, join with the tendency for the knowledge provided by God to be more exclusively related to believers. With this pattern, moral guidance often takes the rigorous form of a "higher law." Conscientious obedience is expected, and there is little likelihood of dialogue with persons outside the religious community about the form and content of guidance. The guidance offered may be directed primarily towards the inner religious life, though necessarily cast in outward form, e.g., a vow of obedience to a religious superior; or the guidance may be more overtly moral, though obedience springs from the heart, e.g., not swearing in court.

A variation in this pattern occurs if the tendency to oppose the world takes the form of seeking to overthrow it. The rigorous content of the moral guidance may then become more militant and conscientious obedience is still expected, e.g., launching a violent crusade against an enemy. If the tendency to oppose the world is not explicitly violent, but nonetheless expresses an intention to change the world, moral guidance is likely formed in relation to selected sources of knowledge available in the world.

In the second pattern, the vision of God views the extent and location of evil as more universal and radical. Lacking a thoroughgoing dualism, it includes an affirmative posture toward the world and assumes that moral knowledge is more universally distributed. With this pattern, the form of moral guidance is less rigorous in the sense that it more likely compromises with various aspects of life in the world. Guidance is more responsive to the demands of culture and society, and is directed to both the religious community and the world. Dialogue about the form and content of this guidance is possible in principle and practice. The more explicit purposes of moral guidance depend in part on the virulence of evil in the world and range from the restraint of evil to more positive directives. If evil is so virulent that little positive good can be accomplished, restraint is emphasized; if possibilities for human flourishing exist, more positive forms of guidance emerge.

The well-known debate about "uses" of the law in the sixteenth century illustrates the purposes of guidance in this second pattern. The commandment "Do not kill" is a form of moral guidance with particular content. For John Calvin,[15] its first use is theological, that is, to convict of sin and perhaps prepare the way for repentance. So the command is radicalized to include anger in the heart, an inner disposition. The second use is political, that is, to restrain evil. A murderer is a killer and a menace to society who must be punished by the state, an outward deed. The third use provides moral guidance which is grounded in the heart and expressed in outward form. The positive intention of the prohibition not to kill is to respect human life. More exact formulations come with dialogue. Unlike Calvin, some theologians endorsed only the first two uses; for these latter, the primary purpose of guidance in the world is the restraint of extremely virulent evil. It may be noted that in the pattern of thought where the tendency is to oppose the world, the commandment not to kill may take the form of a "higher law" and stand as a prohibition in the religious community against all lethal violence. If the tendency toward the world is seeking to overthrow it, this command may be superseded by a different form of "higher law," namely, the call to violent revolution.

Once again, these generalizations are regrettably abstract, and once again, historical instances do not exactly conform. However, the central points about guidance in the form of moral principles should not be lost. Moral principles in a religious context presume a relation between inner and outer dimensions of existence. Their form and content are likely to be more rigorously conscientious or more responsive to the demands of culture and society. They also serve certain purposes. These three features of guidance, in turn, are informed by the religious vision and conditioned by perceptions of good and evil, estimates of reliable sources of knowledge, and different tendencies in religious participation. The factors in religious belief are complex and mutually conditioning.

Summary

Religion is a way of life grounded in a vision of God, and one response to this vision is articulating beliefs. Believing is part, but only part, of walking a way. To analyze religious beliefs is to discern that a religious vision specifies the relation of God to the world by dealing with four distinct yet related factors. Each is important, and each displays its own qualities. To take religious participation as an example, its roots are found in faith and piety which nurture, express, and condition its shape. It is also influenced by the form of a religious association, e.g., a denominational congregation, and it embodies one of the tendencies which belong to this factor, namely, to dissociate from, oppose, or affirm the world. These characteristics blend to compose the distinctive quality of religious participation. This factor, in turn, conditions and interacts with the other factors, each with its own qualities. When informed by a vision of God, the qualities of these four factors form a more or less integrated pattern. This complex and interacting whole provides resources which are brought to everyday life, including the medical arena. Every pastor and physician is aware that those informed by a religious vision respond out of the resources provided by a way of life, sometimes courageously in the face of tragedy and sometimes in despair.

THE ELEMENTS OF DECISION MAKING

An analysis of religion's role in the medical arena could begin inductively by examining the actual responses of believers to illness and health. This paper, however, inquires about the interaction of religion and morality in the medical arena by first setting forth the elements of decision making. Just as the integrity of religion is not well served if reduced to decision making, so the elements of morality deserve their own consideration. Indeed, to ask about the interaction of religion and moral decisions assumes that the latter stands somewhat independently of the former. Yet differing views of morality are conditioned by perspectives which are either more or less comprehensive, and religion presses for a broader, more comprehensive, view. Morality retains its relative independence, but is conceived broadly enough to interact fully with the factors of religion which, again, have nonreligious counterparts; the wider conception is not a product of a religious view only.

This section of the paper states four distinct but related components of decision making, and together, these elements define the subject matter of morality.[16] I do not mean to imply that all religious persons share this understanding, but stating these elements is a basis for inquiring about their relation to religion. Two of the components, moral values and situational analysis, are the common coin of contemporary moral discourse. A third element, loyalties, is more often neglected. The final element is human agency. These components are formal in the sense that different clusters of content are attracted to each.

Moral Values and Situational Analysis

A strong consequentialism is present in biomedical decision making because interventions in the natural life process are undertaken with the expectation that certain results will follow. But will they? And are the predicted results truly beneficial or good? These questions point to two important issues. One concerns facts and values, and the other concerns the adequacy of the method of calculating consequences for ethics. Consideration of these two issues raises a third, namely, the place of purpose in this component of decision making.

The vast literature about the relation of facts and values illustrates that different types of evidence count in making decisions. A division between facts and values presupposes a model in which one type of evidence consisting of pure moral values is applied to another type of evidence consisting of factually delineated situations. This model is endorsed in the important writings of Paul Ramsey.[17] For Ramsey, when a medical team considers resuscitation, it first "reads the situation" by determining whether the patient is dying or nondying. This assessment is a matter of medical fact, and a patient's condition is such that resuscitation will either restore health or prolong the dying process. Once this situation is comprehended, the moral value of "care, but only care" is applied. Care requires informed consent. Care also requires an intervention to restore health, as may be possible, if the consenting patient is nondying. If the patient is dying, however, the obligation "only to care" does not require resuscitation, which would only prolong the dying process, but a ministry to suffering, pain, and loneliness, and the patient is allowed to die. Whether or not patients are always described adequately as either dying or nondying, the two kinds of evidence posit a division of labor. Medical science provides the facts and morality supplies the values to be applied.

This matter, I think, should be treated more subtly. Are "dying" and "nondying" purely factual terms? Any conception of death includes some notion of what is valued about life which, when lost irreversibly, enables the judgment that a person is in fact dead.[18] Similarly, it may be asked whether "care" is a purely moral value which stands independently of factual material. Kubler-Ross's famous studies of the stages of death, for example, emerged out of value-laden observations about what takes place in the processes of dying, and this material shaped notions of care.[19]

Concepts like justice and stealing include and combine different types of evidence. Notions of distributive justice, for example, are formulated by paying attention to situations in which competition exists for scarce resources. Certain situations which otherwise would not be understood are properly described as stealing. These observations do not erase the conceptual distinction between moral values and situational analysis, though the two may coalesce. Rather each of these components combines different types of evidence. So one comprehends the significance of situations in value-laden ways, and moral values are informed by data from the world.

The second issue is whether to modify or erase consequentialism, a question also introduced by Ramsey who argued that the business of morality is to provide rules of right conduct, not to calculate consequences. For Ramsey, it would be morally wrong to assume that death is always a bad consequence; this would tempt us to seek the better result of preserving life at any cost. As a rule of right conduct which does not calculate consequences, the canon of care does not prolong the dying process but allows the patient to die.

Still, Ramsey's stance presupposes that mere survival is not the purpose of human existence. If the "good" of health is assumed to be mere physical existence, care as a rule of right conduct might well support preserving life at very high costs, even in dying patients. The deep problem here is to understand health in relation to the purposes of human existence.[20] If health is the central purpose of existence, it likely will be identified with survival or mere existence. On the other hand, if health is only one aspect of human purpose and a condition for its other aspects, mere existence is not so highly prized. Understanding the good of health in relation to other human purposes is not determined by moral principles; rather, moral principles are placed in their service, in either more or less consequential ways.

With respect to the question of method, my own judgment is that rules of right conduct and calculating consequences are both necessary. A better way to say this is that human conduct is evaluated by referring to the kind of activity it constitutes and in terms of its consequences. Sole reliance on either flounders, if only because of the former's unwillingness to take into account adequately what can be known about the future, and the latter's ultimate inability to foresee the future.

Human purposes condition each of these crucial elements and their interaction. The evidence for reading situations perceptively varies, and the forms of situational analysis range from intuitive perceptions to highly disciplined inquiries informed by different fields of learning. These forms and their content are judged more or less adequate in terms of their purpose. Again, the evidence which counts in formulating moral values varies, and the forms of moral values also vary, including everything from rules of thumb to ethical principles. The adequacy of these forms, as well as the adequacy of their content, is conditioned by their purposes. In sum, the uses of situational analysis and moral values in decision making inevitably serve human purposes. These purposes are set in relation to human capacities and needs in interaction with the structures of society and cultural norms.

Loyalties

"Loyalties" is shorthand to refer to objects of human desire, expectation, and trust. When affirmed, these objects receive our allegiance, hence the term loyalties.[21] The nation is a potential object of devotion, for example. One may desire to be a citizen of a particular country and actively participate in its civic life. One may expect a country to provide protection and guarantee certain rights, and one may expect to participate actively in the processes of ruling and being ruled. If these desires and expectations are fulfilled in some fashion, enough trust develops that an allegiance is formed. Though the process is more complicated than indicated here, the result is that the loyalty of patriotism emerges, and this, in turn, shapes those who hold it.

Loyalties perform three functions, those of orienting, motivating, and providing a general direction. As orientation, patriotism provides a perspective from which to view and interpret life. As motivation, it provides reasons of heart and mind to participate in civic society. The political form of a country, e.g., a constitutional democracy, provides a general direction for at least one aspect of life.

The exact meaning of particular loyalties is discussed and debated, and different loyalties demand different allegiances which interact in various combinations. For example, the family is a potential object of desire, expectation, and trust, and so may become a loyalty. Parenthood provides orientation, motivation, and direction. Conflict in motivation is experienced if the demands of patriotism fail to agree with the perspective and direction of parenthood. Persons form many allegiances and in turn are shaped by them, e.g., economic prosperity and health, so the adjudication of interacting loyalties is perennial.

Loyalties take institutional form and embody cultural values.[22] For the parent, institutional forms of the family embody the values of parenthood. For the patriot, institutional forms of government embody the values of democracy. For the physician, different institutionalizations of care embody the values of health. For the entrepreneur, institutionalizations of business embody values like hard work and success. These and other loyalties form identity because they are purposive. They exist for a reason, and these reasons are brought to bear on decision making. Why go to war? In part because one is a patriot. Why not go to war? In part because patriotism itself may give reasons to do otherwise. Why nurture children? In part because one is a parent. Why provide care? In part because one is a physician.

The interaction of different institutions with cultural norms helps shape a general ethos which is more or less diverse and demanding. This ethos exists in the present, but is deeply conditioned by recollections of the past and expectations of the future. As background and frame of reference, this ethos itself conditions decision making in society, and when ethos changes, existing practices will erode, gain support, or be enriched.

Human Agency

Stated briefly, assumptions which guide conduct are made about the capabilities of human agents, their motives, and their possibilities and limitations within the courses and workings of nature, history, culture, and society. Human beings are a highly diverse lot equipped with a remarkable range of capabilities. People differ according to their genetic endowment and their psychological development, as well as their settings in time and space, and different people have differing motives and intentions. They have different capacities for action and different inclinations toward moral deeds.

Nevertheless, they share a common nature.[23] Human agents are more or less integrated creatures with certain limits and possibilities. Within the context of culture and society, people are formed as their natural endowments develop and interact with the historical formation of dispositions, intentions, and basic convictions. In their varied forms, the motives and intentions of agents are shaped by historic convictions and expressed in conduct. The different motives and intentions of different persons, then, must be taken into account.

Human agency is expressed and embodied in a way of life, one important dimension of which is character.[24] Character refers to the Greek word *hexis,* as in Aristotle, which was translated into Latin as *habitus,* as in Thomas Aquinas, and became the term "habit" in English. A habit or disposition is a readiness to act in a consistent manner, like reading or writing, or a persisting tendency to do things in fairly predictable ways, like driving a car or playing the piano. These skills are not endowed directly by nature, but are acquired over time when training and practice are offered by communities like the family, school, or synagogue. When habits are deemed moral, they are called virtues. Honesty, for example, is a disposition which characterizes some people; we observe, "They are as honest as the day is long," which means at least that they are not tempted to steal every time they go through a checkout counter. The acquisition of habits and dispositions forms identity. A child who learns to read is identified as a "reader" just as an adolescent who learns to drive is known as a "driver." Similarly, practitioners of medicine and those who repair automobiles are identified correctly as physicians and mechanics. These and other identities display the character of a social roles, though these admit a wide variety of expression since they are filtered through individuals. Still, physicians are expected to care and auto mechanics are expected to tell the truth. Character is necessary, both individually and in social roles, if agents are to sustain identity over time. Agency may also take corporate forms, but enough has been written to suggest that it is shaped by a variety of factors which are not readily reducible to a concept like freedom.

Assumptions about character as well as other aspects of agency "fit" the other elements of decision making, both in the sense that they influence them and in the sense that these other elements also shape these assumptions. The moral principle "Do not kill" fits humanity; the commands typically given to other animals, like dogs, do not. Situational analysis is conditioned by these assumptions, and differing assumptions about human nature make differences in how situations are described. The apprehension and statement of the purposes of life in the form of loyalties also fit perceptions of humanity. These interactions are reciprocal.

Summary

One neutral way to pose the moral question is to ask, What ought I to do? Answers are given in the form of judgments, acts, and policies. When judgments are made, acts performed, or policies enacted, they may be challenged. These answers to the moral question are then defended or discussed by giving "reasons" which support them, and these reasons take their form and content from the four components of morality.

Should the patient be resuscitated? If the answer is a judgment, "No," and this judgment is questioned, reasons are given to justify it. One reason appeals to situational analysis: The patient is irreversibly in the process of dying and attempts at resuscitation would only prolong the dying process. A second reason appeals to a moral value. The obligation of the medical team is to care for the patient, but only to care. This means that the patient will be allowed to die, but requires that pain, loneliness, and suffering be attended. A third reason appeals to loyalties: Health is a human good, but not an end in itself. Since health is a condition for other aspects of human flourishing, and these aspects are now beyond attainment, there is reason to allow the patient to die. A fourth reason appeals to human agency: Allowing a person to die accords with the finite nature of humanity and, one presumes, coheres with the dying patient's motives and intentions.

The four reasons are distinct, but together form a larger pattern which coalesces with the complex interaction between judgments, acts, and policies. If the judgment is followed by an act, for example, the patient is not resuscitated. We respond to similarly situated cases in the same way, if only because of the demand of fairness. The result is a policy which, when adopted, becomes a practice which defines, embodies, and expresses the meaning of medical care and gains the support of an ethos.

The interacting reasons of the four components of decision making are in turn conditioned and influenced by the factors of religious belief, or if not them, by their nonreligious counterparts. What is the extent, location, and relation of forces of good and evil? How relate to those who differ in some significant respect? What sources of knowledge are reliable? What types of guidance aid in facing the demands of life? To the degree that a vision of God informs answers to these questions, religious belief interacts with biomedical decision making. The possibilities are multiple.

INTERACTIONS

The multiple possibilities are too rich to be explicated fully here. The whole is a complex and dynamic field of interaction in which a vision of God and the factors of religious belief mutually condition each other and each of the elements of decision making *and* vice versa. I shall illustrate some of these interactions, but first comment on the relation between loyalties and a religious vision.

Vision and Loyalties

The interaction between a vision of God and human loyalties is important, though frequently neglected. Recall that loyalties are objects of human desire, expectation, and confidence which form allegiances like patriotism and parenthood. These are embodied in institutional forms which express cultural values, and so are causes which serve human purposes and shape identify. Loyalties *change* in content over the course of time, *interact* with other allegiances, and require *adjudication*. That is, they are constantly reformulated, related to other loyalties, and so ordered. This ordering is done by a *center of value,* a perspective which relates the demands of differing allegiances and aids in formulating their content.[25] These interactions have inner dimensions insofar as desire, expectation, and trust are coordinated into a whole; they have outer dimensions insofar as the contending demands of external allegiances are ordered coherently. A result is the formation of identity as a pattern of life which orients, motivates, and directs agents in the world.

When a religious vision interacts with human loyalties, its basic import is to distinguish the ultimate from the proximate by subordinating other allegiances to devotion to God. This matter stands at the heart of religious life as the problem of idolatry. To have no other God does not eliminate other human loyalties; it requires they be apprehended as nonultimate. Proximate values in a religious vision range from those which are not worthy of esteem to causes worth serving even to the point of death, e.g., martyrdom on behalf of one's family. Devotion to God as the center of value orders the relative worth of these proximate allegiances in inner and outer dimension. The inner dimension is that the religious vision elicits human trust, expectation, and desire, and transfers them to God. To use traditional Christian language, they are transformed so that trust as faith in God, expectation as hope in God, and desire as love of God, characterize inner devotion to an ultimate cause. *What* is believed about God as the object of faith, hope, and love has important external dimensions. As the center of value, these beliefs deal with the contending demands of the world by helping to order, relate, and formulate the proximate meaning of other human allegiances. When these inner and outer dimensions coalesce, an integrated pattern of life emerges which provides identity as orientation, motivation, and direction for walking a way.

The possibilities considered by Paul Ramsey when he wrote about the meaning of care illustrate the interaction between a vision of God, other human loyalties, and the prospect of intervening in the natural life process. For a patient with appendicitis who is not irreversibly dying, for example, a medical intervention is likely to restore health; otherwise, premature death may result. Suppose, however, that intervention is opposed because it "plays God" by usurping the deity's sovereign rule. God is conceived as the *direct* giver and "taker" of life since the divine presence in the world is identified with the natural life processes of cause and effect. A loyalty to health as physical existence is of little worth when ordered in relation to this center of value.

On the other hand, if an intervention is sanctioned which restores health, God's presence as sustainer of life may be discerned indirectly through a surgical procedure which at the same time mediates God's ordering power. As the center of value, belief in God correlates with a loyalty to health which esteems the gift of physical existence more highly than when intervention is foregone. This latter stance, of course, avoids a "God of the gaps" position in which scientific notions of cause and effect are antithetically juxtaposed with beliefs about the deity If God is conceived as an active power whose presence in the world is mediated in time and space, then what actually takes place in the world must be related in some way to this belief. Vision, loyalties, and the possibility of intervening are interacting variables; knowledge of God is admittedly conditioned by perceptions of the world, not only ideas about health but also notions of cause and effect.

The case of the patient who is irreversibly dying also illustrates the interaction of these variables and the influence of belief in God as the center of value. A medical intervention prolongs the dying process. This intervention correlates with a conception of health as mere physical existence, for the point can only be to "respect" life by preserving it as long as possible. When the limits of technology are not acknowledged, conceptions of God's power to sustain life transcend or remain independent of cause and effect processes.

If no intervention is undertaken, on the other hand, the patient is allowed to die. Lack of intervention correlates with a conception of health as a condition for other aspects of human flourishing, and when these aspects are beyond attainment, mere existence is not so highly prized. God as the center of value is imaged as the indirect giver of life, and also as an ordering power whose purposive presence is mediated in and through the various arenas of life. When these divine purposes, which correlate with other aspects of human flourishing, are no longer attainable, the importance of health as mere survival diminishes. Moreover, a distinction between God and creaturely existence is upheld. So again, the religious vision is the center of value which orders other human loyalties, and this center gains specificity by the way it interacts with the ways things are in the world, in this case, perceptions of health and notions of cause and effect.

The Other Factors of Belief

Loyalties and the vision of God do not stand alone. Their interaction with possibilities for intervening are conditioned by the factors of religious belief, and these, in turn, influence the other components of decision making and vice versa. A religious stance with a thoroughgoing dualism which opposes the world, uses exclusive sources of knowledge, and offers rigorous guidance to the religious community, for example, differs considerably from one which moderates a thoroughgoing dualism, affirms the world, uses inclusive sources of knowledge, and offers guidance to the world. Keyed to distinctive beliefs about God, these and other stances qualify the components of morality differently.

Some of these differences may be illustrated briefly by reverting to the case of the irreversibly dying patient where attempts at resuscitation prolong the dying process. In respect to good and evil forces, a thoroughgoing dualism could view the end of life as the central locus of evil and set human existence over against death as good. The extent and location of evil are not universal or radical but confined to life and death issues, a position which could be elaborated by an eschatology which protests or rebels against human finitude. With respect to religious participation, opposition to the world could be expressed in a refusal to accept the limits of technological innovations, and with it, a failure to recognize the limitations of the medical segment of society. With respect to sources of knowledge, a more exclusive stance could ignore scientific accounts of cause and effect and object to the statement that a patient is irreversibly dying. With respect to moral guidance, conscientious obedience to a rigorous higher law could instruct the religious community to disregard the limits of technology and foster attempts to always preserve life.

Each of these factors is keyed to a vision of God's power to sustain life

which transcends or remains independent of cause and effect processes.
Together, they reinforce the interaction between a vision of God, a conception of health as mere existence, and attempts to preserve life as long as
possible. This combination of factors, moreover, counters the moral reasons which would allow a patient to die, though in ways too intricate to
enumerate here in detail. Still, health is not conceived as a condition and
one aspect of human flourishing, but as physical existence. Human finitude is not accepted but protested. Instead of the canon of care, emphasis
is placed on the moral value of preserving life, and instead of saying that
the patient is irreversibly dying, it could be said that the patient is temporarily ill.

Allowing an irreversibly dying patient to die, on the other hand, may
also be supported by the factors of religious belief. With respect to good
and evil forces, a moderated dualism could discern God's ordering presence in the world amid these interacting powers, though the divine purposes of existence in the varied arenas of life are beyond attainment for the
patient. The gift of life could be acknowledged as a finite good to be
received with a gratitude expressed properly to both its proximate and
ultimate sources, a position which could be elaborated by an eschatology
which affirms the goodness of God and the value of life even in the face of
finitude and death. With respect to religious participation, affirmation of
the world could be expressed by accepting the limits of technological innovation, and with it, a recognition of the limitations of the medical segment
of society. With respect to sources of knowledge, a more inclusive stance
could accept scientific accounts of cause and effect and endorse the statement that a patient is irreversibly dying. With respect to moral guidance
more responsive to the demands of culture and society, the canon of care,
but only care, could be affirmed.

Each of these factors is keyed to a vision of God as the indirect giver of
life and an ordering power whose mediated presence is discerned in the
various arenas of life. Together, they reinforce the interaction between a
vision of God, a conception of health as a condition and aspect of human
flourishing, and a willingness to forego attempts at resuscitation. This
combination of factors, moreover, supports the moral reasons which would
allow a patient to die in ways which, I hope, are clear in basic outline.

The factors of religious belief do not entail or precisely determine the
exact qualifications of the components of moral decision making, which
retain their relative independence, yet profoundly condition and influence
them. The result is that a vision of God and the factors of belief interact
with the elements of morality to form a way of life. The qualities of each of
the factors of religious belief, we have seen, join with a vision of God to
form a pattern, and these, in turn, link with qualifications of the components of decision making to fashion a way of walking in the world.

The image of a journey draws to attention that a way of life does not always move from a vision and the factors of belief to moral problems, but often the reverse.[26] No journey is complete at its beginning, but continues through encounters with problems which may be viewed as pitfalls, dangers, and temptations. These provide the occasion for seeking guidance, acquiring skills, and forming identity in community. Venturers are thereby oriented, motivated, and directed to walk a way in the world. Depending on the vision, and, no doubt, the character of the travelers, encounters in the world may also be viewed as challenges and opportunities. Perhaps a paradox in the vitality of religious belief is found at this point. The deepest convictions of life are often religious, so there are reasons to hold them firmly. If held defensively, for whatever reason, encounters in the world are viewed only as temptations, dangers, and pitfalls. Yet firmness of belief may also bring something like the "cosmic optimism" Perry Miller attributed to the Puritans, a certain confidence in the vision which provides encouragement for the journey of life.[27] Venturers are then challenged to respond to encounters as opportunities to clarify the meaning of existence in the world in relation to the vision.

Prophetic Protest, the Status Quo, and Apocalypticism

More could be said about the rich interaction between a religious vision, the factors of religious belief, and the elements of decision making, but enough has been written to provide a partial basis for explaining how religion sometimes functions as a cover for other interests.[28] The essence of the process is an inversion at the point of loyalties so that beliefs about God become a function of other allegiances which are the actual center of value. The phenomenon is as old as Western religion and stands at the heart of prophetic protests against "priestly" religion, that is, the type of religion sometimes endorsed by the leaders of congregational religion. Prophets typically use moral language to criticize false forms of worship, e.g., "I take no delight in your solemn assemblies . . . let justice roll down like waters" (Amos 5:21, 24). What is centrally at stake, however, is specifying God's relation to the world with respect to a way of life. In congregational religion priests are responsible for leading worship and interpreting the religious message. Trained by an establishment, these leaders may be conservative in two senses: first, they set forth a religious message from the past in the context of worship, and second, along with influential laity, they have a stake in maintaining the status quo. By contrast, the urgency of a prophetic message objects to liturgical practice when it sanctions a way of life unresponsive to God's active presence and provides moral guidance in the form of moral principles which point to a true way of life in the world.

The religious participation of "priestly religion" opposes any change in the status quo, and its use of moral principles reflects this interest. Repeating an unrevised religious message in a liturgical setting, priests insist that the exclusive source of reliable knowledge is the authoritative tradition in which they have been trained and overlook what is actually taking place in the world. They know with scholastic assurance that true belief is cognitive assent to intellectual propositions.[29] The forces of good are located in the status quo, and evil is defined as threats or challenges to this same order. These priests do not provide a religious construal of existence which leads to a way of life responsive to God's active presence. The heart of the matter is an inversion at the point of loyalties, so that beliefs about God function as a cover for other interests which are the actual center of value.

Prophetic criticism of priestly religion can depart from discerning God's ordering presence in the world and focus more completely on the way the world ought to be in the future. The moral urgency of apocalyptic messages is directed toward a new order. Guidance no longer takes the form of moral principles but endorses those inner attitudes deemed necessary for the emergence of a new world. Religious participation does not endorse the existing order but opposes it by fleeing, protesting, seeking change, or attempting to overthrow it. Reliable knowledge is drawn selectively from authoritative texts and other sources which point to a new order. God's relation to the world is specified in terms of what should be rather than what is, though foretastes of the new order may be seen in the present. Judgments must then be made about whether allegiance to a new order is the actual center of value, so that religion functions as a cover for this interest, or whether belief in God actually demands this proximate loyalty. The criteria used to test these judgments are drawn from the religious vision, the factors of belief, and the components of decision making.[30]

Summary

These comments provide the occasion for a summary which focuses on the link between forms of religious participation and beliefs about God's ordering presence in the world which, in turn, interact with the ethos which supports medical practice. Again, the patterns delineated are regrettably abstract. One pattern of religious participation dissociates from the world. With this pattern, God's active presence is not discerned in the world, and interaction with ethos is minimal; medical practice, in all probability, is ignored and sustained by benign neglect.

A second pattern of religious participation opposes the world. When opposition takes the form of protest, God's ordering power as a positive presence in the world is largely absent. Protest may erode the ethos which supports medical practice or perhaps lead to change. When opposition takes the form of change, God's ordering presence in the world is allied with selective tendencies in the culture. The result creates tension in the supporting ethos which perhaps leads to modifications in medical practice, or, if change is not successful, to erosion. When opposition attempts to overthrow the world, ethos is not supported; medical practice may change, remain unchanged, or erode.

The third pattern affirms the world. When affirmation takes the form of virtual embrace, God's ordering presence is identified with the existing order. Ethos, as well as medical practice, is sustained. When affirmation takes the form of an inevitable necessity, God's restraining order is perceived in a world continually threatened by chaos. The ethos which supports medical practice is endorsed to the extent that it continues to limit threats to chaos. When affirmation takes the form of critical acceptance, God's ordering of the world includes sustaining and judging dimensions, and also prospects for new possibilities. The ethos which supports medical practice may be enriched or modified.

CONCLUDING OBSERVATIONS

I conclude with four observations. First, the conception of religion in this paper presses for a broader, more comprehensive, view of morality. It is uneasy with more restrictive views that split fact from value, focus on applying purely moral principles to purely factual situations, conceive agency as moral only to the degree it is free from historical and other forms of conditioning and neglect the importance of human purposes. The primary reason offered in this paper for a broader view is theological. A vision of God is articulated only when the factors of religious belief aid in specifying the deity's relation to the world, and this vision requires a conception of morality responsive to its concerns. Since the factors of religious belief are not always qualified from an explicitly religious point of view, nonreligious reasons could also be adduced for a broader view.

Second, contributions by religion to biomedical decision making are more likely when religious participation is more affirmative, sources of knowledge are more inclusive, moral guidance is directed toward the world, evil is conceived as universal and radical, and God's active presence in the world is discerned in an interacting field of good and evil forces without a thoroughgoing dualism. There is room for caution even here, however. For example, medical practice has learned from those whose religious stance is quite different about respecting persons who refuse medical treatment.

Third, not the least of God's mercies is that the whole scheme outlined in this paper does not have to be used every time a decision is made. Most decisions in ordinary life are a product of informed intuitions, habits, and

practices; an analytical framework certainly does not guarantee better decisions. Moreover, if one's religious stance is more affirmative on participation, more inclusive on sources, more worldly in moral guidance, and so
forth, theological reasons exist for not having to articulate an understanding of God for every decision. Indeed, theologians may participate in good
conscience in public decision making without referring explicitly to their
deepest convictions about God, and my suspicion is that something like
this stance is often adopted by theologians who serve on public commissions. Readers of this paper will have observed that the description of the
moral components of decision making is not theological, though they could
be qualified more directly by religious content than I have indicated.

On the other hand, I am persuaded that the factors of religious belief
deeply condition decision making, whether qualified by religious or nonreligious perspectives. When explicit or implicit assumptions about these
factors are divisive, which is more often than we usually care to acknowledge, they require explicit attention, and it may well be helpful to call
attention to them even when implicit agreement appears to be present.
They are, after all, at the heart of some of the deepest of human convictions. One would think, moreover, that theologians who serve on public
commissions would be expected to contribute to discussions from a religious perspective.

Fourth, all knowledge is historically conditioned and so perspectival in
at least two senses.[31] What one sees and knows depends on where one
stands, for example, twentieth-century America in contrast to first-century
China. What one sees and knows depends also on the glasses or lenses
used to view the world, for example, common sense, one or more of the
sciences, theology, or whatever. Since no neutral standing point or privileged perspective exists, a theologian may be forgiven for observing that a
"confessional" dimension inevitably enters discourse. The four factors of
religious belief profoundly condition decision making, and no point of
view exists from which to qualify them which is not historically conditioned
and perspectival.

Those persuaded of the reality of historical conditioning are uneasy
with notions of what is "public" if they imply the absence of a point of view,
as if, for example, religion represents a private domain set over against
more publicly accessible knowledge. Even science is not public in the
sense that it is unconditioned by perspectives and history. Those trained in
physics often use mathematics in ways which are not easily accessible to
biologists, and chemists sometimes have difficulty conversing with biologists, not to mention paleontologists. I agree with James M. Gustafson that
"there is no scientific public, except perhaps on very, very generalized or
abstract grounds."[32] As one historically conditioned point of view among
others, religion has its own perspective. Its potential contribution to biomedi-

cal decision making is not privileged, of course; judgments must be made on the basis of its arguments, the evidence it cites, its willingness to learn in dialogue from other points of view, and its cogency in open forums.

NOTES

1. See especially, Max Weber, *Economy and Society*, 3 vols., ed. Guenther Roth and Claus Wittich (New York: Bedminster Press, 1968), vol. 2, pp. 399–640, and Ernst Troetsch, *The Social Teaching of the Christian Churches*, 2 vols., trans. Olive Wyon (Louisville: Westminster/ John Knox Press, 1992).

2. James M. Gustafson, *Ethics from a Theocentric Perspective*, 2 vols. (Chicago: The University of Chicago Press, 1981, 1984), vol. 1, *Theology and Ethics*, pp. 209–225. Gustafson also mentions "the self." An enormous literature seeks to describe the modern world, e.g., Niklas Luhmann, *The Differentiation of Society*, trans. Stephen Holmes and Charles Larmore (New York: Columbia University Press, 1982). For suggestive summaries in a theological context, see Max L. Stackhouse, *Public Theology and Political Economy: Christian Stewardship in Modern Society* (Lanham: University Press of America, 1991), pp. 163-174, and Douglas F. Ottati, "The Contemporary Situation for Mainstream Theology and Ministry," *Affirmation*, vol. 4, no. 1 (Spring 1991), pp. 1–24.

3. The two basic questions of theology are, Who is God and how is God related to the world? The central traditions of Christianity answer the first question by saying trinity, and the second by saying creator, governor, and redeemer (the term "governor" includes images of ordering, sustaining and nurturing, preserving and restraining, and judging). The first answer distinguishes Christianity from Judaism, but the two traditions share at least some common ground in answers to the second, which in theology is known as the "nature-grace" issue. This paper concentrates on answers to the second question.

H. Richard Niebuhr in *Christ and Culture* (New York: Harper and Brothers, Harper Torchlight Books, 1951) shows how answers to both questions are related in Christianity, and his reflections are informed by the study of Charles Norris Cochrane, *Christianity and Classical Culture: A Study of Thought and Action from Augustus to Augustine* (New York: Oxford University Press, A Galaxy Book, 1957). I regret that I am not competent to take into account the literature of Judaism and Islam in this paper.

4. These four issues, along with answers to the two questions in the previous endnote, are elements central to a systematic theology. My treatment of these matters is informed by H. Richard Niebuhr's *Christ and Culture*, itself a response to Troeltsch's *The Social Teaching*.

5. Weber, Max, "Politics as a Vocation," in *From Max Weber: Essays in Sociology*, trans. and ed. H. H. Gerth and C. Wright Mills (New York: Oxford University Press, 1958), pp. 122–124.

6. For examples, see Mary Midgley, *Evolution as Religion: Strange Hopes and Stranger Fears* (New York: Methuen, 1985) and *Science as Salvation: A Modern Myth and Its Meaning* (New York: Routledge, 1992); see also James M. Gustafson, "Sociobiology: A Secular Theology" [a review of *On Human Nature* by Edward O. Wilson], *Hastings Center Report*, vol. 9, no. 1 (February 1979), pp. 44-45.

7. Weber, Max, *Economy and Society*, vol. 2, pp. 452–468.

8. Adams, James Luther, "Mediating Structures and the Separation of Powers," *Voluntary Associations: Socio-cultural Analyses and Theological Interpretation*, by James Luther Adams, ed. J. Ronald Engel (Chicago: Exploration Press, 1986), pp. 217–244.

9. Troeltsch's well-known typology of church, sect, and mysticism, appears in *The Social Teaching*.

10. See Adams, "Mediating Structures," and his "The Voluntary Principle in the Forming of American Religion," *Voluntary Associations: Socio-cultural Analyses and Theological Interpreta-*

tion, pp. 171-200. See also, James M. Gustafson, "The Voluntary Church: A Moral Appraisal," *Voluntary Associations: A Study of Groups in Free Societies*, ed. D. B. Robertson (Richmond: John Knox Press, 1966), pp. 299–322.

11. Roof, Wade Clark and William McKinney, *American Mainline Religion: Its Changing Shape and Future* (New Brunswick: Rutgers University Press, 1987).

12. I cannot locate an exact quotation, but see H. Richard Niebuhr, *The Responsible Self: An Essay in Christian Moral Philosophy* (New York: Harper & Row, 1963), pp. 47–68.

13. Normative and descriptive studies exist. For Protestantism, Paul Ramsey, *Who Speaks for the Church? A Critique of the 1966 Geneva Conference on Church and Society* (Nashville: Abingdon Press, 1967) initiated a continuing debate. See also James M. Gustafson, *Protestant and Roman Catholic Ethics: Prospects for Rapprochement* (Chicago: University of Chicago Press, 1978), pp. 126-137. For Roman Catholicism, a place to begin is *Readings in Moral Theology No. 3, The Magisterium and Morality*, ed. Charles E. Curran and Richard A. McCormick (New York: Paulist Press, 1982). See also *The Crisis in Moral Teachings in the Episcopal Church*, ed. Timothy Sedgwick and Philip Turner (Harrisburg: Morehouse Publishing, 1992), and Todd Whitmore, "Reason and Authority in Church Social Documents: The Case for Plausibility and Coherence," *Ethics in the Nuclear Age: Strategy, Religious Studies, and the Churches*, ed. Todd Whitmore (Dallas: Southern Methodist University Press, 1989), pp. 181–231. Descriptive accounts are found in a number of social studies.

14. Cahill, Lisa Sowle, *Between the Sexes: Foundations for a Christian Ethics of Sexuality* (Philadelphia: Fortress Press, 1985), p. 5. Cahill's statement should be compared with Gustafson's four sources in *Protestant and Roman Catholic Ethics*, p. 142.

15. Calvin, John, *Institutes of the Christian Religion*, 2 vols. (Philadelphia: Westminster Press [Library of Christian Classics, vol. 20, ed. John T. McNeill], 1960), trans. Ford Lewis Battles, vol. 1, pp. 348–366. The impact of these formulations had far-ranging consequences on the Puritans and in America. For a fascinating but neglected study, see David Little, *Religion, Order, and Law: A Study in Pre-Revolutionary England* (New York: Harper Torchbooks, 1969 [reprint, University of Chicago, Midway Press, 1984]).

16. Four components of decision making are cited by a number of different authors, though in differing forms, e.g., Ralph B. Potter, *War and Moral Discourse* (Richmond: John Knox Press, 1970), pp. 23–24, James M Gustafson, *Protestant and Roman Catholic Ethics*, pp. 139–141, and Gustafson, *Ethics from a Theocentric Perspective*, vol. 2, *Ethics and Theology*, p. 143. My views are informed by Gustafson though I think he collapses proximate loyalties into his "theological base." The usefulness of the four components for analytical purposes is illustrated in Harlan Beckley, *Passion for Justice: Retrieving the Legacies of Walter Rauschenbusch, John A. Ryan, and Reinhold Niebuhr* (Louisville: Westminster/John Knox Press, 1992). This latter book, incidentally, shows that theological convictions can be important in formulating conceptions of justice and demonstrates that theologians from different Christian denominations contributed to the "public" moral discourse in twentieth century America.

17. Ramsey, Paul, *The Patient as Person* (New Haven: Yale University Press, 1970), pp. 113–164.

18. Veatch, Robert M., *Death, Dying, and the Biological Revolution: Our Last Quest for Responsibility*, rev. ed. (New Haven: Yale University Press, 1989), pp. 15–44. The literature is extensive.

19. Kubler-Ross, Elisabeth, *On Death and Dying* (New York: Macmillan Company, 1969). See also, Milton Mayeroff, *On Caring* (New York: Harper & Row, Perennial Library, 1971).

20. See Leon R. Kass, "The End of Medicine and the Pursuit of Health," *Toward a More Natural Science: Biology and Human Affairs* (New York: Free Press, 1985), pp. 157–186.

21. Augustine's treatment of loyalties remains influential, perhaps especially the nineteenth book of *Concerning the City of God Against the Pagans*, trans. Henry Bettenson, intro. David Knowles (Baltimore: Penguin Books, 1972), pp. 843–894.

22. John Rawls writes about practices in "Two Concepts of Rules," *Philosophical Review*, vol. 64, no. 1 (January 1955), pp. 3–32, an article cited by James M. Gustafson in *The Contributions*

of Theology to Medical Ethics (Milwaukee: Marquette University Theology Department, 1975). On practices, see also Alasdair MacIntyre, *After Virtue: A Study in Moral Theory* (Notre Dame: University of Notre Dame Press, 1981).

23. My abbreviated account is informed by Gustafson, *Can Ethics Be Christian?* (Chicago: University of Chicago Press, 1975), pp. 25–47. Theological construals of human nature inevitably presuppose a philosophical account. Both Mary Midgley, *Beast and Man: The Roots of Human Nature* (Ithaca: Cornell University Press, 1978) and Melvin Konner, *The Tangled Wing: Biological Constraints on the Human Spirit* (New York: Holt, Rinehart and Winston, 1982) show that a dualism between nature and spirit, or between phenomenal and noumenal aspects of agency, cannot be sustained in light of contemporary knowledge of biology.

24. My brief account of character is informed loosely by Aristotle, Thomas Aquinas, James M. Gustafson, and Stanley Hauerwas.

25. Niebuhr, H. Richard, *Radical Monotheism and Western Culture: With Supplementary Essays* (New York: Harper & Brothers, 1943, 1952, 1955, 1960), uses the term "center of value." Both Niebuhr and Gustafson are informed by Augustine as well as Josiah Royce. Gustafson explicitly mentions faith, hope, and love, as well as desire, expectation, and confidence, in *Ethics from a Theocentric Perspective*, vol. 1, *Theology and Ethics*, pp. 224–225, and like Niebuhr, distinguishes faith as confidence from faith as fidelity.

26. Augustine, "The Way of Life of the Catholic Church," *The Catholic and Manichean Ways of Life*, trans. Donald A. Gallagher and Idella J. Gallagher (Washington, D.C.: Catholic University Press, 1966), pp. 3–61, has had an enormous influence in Christianity. The classic delineation of religion as a way of life in sociology is Max Weber, *Economy and Society*, vol. 2, pp. 399–640. See also, Paul M. van Buren, *A Theology of the Jewish-Christian Reality*, Part I, *Discerning the Way* (San Francisco: Harper & Row, 1980).

27. Miller, Perry, *The New England Mind*, vol. 1, *The Seventeenth Century* (Boston: Beacon Press, 1961), p. 18.

28. Roof, Wade Clark, *Community & Commitment: Religious Plausibility in a Liberal Protestant Church* (New York: Elsevier, 1978), delineates "local" and "cosmopolitan" outlooks as variables of religious meaning and belonging. Religion as a "function" of other interests is a well-worn topic in sociology.

29. Observations about a scholastic religious response to modernity are found in Clifford Geertz, *Islam Observed: Religious Development in Morocco and Indonesia* (New Haven: Yale University Press, 1968).

30. For two discussions of criteria, see Douglas F. Ottati, "Christian Theology and Other Disciplines," *Journal of Religion*, vol. 64, no. 2 (April 1984), pp. 173–187, and James M. Gustafson, *Can Ethics Be Christian?*, pp. 130–143. Stackhouse's more intuitive appeal to evidence from "the world" and from "the Word" is of interest; see *Public Theology and Political Economy*.

31. A literature that began more than thirty years ago stresses the importance of a point of view in science. See Norwood Russell Hanson, *Patterns of Discovery: An Inquiry into the Conceptual Foundations of Science* (Cambridge: Cambridge University Press, 1965; originally 1958); Michael Polanyi, *Personal Knowledge* (New York: Harper and Row, 1964; originally 1958); Stephen Toulmin, *Foresight and Understanding* (New York: Harper and Row, 1961); and Thomas S. Kuhn, *The Structure of Scientific Revolutions*, 2d ed. (Chicago: University of Chicago Press, 1970; originally 1962). A philosophically aware and clear discussion of these matters is Harold I. Brown, *Perception, Theory and Commitment: The New Philosophy of Science* (Chicago: University of Chicago Press, 1979). See also, Stephen Toulmin, *Human Understanding: The Collective Use and Evolution of Concepts* (Princeton: Princeton University Press, 1972).

32. Gustafson, James M., "Response to Francis Schussler Fiorenza," *The Legacy of H. Richard Niebuhr*, ed. Ronald F. Thiemann (Minneapolis: Fortress Press, 1991), p. 79. My previous sentence is drawn from this article.

Trust, Honesty, and the Authority of Science

STEVEN SHAPIN, Ph.D.
Professor of Sociology and Science Studies,
University of California, San Diego

There is as much modern uneasiness about putting scientists in a position to make ethical decisions as there is about releasing them totally from such responsibilities. On the one hand, many contemporary areas of ethical choice implicate such technical knowledgeability that few but the possessors of relevant expertise can hope competently to address the issues involved, while, on the other, it is not now supposed that those who have expert knowledge are ethically privileged or more likely to make virtuous decisions than anybody else in our society. In dominant sensibilities, to know more than other people about human respiration is quite a different capacity than knowing when it is right to turn off the respirator.

That, indeed, is a way of stating the problem. If these sensibilities did not obtain, then there would be widespread contentment that doctors should disconnect life-support systems and molecular biologists should determine the nucleotide sequence of the entire human genome without any intervention by "ethical experts" or those trusted to represent the concerns and preferences of interested parties. But there is no such contentment. Authority to speak on what is true is disengaged from authority to speak on what is good.

As a lay member of late-twentieth-century American society, I recognize that sentiment and have found myself endorsing it frequently enough. I have not routinely imputed special virtue to scientists and physicians, just as I am sure that few modern scientists regard themselves, or wish to be regarded, as moral paragons, with all the attendant responsibility. I have no very clever ideas about how the relationship between morality and expertise ought to be managed, and, while in general I like the idea of opening up decision-making processes to a range of interested parties, I am not comfortable with the notion of ethical expertise. For all that, I do not expect that my personal views on such matters ought to be of the slightest interest to anyone.

It is, rather, as an historian of early modern science and as a sociologist of scientific knowledge that I feel I might have something to contribute to contemporary debates over science and ethics. I want to draw attention to how the modern state of affairs just outlined came to be. Historical perspectives occasionally have the capacity to encourage a more disengaged look at present predicaments, while the fact that the divorce between expertise and virtue is, as I shall indicate, a strikingly recent one can prompt the thought that there may be some point in seeking to "unwind" a bit of history. There is nothing inherently "natural" about the late-twentieth-century distinctions between virtue and scientific knowledgeability. The historical record offers a vision of alternative arrangements. Moreover, the same historical perspective can suggest that the modern disengagement between virtue and expertise may be more in the appearance than the reality. To the extent that we accept such a disengagement as real, right, and proper, I suggest that we are storing up problems not just for scientists' moral authority but for their credibility.

Indeed, I want to approach the problem of scientists' moral authority by way of an historical inquiry into their *credibility,* the grounds on which scientists' pronouncements about the natural world are taken as true, objective, or reliable. Just because personal morality and knowledgeability are so widely considered as distinct in the modern condition, I start by outlining a scheme of things in which they were not reckoned to be so in the past. I shall describe a culture in which the credibility of scientific claims and the moral standing of those who make the claims are intertwined. Specifically, I mean to describe a relationship between credibility and virtue by drawing attention to the importance of *trust relations* in the making of scientific knowledge. I suggest that while those trust relations continue to be vitally important in modern science it has become harder and harder to appreciate them. One consequence of the invisibility of trust is the very attitude towards the disengagement between virtue and expertise which gives our modern dilemma its basic shape.

WHAT IS THE BASIS OF SCIENTISTS' CREDIBILITY?

Why do we believe what scientists tell us about the natural world? Why do we trust them to tell the truth? The fact of that trust, as well as its enormous extent and consequences, should be in no doubt. Most of our formal knowledge of the natural world is derived from no other source than what scientists tell us, or, more precisely, from what is told us by their apparent spokespersons: those who teach science, those who are represented as applying it in our personal domains, those who write or speak about it in the public culture. That we *have to* trust them for almost all aspects of our formal natural knowledge should also be in no doubt. For practical reasons alone we are unlikely to subject scientists' claims to effective personal skepticism. If indeed we know these things at all, we take *on faith* the principles of aerodynamics and hydrostatics, the role of DNA in heredity and development, the chemical structure of benzene. And the public "we" includes scientists as well as the laity, for scientists are largely in the position of laypersons when it comes to the specialist knowledge of other types of scientists.

Just noting the extent of the trust-dependency of our natural knowledge is enough to set some current worries about "antiscience" into perspective. The homage paid to science is best evident in the very existence of a public stock of formal natural knowledge. All those who believe that the earth goes around the sun, that DNA is the genetic substance, that there are such things as electrons, and that light travels at 186,000 miles per second are, by so believing, doing scientists honor. Nor is that honor restricted to blind acceptance. Many of those who *doubt* that CFCs are the cause of a shrinking ozone layer, that the burning of fossil fuels is raising global temperatures, or that organic change is accounted for by natural selection of small continuous variations, may likewise be regarded as doing science honor. Here, skeptics may be questioning *where the real scientists are* in disputed territory, or whether, indeed, any of the claims in question have the legitimate status of "science." Yet in so doing they reinforce the notion that there is such a thing as real science—objective, true, and powerful. Similarly, legitimate concerns over the "use" and "consequences" of scientific knowledge do not affect the honor paid to science: the very problems that science is said to generate flow from the recognition of its potency.

The point to which I wish to draw attention here is not whether the public trusts science, or trusts it enough. Opinions can legitimately differ about whether there is a problem of insufficient public confidence and respect for some group of scientists or some corpus of scientific knowledge. Rather, starting from the observation that public trust in science *is* enormous, I want to pose some questions about the basis of that trust. On what grounds, on the basis of what understandings, do we trust scientists to tell the truth about the natural world, as opposed to some other group of practitioners like psychics or captains of industry? I will argue that an important element of our response to the question "Why trust scientists?" proceeds from an understanding of what *kind of people* scientists are and how they relate to the sources of their knowledge and to other members of the scientific community. Are scientists thought to be exceptional in respect of their personal morality, their rugged individualism, the extent of their disinterestedness, their skepticism? And are any or all of those personal traits regarded as sufficient to ground our confidence in scientific reliability and truthfulness? Or are scientists understood to be ordinary people whose extraordinary knowledge is guaranteed by characteristics of the institutions in which they are placed? We trust science, in large part, through having some sort of understanding of what scientists are like, individually and collectively.

This paper is in four parts: (1) I argue the importance of trust relations among scientists as a general matter, and I describe the historical development of a sensibility which makes it hard for those trust relations—and hence the role of virtue in the scientific community—to be appreciated; (2) I describe the pre- and early modern culture which forged a publicly recognized link between the integrity of individuals, on the one hand, and their ability and willingness to speak the truth, on the other; (3) I note some evidence that this traditional relationship between understandings of individual virtue and of intellectual honesty may be breaking down, and that the public is increasingly being offered a different view of the bases of scientific truthfulness; (4) I argue that this emerging new view of the bases of scientific credibility—one which takes as a matter of course the divorce between expertise and virtue—is just the framework which makes the idea of scientists' moral authority so problematic. I suggest that it is ultimately a misguided view and that an understanding of the nature of scientific work which does not recognize and enforce a degree of individual virtue threatens the moral economy in which scientific knowledge itself is created and maintained. Virtue and credibility, I will conclude, cannot stably be so disengaged as present-day sensibilities seem to accept. I suggest that a reinspection of the cultural patterns outlined in (2) can inform the present debates over the ethical authority of science and ethical conduct in science.

I mean to focus upon scientists' honesty or sincerity as an element in the public credibility of their knowledge.[1] However, I need to make a caveat against seeming to claim too much for such considerations. Suppose we say that there are three main features endemically implicated in assessments of what we are told, whether by scientists or others: the plausibility of the claim; the intellectual entitlement of the source; and the honesty of the source.[2] First, all things being equal, we are likely to believe claims that accord with what we already know about the world, even if they are told us by people whose knowledgeability or expertise in the matter is slight. Just for that reason plausibility may be a trouble, rather than a positive resource, in fostering public trust in science, at least to the extent that novel or noncommonsensical claims are at issue. How can scientists hope radically to revise or add to the public stock of knowledge unless there is some other basis for belief than plausibility?

Second, we are more likely to accept claims from sources of recognized expertise and knowledgeability than from those considered to lack these entitlements. This too is a fully general maxim of assent. Specialized scientific expertise is no invention of the modern era: even in antiquity practitioners of the mathematical sciences—astronomy, optics, and statics, as well as pure mathematics itself—were understood to possess arduously acquired special knowledge and skills which set them apart from the common culture, with the consequence that only other specialists were in a position adequately to assess knowledge-claims in these domains.[3] The view that there exists a special, universal, and efficacious "scientific method," though intermittently denied by eminent scientists as well as historians and sociologists of science, represents a particular form of the attribution of expertise, and we ought to have a better understanding of what the public believes about "method" in science and its potency. Scientific specialization has, of course, vastly increased in modern times, but the problems that specialization poses for public belief are far from new.

Third, just because we are unlikely to be in a position directly to verify expert knowledge-claims, we must have some other warrants for believing them. Even our recognition that *these people are experts* has to be grounded on something other than our independent knowledge of their expertise, for example, upon our belief in the honesty of those who, directly or indirectly, vouch for their expertise. Accordingly, the acknowledgment of expertise is embedded within the recognition of honesty: experts have honestly reported how matters stand in the world; their legitimate possession of expertise has been honestly represented and vouched for. In this sense, the recognition of practitioners as truthful—individually or collectively—is a fundamental basis of public credibility. Other inducements to credibility must pass through a judgment that those who speak do so honestly.[4] That is to say, against much modern sensibility, that scientists' authority to say what is true implicates some conception of virtuous behavior.

TRUST AND THE QUALITY OF SCIENTIFIC KNOWLEDGE

I want briefly to describe the historical development of a picture of scientists' relations with the natural world and with each other which has made the role of trust difficult to see and to value. I will suggest that this picture is systematically misleading, and later I will argue that it has come to constitute a major problem for an informed public view of what an honest scientist is and does, and, by extension, for the moral authority of science. Failure to appreciate the trust-dependency of science therefore endangers not only the public credibility of science but also, indirectly, the economy in which scientists can continue to produce credible knowledge and to take a role in debates over the proper uses of science.

The sentiment that regards trust and authority in the guise of potential *problems* for genuine scientific knowledge has the most spotless of philosophical pedigrees. It is as old as modernity itself. The seventeenth-century "moderns" enjoined those who would reform traditional natural knowledge and set it upon proper foundations to reject reliance upon authoritative ancient texts and the hearsay testimony of other people. In one formulation, experience was to be preferred to authority, the Book of Nature to the texts of Aristotle and "old wives' tales." In another, rationally disciplined self-inquiry was deemed superior to the whole stock of Scholastic knowledge. Bacon and the English empiricists embodied the first tendency, Descartes and the Continental rationalists the other. Descartes locked himself up alone in his stove-heated room in order to set aside the authoritative knowledge he had acquired from the Schools, "resolving to seek no other science than that which could be found in myself." An individual, equipped with right method, need not rely for his knowledge upon any intellectual tradition, or upon the relations of any other person.[5] In John Locke's view: "We may as rationally hope to see with other men's eyes, as to know by other men's understandings. So much as we ourselves consider and comprehend of truth and reason, so much we possess of real and true knowledge. . . . In the sciences, every one has so much as he really knows and comprehends. What he believes only, and takes on trust, are but shreds."[6] In their different modes, both sets of "moderns" viewed reliance upon traditionally trusted sources as an inadequate basis for proper knowledge. The role of trust and authority was shown to stand against the very idea of science. Knowledge was supposed to be the product of a sovereign individual confronting the world. Our knowledge was said to be secure insofar as its producers were conceived as solitary. That sentiment is at the root of the modern disengagement between truth and the social virtues. So far as truth-making is concerned, the social virtues may even be treated as an impediment.

Seventeenth-century moderns placed the solitary knower at the center of a scientific stage where he has remained—minority academic voices notwithstanding—until the present day. From those moderns we inherit the legacy of epistemic individualism, a legacy which makes the constitutive role of trust and authority in the making of knowledge hard to see and harder still to appreciate as a virtue. Yet all forms of collectively held natural knowledge, including the most valued bodies of modern scientific knowledge, are utterly trust-dependent. The seventeenth-century modern rhetoric which rejected trust and authority signaled skepticism about ancient authority and credulous acceptance of hearsay testimony. It did not, in practice, mean the wholesale rejection of trust in other people's narrations as an adequate basis for empirical scientific knowledge. The Royal Society's motto—*Nullius in verba*—meant, in operational terms, *Do not give ancient authority or indirect testimony your whole and unconditional trust.*

The new empirical and experimental practitioners of the seventeenth century relied massively upon trust in human testimony about the natural world, and, indeed, it is impossible that they could have produced any recognizable body of natural knowledge had they not done so. The "public" experiments so vigorously advocated by Royal Society publicists were rarely witnessed by more than a handful of practitioners, and more rarely still replicated by distant others. Experimentally produced phenomena became part of the stock of collective knowledge largely through the testimony of trusted authors. The experiment—called "crucial" by Robert Boyle—in which a barometer was carried up the Puy-de-Dôme in France in order to show that we lived at the bottom of an ocean of air yielded knowledge for Boyle insofar as he trusted Blaise Pascal, who narrated the experiment, who in turn trusted his brother-in-law, who carried the apparatus up the mountain and reported that the mercury level fell.[7] Natural historical knowledge of distant phenomena similarly relied upon the narrations of trusted travelers: scientists who remained the whole of their lives in the south of England knew that the world contained polar bears, icebergs, regularly spouting geysers, and men "whose heads do grow beneath their shoulders" on no other basis. Many naturally occurring phenomena were accessible only to individuals privileged by space and time to see them, but knowledge of them became widespread through these persons' credible testimony. Those who never themselves witnessed the comet of 1664 knew its apparent motion through the heavens by trusting those who had, while the very notion of a comet's path only existed through trust relations since no one individual observed all of its positions.[8]

Late-twentieth-century science is no less trust-dependent, and arguably it is more so. The great specialization of modern science means in a very obvious way that individual scientists do not hold the whole of their own discipline's knowledge, and still less that of science in general, in their heads. The chemical knowledge needed by biologists to conduct an assay, like the physical knowledge embodied in their instruments, is largely taken on trust and, often literally, "off the shelf." This much has been intermittently noted by modern scientists and commentators upon science. As Michael Polanyi observed in 1958, "The overwhelming proportion of our factual beliefs [are] held at second hand through trusting others."[9]

Modern scientists, no less than the laity, hold the bulk of their knowledge, even the knowledge of their own disciplines, so to speak, by courtesy. As students they acquire their knowledge from authoritative sources, and as mature practitioners they rely upon the trustworthiness of other expert sources. The sociologist Barry Barnes points out that to say that a society "knows" something which no one individual in that society knows is proper speech only by virtue of recognizing the role of trust relations in constituting knowledge:

> If an individual knows Euclid's geometry up to the twentieth theorem we can straightforwardly say that he is in a position to prove the twenty-first theorem: he knows all it is necessary to know. But imagine that this knowledge is spread over the members of a society, some known by some individuals, some by others. We cannot say of this society that it knows enough to prove the twenty-first theorem. To think of the society as an individual writ large in this way would be quite misconceived. Suppose that the different individuals, with the different necessary bits of knowledge, did not know each other, or how to find each other. Or suppose they did not trust each other, or know how to check on each other's trustworthiness. In both cases, the twenty-first theorem would remain unproven. The technical knowledge would have been present in the society, but not the necessary internal ordering—the necessary social relationships—for the proof to be executed. Individuals would have known enough mathematics, but not known enough about themselves.[10]

Trust appears as a "problem" in formal commentary on science just because its constitutive role is so rarely recognized and is so often vigorously denied. To judge that one holds one's knowledge at "second hand," as Polanyi himself says, is reckoned to identify its potential inadequacy.[11] It is right to draw attention to the quantity of knowledge which scientists hold on no other basis than what they are told by trusted sources. Yet it is not right, save in a restricted sense, to juxtapose trust-dependency to more direct warrants for knowledge. Scientists *are* sometimes skeptical of relevant claims, and they *do* sometimes aim to replicate claims or subject them to independent scrutiny, though the extent of such skeptical replication has undeniably been grossly exaggerated in popular portrayals of scientific practice. However, the ineradicable role of trust is as apparent in acts of skepticism as it is in routine trust.

Suppose that a molecular biologist, declining to accept what authoritative sources claimed, was skeptical that the HIV virus contained RNA. Such a scientist might indeed secure an independent supply of the virus and subject it to analysis, and in so doing might rightly be said to be rejecting trust and seeking personal verification. But that act of focused doubt would only be possible if the skeptical scientist took on trust *almost everything else* relevant to the act: the identity of the virus sample with which he or she had been supplied, the identity and claimed purity of the reagents used in the assay, the labeled speed of the centrifuge and the proper working of other instruments, and the honesty of technicians and of the authors of papers and manuals functioning as necessary resources in performing this act of skeptical checking. It should, therefore, be evident that each act of distrust would be predicated upon an overall framework of trust, and, indeed, all distrust presupposes a system of takings-for-granted which make *this instance* of distrust possible. Distrust is something which takes place on the *margins* of trusting systems.[12]

HONOR, HONESTY, AND FREE ACTION
IN EARLY MODERN SCIENCE

I have sketched a general argument that trust is constitutive of the very idea of knowledge and that, despite much seventeenth-century and present-day rhetoric to the contrary, the empirical knowledge of natural scientific communities is no less trust-dependent than other cultural practices whose knowledge is less highly valued. There must always be some practical solution to the question "Whom to trust?", while the content of the answer to that question varies from setting to setting and time to time.

Seventeenth-century answers to the question "Whom to trust?" in science do overlap considerably with those familiar to late-twentieth-century moderns. Early modern practitioners were, for example, more likely to believe the observation-reports and interpretations of skilled astronomers than of those with no such entitlements. Indeed, contemporary culture possessed rich resources for identifying the limitations and inadequacies of common sense, the unreliability of uninstructed observation, and the liability of "the vulgar" towards delusion and credulity. The same "modern" tendency which insisted upon direct observation as a bulwark against trust in ancient authority also cautioned that not everyone was capable of reliable observation and that experience always needed to be instructed by educated reason. Consequently, as I have already indicated, the recognition of expertise has always been a powerful inducement to assent.

I have also noted that experts will not be believed unless their honesty in reporting what they know to be the case is also granted. How, then, were sincerity and truthfulness recognized at the origins of modern science? Here there was a variety of answers to the questions "Who told the truth about the world?" and "On what bases did they tell the truth?" In ancient Greece the role of the *philosopher* was defined around his love of truth. The philosopher was that exceptional person, set apart from civil society, who spurned worldly rewards and pleasures and dedicated himself solely to truth.[13] He not only needed less of the world's goods and applause to produce his cultural goods, he positively needed disengagement from the mundane system of material rewards to seek truth and to be seen to do so. Only he who was free from worldly motives was free to conduct disinterested inquiry and to find truth. As the ancient story has it, when the philosopher Diogenes was asked by Alexander whether there was anything he wanted, the philosopher replied, "Yes, I would have you stand from between me and the sun."[14] Socrates prided himself on "how many things there are which I do not want." The integrity of the traditional philosopher's knowledge was recognized to flow from the special integrity of his person. By his love of truth alone the philosopher was understood to imitate God, the source of all truth.[15]

That ancient cultural appreciation of the philosopher's identity and its guarantee of his honesty persisted for many centuries, modified and reinforced by patterns of Christian intellectuality. In 1690 John Locke merely echoed Greek philosophical sentiments in announcing: "He that would seriously set upon the search for truth, ought in the first place to prepare his mind with a love of it. For he that loves it not, will not take much pains to get it; nor be much concerned when he misses it."[16] However, by the seventeenth century another type of social figure was increasingly participating in formal intellectual inquiry, bringing with him a different warrant for truthfulness. This figure was the *gentleman*. In the sixteenth century, humanist writers were urging that learning not be left to professional scholars and that gentlemen would increase their virtue as well as their social utility if they too participated in the life of the mind. By the end of the sixteenth century and the early seventeenth century such writers as Francis Bacon were offering influential arguments for the special civic utility of scientific studies and their special suitability for gentle participation.[17] The founding of the Royal Society of London in 1660 is witness to the impact of those arguments, and the person of its most eminent member—the Honourable Robert Boyle, son of the Earl of Cork—embodied the conjunction of scientific inquiry and gentlemanly virtue. The Society's first historian aptly described the early Royal Society as an organization predominantly made up of "Gentlemen, free, and unconfin'd."[18] The culture surrounding the seventeenth-century gentleman offered a quite special appreciation of the bases of gentle truthfulness. Gentlemen were said to tell the truth because they were free of any inducements to do otherwise. He who lied revealed his servility, baseness, and cowardice: he was, as both Montaigne and Bacon said, brave towards God and a coward to his fellow man.[19] Within a traditional honor culture, the imputation of fear and baseness was a grave act. Truthfulness was a measure of honor, and to represent another as mendacious was precisely to dispute his identity as a man of honor, a gentleman. Accordingly, it was only the accusation that a man *lied* which, in early modern society, could reliably provoke a challenge to a duel.

Reputation for truthfulness was, therefore, basic to the identity of a gentleman, while early modern English gentle culture offered a rich repertoire of appreciations of *why* the gentleman was a reliable truth-teller. On the surface, these accounts look different from those explaining philosophical veracity. They were, for the most part, secular in idiom. Among the most important understandings of the gentleman's truthfulness was an attributed causal link between the integrity of his social and economic circumstances and the integrity of his word. It was not that the gentleman was he who possessed the most money or the most power: the king and the great courtiers had more of those commodities. But those who had need to flatter, or those who were duty bound to represent their country's interests, might be under an obligation to deceive. On the other hand, those who possessed very *little* money or power were routinely in a position where they needed to seek advantage, or, if servants, were required to submerge their integrity in their masters' interests. Hence, both want or need, and very great power, induced departures from truthfulness. However, the English gentleman liked to see himself at the "golden mean" of the social order, and this was considered to be the position where integrity was unconstrained.

The gentleman told the truth *because no influences worked upon him to shift his narratives out of correspondence with what he believed to be the case.* His integrity was recognized to flow from his capacity for free action, and that same free action underwrote the truthfulness of his word. Conceptions of innate honor were, in that culture, bound up with notions of free action, gentle identity, and truth-telling. Understandings of the philosopher's and the gentleman's truthfulness therefore differed. But they concurred in two respects: (1) the truthfulness of both the philosopher and the gentleman emerged out of the acknowledgment that these were quite special sorts of persons, and (2) for both, the virtue of the person underwrote the veracity of his narratives.

FROM VIRTUE TO VIGILANCE

The culture which thus tied intellectual veracity to personal virtue persisted in European and, later, in American culture. In particular, the special reliability and objectivity of the scientist's testimony continued strongly to be associated with the special virtues of the scientist's personality. What was said of Boyle and Newton in the late seventeenth century continued to be applied to heroic scientific truth-seekers. When Boyle died in 1691 the funeral sermon advertised the spotless character of a "Christian Virtuoso": "He could neither lie, nor equivocate."[20] In 1725 the editor of his works wrote of Boyle's "candour" and "fidelity" as adequate grounds for belief, even in the most philosophically implausible claims: "We may certainly depend upon this, that what Mr. Boyle delivers as an experiment or observation of his own, is related in the precise manner wherein it appeared to him: no one ever yet deny'd, that he was a man of punctual veracity." Into the nineteenth century, commentators on Isaac Newton insisted upon the relationship between his genius and his moral makeup. In 1857 the philosopher and historian of science William Whewell wrote that "those who love to think that great [scientific] talents are naturally associated with virtue, have always dwelt with pleasure upon the views given of Newton by his contemporaries; for they have uniformly represented him as candid and humble, mild and good."[21]

In eighteenth-century England the chemist Joseph Priestley wrote that "A Philosopher ought to be something greater, and better than another man." If the scientist was not already virtuous, then the "contemplation of the works of God should give a sublimity to his virtue, should expand his benevolence, extinguish everything mean, base, and selfish in [his] nature," and such sentiments were standard in the British natural theological tradition well into the nineteenth-century.[22] Dorinda Outram's splendid biography of the early-nineteenth-century anatomist Georges Cuvier shows how the French public was given to understand the causal relationship between special scientific gifts and special personal virtues, and how objectivity was seen to flow from personal authenticity.[23] And Charles Paul describes how the *eloges* delivered to the eighteenth-century Paris Academy of Sciences repeatedly pointed to the special personal virtues of great scientists: simplicity, righteousness, modesty, candor, frankness, and sincerity.[24]

Great nineteenth-century scientists were widely advertised as moral heroes. The experimental biologist Claude Bernard influentially portrayed the special personal kindliness and modesty of those pursuing experimental truth. Such self-denial was necessary to preserve that "absolute freedom of mind" which allowed the experimentalist to be skeptical even of his own favored theories and to submit himself to truth alone.[25] Celebration of scientific heroism and virtue arguably reached its apogee in accounts of the life of Louis Pasteur: "Like his scientific prowess, Pasteur's moral fiber was incomparable. . . . [His] spiritual life was imbued with lofty ideals: sincerity, honesty, decency, and affection for truth."[26] In early-twentieth-century Germany, Max Weber's essay on "Science as a Vocation" advertised the intensely self-denying "passionate" and "inner devotion" necessary to pursue the life of modern specialized research.[27] For many educated Americans Sinclair Lewis's characters of Max Gottlieb and Martin Arrowsmith (1925) came to represent the very special nature of the scientist's vocation:

> To be a scientist [says Dr. Gottlieb]—it is not just a different job, so that a man should choose between being a scientist and being a bond-salesman . . . It makes its victim all different from the good normal man. The normal man, he does not care much what he does except that he should eat and sleep and make love. But the scientist is intensely religious—he is so religious that he will not accept quarter-truths, because they are an insult to his faith.[28]

   A picture of scientists as moral heroes, and an appreciation that their virtuous heroism underwrote the truthfulness of their claims, thus persisted well into this century. Yet some time around the 1930s—one ought to be no more precise than that—a quite different understanding of the scientist's character, and a different view of what guaranteed the truth of scientific knowledge, began to be made available to the public. One of the most interesting sites in which this view surfaced was closely associated with the origins of the academic discipline known as the sociology of science.

   By the late 1930s and 1940s Robert K. Merton, one of the most influential American sociologists, was presenting it as a *matter of course* that scientists "were as other men," and that the production of objective knowledge could not possibly be underwritten by the dispositions and temperaments of individual practitioners. Disinterested and objective knowledge was produced by interested and, occasionally, irrationally acting individuals: "A passion for knowledge, idle curiosity, altruistic concern with the benefit to humanity, and a host of other special motives have been attributed to the scientist. The quest for distinctive motives appears to have been misdirected." There is no satisfactory evidence that scientists are "recruited from the ranks of those who exhibit an unusual degree of moral integrity" or that the objectivity of scientific knowledge proceeds from "the personal qualities of scientists." Rather, what underpins scientific truthfulness was said to be an elaborated system of institutional norms, whose "internalization" guarantees that transgressions will generate psychic pain and whose implementation by the community guarantees that transgressors will be found out and punished.[29]

   Of course, such arguments against the so-called "motivational level of analysis" served important disciplinary purposes: they demarcated sociology from psychology and showed the legitimacy of social-structural answers to questions about scientific objectivity. Nevertheless, these and similar appreciations of the scientist's personality and communal relations fed into a public culture which was, in any event, increasingly being made aware from a variety of sources that the scientific "vocation" was rapidly changing from a "calling" to a "job." The scientist was not understood as "called" to a passionate search for truth but to be doing a job like any other, except that its products counted as truth. Meanwhile, a small number of psychological studies of scientists broadly supported that understanding while pointing out that scientists were not notably competent in their individual command of the formal principles of logical reasoning.[30] When James Watson's *The Double Helix* (1968) caused such apparent public delight (and mock consternation) about the all-too-human face of modern science, Robert Merton was joined by a number of leading statesmen of science in saying, in effect, "I told you so." John Lear described Watson's book "as therapy for those who think of science as a realm permeated with unalloyed idealism and of scientists as plumed knights searching always and exclusively for truth."[31]

Thus, by the middle of the twentieth century it appears that the causal link posited by early modern gentlemanly culture between truth-telling and virtuous free action had been turned upside down. In fact, we still know relatively little about current lay attitudes towards science and scientists, and we ought to know much more, yet it is not unreasonable to assume substantial overlap between what the public is persistently told about science and scientists and what they may come to believe.[32] And what the public is pervasively told is that objective scientific knowledge is not now guaranteed by the participation of virtuous "Gentlemen, free, and unconfin'd," but by institutions which most vigilantly *constrain* the free action of their members. Robert Merton was, accordingly, well aware of apparent *lese majesty* in declaring that "the activities of scientists are subject to rigorous policing, to a degree perhaps unparalleled in any other field of activity."[33] The modern place of knowledge here appears not as a gentleman's drawing room but as a great Panopticon of Truth.

"AFTER VIRTUE" AND ITS EFFECTS

I want to sketch some possible consequences of this changing appreciation of the grounds of scientific credibility, drawing out the link between credibility and moral authority outlined at the beginning of this paper. These notes are frankly speculative, intended not as definitive conclusions but as promptings to reflect on the nature of the modern predicament and, from this somewhat unfamiliar historical and sociological perspective, to consider anew what might be done about it.

As an historian and sociologist, I am unaccustomed to making recommendations about what scientists and policymakers "ought to do." (That is to say, my academic community tends to have its own institutional separation between our expert knowledge and our moral authority.) Nevertheless, I feel that the historical understandings outlined above license a suggestion that some present-day initiatives for dealing with alleged problems of ethical behavior in science are in danger of getting it quite wrong.

If what I have had to say about the fundamental and ineradicable role of trust in science is broadly correct, then systematic attempts to subject the conduct of the scientific community to vigilant policing are more likely to kill the patient than to cure the disease. Vigilance can do serious damage to science for the reason that *trust relations* among scientists are constitutive of the making, maintenance, and extension of scientific knowledge, that is, to the capacity of the scientific community to produce consensual knowledge upon which others may rely. Only when that trust dependency is ignored or seen solely as a *problem* for science do vigilance models possess their apparent appeal. Vigilance as a solution to problems of dishonesty amounts in practice to the enforcement of skepticism and distrust among scientists. Scientific reports may be fraudulent, so scientists are enjoined more and more systematically to replicate others' experiments and observations, and to ensure that their own reports will stand up to others' more vigorous skeptical scrutiny. Inference from evidential findings is to be more tightly controlled, so scientists are recommended more thoroughly to report exactly what was done and exactly how it was done. And if they will not do so, then, it is said, external means must be put in place to ensure skepticism and distrust.

To suggest that skepticism and distrust should be very much more common in science is, in effect, to take the position that much of our modern structure of scientific knowledge should be unwound, put into reverse, and ultimately dismantled. Instead of laboratories for the production of new knowledge, we should build great facilities for the close re-inspection of what is currently taken to be knowledge. Grants will be given for checking routine findings; published reports will look more and more like laboratory notebooks; libraries will have to be expanded to house an unimaginably vast literature reporting upon acts of distrust; relations between scientists will become uncoordinated, unproductive, and unpleasant. No one actually defends such consequences, largely because those effects of enforced skepticism have not been clearly foreseen. Nor would anyone seriously advocate measures that might lead to anything like these consequences if the constitutive role of trust in making scientific knowledge were more widely recognized. It needs to be understood that trust is a *condition* for having the body of knowledge currently called science. As Hardwig puts it, "the alternative to trust is . . . ignorance."[34]

No doubt, those who argue for such measures do so in good faith, convinced that skepticism and distrust are the very essence of what it is to be scientific. In this respect, they endorse the seventeenth-century "modern" rhetoric of epistemic individualism. Yet, as I have sought to show, individualistic rhetoric, however important as a cultural *evaluation* of how proper knowledge ought to be secured, fails to represent the realities of scientific practice. Science is a trusting institution. Trust is not an epistemic *problem* for science; it is—if one wants to engage in such evaluations—an evident epistemic virtue. It is only by trusting others that scientists hold the vast bulk of their knowledge, that their knowledge has scope, that they can know things they themselves have not experienced, and, indeed, that they can be effectively skeptical when they wish to be. The very existence of highly interdependent, specialized, and differentiated knowledge-communities testifies to the real extent of that trust-dependency.

The point is not that vigilant policing is incapable of controlling some forms of undesirable behavior in science. Of course, the policing of science does in principle have that capacity, just as it does in financial circles or in everyday life. The question to be asked before embarking upon such policing is whether the nature of the practice is likely to be distorted or destroyed by enforced skepticism, whether that for which the practice is valued, and supported, by society is itself critically dependent upon trust rather than its opposite. Put another way, are there any *special reasons* for exempting science from the sort of policing to which many other areas of everyday life are routinely subject?

I have suggested that there are such reasons. Take any institution in modern society with whose workings and products we are broadly satisfied. Then come to a reflective appreciation of the extent to which those workings and those products are trust-dependent and liable to be eroded by the imposition of vigilant skepticism. If we are on the whole satisfied with the quality of scientific knowledge, and if we understand that science is fundamentally a trusting institution, then we have adequate grounds for the exemption in question. I know more about science than about other modern specialized institutions, but I do not doubt that there are others that meet the conditions for exemption: one thinks of sectors of the financial system and the civil service. Policy in such matters ought to be informed by our best current understandings of the conditions in which geese lay golden eggs. My fear is that the historical and sociological understandings that currently seem to inform the relevant policy debates are not as good as they ought to be.

If what I have had to say about the fundamental role of trust in science is broadly correct, then some aspects of the modern sensibility that separates virtue and credibility can be usefully reassessed. In that sensibility, what is agreed upon among scientists as "the facts of the matter" is widely considered an unproblematic element in any potential discussions over "what then ought to be done" as a morally relevant decision. That is just a way of phrasing the disengagement between expertise and virtue which lies at the heart of the modern sensibility.

Yet, insofar as trust is critical to the making and maintenance of scientific knowledge, then the attribution of expertise—specialized knowledge of what is true—cannot be divorced from the practical recognition of virtue—in this case, of integrity and honesty. Agreement about the "scientific facts" is itself a moral matter. Being "trust-dependent," such agreement is no less interesting and no less problematic than "the ethical application" of agreed-upon facts. Our technical knowledge is only as secure as the moral economy in which it is produced. The "scientific portion" of any ethical decision contains institutionalized moral judgments, and the fact that we do not recognize them as such is itself an aspect of the modern condition.[35] We just do not yet have a very satisfactory understanding of the processes by which scientists come to agree, or agree not to disagree, and hence how the "facts of the matter" come to appear an unproblematic element in ethical decision-making.

It is the "vigilance model" of scientific objectivity that seems to generate some of our fundamental current dilemmas about the moral authority of science. Scientific knowledge will be seen as reliable insofar as scientists are subject to internal and external vigilance and, in that sense, the relevant invigilated experts will inevitably take part in ethical decisions involving specialized knowledge. Yet, if scientists are seen as no more honest and selfless than anyone else, then it follows that they will not be accorded any more moral authority than anyone else. The result may be a strange and an unsatisfactory situation in which those most intimately familiar with the "facts of the matter at hand" will neither be given, nor encouraged to take, any special role in the moral disposition of "the matter at hand." That we can contemplate this situation with equanimity is an expression of modern sentiment that holds the divorce between knowledgeability and virtue to be "natural," to be accepted as a matter of course. If, however, history holds any lessons, it is that the relationship between the two is a contingent matter. And what is historically contingent is historically revisable.

What is to be done? Again, I pretend to no special authority to participate in such discussions. Yet, as I suggested, the disengagement afforded by an historical perspective can loosen up our sense of possibilities. One idea would take seriously as a problem the link between questions of scientific honesty and moral authority introduced at the outset. If our current appreciation of the former leads to problems with the latter, then the remedy can only be to try to reconstitute an appreciation of the scientist as "more virtuous" than other people, and to disseminate that appreciation, without embarrassment, in the wider culture.

The moral philosopher Alasdair MacIntyre distinguishes between a "practice" and an "institution."[36] A practice is an organized form of human activity which provides its members "internal goods," rewards which can only be secured by accepting the standards of excellence that belong to that practice and to it alone. By contrast, there are coherent social institutions which offer their members "external goods," those available through participation in the institution, but which do not differentiate that institution from others and which may even be had without accepting its internal standards. So, a person may, indeed, get money by cheating at chess or at science: chess or science may be widely seen just as a way of getting money. But then they do not have the status of practices. Chess and science are practices insofar as participants actually desire those internal rewards which can only be had by wanting to solve problems or extend understanding, and then doing so.

The extent to which that idea seems embarrassing and old-fashioned is the extent to which we have a problem of scientific honesty and, therefore, of moral authority. The Greeks had the notion of a philosopher as someone who loved truth and would not tell a lie, and the early modern English had their understanding of a gentleman as someone who valued the integrity of his word as he valued his sense of honor. If we are in fact serious about addressing problems of intellectual dishonesty and the erosion of moral authority, I doubt very much whether we can do better than try, over a long period, to revive and reinstill some such culture of virtue. This is not a "quick fix," but, at the end of the day, it may well be our only stable "fix." The Greeks and the early moderns understood that virtue had to be practiced and that it could be taught. Efforts at ethical education, if seriously intended and well-designed, are likely to have an effect. However, nothing can be as effective as the daily visibility of respected individuals who are seen to be doing science "for the love of truth," "for the pleasure of solving puzzles and getting it right," and not "for the love of lucre." Such individuals would be understood not to lie because nothing they wanted could be gained from a lie. The proposed solution must be recognized as having two sides. Just as one is saying that we ought specially to trust scientists, so one is saying that scientists ought to *deserve* to be regarded as specially trustworthy people.

And such individuals might, for that reason, possess a useful form of moral authority. There should be no illusions about the nature of the moral authority which the scientist-restored-to-virtue might have. It would be of a very general sort. If there really are such people as "ethical experts" in our society, then this scientist would not be one. Rather, he or she might have whatever general moral authority still attaches to someone reputed to be honest and selfless, to possess integrity, to love truth more than lucre. More than that cannot, I think, be reasonably hoped for in our society. Less than that should be considered unacceptable.

NOTES

1. I appreciate that the present committee is not primarily interested in questions of scientific honesty or dishonesty, but I shall be trying to show why—properly conceived—such questions are indeed germane to some of this committee's concerns about the moral authority of science.

2. This is a simplified version of an account of maxims of credibility developed in Steven Shapin, *A Social History of Truth: Civility and Science in Seventeenth-Century England* (Chicago: University of Chicago Press, 1994), ch. 5.

3. Thomas S. Kuhn. "Mathematical versus Experimental Traditions in the Development of Physical Science," in idem, *The Essential Tension: Selected Studies in Scientific Tradition and Change* (Chicago: University of Chicago Press, 1977), 31–65, esp. pp. 35–37.

4. This point has recently been nicely summarized in a philosophical idiom by John Hardwig, "The Role of Trust in Knowledge," *Journal of Philosophy* 88 (1991), 693–708, esp. pp. 700–701.

5. Rene Descartes, "Discourse on the Method," in *The Philosophical Works of Descartes*, eds.

and trans. Elizabeth S. Haldane and G.R.T. Ross, 2 vols. (New York: Dover, 1955; orig. publ. 1637), I, 79–130, quoting p. 86.

6. John Locke, *An Essay Concerning Human Understanding,* ed. Alexander Campbell Fraser, 2 vols. (New York: Dover, 1959; orig. publ. 1690), I, 115.

7. Robert Boyle. "A Defence of the Doctrine Touching the Spring and Weight of the Air," in idem, *Works,* ed. Thomas Birch, 6 vols. (London, 1772; text orig. publ. 1662), I, 118–185, on p. 151. For studies of experimental performances and replication in seventeenth-century England, see S. Shapin, "Pump and Circumstance: Robert Boyle's Literary Technology," *Social Studies of Science* 14 (1984), 481–520; Shapin and Simon Schaffer, *Leviathan and the Air-Pump: Hobbes, Boyle, and the Experimental Life* (Princeton, N: Princeton University Press, 1985), esp. chs. 2 and 6.

8. The management of empirical testimony in seventeenth-century England is treated in detail in Shapin, *A Social History of Truth,* esp. ch. 6.

9. E.g., Michael Polanyi, *Personal Knowledge: Towards a Post-Critical Philosophy* (Chicago: University of Chicago Press, 1958), esp. 207–208, 216, 240–241, 375, quoting p. 208. For a more recent, albeit limited, philosophical appreciation of trust in science, see, e.g., Philip Kitcher, *The Advancement of Science: Science without Legend, Objectivity without Illusions* (New York: Oxford University Press, 1993), ch. 8; also Michael Welbourne, *The Community of Knowledge* (Aberdeen: Aberdeen University Press, 1986); and the more full-bloodedly sociological Hardwig, "The Role of Trust in Knowledge."

10. Barry Barnes. *About Science* (Oxford: Basil Blackwell, 1985), 82 (and see ch. 3, *passim,* for an excellent sociological appreciation of the role of trust and authority in science). As Hardwig ("The Role of Trust in Knowledge," 697) nicely puts it: "Knowing [is] not a privileged psychological state. If it is a privileged state at all, it is a privileged social state."

11. Accordingly, while pointing to the central role of trust in modern science Polanyi (*Personal Knowledge,* 217) described an ideal chain of skepticism whereby members of specialized scientific communities might validate each other's knowledge: even though scientist A was obliged to take the knowledge of scientist C on trust, he or she was able directly to check over the knowledge of B, who was, in turn, competent to assess C.

12. See Barry Barnes' concise account of the knowledge-dependency of skepticism with respect to anomalous scientific findings: *About Science,* 59–63, and, for practical trust in the "black-boxed" knowledge and routines of modern science, see Kathleen Jordan and Michael Lynch, "The Sociology of a Genetic Engineering Technique: Ritual and Rationality in the Performance of the 'Plasmid Prep' in *The Right Tools for the Job. At Work in Twentieth-Century Life Science,* eds. Adele Clarke and Joan H. Fujimura (Princeton, NJ: Princeton University Press, 1992), 77–114, esp. pp. 93, 102.

13. The "apartness" of the philosopher as a pervasive cultural trope is discussed in S. Shapin, 'The Mind is Its Own Place': Science and Solitude in Seventeenth-Century England," *Science in Context* 4 (1991), 191–218, esp. pp. 192–198, and, for classic treatment of the *vita contemplativa,* see Hannah Arendt, *The Human Condition* (Chicago: University of Chicago Press, 1958). See also Owsei Temkin, "Historical Reflections on a Scientist's Virtue," *Isis* 60 (1969), 427–438, esp. pp. 427–428.

14. Plutarch, *The Lives of the Noble Grecians and Romans,* trans. John Dryden and rev. Arthur Hugh Clough (New York: Modern Library, [1932]), 810.

15. Classic sources for these sentiments include Diogenes Lartius, *The Lives and Opinions of Eminent Philosophers,* trans. C.D. Yonge (London: Henry G. Bohn, 1853), quoting p. 66, and Thomas Stanley, *The History of Philosophy,* 3 vols. (London, 1655–1660).

16. Locke, *Essay Concerning Human Understanding,* II, 428.

17. S. Shapin. "'A Scholar and a Gentleman': The Problematic Identity of the Scientific Practitioner in Early Modern England," *History of Science* 29 (1991), 279–327, esp. pp. 282–299; Julian Martin, *Francis Bacon, the State, and the Reform of Natural Philosophy* (Cambridge: Cambridge University Press, 1992), ch. 6.

18. Thomas Sprat. *The History of the Royal Society* (London, 1667), 67; also 405–407. For the scientific significance of the gentlemanly wake-up of the early Royal Society, see Steven Shapin, "The House of Experiment in Seventeenth-Century England," *Isis* 73 (1988), 373-404, and, for Boyle as gentleman-scientist, see Shapin, *A Social History of Truth*, ch. 4. I draw attention here to the special significance of gentlemanly codes for early modern *English* science. I argue that those codes were influential for the subsequent development of the natural sciences while recognizing that Continental patterns showed significant difference.

19. Michael de Montaigne. *The Complete Essays of Montaigne*, trans. Donald M. Frame (Stanford, CA: Stanford University Press, 1965), 505; Francis Bacon, "Of Truth," in idem, *The Moral and Historical Works of Lord Bacon, Including His Essays . . .*, ed. Joseph Devey (London: Henry G. Bohn, 1852; orig. publ. 1597), 1–4.

20. Gilbert Burnet. "Character of a Christian Philosopher, in a Sermon Preached January 7, 1691–1692, at the Funeral of the Hon. Robert Boyle," in idem, *Lives, Characters, and an Address to Posterity*, ed. John Jebb (London, 1833), 368.

21. Peter Shaw. "General Preface," in idem, ed., *Boyle's Philosophical Works* (London, 1725), ix-xv.

22. William Whewell. *Selected Writings on the History of Science*, ed. Yehuda Elkana (Chicago: University of Chicago Press, 1984), 63. In this connection, see especially Richard Yeo, "Genius, Method and Morality: Images of Newton in Britain, 1760–1860," *Science in Context* 2 (1988), 257–284. Recent historical work on Newton's character has been notably more harsh.

23. Joseph Priestley. *The History and Present State of Electricity*, 2 vols., 3rd ed. (London, 1775), I, xxiii.

24. Dorinda Outram, *Georges Cuvier: Vocation, Science, and Authority in Post-Revolutionary France* (Manchester: Manchester University Press, 1984), esp. 63–64, 79, 94, 117.

25. Charles B. Paul. *Science and Immortality: The Eloges of the Paris Academy of Sciences (1691–1799)* (Berkeley: University of California Press, 1980), esp. 92–109.

26. Claude Bernard. *An Introduction to the Study of Experimental Medicine*, trans. Henry Copley Greene (New York: Dover, 1957; orig. publ. 1865), esp. 28, 35–39, quoting p. 35.

27. P. Vallery-Radot. *Louis Pasteur: A Great Life in Brief*, trans. Alfred Joseph (New York: Alfred A. Knopf, 1966; orig. publ. 1885), vi. As with Newton, recent historical work has taken Pasteur's reputation for personal virtue down several pegs.

28. Max Weber. "Science as a Vocation," in idem, *From Max Weber: Essays in Sociology*, eds. and trans. H.H. Gerth and C. Wright Mills (London: Routledge, 1991; essay orig. publ. 1919), 129–156, quoting pp. 135, 137. For useful treatment of the nineteenth- and early twentieth-century German scientist as moral exemplar and producer of *wertfrei* knowledge, see Robert N. Proctor, *Value-Free Science? Purity and Power in Modern Knowledge* (Cambridge, MA: Harvard University Press, 1991), chs. 5–10.

29. Sinclair Lewis. *Arrowsmith* (New York: Signet, 1980; orig. publ. 1925), 267. For the cultural significance and scientific model of the character of Martin Arrowsmith, see Charles E. Rosenberg, "Martin Arrowsmith: The Scientist as Hero," in idem, *No Other Gods: On Science and American Social Thought* (Baltimore, MD: Johns Hopkins University Press, 1976), 123–131.

30. Robert K. Merton. *The Sociology of Science: Theoretical and Empirical Investigations*, ed. Norman W. Storer (Chicago: University of Chicago Press, 1973; quoting art. orig. publ. 1942), 275–276; see also 259, 290–291; idem, *Sociological Ambivalence and Other Essays* (New York: Free Press, 1976; art. orig. publ. 1963), 34–35. The conclusion that scientists, even the great ones, "were as other men" was evidently being argued, against residual tendencies to the contrary, within the scientific community at the time: see, for example, G.H. Hardy, *A Mathematician's Apology* (Cambridge: Cambridge University Press, 1992; orig. publ 1940), 78: "Ambition has been the driving force behind nearly all the best work. . . . We must guard against a fallacy common among apologists for science, the fallacy of supposing . . . that physiologists, for example, have particularly noble souls."

31. This work is usefully assessed in Michael J. Mahoney, "Psychology of Scientists: An Evaluative Review," *Social Studies of Science* 9 (1979), 349–375, esp. pp. 354–356.

32. Robert K. Merton. "Making It Scientifically," in James D. Watson, *The Double Helix: A Personal Account of the Discovery of the Structure of DNA: Text, Commentaries, Reviews, Original Papers,* ed. Gunther S. Stent (New York: W.W. Norton, 1980; orig. publ. 1968), 213–218; John Lear, "Heredity Transactions," ibid., 194–198 (quoting 194–195); see also reviews by Richard C. Lewontin (pp. 185–187, for comparisons with Martin Arrowsmith), Mary Ellman (pp. 187–191), P.B. Medawar (pp. 218–224): [Watson's book ought to prevent anyone from going] "on believing that The Scientist is some definite kind of person." Some scientist-reviewers, to be sure, found Watson's portrayal of normal scientific practice both wrong and damaging to the reputation of science. At about the same time, Daniel S. Greenberg's *The Politics of Pure Science* (New York: New American Library, 1967) and his journalism for *Science* magazine did much to form a public awareness of scientists as entrepreneurs "on the make." Indeed, Greenberg's semi-fictional "Dr. Grant Swinger" was somewhat *more* merely human than the average stockbroker.

33. For reflective study of the public credibility of science and its bases, see, e.g., Brian Wynne, "Public Understanding of Science Research: New Horizons or Hall of Mirrors?" *Public Understanding of Science* 1 (1992), 37–43; idem, "Misunderstood Misunderstanding: Social Identities and Public Uptake of Science," ibid., 281–304, esp. p. 298; also Marcel C. LaFollette, *Making Science Our Own: Public Images of Science, 1910–1955* (Chicago: University of Chicago Press, 1990).

34. Merton, *The Sociology of Science,* 275–276.

35. Hardwig, "The Role of Trust in Knowledge," 707; also Shapin, *A Social History of Truth,* ch. 1.

36. The sociologist H.M. Collins has studied episodes of "extraordinary science," in which scientists cannot effectively appeal to "the facts of the matter" to settle disputes, since it is those facts which are being contested. In such episodes, scientists may invoke characterizations of participants' basic competence and morality in attempts to achieve resolution: Collins, *Changing Order: Replication and Induction in Scientific Practice,* 2nd ed. (Chicago: University of Chicago Press, 1992).

37. Alasdair MacIntyre. *After Virtue: A Study in Moral Theory,* 2nd ed. (Notre Dame: I: Notre Dame University Press, 1984), esp. chs. 13–14. MacIntyre's views are brought to bear upon the problem of fraud in science by C. J. List, "Scientific Fraud: Social Deviance or the Failure of Virtue?" *Science, Technology and Human Values* 10, 4 (1985), 27–36, esp. 30–32.

Institutional Ethics Committees: Local Perspectives on Ethical Issues in Medicine

ELIZABETH HEITMAN, Ph.D.

Assistant Professor, University of Texas School of Public Health

THE HISTORICAL DEVELOPMENT OF INSTITUTIONAL ETHICS COMMITTEES

Institutional ethics committees (IECs) have evolved over the past two decades in the United States and Canada as health care professionals, hospital administrators, regulatory agencies and legal authorities, and patients and their families have struggled to make good decisions about applying resuscitative and life-sustaining technologies. Much of the history of the IEC parallels the development of medical ethics as an academic and, more particularly, clinical discipline. However, the practical nature of clinical ethics and constraints of law and institutional policy have also led IECs to a theory and practice distinct from academic ethics.

The first public call[1] for an advisory body on clinical ethics[2] came in 1971 from the Catholic Hospital Association of Canada (CHAC) and the Canadian Catholic bishops.[3] Their *Medico-Moral Guide* (1), a handbook on the application of the Roman Catholic teachings known as the *Ethical and Religious Directives for Catholic Hospitals*, recommended that Catholic institutions establish special committees to: (a) educate the hospital community on the moral dimensions of life-sustaining technologies; (b) provide a forum for interdisciplinary dialogue on their appropriate use; (c) make institutional policy on the application of the CHAC's guidelines in treatment; and (d) serve as a legislative watchdog for Catholic interests.

The first mention of such committees in the United States appeared in a 1975 article on the highly publicized nontreatment of a newborn with Down's Syndrome at Johns Hopkins Hospital (2). Physician Karen Teel

409

observed that doctors often hesitated to make difficult medical decisions because of the perceived threat of legal action against them. She suggested that an institutional sharing of responsibility for morally charged treatment decisions might make it easier for physicians to take appropriate action. Teel recommended that multidisciplinary committees analyze treatment options for deformed infants in light of their legal, ethical, and social aspects, and support physicians in their implementation.

In 1976 the New Jersey Supreme Court cited Teel's work in its ruling *In re Quinlan* (3). Although the Court assumed jurisdiction over the issue of surrogate decision making and awarded Karen Ann Quinlan's father guardianship for the express purpose of consenting to the withdrawal of her ventilator, it contended that the court was not the proper site for such decisions. Instead, it declared that the authority of an incompetent patient's guardian included decisions to limit or refuse life support, and that such decisions should be made in consultation with an "ethics committee," as described by Teel, or a "reasonable counterpart." The Court understood the committee's role more in terms of assessing the patient's prognosis than resolving the ethical dilemmas of treatment, and mistakenly assumed from Teel's comments that hospitals commonly had such committees. The state then issued guidelines for such prognostic bodies, consisting of physicians from varied specialties, and for their role in decisions to withdraw life support (4). In 1977, the Hastings Center held a conference on the actual and potential roles and responsibilities of IECs. Participants' experience of the roles and constitution of such bodies differed, but they generally agreed that multidisciplinary committees, well versed in the ethical issues of medicine, could serve in a valuable advisory capacity to physicians and families confronted with difficult treatment decisions (5).

In 1983, the President's Commission for the Study of Ethical Issues in Medicine and Biomedical and Behavioral Research issued its report on the ethical, medical, and legal issues in decisions to forego life-sustaining treatment (6). The report focused on the creation of procedures for such decisions, and examined the role of public and private organizations in establishing and governing the process. The Commission recommended that hospitals formulate specific policies on withholding and withdrawing life support for competent and incompetent adults, and children and infants. In evaluating procedures for surrogate decision making, they rejected the practice of seeking formal judicial review as too cumbersome, too adversarial, too expensive, too public, and too harmful to the process of patient care (6, 159). They concluded that institutions should establish institutional procedures to "promote effective decisionmaking for incapacitated individuals" (6, 160), including neonates (6, 227); one such procedure was review by a hospital ethics committee (6, 439–442).

As envisioned in a model bill included in the report (6, 439–442), institutional ethics committees could serve to: (a) confirm the patient's diagnosis and prognosis; (b) provide a forum for discussing the social and ethical issues that a particular case might raise; (c) educate staff on the identification and resolution of ethical problems; (d) formulate institutional policy and procedural guidelines on decision making; (e) review treatment decisions made for specific patients by doctors and surrogates; and (f) mediate conflict over patient care between health care professionals, patients, family members, and the institution. They recommended a multidisciplinary committee that would be available to staff and patients and their families, and that would operate formally, keeping minutes and placing consultation records in patients' charts.

The Commission's survey of hospitals found that few had established formal institutional structures, and those that had reported them to have widely divergent functions and composition (6, 443–457). While the Commission concluded that IECs offered an appropriately sensitive, rapid, and private approach to safeguarding the interests of incompetent patients, it cautioned that there needed to be more study of their use and outcomes before their adoption could be recommended, much less required. It further suggested that both the American Hospital Association (AHA) and the Joint Commission on the Accreditation of Hospitals (JCAH) examine the formation and varied functions of IECs.

In 1983, when the federal government established guidelines equating nontreatment of severely impaired newborns with discrimination against the handicapped, known as the Baby Doe rules (7), both the AHA and the American Academy of Pediatrics (AAP) challenged the regulations on the grounds that local ethics review would be more valuable than federal oversight. The AHA, AAP, and American Medical Association (AMA) filed suit to have the rules invalidated, and later that year, the AAP issued guidelines for the establishment of multidisciplinary "infant bioethics committees" to review the proposed nontreatment of severely impaired infants using a best-interests standard that recognized the limits of technological intervention (8).

When the regulations were overturned in early 1984, a judgment subsequently affirmed by the U.S. Supreme Court (9), Congress attempted "compromise legislation" that made the withholding of "medically indicated" treatment a form of child abuse or neglect (10). An essential part of this legislation was the requirement that hospitals with neonatal intensive care units (NICUs) have a multidisciplinary Infant Care Review Committee (ICRC) to assist in the determination of appropriate intervention for affected infants, in keeping with the AAP guidelines. Also in 1984, the AMA (11) and AHA (12) each called for the formation of voluntary ethics committees in hospitals and other inpatient institutions to "consider and assist in resolving unusual, complicated ethical problems" in such areas as quality of life, terminal illness, and the use of limited resources (11). The AHA suggested that the IEC could serve to establish policies on withdrawing and withholding treatment at the end of life; to educate staff, patients, and the public on the medico-moral aspects of caring for terminally ill and/or severely deformed infants; and to provide consultation to doctors, other health professionals, patients, and families in situations where the use of medical technology created ethical conflict (12).

In 1987, the state of Maryland enacted legislation requiring hospitals to establish IECs to advise caregivers, patients, and family members on ethical aspects of the treatment of terminal illness (13). The law also suggested that committees review and formulate institutional policy on the use of life support as well as conduct educational programs for hospital staff and patients and their families on ethical issues in medical decision making. The Act specified standards for the IEC's composition, as well as a variety of procedural aspects, including that it: (a) notify all patients of its existence and their right to seek an advisory opinion; (b) consult all caregivers, the patient, and the patient's family in its deliberations; (c) and keep written, but confidential, records and place its formal recommendation in the patient's chart. The Act also freed the IEC from legal liability for recommendations given in good faith.

In 1990, the U.S. Supreme Court affirmed Missouri's right to impose a strict standard of evidence of patients' wishes regarding withholding and withdrawing treatment (14), ruling in the case of Nancy Cruzan, a permanently unconscious woman whose family sought to discontinue her tubal feeding. As *Cruzan* was unfolding, Missouri Senator John Danforth, intent on preventing the need for court intervention in treatment decisions, proposed legislation to require hospitals and other inpatient institutions to inform patients about their state's law on the use of life-sustaining treatment, and to ask patients upon admission whether they had an advance directive. The initial version of the federal Patient Self-Determination Act (PSDA) called for the creation of IECs to educate caregivers, patients, and the public about advance directives, and to consult on difficult treatment decisions. This provision was dropped in the final version of the bill (15), however, because of widespread concern that IECs were relatively new and their effectiveness unknown (16).

While the federal government ultimately did not mandate the creation of ethics committees, the Joint Commission on the Accreditation of Healthcare Organizations (JCAHO, formerly JCAH) did so in late 1990 in its 1992 *Accreditation Manual for Hospitals* (*AMH*) (17). JCAHO's new accreditation standards on patient rights included a requirement for a "mechanism(s) for the consideration of ethical issues in the care of patients and to provide education to caregivers and patients on ethical issues in health care" (17, 156). As of January 1, 1992, these standards require U.S. hospitals to have an IEC or a similar body or process as a condition for accreditation and eligibility for Medicare payments.

There has been tremendous growth in the numbers of IECs in the last decade, although their actual prevalence has been difficult to assess. In 1982, the President's Commission survey of 602 hospitals found that only 3% had an IEC or other organizational body that might be involved in medical decision making; all were in hospitals with over 200 beds (6, 439–457). A 1983 national survey by the AHA's National Society for Patient Representatives found that 26% of hospitals responding had an IEC; by 1985 that number had grown to 60% (18). The most likely hospitals in the survey to have an IEC were large, teaching hospitals; surprisingly, the number of nonteaching hospitals with an IEC dropped almost 10% in the two years between the surveys. In a study of the effects of Maryland's 1987 law requiring IECs two years after the Act's passage, 55 of the 63 hospitals surveyed responded that they had an IEC, compared with 14 of 18 in the District of Columbia and 29 of 114 in Virginia (19). Hospitals with fewer than 250 beds were not likely to have an IEC, and many of the administrators of hospitals in the District of Columbia and Virginia commented that they did not perceive a need for such a committee.

Although considerable time has passed since JCAHO's patient rights standards were proposed, there are still hospitals with no formal mechanism in place, particularly small private hospitals and those in rural areas. Despite an extensive literature in clinical and hospital ethics and the availability of several handbooks on IECs (20–25), many hospital administrators are unsure of what is required of them or where to turn for information. Even in hospitals with established IECs, committee members may be uncertain about the committee's purpose, as well as their own roles and the adequacy of their knowledge in ethics, law, or medicine (19; 26; 27). This uncertainty, coupled with the fact that JCAHO instituted the requirement for IECs at the same time as a host of other changes, suggests that hospitals that create IECs primarily to conform to the *AMH*'s standards are unlikely to have active committees for some time to come (19).

ROLES OF THE IEC

As described above, the IEC has three typical roles, which are complementary and mutually sustaining: (a) the recommendation or creation of policy on ethical issues in patient care; (b) the education of hospital staff, patients, family members, and the community on ethical issues and the philosophy and policies of the institution; and (c) the consideration of and consultation on ethical issues in patient care generally and questions about the treatment of specific patients. Not every IEC is involved in all of these activities, and some have additional responsibilities. JCAHO standards require only that committees provide education on ethical issues and a forum for their discussion (17).

Policy

Much of the uncertainty that surrounds difficult treatment decisions can be prevented with well-written, comprehensive institutional policies governing the areas where conflict is most likely. Since IECs were first conceived, their primary responsibility in the area of policy has been to define institutional guidelines and procedures for the withholding and withdrawing of resuscitative and life-sustaining treatment, as recommended by the President's Commission.

Although they do not stipulate that the IEC be responsible for making policy, JCAHO's standards on patient rights (17) also outline requirements for institutional policy in several areas where the IEC may have considerable interest, and where its advice or leadership may be valuable (28):

- The objectives, procedures, and jurisdiction of the IEC;
- Resuscitative services and the use of do-not-rescuscitate (DNR) orders;
- Informed decision making and informed consent;
- Advance directives and their implementation, and withholding and withdrawing life-sustaining treatment generally;
- Surrogate decision making for incompetent patients, including infants, children, and the unconscious;
- Assessment and management of pain;
- Transfer of patients to other facilities; and
- Respect for patients' religious and cultural preferences.

The IEC should be sufficiently familiar with existing policies and procedural guidelines and state and federal law, to clarify, rather than complicate, the standards of clinical practice.

Education

It takes an educated committee to write good policy and provide meaningful consultation, educated caregivers to carry out policies and recommended courses of action, and educated patients and families to appreciate the institution's policies and make meaningful personal choices. While the necessary scope of IEC members' background in medicine and ethics is controversial, they certainly need a foundation in clinical ethical theory and practice, medical law relevant to issues of treatment at the end of life, and the process and techniques of mediation (22–27; 29–31). Education in clinical ethics, as in medicine, is an ongoing process, as new issues may arise that require committees to reevaluate "settled" questions (30). Turn-over of committee membership implies a need for introductory materials for new members and ongoing committee education to ensure that the members have a common framework, without which the committee risks inconsistency in policymaking and consultation.

Physicians and hospital staff need ongoing education on the insti-tution's policies and relevant law on such issues as DNR orders, advance directives, withholding and withdrawing treatment, and surrogate decision making. These elements are frequently omitted from the orientation of new personnel, and where physicians practice in more than one facility differing policies among institutions can lead to confusion and conflict. Routine medical staff education is also essential in teaching hospitals where house staff and faculty trained in other states may incorrectly assume that laws and policies are national. Many younger health professionals have some education in ethics; however, caregivers need continuing ethics edu-cation to avoid the well-intentioned application of theories and laws that have been modified or superseded (23). Finally, staff members must learn how to contact the IEC to clarify questions of policy or law or to request consultation.

Under the PSDA and the JCAHO standards, hospitals and other inpa-tient institutions are required to provide education to patients, their family members, and the community on their rights to make certain treatment decisions, including the right to formulate advance directives, and on the institution's mechanism for resolving conflict over treatment. Such educa-tion should involve meaningful discussion of the goals and real limits of medical intervention (32), so that lay people truly understand the nature of the decisions that they are called to make. Lastly, patients and their families need information about the IEC, its purpose, and how to use it; unfortunately, even in hospitals with well-established committees, most patients and family members still know nothing about the IEC (19; 33; 34),

Consultation

Consultation is the IEC's most controversial role, as some physicians question the need for ethics consultation. Where consultation does take place it assumes numerous forms (29; 34–41). There remains no real consensus on some important aspects of consultation, even after almost a decade of discussion and experience. The primary issues include:

Who may seek consultation? The President's Commission and JCAHO call for the IEC to be available to all members of the institutional community, including physicians, nurses, allied health professionals, patients, family members, and potentially even outsiders. However, some IECs that operate on a conservative interpretation of the AMA guidelines (11) limit consultation to physicians; the JCAHO standard on universal access to consultation will likely meet with resistance in such hospitals. In some facilities, this limitation has led to the creation of parallel "nursing ethics committees," where nurses seeking advice or interpretation of policy may get an answer directly; often their issues involve conflict with physicians (42). Clinical ethicists typically advocate broad access to a central IEC, concerned that nursing committees marginalize nurses and compartmentalize institutional issues along disciplinary lines.

Who may attend meetings, participate in discussion of cases, and attend a consultation? Closely related to the issue of who may seek consultation is whether meetings and case discussion are open only to members or to the hospital at large (40; 43). The openness of regular business meetings is typically less a problem than is the open discussion of cases where both the patient's confidential information and the caregivers' insecurities may be exposed. Many committees hold open business meetings, particularly in teaching hospitals. Some IECs permit anyone to attend a consultation who is involved in the relevant patient's care, but hold formal deliberation privately. Others hold closed business meetings and case review, admitting nonmembers only by invitation. Some critics have argued that too many committees exclude even the patient and their surrogates, denying them due process (34; 35) and violating confidentiality (29; 35; 40; 44). IECs need to distinguish between concern for protecting confidentiality and the risk-averse desire for secrecy before the question of openness can be resolved.

How formal a consultation is necessary for different levels of advice? A number of levels of consultation are possible, from the quick telephone call to confirm the meaning of a policy, to the bedside consultation by an ethics consultant or IEC subcommittee, to the convening of the entire IEC for formal presentations and extensive discussion. The level of formality varies with the information needed, the patient's condition, and the complexity of the issue, including the duration of the controversy and the roles of the caregivers and family members involved (41). Most clinical ethicists now agree that, except in straightforward cases of defining policies, the consulting ethicist or a representative of the IEC should see the patient (33–36; 38; 39). For some this visit is intended to confirm the patient's diagnosis and "gather . . . a clinical database" (39); for others it is to talk with the patient and the family firsthand about the issues (34; 35).

Much, and by some accounts most, of the apparent conflict that prompts a call for ethics consultation is the result of poor communication (22, 241–243; 31). Consequently, the best type of consultation may depend on the severity of the miscommunication or the format most likely to resolve the particular communication problem. A formal meeting of the entire committee can seem adversarial to some patients or family members, who may feel threatened or inadequate before a large group of "hospital authorities"; physicians may also become anxious in a setting that looks too much like a peer review hearing (40). However, a full committee consultation may be quite effective when communication is the real problem, as the committee's need for a complete picture also affords the principals an opportunity to hear others' perspectives. Although the IEC can promote comprehensive communication among caregivers, the patient, and family members, an IEC consultation is neither the only nor the best format for achieving such results; multidisciplinary family conferences can be equally effective in many instances.

Who is told of the IEC's recommendation? How? When? The IEC's recommendation will vary in its specificity and formality in part according to the format of the consultation. Clearly the person requesting the consultation should be informed of the IEC's recommendation, as should the other principals, including the patient and attending physician (33–35). At some point, too, others involved in the patient's care will need to be informed of any changes in the treatment, and their rationale. The question of how and by whom the information should be relayed is tied into:

What documentation should be kept, and where? The President's Commission and most other bodies with guidelines on the conduct of IECs call for a consultation record to be put in the patient's chart in much the same way that other consultations generate chart notes; additional copies of the recommendation could be provided to the attending physician, patient, or person seeking the consultation, as needed. This format works very well in many institutions.

However, many hospital attorneys and many more physicians are leery of formal records, worried that a patient who is the subject of an IEC consultation is likely to become the focus of litigation (23; 27; 44). Some fear that a formal IEC note—or even a mention of the IEC's involvement—in the patient's chart might heighten a malpractice attorney's curiosity about any physician wrongdoing; in some hospitals, the consultation notes are kept only in the IEC's files, ostensibly to protect them from discovery. The committee's chair or another member confers with the attending physician and the patient or family to relate, and if necessary interpret, the IEC's opinion; the physician is then responsible for writing orders that reflect treatment plans in light of the recommendation. Unfortunately, this practice offers physicians none of the benefits of the "institutional sharing of responsibility," and may confuse other staff who must rely on word-of-mouth information to learn about the IEC's perspective. Moreover, in the few cases where litigation is pursued, the absence of an IEC record in the chart may generate interest in "undiscoverable" material that otherwise might be left alone.

What if the attending physician disagrees with the IEC's recommendation?

Most IECs consider even their formal opinions to be advisory only, and as with other clinical consultations, the physician is free to follow all, part, or none of the IEC's advice. Although IEC recommendations are typically the product of a consensus in which the physician has participated, doctors are suspicious of formal consultation because they fear that the IEC will "rule" against them, and that disagreeing with the IEC will create a risk of litigation (23; 27; 44; 45). Some have argued that, in practice, even informal recommendations may function as binding decisions (46). Where the IEC is not able to resolve a conflict between doctor and patient or family, the IEC typically informs the patient or family that they may seek another physician, and reminds the physician of the professional (and in some states legal) duty to facilitate a transfer should the patient or surrogate decision maker request it.[4]

What if the patient or family disagrees? Including the patient or family in discussion and planning of treatment typically prevents conflict, and the communication that the IEC facilitates often results in compromise and consensus that includes patients' or family members' views. Often the question involves conflict among family members that may have nothing to do with the patient's care; here it is more important to determine who has decision-making authority than to achieve consensus. If a patient or family member with decision-making authority disagrees with the IEC's recommendation and the attending physician's advice, the patient may request to be transferred to another physician or hospital, and the physician should facilitate the transfer, if possible.

Increasingly, such situations have involved family members' requests for treatment that physicians and IECs contend are unduly burdensome for the patient, inappropriate to the goals of treatment, or "futile" (34; 47–49). Many hospitals claim to follow the guidelines of the Society of Critical Care Medicine (34; 48), which state that the attending physician is under no obligation to provide treatment that "has no chance of achieving benefit" (50). However, determinations of medical futility have become quite controversial in light of two court rulings that appear to have given patients a right to "futile" treatment that the physician and hospital sought to discontinue (51; 52). This question is likely to remain unresolved for some time, as the clinical issues converge with the social debate on the right to health care and the value of life in any form (32; 53; 48; 49).

ADMINISTRATIVE ASPECTS

Despite its broad mandate, the IEC is a hospital committee with the same administrative considerations as other committees, many of which are shaped more by the general practices and culture of the institution than by the IEC's formal charge. Several of the proposed guidelines for

IECs attempt to define administrative structures and processes (11; 20–25). JCAHO's standards are exceptionally open, in keeping with its Principles of Quality Improvement, which are intended to support institutions' efforts to tailor guidelines to their own needs (17). Some basic administrative questions to be resolved at the institutional level include:

Should the IEC be under the jurisdiction of the medical staff, administration, or governing board? A number of aspects of the committee's structure and function may be influenced by its place in the hospital's administrative structure. The IEC's authority, accountability, leadership, membership, and length of terms may all be defined by its location in the institutional hierarchy. The AMA recommends that the IEC work under the Medical Executive Committee, primarily to ensure that physicians have a prominent voice in policy (11), but some would argue that such IECs might not have the independence necessary to question physicians' practice (29). Others place the committee under the administration, as administrators are typically responsible for what may be perceived as the risk-management and policy aspects of the committee's work. However, such placement may marginalize the committee in clinical practice if physicians do not have a sense of ownership (29). Placement under the governing board can give the IEC the authority and political freedom to work effectively throughout the institution, but requires strong committee leadership, and a self-critical sense of purpose among the members. The IEC's budget and the availability of support staff, meeting rooms, and other essentials may also be defined by its relationship to particular offices. These considerations are especially important in smaller hospitals, and where staff and facilities are overburdened owing to financial constraints.

The maintenance, availability, and discoverability of the IEC's records may also be affected by its placement in the hospital's administrative structure (22; 23; 27; 29; 45). The IEC's minutes and case reports might be safeguarded like quality assurance materials if the IEC is an administrative committee; records might come under peer review protection if the IEC is a medical staff committee. However, neither of these assumptions has been tested, and there is no consensus of legal opinion about the protection of IEC documents or the potential testimony of IEC members in litigation. Moreover, preoccupation with secrecy is not consistent with the publicly projected image of the IEC as a means of ensuring the accountability of health care professionals and institutions in decision making.

Who should chair the IEC? Leadership is crucial to the proper functioning of any group, especially one that has a potentially controversial role. The head of the IEC must have the respect of the hospital community for the committee to be effective (22; 23; 29). Some guidelines suggest that the chair have a highly visible position of authority within the hospital; elsewhere, experience suggests that a chair's high profile may limit the

IEC's effectiveness (53). Practically, the chair should be someone to whom people already turn for advice. In the beginning, he or she must be able to recruit others to participate, create enthusiasm and a sense of accomplishment among the members, and establish the IEC's place and value in the institution. The chair needs to know enough about clinical ethics and institutional processes to guide the committee's self-education and the creation of policy, as well as to determine what problems will be appropriate "cases" for the IEC to address. Later, he or she must be able to facilitate discussion of emotionally charged issues in a way that mitigates power struggles and leads to specific resolution. Because very few individuals have the time or talent to do all these things in addition to their primary professional work, IECs may have co-chairs or a chair and an administrative or consultation coordinator. The rotation of leadership varies greatly among institutions, again dependent on structural and personal variables as much as administrative order.

Who should be members? Members need to be respected members of the hospital community, who can both represent their colleagues to the IEC and represent the IEC to their colleagues (23; 29). Official guidelines and handbooks on IECs unanimously stress the importance of a multi-disciplinary membership, able to address the varied issues that policy-making and consultation may raise. Members also need good skills in reflective analysis and communication, compassion and emotional stability, open-mindedness and humility, integrity and courage of their convictions, and the willingness to spend time reading and thinking about topics outside their own areas of expertise.

Ultimately, the committee's membership reflects the question of who the IEC is intended to serve: the hospital's administration or corporate interests, physicians, nurses, patients and their families, or some other entity. The need for a diverse professional membership is widely acknowledged, as the IEC's ability to recognize and address the problems and options that particular situations may entail is enhanced by its members' broadly based professional expertise. The need for diversity of age, gender, ethnicity, and socioeconomic status, characteristics that shape members' values and perspectives on the meaning of specific practices, has been less well addressed in theory or practice.

Typically, IEC membership may include:

Physicians of various specialties, particularly critical care for expertise in life support and resuscitation; neurology for expertise in states of consciousness; psychiatry for expertise in decision-making capacity, competence, and the mental consequences of physical illness and its treatment; gerontology, to provide a comprehensive view of elderly patients; and other specialties that may be important in the individual institution.

From the beginning, physicians have been skeptical about the value of an IEC, and have been worried that the committee would be looking constantly over doctors' shoulders, telling them how to practice medicine (22; 29). While some of this initial hesitance has abated, especially among younger doctors, some physicians are unwilling to serve on what they perceive will be a meddlesome committee, or are fearful of the political consequences of appearing to sit in judgment of their peers (29). Others do not want to participate in a multidisciplinary IEC because they are unaccustomed to working with nonphysicians, or they may object to the implication that others can adequately assess the ethical dilemmas that doctors face. However, some IECs have found that critics of the committee can become its champions if they are invited to share their opinions as members.

Nurses of various specialties, including floor nursing, critical care, and administration. Nurses are especially important because of their experience in carrying out treatment orders in controversial situations and their appreciation of the more personal responses of patients and families to serious illness. Moreover, they often recognize the political issues at stake in both policy and practice, and know how to negotiate them. In most institutions, nurses are eager to take part in the IEC, and it may be difficult to determine who among a number of qualified candidates should serve. Some nurses hope that the IEC will provide an opportunity to redress injustices that nurses have suffered in the past; but just as physicians must work with others, nurses must be willing to work with doctors.

Social workers, patient representatives, and discharge planners, valuable because they are often called upon to handle the problems of "difficult" patients, whose "trouble making" may be the result of conflicting ethical or sociocultural values. They typically know both how to recognize the sources of conflict among caregivers, patients, and family members and often how to present options to resolve the conflict. Social workers and discharge planners can be central to the strategic aspects of an IEC's consultation, as they know what options are possible and how to use community resources to support patients' and families wishes for care that cannot be provided in the hospital.

Physical and respiratory therapists, seldom included in lists of prospective members, but whose familiarity with the care of the chronically ill and comatose, as well as knowledge of the stresses and rewards of rehabilitation, make them invaluable to some committees. They, like nurses, typically implement treatment orders for patients likely to fall under IEC policies, and they see the long-term consequences of critical care. They can be helpful in case consultation because they often give social and emotional support to patients and families, and their teaching skills often enable them to communicate complex medical concepts to lay people.

Clergy, whether hospital chaplains or clergy from the community, who can assist the IEC in appreciating the religious meaning that both health professionals and lay people may find in illness and medical care, and in identifying symbolic issues that can complicate decision making. Clergy can offer reassurance and reinterpretation of religious teachings to patients, family members, and staff who mistakenly fear that their intended actions are prohibited within certain religious traditions. Many clergy are trained in moral analysis, and although the perspective of their particular denomination may not be immediately applicable, their ability to identify central ethical themes and questions can be quite useful to the consultative process. Community-based clergy can be particularly helpful when they are familiar with the values, experiences, and daily life of the hospital's patient population.

Hospital administrators, who are often responsible for drafting and implementing hospital policy that may affect the IEC. As committee members they may both facilitate the IEC's work in policy and learn lessons from the IEC's experience that will make hospital policy more appropriate to clinical needs. The presence of the hospital's CEO or other upper management on the IEC can also lend authority to its work. Administrators, like physicians, however, must appreciate the necessary collegial nature of the IEC and its deliberation, and refrain from imposing top-down decisions based on business criteria.

Community representatives, including former patients or their family members who can provide important insight into the lay person's perspective on medical issues, and represent the committee and the hospital outside the institution. In case consultation they may be able to translate the language of health professionals into words and ideas more familiar to patients, and offer reassurance that the conflict over care is not a medical conspiracy. Community representatives are typically the most difficult for IECs to recruit and retain, often not because community members are unwilling to serve, but because the professional staff does not know whom to recruit. To identify potential community members, the IEC must know its patient population and what characteristics might be representative. Where community members are not effective representatives of the hospital's patient population, patients and their families may perceive the IEC to be simply another way in which the hospital protects its self-interest (29; 33).

Attorneys and ethicists, who may be found on the IECs of larger, urban hospitals, especially university-affiliated institutions with a program in medical ethics or medical humanities. Many of the country's first IECs were started in collaboration with faculty from such programs. Some university-affiliated hospitals now have clinical ethics programs that offer ethics consultation services, as part of or independent of the IEC. Attorneys and ethicists have analytic skills and knowledge of tradition and contemporary standards that can strengthen the IEC's confidence and effectiveness. The place of lawyers and ethicists on the IEC has been debated, however, and many hospitals have no opportunity to include experienced professionals in health law or clinical ethics in their committees.

Lawyers and theoretical ethicists, with no clinical experience may misunderstand the issues and mislead the IEC with information and perspectives that, while technically correct, are inappropriately applied (22; 27; 54). Hospitals with an attorney on retainer are often hesitant to pay to have legal counsel attend committee meetings, and few nonuniversity hospitals contract for an ethicist's ongoing professional services. Small hospitals in large for-profit chains may work primarily with lawyers at a corporate headquarters who know little about the specific institution. Attorneys who see their single role as protecting the hospital from liability may encourage the IEC to become a risk-management committee; ethicists who see themselves as the patient's only advocate may put off the very caregivers who most need consultation; both may hamper the effectiveness of the IEC in consultation and the creation of policy.

Some handbooks written by clinical ethicists concede that there is no need for a staff ethicist on many IECs, but note that committees should attempt to include professional ethicists among their educational speakers (22; 23). However, the continued growth of this discipline and the educational opportunities in clinical ethics will almost certainly increase the prominence of clinical ethicists in the hospital setting.

Since the publication of its patient rights standards, JCAHO has taken interest in the makeup of IECs, and has begun to consider standards for IEC membership and ethics consultation (55). JCAHO's interest comes at a time when there is already a spirited discussion among clinical ethicists about the value of professional certification (56). Ethicists themselves are far from agreed on whether clinical ethics consultation is a profession, and if so what level of education, training, and expertise should be expected of its members. JCAHO is interested in the practice and credentials of clinical ethicists, but is particularly concerned about the quality of IECs in small and rural hospitals where ethicists are virtually nonexistent and few caregivers are likely to be proficient in clinical ethics. JCAHO is currently observing the creation of ethics committee networks in Virginia, with the hope that similar affiliations elsewhere could serve as cooperative regional ethics committees for institutions unable to create IECs individually (E.M. Spencer, personal communication).

Over the past several years, a number of local and statewide IEC networks have evolved across the country (57). Typically networks develop as members of newly formed IECs seek advice from other institutions, particularly in the areas of policy and consultation. Some networks have worked on standardized forms for DNR and supportive care orders, and others have defined community standards for withdrawing treatment; even informally, networks provide a means of establishing community standards for IECs by informing members about the operations and activities of other committees against which they may measure their own work. Some networks coordinate public educational efforts; others provide committee education or review difficult cases. With the implementation of health reform, such administrative umbrellas are likely to be increasingly important in facilitating the integration of IECs within health alliances, and safeguarding the ethical quality of care from the potential negative consequences of managed competition.

ISSUES ON THE HORIZON

As many new IECs become established, others are entering their second decade. The future of ethics committees will be difficult to predict, as much remains unknown about them currently. Some issues on the horizon include the development of IECs in long-term care facilities; the liability of IECs and their members for their consultation; the role of IECs in cost containment; and the need for formal evaluation of IECs and their varied roles.

IECs in Long-Term-Care Facilities

Although nursing homes and other long-term care facilities are subject to the PSDA and required to meet JCAHO standards in order to receive Medicare payments, there has been little study of IECs in such institutions. Some research and anecdotal evidence suggests that many do not inform patients or their families about their right to an advance directive or their options for treatment, and few have established IECs (58–61).

For many hospital IECs, nursing homes and other long-term care facilities are a source of ethical problems, as their residents are repeatedly hospitalized for the treatment of strokes, infections, and fractures from which they will neither recover nor die. Most patients come from such facilities to the hospital unable to make their own decisions, and many have no available family member or other surrogate decision maker (59; 61). However, hospitals often discharge patients to long-term care rather than face difficult questions of appropriate intervention in the treatment of comatose or otherwise incompetent patients whose quality of life is limited. Typically there is little communication between hospitals and long-term care institutions over advance directives, DNR orders, and the goals of treatment, which itself may contribute to ethical conflict in such patients' care. IECs in nursing homes will be increasingly important in the coming years, as the population ages and hospitals and health policymakers re-evaluate the use of acute care facilities and life-sustaining interventions. Long-term care facilities present many of the same institutional challenges as hospitals in terms of education in clinical ethics and policymaking; their higher turnover and typically less well-trained personnel make ongoing education and clear policies even more important. The prevalence of incapacitated patients means that surrogate decision making may be the norm, and the low rate of reimbursement for physician visits may make doctors less willing to spend time with patients and their families for advance planning. The role for IECs in long-term care facilities must be one aspect of a comprehensive assessment of the care of the elderly and severely disabled under health care reform.

IECs' Liability for Malpractice and Other Legal Action

Ethics committees were first suggested as a forum for resolving the conflicts that might lead to a court's intervention; both the New Jersey Supreme Court and Congress anticipated that IECs would help to keep medical decisions out of the courtroom (3; 16). Good policies should prevent hospitals and physicians from needing a court's opinion in all but extreme cases, and IEC consultation should reduce the risk of malpractice litigation against physicians as evidence that "due care" was used in decision making (29). Moreover, most malpractice suits stem from poor communication between patient and from physician, and patients' or families' perceptions that their opinions did not count (62). By actively including patients and their families in controversial decisions, taking their views seriously, and mediating conflict, IECs should prevent the resentment that typically leads to suit.

There remains the possibility, however, that IECs themselves could become the target of litigation, either from a patient or family member who is dissatisfied with the consultative process or advisory opinion, or from a physician sued after relying on an IEC's recommendation. While Maryland law makes ethics committees immune from legal action, IECs in other states have no such protection (63). In 1986, an IEC in California was sued by Elizabeth Bouvia for its role in supporting a physician's decision to force-feed her through a nasogastric tube (64). That conflict was ultimately resolved without going to trial, and there have been no such suits since. However, there are a number of gray areas in which an IEC might recommend action that could be considered to violate the patient's legal rights: the discontinuation of "futile" life-sustaining treatment against a surrogate's wishes is a likely possibility. Where the IEC makes binding rulings or "optional" recommendations that are not really optional (46), a physician sued for following the IEC's advice might seek damages from the committee or its individual members.

In either situation, the IEC would need to demonstrate the duty of care that ethics committees have to patients, and establish that it had not breached that duty. In a case of a recommendation on a controversial issue, it would have to show how it arrived at the conclusion, and that it followed the standard of practice that similar bodies would accept in reaching a conclusion. Individual members would need to show that they had the knowledge and exercised the skill and judgment of a reasonable member of an IEC in deliberating and reaching a recommendation. Records supporting the ICE's position would be crucial, as would evidence that documented the process.

Because there are no well-established standards for IECs, including criteria for membership and appropriate process, a committee under public scrutiny might find it difficult to prove that it met a standard of care. Moreover, as some committees keep only minimal records, documenting the decision-making process could be even more troublesome. In the unlikely, but equally possible, case that an IEC came under criminal investigation for such crimes as conspiracy to commit murder or child or elder abuse, the existence of formal measures and the availability of records would be even more important. While IECs will likely always face some risk of legal action, clear professional and institutional standards for their constitution and operation would reduce that risk.

IECs and Cost Containment

For many caregivers, questions of appropriate intervention become ethical questions when the patient cannot pay for care. In a recent nonfiction book portraying the work of an IEC in a large urban hospital, economic issues lie behind every treatment decision (65). Although the IEC never discusses the cost of care, the book is laced with descriptions of caregivers and other institutional bodies considering the financial impact of the intensive care and technological intervention provided to indigent patients. Ethics committees have typically focused as a matter of principle on serving the patient's best interests. They have sought to remain above the debate about cost containment and allocation of resources.

Increasingly, the inequalities of access to care, the inequalities of care once accessed, and the high cost of many life saving interventions—some in short supply—are likely to force IECs into the discussion of costs, especially in light of health care reform. The question of *how* IECs should participate in the discussion and how they should use financial information in their consideration of patient care and policy remains unanswered (65–68). IECs should know what role their individual institutions expect them to play in the hospital's larger agenda, and ensure that the ethical criteria for its policies and practices are not subverted by other interests. The IEC can promote the hospital's healing mission where others serve the bottom line, and it can examine head-on the issue of cost containment in selective policy and case review, providing the institution with a clear understanding of the difference between ethics and economics.

On a societal level, IECs and ethics committee networks can consider the Canadian Catholic bishops' suggestion that they observe and respond to governmental efforts to address health care (1), safeguarding the interests of patients and caregivers in the process of health care reform by sharing with policymakers their ethical expertise and practical experience.

Measuring the Effects of IECs

In the more than ten years that professional organizations and licensing and accrediting bodies have recommended or required the establishment of IECs, a number of manuals have offered guidelines on their self-assessment, and there have been many calls for substantive evaluation of their effects (5; 6; 16; 21–23; 31; 43; 53; 70–73). To date, assessment has been confined to a few academic articles, workshops at professional meetings, and the informal shoptalk of clinical ethicists. Given the limited degree to which *any* technology is evaluated before its widespread diffusion into clinical practice (72), and the limited funds available for health services research, this uncritical adoption of IECs is not surprising. Assessment of the effects of IECs is also complicated by the fact that these committees are intended to serve a variety of purposes, not all of which have been clearly defined even among practicing clinical ethicists.

Establishing what is meant by "success," the standards by which IECs should be measured, and the rationale for these definitions is essential before meaningful assessment can take place (53; 69; 70; 72). As JCAHO surveyors gain experience with IECs in their varied formats, it is likely that the *AMH* will set more specific standards and assessment criteria for their composition and function. The establishment of formal standards should not be left to JCAHO alone, however, but should involve the ethicists, clinicians, and policymakers whose work has led to the growth of clinical ethical theory and the rise of active IECs, and the individual committees themselves.

Anecdotal evidence suggests that IECs have been successful at the widely claimed goal of limiting court intervention in treatment decisions. It is less clear whether this effect is truly due to the IECs' mediating capacities, their occasional tendency to function as risk-management committees, the effectiveness of staff and patient education on ethical issues, or a growing social consensus about appropriate treatment at the end of life.

Each of these questions is worthy of study, and should provide valuable insight into the future direction of IECs.

NOTES

1. Some discussions of the development of IECs find important parallels to institutional review boards (IRBs) governing biomedical research with human subjects and/or Seattle's dialysis allocation committee of the 1960s. Like the IRB, hospital ethics committees are intended to safeguard patients' interests and right to informed consent; like Seattle's "God Committee," IECs may deliberate on the appropriate use of advanced life-sustaining treatment. However, neither of these bodies is truly similar to the IEC. Its mandate has been much broader than that of the other structures, and was derived primarily from the need to define whether and how to *end* treatment that physicians might construe as being in the *patient's* interests.

2. For simplicity, all such institutional structures and processes will be referred to here as IECs.

3. Clinical ethics has developed as a field in Canada in parallel with the United States; although under somewhat different guidelines, IECs serve much the same purposes there as here.

4. In a some instances, however, patients and families will not seek transfer and doctors do not seek to remove themselves from the patient's case. Although this phenomenon has not been explored, it appears to be more common in community hospitals and where the physician and patient have had a long-term relationship. For patients, families, and doctors faced with a life-threatening situation, conflict in a familiar relationship may be preferable to the anxiety and unknown outcome of change.

REFERENCES

1. Catholic Health Association of Canada. Medico-Moral Guide. Ottawa, ON: CHAC, 1971.

2. Teel, K. "The physician's dilemma: A doctor's view: What the law should be." *Baylor Law Review*, 1975, 27, 6, 8–9.

3. *In re Quinlan*, 70 N.J. 10, 355 A. 2d 647, *cert. denied*, 429 U.S. 922 (1976).

4. New Jersey Health Department. "Guidelines for health care facilities to implement procedures concerning care of comatose, non-cognitive patients," 1976. Cited in E.J. Leadem, "Guidelines for health care facilities to implement procedures concerning care of comatose, non-cognitive patients — A perspective," *Hospital Progress*, 1977, 58 (March), 9–10.

5. Levine, C. "Hospital ethics committees: A guarded prognosis." *Hastings Center Report*, 1977, 7 (June), 25–27.

6. President's Commission for the Study of Ethical Problems in Medicine and Biomedical and Behavioral Research. *Deciding to Forego Life-Sustaining Treatment: Ethical, Medical, and Legal Issues in Treatment Decisions.* Washington, DC: U.S. Government Printing Office, 1983.

7. "Nondiscrimination on the basis of handicap: Procedures and guidelines relating to health care for handicapped infants." *Federal Register*, Jan. 12, 1984, 49, 1622–1654.

8. American Academy of Pediatrics, Infant Bioethics Taskforce and Consultants. "Guidelines for infant bioethics committees." *Pediatrics*, 1984, 74, 306–310.

9. *United States v. University Hospital*, 729 F. 2d 144 (CA2) (1984), and *Bowen v. American Hospital Association et al.*, 476 U.S. Supreme Court 610 (1986).

10. Child Abuse Prevention and Treatment Act, 42 U.S.C., Section 5101-05 (1984).

11. Judicial Council, American Medical Association. "Guidelines for ethics committees in health care institutions." *Journal of the American Medical Association*, 1985, 253, 2698–2699.

12. American Hospital Association. *Guidelines: Hospital Committees on Biomedical Ethics*. Chicago, IL: AHA, 1984.

13. Patient Care Advisory Committee Act of 1987, Maryland Health Gen. Code Ann. 19-370-19374.

14. *Cruzan v. Director of Missouri Department of Health*, U.S. Supreme Court 58 LW 4916, 1990.

15. The Patient Self-Determination Act, Omnibus Budget Reconciliation Act of 1990, P.L. 101-508, Nov. 5, 1990.

16. McCloskey, E.L. "The Patient Self-Determination Act." *Kennedy Institute of Ethics Journal*, 1991, 1, 163–169.

17. Joint Commission on Accreditation of Healthcare Organizations. *Accreditation Manual for Hospitals*. Oak Park, IL: JCAHO, 1992.

18. Anonymous. "Ethics committees double since '83: Survey." *Hospitals*, 1985, 59 (Nov. 1), 60–61.

19. Hoffman, D.E. "Does legislating hospital ethics committees make a difference? A study of hospital ethics committees in Maryland, the District of Columbia, and Virginia." *Law, Medicine, and Health Care*, 1991, 19, 105–119.

20. Cranford, R.E., and Dudera, A.E., eds. *Institutional Ethics Committees and Health Care Decision Making*. Ann Arbor, MI: Health Administration Press, 1984.

21. Craig, R.P., Middleton, C.L., and O'Connell, L.J. *Ethics committees: A Practical approach*. St. Louis, MO: Catholic Health Association, 1986.

22. Hosford, B. *Bioethics Committees: The Health Care Provider's Guide*. Rockville, MD: Aspen Systems Corporation. 1986.

23. Ross, J.W., Bayley, C., Michel, V., and Pugh, D. *Handbook for Hospital Ethics Committees*. Chicago, IL: American Hospital Publishing, Inc., 1986.

24. The Hastings Center. *Guidelines on the Termination of Life-Sustaining Treatment and the Care of the Dying*. Bloomington, IN: Indiana University Press, 1987.

25. Macklin, R., and Kupfer, R.B. *Hospital Ethics Committees: Manual for A Training Program*. Bronx, NY: Albert Einstein College of Medicine, 1988.

26. Ross, J.W. "What do ethics committee members want?" *Ethical Currents*, 1991, 3, 7–8.

27. Cohen, M., Schwartz, R., Hartz, J., and Shapiro, R. "Everything you always wanted to ask a lawyer about ethics committees." *Cambridge Quarterly of Healthcare Ethics*, 1992, 1, 33–39.

28. Heitman, E. "Meeting the JCAHO Standards on Patient Rights: A proactive role for the institutional ethics committee or clinical ethicist." *Trends in Health Care, Law, and Ethics*, 1993 8(4), 8–12.

29. Fost, N., and Cranford, R.E. "Hospital ethics committees: Administrative aspects." *Journal of the American Medical Association*, 1985, 253, 2687–2692.

30. Bayley, C., and Cranford, E.E. "Techniques for committee self-education and institution-wide education", in R.E. Cranford and A.E. Dudera (eds.), *Institutional Ethics Committees and Health Care Decision Making*. Ann Arbor, MI: Health Administration Press, 1984, 139–156.

31. West, M.B., and Gibson, J.M. "Facilitating medical ethics case review: What ethics committees can learn from mediation and facilitation techniques." *Cambridge Quarterly of Healthcare Ethics*, 1992, 1, 63–74.

32. Brennan, T.A. "Physicians and futile care: Ethics committees to slow the momentum." *Law, Medicine, and Health Care*, 1992, 20, 336–339.

33. Youngner, S.J., Coulton, C., Juknialis, B.W., and Jackson, D.L. "Patients' attitudes toward hospital ethics committees." in R.E. Cranford and A.E. Dudera (eds.), *Institutional Ethics Committees and Health Care Decision Making*. Ann Arbor, MI: Health Administration Press, 1984, 73–84.

34. Wolf, S.M. "Toward a theory of due process." *Law, Medicine, and Health Care*, 1992, 20, 278–290.

35. Fletcher, J.C. "Ethics committees and due process." *Law, Medicine, and Health Care*, 1992, 20, 291–293.

36. Cohen, C.B. "Avoiding 'Cloudcuckooland' in ethics committee case review: Matching models to issues and concerns." *Law, Medicine, and Health Care*, 1992, 20, 294–299.

37. Singer, P., Pellegrino, E., and Seigler, M. "Ethics committees and consultants." *Journal of Clinical Ethics*, 1990, 1, 263–267.

38. Lowey, E.H. "Ethics consultation and ethics committees." *Hospital Ethics Committee Forum*, 1990, 2, 351–359.

39. LaPuma, J., and Schiedermayer, D.L. "Must the ethics consultant see the patient." *Journal of Clinical Ethics*, 1990, 1, 56–59.

40. Agich, G., and Youngner, S. "For experts only? Access to hospital ethics committees." *Hastings Center Report*, 1991, 21 (Jan./Feb.), 17–24.

41. Ross, J.W. "Why cases sometimes go wrong." *Hastings Center Report*, 1989, 19 (Jan./Feb.), 22–23.

42. Edwards, B.J., and Haddad, A.M. "Establishing a nursing bioethics committee." *Journal of Nursing Administration*, 1988, 18 (March), 30–33.

43. Lo, B. "Behind closed doors: Promises and pitfalls of ethics committees." *New England Journal of Medicine*, 1987, 317, 46–50.

44. Veatch, R.M. "Advice and consent." *Hastings Center Report*, 1989, 19 (Jan./Feb.), 20–22.

45. Capron, A.M. "Legal perspectives on institutional ethics committees." In B. Weinstein (ed.), *Ethics in the Hospital Setting*, Morgantown, WV: West Virginia University Press, 1985, 66–84.

46. Ritchie, K. "When it's not really optional." *Hastings Center Report*, 1988, 18 (Aug./Sept.), 25–26.

47. Smith, D.G. "Committee consultation to override family wishes—Commentary," *Hastings Center Report*, 1989, 19 (Sept./Oct.), 24–25.

48. Rie, M.A. "The limits of a wish." *Hastings Center Report*, 1991, 21 (July/Aug.), 24–27.

49. Callahan, D. "Medical futility: The-problem-without-a-name." *Hastings Center Report*, 1991, 21 (July/Aug.), 30–35.

50. Society for Critical Care Medicine. "Consensus report on the ethics of foregoing life-sustaining treatments in the critically ill." *Critical Care Medicine*, 1990, 18, 1435–1439.

51. *In re Helga Wanglie*, 4th Judicial District (Dist. Ct., Probate Ct. Div.) PX-91-283, Minnesota, Hennepin County.

52. *In re Baby K*, Civil Action No. 93-68-1 (Julyy 1, 1993). Discussed in L. Greenhouse, "Hospital appeals decision ordering treatment for baby missing a brain." *New York Times*, Sept. 24, 1993, A8.

53. Scheirton, L.S. "Determinants of hospital ethics committee success." *HEC Forum*, 1992, 4, 342–359.

54. Mitchell, S.M., and Swartz, M.S. "Is there a place for lawyers on ethics committees? A view from inside." *Hastings Center Report*, 1990, 20 (March/April), 32–33.

55. Schuyve, P.M. "A systems perspective on individual competence in ethics consultation." *Newsletter of the Society for Bioethics Consultation*, 1993, Winter, 1, 4–6.

56. Fletcher, J.C. "Training program in ethics consultation: The time is now." *Newsletter of the Society for Bioethics Consultation*, 1992, Spring, 1, 6.

57. Kushner, T. "Networks across America." *Hastings Center Report*, 1988, 18 (Feb./March), 14.

58. Brown, B.A., Miles, S.H., and Aroskar, M.A. "The prevalence and design of ethics committees in nursing homes." *Journal of the American Geriatric Society*, 1987, 35, 1028–1033.

59. Glasser, G., Zweibel, N.R., and Cassell, C.K. "The ethics committee in the nursing home: Results of a national survey." *Journal of the American Geriatric Society*, 1987, 36, 150–156.

60. Zweibel, N.R., and Cassell, C.K. "Ethics committees in nursing homes: Applying the hospital experience." *Hastings Center Report*, 1988, 18 (Aug./Sept.), 23–24.

61. Eubanks, P. "Nursing homes seek advance directives." *Hospitals*, 1990, 64 (22), 52–54.

62. Press, I. "The predisposition to file claims: The patient's perspective." *Law, Medicine, and Health Care*, 1984, 12, 53–62.

63. Merritt, A.L. "Assessing the risk of legal liability for ethics committees." *Hastings Center Report*, 1988, 18 (Feb./March), 13–14.

64. *Bouvia v. Glenchur*, L.A. Superior Court, C583828, Oct. 7, 1986.

65. Belkin, L. *First, Do No Harm.* New York: Simon Schuster, 1992.

66. Wikler, D. "Institutional agendas and ethics committees." *Hastings Center Report*, 1989, 19 (Sept./Oct.), 21–23.

67. Brock, D. "Ethics committees and cost containment." *Hastings Center Report*, 1990, 20 (March/April), 29–31.

68. Cohen, C.B. "Ethics committees as corporate and public policy advocates." *Hastings Center Report*, 1990, 20 (Sept./Oct.), 36–37.

69. Povar, G.J. "Evaluating ethics committees: What do we mean by success?" *Maryland Law Review*, 1991, 50, 904–919.

70. Keffer, M.J., and Keffer, J.L. "U.S. ethics committees: Perceived vs. actual roles." *Hospital Ethics Committee Forum*, 1991, 3, 227–230.

71. van Allen, E., Moldow, D.G., and Cranford, R. "Evaluating ethics committees." *Hastings Center Report*, 1989, 19 (Sept./Oct.), 23–24.

72. Rosner, F. "Hospital medical ethics committees: A review of their development." *Journal of the American Medical Association*, 1985, 253, 2693–2697.

73. Greer, A.L. "The state of the art versus the state of the science: The diffusion of new medical technologies into practice." *International Journal of Technology Assessment in Health Care*, 1988, 4, 5–26.

The Ethical, Legal, and Social Implications Program of the National Center for Human Genome Research: A Missed Opportunity?

KATHI E. HANNA

Science and Health Policy Consultant, Washington, D.C.

ELSI is not a guarantee that all is well in the Genome Project, that all moral problems will be neatly anticipated, dissected, and managed. It is ludicrous to think that a handful of scholars and clinicians who comprise [sic] the ELSI Working Group are capable of such heroic wisdom and foresight, or even to believe that the many scholars whose independent work is being funded through the ELSI program can do the same. The ELSI Working Group is not a commission or regulatory agency empowered to speak for the public or to exercise control in the public interest. Experts in medicine or ethics or law, although they may clarify issues and offer useful critiques of public policy, lack the moral and political authority to decide what ought to be done.

There are dangers here. The public, including public officials, must not be misled about what ELSI can do, lest it let down its guard.

> Thomas H. Murray,
> member of the ELSI Working Group (1992)

The Human Genome Project of the National Institutes of Health (NIH) and the Department of Energy (DOE) was initiated in fiscal year 1988 as a line item in the federal budget to map and sequence the entire complement of genetic information in the human genome. The project, the first major federally funded biology initiative, is expected to take 15 years at a cost of approximately $3 billion. Simultaneously hailed as the search for the biological "holy grail" (Hall, 1990) and big science at its worst (Lewin, 1986a, 1986b; Walsh and Marks, 1990), the human genome project is unprecedented in many ways. Besides being "big biology," the research alliance between NIH and DOE was also a first (see Cook-Deegan, 1991; NRC, 1988; OTA, 1988), as was the allocation of 3 percent of the research budget for the study of ethical, legal, and social implications of the application of knowledge gained from the mapping and sequencing research enterprise. Never before had the federal government rushed headlong into such an ambitious research program while at the same time supporting efforts that would raise questions about the wisdom, pace, and potential social consequences of its actions.

The knowledge gained from the Human Genome Project is expected to have major impacts on the understanding of disease, both genetic and acquired, for society in general, and for us, as individuals. It is the ability to characterize and profile the genetic information of individuals that has led to speculation and concern about the use and potential abuse of such information in terms of discrimination, stigmatization, and potential medical harm.

Although these concerns are not new—they were previously raised in concert with early genetic diagnostic capabilities such as sickle cell carrier screening and the use of prenatal diagnosis for selective abortion—the debate about the human genome initiative brought many of these issues to the surface once again because of the scale and magnitude of the mapping effort. Whereas ethical, legal, and social concerns were previously addressed on a case-by-case basis, the accelerated pace of new discoveries from the Human Genome Project could render such an approach dangerously obsolete. The genome project will inevitably lead to genetic tests that are faster, cheaper, more accurate, and more applicable to a multitude of diseases. The effects on the conduct of biomedical research and approaches to disease treatment could be revolutionary.

James D. Watson, codiscoverer of the molecular structure of DNA and a early proponent of a federal effort to map the human genome, recognized the need to confront these policy issues early in the project. He reiterated his commitment at a press conference in October 1988 announcing his appointment as the first head of the NIH Office of Human Genome Research:

> Some very real dilemmas exist already about the privacy of DNA. The problems are with us now, independent of the genome program, but they will be associated with it. We should devote real money to discussing these issues. People are afraid of genetic knowledge instead of seeing it as an opportunity [quoted in Roberts, 1989].

Watson felt that the NIH program should spend some of its genome money on pursuing the social, legal, and ethical issues raised by rapid advances in genetic knowledge. This belief led to the creation of the Ethical, Legal, and Social Implications (ELSI) Program, a grant-making and policymaking body within the National Institutes of Health.

Watson continued to defend his surprising and somewhat controversial proposal as the months of debate about federal support for the project went on (Watson, 1988). Because concerns about the social and ethical implications of genetic research were not new in Washington—and, in fact, were the subject of several congressional hearings as well as the work of the National Academy of Sciences, Congress's Office of Technology Assessment, and the President's Commission for the Study of Ethical Problems in Medicine and Biomedical and Behavioral Research (President's Commission)—some argue that Watson was wise to take the bull by the horns and preempt any attempt by policymakers to prematurely inhibit progress through overzealous regulation or legislation.

The fact that the historical leader of modern American molecular genetics would argue so strongly for public funding for social studies of science was welcome news to some observers and suspect to others, who viewed the diversion of funds from science to social research as, at best, an "unavoidable political tax" that the shrewd Watson was willing to pay to accomplish scientific goals (Juengst, personal communication, April 1993). That ethics tax, like any tax, is not without controversy. While it is, at best, encouraging that the Human Genome Project has an ethics component, the value of such an organization in affecting decisions and policy remains to be seen. And some observers are downright skeptical. In the words of Judith Swazey:

> ELSI—an imagistically unfortunate acronym—certainly is being taken seriously by the social scientists, ethicists, lawyers, and assorted other scholars, who have seldom had such financial largesse available to them, and their studies should yield a body of interesting and in some cases practically useful findings and recommendations. But in both the short term and the long run, the significance of the ELSI component will be greatly diminished if the concerns that generated it, and its work and results, are seen by scientists and clinicians as politically necessary but basically irrelevant appendages to the "real work" of the Genome Project [Swazey, 1992].

Those who have worked closely with Watson on the creation of the National Center for Human Genome Research and its ELSI program claim that he truly believes in the need for such analyses and that the policy issues which will arise out of genome research are too important to be left to scientists alone (Cook-Deegan, personal communication, May 1993).

A HISTORY OF BIOETHICAL DISCOURSE IN GENETICS IN PUBLIC POLICY

Major public discussion of the social impacts of genetics date back to 1975, when the National Academy of Sciences (NAS) issued a report on genetic screening (NAS, 1975). In the same year the NAS report was released, scientists met in Asilomar, California, to discuss the safety of proceeding with recombinant DNA experiments. This meeting set off a lengthy debate not only about the safety of such research, but the roles of science in regulating itself and the public in participating in the decision-making process (see Fredrickson, 1991).

The debate would result in the formation of the NIH Recombinant DNA Advisory Committee (RAC), created to oversee and approve the safety of such experiments. The RAC still stands today as testimony to the ability of the scientific community to proceed cautiously in certain areas of research. But the RAC was not designed to monitor the use of the information that would arise from advances in molecular biology (i.e., genetic screening and testing), only the research that would precede such advances.

In the early 1980s, the President's Commission issued reports on gene therapy and genetic screening (President's Commission, 1982; 1983), building on the earlier work of the Hastings Center (Institute of Society, Ethics, and the Life Sciences, 1972; Powledge and Fletcher, 1979) and the National Academy of Sciences (1975).

The Commission's genetic screening report correctly identified issues, but languished until eight years later, when the discovery of the gene for cystic fibrosis (CF) rekindled a national debate about the social, ethical, and legal implications of widespread population carrier screening for CF. In 1990, House congressional committees asked Congress's research agency, the Office of Technology Assessment (OTA), to study the issues raised by the ability to identify carriers in terms of discrimination, stigmatization, access to health care, reproductive planning, and professional and regulatory practice (OTA, 1992). OTA reviewed policy issues and concluded that congressional action was most relevant in the areas of increasing public education and professional training, protecting against discrimination, and ensuring clinical laboratory and medical device regulation.

The gene therapy report of the President's Commission, *Splicing Life* (President's Commission, 1983), served to ground a potentially explosive discussion and to thwart legislation under consideration (Cook-Deegan, 1994). The report was released at a hearing before Albert Gore, Jr., then a member of the House of Representatives. The hearing focused on the implications of human genetics, particularly gene therapy. *Splicing Life* emphasized the distinction between genetically altering somatic cells, which would not lead to inherited changes, and altering germ cells (sperm, egg cells, and their precursors), which would induce inherited changes. This distinction permitted policymakers and others to clearly understand that there were cases of gene therapy that would not be morally different from any other treatment, clearly pointing to some cases where gene therapy might be technically preferable—and morally equivalent—to other treat-

ments. The report moved the debate away from vague speculations about
playing God and how to thwart the technological imperative and towards
prudent policies of research protocol review and processes to formulate
policy (Cook-Deegan, 1994; Walters, 1992).

   Splicing Life recommended that the National Institutes of Health review
progress in gene therapy through its Recombinant DNA Advisory Committee, and that NIH consider the broad implications of commencing gene
therapy. The Recombinant DNA Advisory Committee accepted this recommendation in April 1983 and began to debate the merits of the new
technology and to assess its social implications. A working group on human gene therapy was established later that year. The working group
proceeded to draft "Points to Consider in the Design and Submission of
Human Somatic Cell Gene Therapy Protocols," adopted in 1986 as the key
document in public oversight of the new technology (Fletcher, 1990;
Murray, 1990; Walters, 1992). The working group was later reconstituted
as the current Human Gene Therapy Subcommittee. Thus, the work of the
President's Commission and the Human Gene Therapy Subcommittee has
adequately addressed concerns arising from gene therapy research.

   Splicing Life also noted that there was a need for public debate of
genetic issues, which could be mediated by an ad hoc commission on
genetics or by a standing federal bioethics commission. Representative
Gore was impressed with the report and by the process that produced it.
He subsequently introduced legislation to create a President's Commission
on human genetic engineering, favoring permanent oversight of advances
in human genetics and reproduction. This became the seed for legislation
enacted in 1985 to create the Biomedical Ethics Board and Advisory Committee within the Congress, with a broader mandate than human genetics,
as Gore became convinced that a broader mandate would be more useful.
But the ethics of genetic research arose early on in the short history of the
Biomedical Ethics Advisory Committee[1] (Cook-Deegan, 1994; Hanna et al.,
1993).

   In 1989 the Advisory Committee was pursuing its congressional mandate to report on ethical issues related to "human genetic engineering."
LeRoy Walters of the Kennedy Institute of Ethics testified before the committee as chairman of the NIH subcommittee that oversaw gene therapy.
He cited 17 reports already produced on gene therapy and observed that
there was little need for another one. Furthermore, he testified, there was
already a consensus on gene therapy policy at the NIH and the Food and
Drug Administration. Walters then pointed to genetic tests, saying that
there were many unresolved issues raised by genetic testing and screening,
such as the potential for stigmatization and discrimination, that were in
need of attention (Cook-Deegan, 1991).

   The debate over the need for a national body dedicated to analysis of social, ethical, and legal issues raised by genetic technology persisted. After moving to the Senate, as chair of the Science, Space, and Technology Subcommittee, Senator Gore held hearings in 1989 on the Human Genome Project. The need for a mechanism for addressing social, legal, and ethical issues again surfaced when Senator Gore queried a Department of Energy official about the department's intent to fund an ethical component along with its science agenda. As DOE equivocated on this question over the ensuing months, James Watson warned that if DOE did not directly fund ethics, ". . . Congress will chop your head off" (Cook-Deegan, 1994). At the same hearing, Watson had featured his plans for the ELSI program of the National Center for Human Genome Research in his opening statement before the subcommittee.

Eventually, the ELSI program would be the recipient of 3 percent of the genome budget and, today, 5 percent of the NIH share. Watson has even suggested that spending could rise to the 10 percent level by 1996 (U.S. Congress, House, 1991).

Gore was not alone in Congress in his concern about the use of genetic information. Others voiced concerns about potential misuse or abuse of genetic information gleaned from the Human Genome Project. Senator Orrin Hatch was concerned about increases in prenatal diagnosis and abortion. Senator Barbara Mikulski was concerned about adverse social impacts of advancing too rapidly on the Human Genome Project, and Representative David Obey raised questions about the potential for discrimination by insurers and employers as the ability to diagnosis genetic conditions is magnified through the technological advances of the Human Genome Project (Cook-Deegan, 1991).

Had the BEAC survived (see note 1), issues of genetics and public policy would have been on the top of its agenda. As it was, there was no national public forum in which to analyze, debate, and recommend policy regarding issues raised by the Human Genome Project, even though groups such as the Recombinant DNA Advisory Committee of the NIH, OTA, the Institute of Medicine (IOM), and the congressional hearing process were able to contribute piecemeal to policy debates. The time was ripe for some type of action in this area. The question remains, however, whether the ELSI program the best route to take in facing the social consequences of the Human Genome Project?

The Ethical, Legal, and Social Implications Program

Specific funding for genome research at NIH, in general, began in fiscal year 1988, two years before the establishment of the National Center for Human Genome Research. During that two-year interval, research funds were administered by the National Institute for General Medical

Sciences, and the scientific community advised NIH staff on a configuration for what is now NCHGR (NCHGR, Annual Report 1990). Then NIH director James Wyngaarden assembled a group of scientists, administrators, and science policy analysts to develop an NIH plan for the human genome project.

In 1988, James Watson was named associate director for human genome research and an Office of Human Genome Research was created in the Office of the NIH director. In the following year an advisory committee was named which established working relationships with DOE and other federal agencies. Two members of the advisory committee were to play key roles in the development of the ELSI program, Nancy Wexler, President of the Hereditary Disease Foundation and on the faculty of neurology and psychiatry at Columbia University, and Victor McKusick, a medical geneticist at Johns Hopkins University and keeper of *Mendelian Inheritance in Man,* the largest database in the world of genetic disorders.

When NCHGR was approved and funded by Congress in 1990, the advisory committee and NIH and DOE staff had already developed a five-year scientific plan (NCHGR, Annual Report 1990). Part of the plan addressed ethical, legal, and social considerations, with specific directives to:

• Develop programs addressing the understanding of the ethical, legal, and social implications of the Human Genome Project.
• Identify and define the major issues and develop initial policy options to address them.

The advisory committee, in its initial deliberations, decided to spin off working groups to address specific areas of the project. Nancy Wexler was to become the chair of the ELSI working group, which would eventually serve both NIH and DOE as a Joint working group.

Federal rules concerning working groups are intended to make them temporary. Thus, while Wexler serves as an advisory committee member chairing the Working Group, the other six members are actually ad hoc technical consultants—serving at the pleasure of the director of NCHGR—representing basic and clinical genetics, law, and ethics. If NIH were to charter the working group and make it permanent, it might speak with greater authority. On the other hand, chartering the Working Group would essentially create a commission under the genome project—a move that could both undermine its independence and give the impression of the fox guarding the chicken coop. This last concern might be adequately addressed by ensuring appropriate leadership and broader representation on the working group.

It is not clear what criteria were used in selecting the members but, according to one member of the group, Watson felt strongly that Jonathan Beckwith, a molecular biologist and skeptic about the Human Genome

Project, be named to the group (Cook-Deegan, personal communication, May 1993). The other members had previous experience serving on national bioethics commissions and advisory panels, or as policy analysts.

Since the working group was first selected there have been repeated requests from the disabilities community and genetics disease groups for representation (Cook-Deegan, personal communication, 1993; Juengst, personal communication, April 1993). The response from the Working Group has been to invite an equal number of non-Working Group members to each meeting, depending on its topic. In addition, members of the Working Group have submitted to NIH staff the names of individuals they feel would improve the diversity and representativeness of the group. No action has been taken as of this writing because of the uncertain technical status of the Working Group and because of a wider debate about the need for a national forum for addressing bioethics which could result in a reconfiguration of ELSI in the national bioethics infrastructure.

Development of an Agenda

The Working Group first met in 1989 to define and develop a plan of activities. Meetings are, ostensibly, open to the public but are not publicized. At the first meeting, representatives of the National Science Foundation and the National Endowment for the Humanities were invited to present their programs for research on ethics, science, and society. After discussion, the Working Group operationalized its mission by agreeing to the following activities:

- stimulate research on issues through grant making;
- refine the research agenda through workshops, commissioned papers, and invited lectures;
- solicit public input through town meetings and public testimony;
- support the development of educational materials; and
- encourage international collaboration in this area.

Thus, at the operational level, the Working Group developed realistic and practical goals in the model of data gathering and dissemination. In a sense, their early mission was to study what should be studied, both by policymakers and the public. In terms of policymaking, the group developed the following objectives:

- clarify the ethical, legal, and social consequences of mapping and sequencing the human genome through a program of targeted research;
- develop policy options at professional, institutional, governmental, and societal levels to ensure that genetic information is used to maximize the benefit to individuals and society;

- improve understanding of the issues and policy options through educational initiatives at public, professional, and policymaking levels; and
- stimulate public discussion of the issues and policy options.

Although it is not clear whether the ELSI Working Group was prepared to take on the above listed challenges or assign them elsewhere, specific program objectives were addressed in the original five-year plan.

In addition, specific topics were recommended for research support (see Table 1). In fact, much policy research had already been conducted or was under way on some of the topics listed, such as the use of genetic information by employers (OTA, 1983, 1991), its use in the criminal justice system (NRC, 1992; OTA, 1990), commercialization (Holtzman, 1989; OTA, 1987, 1988, 1989); and genetic testing when no therapy is available (Holtzman, 1989). One wonders whether the Working Group found existing work to be so inconclusive as to warrant repeat attention. Nevertheless, the development of a laundry list for topics to be addressed by future grantees is an expansive, if inefficient, method for setting priorities.

Three sets of issues were identified as particularly important considerations: privacy of genetic information, safety and efficacy of new genetic testing options, and fairness in the use of genetic information. While critical, these issues are narrowly confined to what could be considered a civil liberties orientation. Were the membership of the Working Group more diverse, other equally important issues might have been placed on the agenda, such as the effects of commercial interests on the research agenda, intellectual property rights, conflicts of interest for genome scientists, and quality assurance and control beyond issues of safety and efficacy. According to several members of the Working Group, these issues were "missed" for a variety of reasons, including lack of diversity in the Working Group. Another prominent reason, according to Working Group member Robert Cook-Deegan, is that the group operated on the premise that issues related to commercialization (e.g., conflict of interest, intellectual property, public/private interests) were being handled by other staff within NCHGR. In any case, lack of communication, erroneous assumptions, or poor judgment led to lack of attention to an important social issue that would contribute to the first policy consequence of the Human Genome Project.

The issues addressed by the Working Group in their initial agenda are forward thinking and apply to the transfer of technology into clinical practice, but ignored current concerns that arise within the scientific culture as most of the work is still in the research stage. There is no evidence that the ELSI Working Group ever directly addressed issues related to the effect of the Human Genome Project on the scientific enterprise. Only one grant

TABLE 1 Working Group Topics Suggested for Research Support

Fairness in the use of genetic information
- insurance
- employment
- the criminal justice system
- the education system
- adoptions
- the military

The impact of knowledge of genetic variation on the individual
- stigmatization
- ostracism
- labelling
- individual psychological responses

Privacy and confidentiality
- ownership and control of genetic information
- consent issues

The impact of the Human Genome Project on genetic counseling
- prenatal testing
- pre-symptomatic testing
- carrier status testing
- testing when there is no therapeutic remedy
- counseling and testing for polygenic disorders
- population screening versus testing

Reproductive decisions influenced by genetic information
- effect of genetic information on options available
- use of genetic information in the decision-making process

Issues raised by the introduction of genetics into mainstream medical practice
- qualifications and continuing education of all appropriate medical and allied health personnel
- standards and quality control
- education of patients
- education of the general public

Uses and misuses of genetics in the past and the relevance to the present
- the eugenics movement in the United States and abroad
- problems arising from screening for sickle-cell trait and other recent examples
- the misuse of behavioral genetics to advance eugenics or prejudicial stereotypes

Commercialization of the products of the Human Genome Project
- intellectual property rights
- property rights
- impact on scientific collaboration and candor
- accessibility of data and materials

Conceptual and philosophical implications of the Human Genome Project
- the concept of human responsibility
- the issue of free will versus determinism
- the concept of genetic disease

SOURCE: Adapted from *Understanding Our Genetic Inheritance: The U.S. Human Genome Project: The First Five Years, FY 1991–1995*, U.S. Department of Health and Human Services, Public Health Service, National Institutes of Health, and U.S. Department of Energy, Office of Energy Research, Office of Health and Environmental Research (Bethesda, MD: National Center for Human Genome Research, NIH Publication No. 90-1580, April 1990).

was awarded that was directly related. In 1992, $100,000 was awarded for the study of academic-industry relationships in genetics.

The issues of patenting cDNA and potential conflicts of interest for genome office officials and researchers would eventually bring the genome project's director, James Watson, in direct confrontation with Bernadine Healy, then Director of NIH, and would later contribute to his resignation. Meanwhile, the issue was assigned by Congress for analysis to OTA and by the executive branch to the Federal Coordinating Committee on Science and Technology (FCCSET) committee of the White House Office of Science and Technology Policy.

The representativeness of the Working Group is not sufficiently broad to ensure that priority-setting will be reflective of society. For example, a major mission of the Working Group has been evaluating issues pertaining to genetic information and insurance but there are no representatives on the Working Group of the insurance industry, consumers, employers who self-insure, or their employees. The Working Group's involvement in developing a statement on the Americans with Disabilities Act was initiated despite a lack of representation from disabilities or civil rights groups, although their views were solicited. A report of the House Committee on Government Operations noted: "These interests do not necessarily need to participate in developing a genetic information research agenda. They must be involved in developing a genetic information policy agenda" (U.S. Congress, House, 1992, p. 27).

Beyond setting a research agenda, the NCHGR's ELSI program was assigned the broad goal of "developing the safeguards required as new genetic information is put to practical purposes" (NCHGR, Annual Report, 1990, p. 35). The language of NCHGR literature is filled with ambitious verbiage such as "develop sound policy recommendations that will govern the confidentiality of genetic test results, insure equal access to adequate education and counseling for patients, establish minimum qualifications for clinicians, assure quality control for genetic tests, establish guidelines for genetic testing programs, and define ethical and legal responsibilities of clinicians who perform tests" (NCHGR, Annual Report, 1990). These are awesome goals for an entire government, let alone a working group of seven people. The basic flaw in the design of the ELSI program and its Working Group, to be argued later, is that is has no authority to affect policy and no clear route for communicating the information it gathers to the policy arena. This dilemma has been the subject of debate at virtually every meeting of the Working Group as it has grappled with its role in policymaking and the best route to affect decision making in this area (Cook-Deegan, personal communication, May 1993; King, personal communication, May 1993).

Policymaking Through Extramural Research

What distinguishes ELSI from other national ethics bodies is its mandate to administer a grants program. The ELSI grants programs solicit proposals through the routine program announcements and requests for applications used throughout the federal scientific establishment. At NIH, the Division of Research Grants reviews all grants applications and assigns them to the appropriate study sections. The multidisciplinary review groups consist of bioethicists, educators, genetic counselors, lawyers, theologians, philosophers, psychologists, and geneticists. After study section review, the National Advisory Council for Human Genome Research provides a second round of review. Unlike other NIH study sections, there is no standing ELSI study section. Each grant is reviewed by a different set of reviewers, based on assignment by NIH staff. NIH justifies this practice based on the wide variability in applications (Juengst, personal communication, 1993). While this view might be valid, the practice also militates against consistency and creates a situation where no one has the big picture regarding the quality and substance of grants under review.

The peer-review method of selecting grants might work well for ensuring the quality of the work but cannot guarantee that proper and appropriate attention is being given to important issues. It is not the best way to set a policy agenda because the only citizens with access to the process are those schooled in an academic or professional discipline and capable of responding to the requirements of grant writing. In many ways it is a reductionist process that runs the risk of ignoring the most pressing policy issues. Academicians are not representative of society and can be dangerously naive when it comes to public policy. On the other hand, setting a policy agenda through a bottoms-up approach provides the potential for more long-term analytical approaches to issues that might otherwise be subject to political winds. The President's Commission and the National Commission, however, were able to function appropriately in a nonpartisan manner despite pressures from many political extremes (Hanna et al., 1993). The President's Commission adhered to an open process of hearings and publication, ensuring an opportunity for representativeness that does not exist with the ELSI Working Group. The bottoms-up approach of ELSI can in no way guarantee fair representation of all points of view.

The first set of ELSI grantees, for example, were hardly representative of the general population. They were all specialists in genetics and ethics, having written numerous publications on the topics they proposed to study. The titles of their grants were general and similar: "Legal and Ethical Issues Raised by the Genome Project," "Ethical and Legal Implications of Genetic Testing," "Ethical and Legal Issues in the Diffusion of Genetic Tests." Nearly $900,000 went to eight white, male principal investigators in academic and science policy settings. It is a small universe that directs and benefits from the ELSI grant program (see Table 2 for a listing of sample grants). Analysis of projects funded over the course of the ELSI program reveals that Working Group members have been listed as principal investigators or key personnel on projects, although there is no evidence that members of the Working Group have any influence in the grants process.

In its first year, the ELSI program also undertook the support of four scholarly conferences to "begin the process of developing sound professional and social policy" about these issues. In its first annual report, the program claims to have accomplished four important preliminary goals: (1) inaugurating open discussions of ELSI issues by the public, the scholarly community, and policymakers; (2) initiating a program of research; (3) facilitating the development of professional and social policy; and (4) fostering public education. Indeed, one of the ELSI program's primary goals was to provide for the development of important factual information that is now lacking regarding social policy and genetic information. One can argue about whether developing this information through the process of peer review and grant making is either efficient or productive.

The ELSI program is principally designed to support academic research, and this it does well. In fact, one of the major products of the ELSI program has been articles published by the principal investigators. One principal investigator, for example, lists eight published books and articles resulting from ELSI support. Surely such productivity enhances the scholarly writings in the field, and is consistent with the traditional output of federally funded research, but is it in the public interest? The writings that have arisen from the grant funds appear in peer-reviewed journals and the

TABLE 2   Representative Grants of the ELSI Program

Ethical and Legal Issues in the Diffusion of Genetic Tests ($969,513)
Ethical and Policy Issues in Cystic Fibrosis Screening ($695,696)
The Human Genome Project: Human and Scientific Dimensions ($328,250)
Insurance Implications of a Complete Genome Map ($518,097)
Access to the Genome: Justice at the Frontier of Science ($162,622)
The Human Genome Project and Women ($193,688)
Reassessing Health, Normality, and Confidentiality ($175,494
Ethical and Legal Studies Relating to the Program to Map and Sequence the
    Human Genome ($424,941)
Human Heredity in American Popular Culture ($206,104)
Theological Questions Raised by the Human Genome Initiative ($260,991)
A Paradigm Approach to Ethical Problems in Genetics ($215,510)
Genetic Counselors as Educators on Human Genome Issues ($278,132)

SOURCE: *Funding Status Report*, February 1993, National Center for Human Genome Research, Ethical, Legal, and Social Implications Program.

academic press, hardly accessible to most policymakers and much of the public. There is no mechanism for ensuring that the results of these scholarly pursuits will make their way back to the policy arena unless one relies, in the words of one grantee's abstract, on absorption of the facts by "a general audience of intelligent readers." This lack of feedback from its extramural program into the policy process is perhaps the most troubling aspect of viewing ELSI as a policymaking body. Many credit the success of the President's Commission to its publications, which accurately and readably presented the issues debated by the Commission (OTA, 1993). ELSI has no such mechanism and its deliberations are not publicized. The ELSI process would be greatly improved by adherence to a publication schedule that analyzes and synthesizes its deliberations and the results of its grants program. This lack of an opportunity to synthesize the many inputs into the knowledge base is a missed opportunity.

Congressional Oversight

The lack of a clear mechanism for ELSI input into the policy process has not gone unnoticed by Congress. The following exchange between Representative Bob Wise and NIH Director Bernadine Healy at a 1991 hearing illustrates the lack of clarity in the authoritative power of the ELSI program:

> **MR. WISE:** Suppose that one of the papers or groups that has been commissioned by ELSI contains a valuable legislative recommendation. How does that work its way through the administrative process of the executive branch, eventually getting to Congress? Does the Bush administration, for instance, have to endorse such a proposal before you distribute it?
>
> **DR. HEALY:** No, not at all. In fact, the history of NIH's ventures into these areas—even in some very delicate areas—shows that those reports are independent, and they are available to everyone; and usually incite rather informed and vigorous dialogue. There is nothing hidden or confidential about these recommendations, depending upon what political leadership we have in the executive branch of government.
>
> The President does not involve himself in these activities; he strongly endorses both the Human Genome Project and the process of the ELSI program, but in no way tried to influence the process in a policy sense.
>
> **MR. WISE:** But does the administration, at some point, endorse a proposal? It would seem to me that there does need to be administration leadership at some point if something is to come to Congress, particularly if the administration is going to advocate it.
>
> **DR. HEALY:** There has not been to date, to my knowledge. But if there were a specific recommendation where we needed a legislative action, the executive branch of government, the Department of Health and

Human Services, would review it and would have input and would either disagree or agree. But that same document would, of course, be available to Congress. This is not exclusive advice for the executive branch of government.

MR. WISE: But, presumably, then it would go the Secretary of Health and Human Services—

DR. HEALY: Yes, it would go through Secretary Sullivan, through Dr. Mason, the Assistant Secretary, and there would be a policy debate at that level. Then, if appropriate, it would go on up to the White House.

MR. WISE: Via OMB?

DR. HEALY: Yes. But what I am trying to say is that ELSI is not the genomic OSTP of the Department of Health and Human Services. I mean, this is an independent group that is examining legal and social and ethical implications of human genome research, but it is outside of any particular political ideology. It is quite removed and quite independent [U.S. Congress, House, 1992].

In 1992, the Committee on Government Operations in the House of Representatives released a report calling for the formation of an independent policy review mechanism for exploration of the ethical, legal, and social implications of the Human Genome Project (U.S. House, Government Operations, 1992). The report notes that "neither department [NIH or DOE] has established a clearly defined timetable, goal, or set of priorities for the ELSI programs." The report goes on further, saying, "The ELSI programs do not have the ability to present policy recommendations to the Nation, the Congress, or the executive branch in an effective manner. There is no existing policy process that will use the results of the ELSI research to make recommendations." The scientific and academic approach to addressing social issues has worked against developing timetables or expectations. In testimony before Congress in October 1991, NIH director Bernadine Healy and DOE associate director David Galas gave few clues as to the jurisdiction, scope, or expectations of the ELSI programs (U.S. Congress, House, 1992).

In June 1992, the NIH ELSI program was officially elevated to branch status, a bureaucratic action that formalizes relations between ELSI and NCHGR and elevates the status of the ELSI program within the NIH bureaucracy (*Human Genome News,* July 1992). This action placed ELSI more permanently in the NIH organizational chart, which has both advantages and disadvantages. The advantages are the ability of the program to provide assistance to and participate in similar social issues discussions across NIH and to have some status and authority within NIH. The disadvantage is exactly the concern illustrated in the exchange between Dr. Healy and Representative Wise: the ability of ELSI to make independent policy recommendations free of the politics and bureaucratic hurdles associated with executive management is further diminished.

Because it has never been tested, the ability of the ELSI Working Group to clear any recommendations through the executive branch hierarchy is purely speculative. It is hard to imagine that such recommendations would survive intact the delays and interference inherent in such a process. If, however, ELSI were to produce analytical policy documents, the information would become part of the general debate, not necessarily exclusively for consumption by the executive branch. That contribution alone is worth pursuing.

ELSI's Forays into Policymaking

The controversy over ELSI's role in the policymaking process has followed it throughout its history. Even within the Working Group there is disagreement about its role in policymaking and there have been numerous discussions about the lack of clarity in its mandate (Cook-Deegan, personal communication, May 1993; King, personal communication, May 1993). Although NCHGR literature cites the policymaking role as a mission of ELSI, and appropriations language from Congress has repeatedly prescribed a policymaking function, only recently has proposed legislation codified the role of ELSI in the policy process (S. 1 and H.R. 4). General language charging ELSI with a policy function has not been sufficient in providing a mechanism by which to implement that function. The distraction of the grants program has prevented ELSI staff from having the time or resources to produce policy documents.

If ELSI is to recommend policy in the same manner as the President's Commission, OTA, or IOM, it is ill-equipped to do so in a timely fashion. It lacks diversity, staff, and a clearcut mechanism for transmitting its recommendations. It is impossible to expect that ELSI staff can administer a grants program, organize ELSI meetings, write policy papers, and prepare publications. Instead, the Working Group has chosen a variety of mechanisms to assist in the policy process. The largest effort has been to set policy through the extramural program, as is being done in the cystic fibrosis pilot projects (described below). Less ambitious efforts have been through a lengthy information collecting process that has, in one case, resulted in a policy statement on the Americans with Disabilities Act, and in another a report issued in 1993 on insurance aspects of genetic information. Each effort is described below.

Population Carrier Screening for Cystic Fibrosis

The first singular issue taken on by ELSI involved the use of a new diagnostic test to determine carrier status for cystic fibrosis (CF), a lethal autosomal recessive disorder prevalent in the Caucasian population. The

gene for CF was discovered in 1988 and, initially, the most common muta-
tion could be found in approximately 70 percent of carriers. As more
mutations have been found the ability of the test to detect carriers has
improved to nearly 90 percent, and in some cases, 95 percent. When
widespread carrier screening was first contemplated, policy analysts and
bioethicists saw CF as an important test case for the application of future
genetic tests. The ability of genetic services and the public to assimilate
and interpret this test would provide useful precedential information regarding the introduction of genetic tests developed through the Human
Genome Project.

Opponents of routine CF carrier screening argued that past experiences with genetic screening programs do not adequately address potential
adverse consequences raised by widespread screening, and argued vocifer-
ously for federally funded pilot projects specific to CF. Despite these concerns, federally funded pilot projects were not quick to come (Roberts,
1990). At the urging of James Watson, who urged ELSI to stretch its self-
definition, the Working Group decided to go beyond its reconnaissance
mission and seek funds for pilot projects to assess the impact of wide-scale
population carrier screening for CF (Juengst, personal communication,
April 1993).

To analyze the implications for genome research, the ELSI Working
Group convened a workshop in September 1990, inviting 12 experts from
various sectors of genetic services to discuss the technical status of CF
testing and to outline the policy issues facing the nation (NIH-DOE Workshop Report, 1990).

The Working Group identified the following issues to be considered in
preparing for the introduction of new tests such as CF: (1) the need for
trial testing and screening programs; (2) assessment of how genetic tests
are paid for; (3) professional education; (4) public education; (5) laboratory quality control; (6) informed consent and confidentiality; and 7) discrimination against families at genetic risk. The Working Group was sufficiently concerned about these issues to forward a resolution to the NCHGR
Advisory Committee recommending that NCHGR take a leadership role in
developing support for funding pilot research projects. Meanwhile, OTA
had initiated a study of these issues at the request of two House committees
(OTA, 1992).

In April 1991, NCHGR issued a request for applications (RFA) for
studies of testing and counseling for cystic fibrosis mutations. A series of
questions was presented in the RFA describing the research goals of the
pilot projects, viz., to gather information that can be used to "identify
clinical practices that best increase patient understanding of disease-gene
carrier testing and test results, and best protect individuals and families
from test-related psychological harm, stigmatization and discrimination."

The RFA also stressed the importance of coordination between grantees through workshops to be convened by NIH. Eight clinical research institutions received a total of $1 million in late 1991 to start work in 1992.

This studied approach to understanding the complexities of CF carrier screening is certainly needed and will, no doubt, be useful information in devising strategies for offering future tests. Its timeliness, however, in terms of contributing to the policy debate, is remarkably delayed. The OTA report on CF carrier screening was released in August 1992 citing several policy options to be considered by Congress, including professional and public education, discrimination, and clinical laboratory and medical device regulations. The OTA report concluded that CF carrier screening was quickly entering the realm of genetics practice and saw little need for congressional action other than through oversight and regulation. By early 1993, the cost of CF carrier screening had dropped dramatically, the sensitivity of the test had risen to 90 to 95 percent, and much of the debate about its use had subsided. Any incremental gain that will be gleaned from the federally funded studies will inform the counseling process but is insufficient to a priori prevent routine screening from proceeding (OTA, 1992).

Thus, the pilot studies, unless they reveal unpredictable and surprising results, will contribute little to the policy debate but will provide useful information to the clinical research community and future recipients of new diagnostic tests. Supporting research to address a policy issue is useful around the margins but ineffective if not constrained in time or place. When the consortium does report its results, it is not clear who the policy audience will be. This is not meant to undermine the value of the pilot study process to the clinical genetics community. The lag in time between consideration of the issue and the production of useful results leaves a void for practitioners and attorneys, who must rely on pronouncements regarding the standard of care generated amidst much controversy. And the lack of an authoritative voice leaves room for commercial interests to move ahead unfettered.

In a positive way, however, through the CF pilot studies, the ELSI program established an important professional policy precedent: incorporating assessment of psychosocial impact into clinical studies usually dominated by concerns of medical safety, reliability, and efficacy. Other institutes within NIH would later follow suit, with the National Cancer Institute adding client-centered assessment guidelines in evaluating the clinical use of the p53 genetic marker for increased cancer risk in families (Li et al., 1992). Thus, the ELSI Working Group, through its approach to the CF pilot studies, has had an impact on the practice of clinical investigation, an impact that should be emphasized when assessing ELSI's role in affecting change.

Pedigree Studies Workshop

Another example of the ELSI program's unique ability to assist the Public Health service in developing sound research practices came with a workshop it cofunded with the National Institute of Mental Health (NIMH) and the Office for Protection from Research Risks (OPRR) of NIH. The workshop was convened to discuss the special considerations needed when conducting genetic research on extended families. Issues such as discrimination and stigmatization and the need to ensure confidentiality while recruiting family members for study fall directly in the domain of NIMH and OPRR.

These issues were initially raised by genetic disease support group representatives at an ELSI Working Group workshop on privacy issues in 1991 and confirmed as important at an ELSI-funded conference in 1992. In response NCHGR and OPRR collaborated to convene yet another working group to develop guidance for investigators and research review boards considering genetic studies of families. The guidance was to be available sometime in 1993 (NCHGR, 1993 draft annual report). Although the bureaucratic response can be painfully slow, the final result will be better guidance for investigators and, presumably, better protection for families with genetic disease.

Insurance Task Force

Since its inception, the joint NIH-DOE Working Group focused on its concerns regarding the insurability of individuals diagnosed with genetic disease, or predisposition or susceptibility to disease. The Working Group has also made the fair use of genetic information by employers a priority issue. In January 1991, the Working Group formed the Task Force on Genetics and Insurance to gather information and prepare a report of policy options to prevent discriminatory use of genetic information by insurance companies and policy purchasers. The Task Force includes representatives from the insurance industry, corporate benefit plans, consumer and health voluntary groups, and scholars researching insurance issues (NIH-DOE, 1993). This group plans to formulate principles and policy options for addressing the major issues identified by the group. These issues have been identified through several information-gathering meetings.

A draft of the Task Force's final report written by NIH staff was circulated for discussion at a November 1992 meeting of the Insurance Task Force. Another meeting to discuss the draft report and policy options was held in early 1993 and the final report was published in May 1993.

Several additional federal and private sector efforts aimed at studying the insurance and discrimination consequences of the Human Genome Project have been initiated, resulting in a variety of products. These efforts include projects of IOM (funded through ELSI), OTA, American Council of Life Insurance (ACLI) and the Health Insurance Association of America (HIAA) Task Force on Genetic Testing. Thus, ELSI was not the first or the only group to tackle these issues.

In addition to the work of the ELSI Insurance Task Force, several projects pertaining to insurance and genetic information have been funded through the ELSI grant-making mechanisms. These range from conferences with sessions devoted to insurance issues to interdisciplinary, multi-year projects focused solely on insurance issues, resulting in journal articles and conference proceedings.

Policies regarding genetics and insurance are difficult to tackle because of the diffuse and complex nature of insurance. One wonders what impact ELSI can have other than participating in the debate and ensuring that the appropriate parties are invited to the table. In fact, the insurance industry has already moved to address these issues internally. The major trade associations of the health and life insurance industries (HIAA and ACLI) have embarked on several initiatives related to genetic information and insurance. A CEO-level joint task force on genetic testing was formed to assess the public policy implications of the emerging technology. In late 1992, the task force issued a report on genetic testing with recommendations on the industry response (ACLI/HIAA, 1991). The report encourages industry to deal with the genetic testing issue now, while the technology is still emerging and public opinion is not yet set (Chase, 1992).

A report of the ACLI's Subcommittee on Privacy Legislation accompanied its task force report on genetic testing. This report encouraged insurers to adopt voluntary confidentiality programs at the corporate level as well as support uniform state privacy legislation. It also contained specific recommendations regarding the privacy of genetic information.

A conference for insurance medical directors on genetic issues in insurance medicine" was held in February 1993, cosponsored by the American Academy of Insurance Medicine, ACLI, HIAA, and the American Society of Human Genetics. The conference addressed current genetic technology as it applies to insurance risk assessment. Similar conferences have been held for insurance medical directors in the past on new medical developments.

Again, the fact that other groups have already been assembled, collected information, and issued reports with recommendations is evidence that the ELSI process, as currently configured, is inadequate for making policy because in order to be most effective, ELSI must be in front of, not behind, an issue. Perhaps ELSI's academic approach to policymaking reflects its unease with its perceived lack of authority to assemble the findings of the research, identify the values involved, and offer a coherent set of recommendations. Perhaps it merely reflects a lack of adequate staff and resources. Whatever the outcome of the Insurance Task Force deliberations, it is hard to imagine an entire community of insurers, employers, labor unions, civil liberties groups, and health care providers accepting the recommendations of a small group of individuals with no clear authority when their respective parent organizations have already taken a stand. At best, the Task Force report can be marketed as a voice of moral authority that can guide ongoing debates.

Statement on Americans with Disabilities Act

In April 1991 the ELSI Working Group convened experts from law, the humanities, genetics, and voluntary health organizations to discuss the Americans with Disabilities Act (ADA) to determine the effect of the law on individuals with identified disease or susceptibility genes. This meeting resulted in an ELSI statement to the Equal Employment Opportunity Commission identifying three areas in which significant changes to the EEOC regulations should be made to improve ADA's protections against genetic discrimination in the workplace (Joint Working Group, 1991):

- discriminatory actions based on genotype, including the possibility of having affected children, should be covered by the ADA;
- post-offer, employment entrance medical examinations should be limited to assessing job-related physical and mental conditions; and
- limits should be enacted to protect the genetic privacy of employees.

The EEOC responded to the concerns raised by the Working Group but none of the recommendations were incorporated into the final EEOC regulations implementing the ADA. However, this should not be considered a diminution of ELSI's efforts. This type of direct communication between two federal bureaucracies is beneficial and noteworthy and perhaps one of the best uses of the information gathered by ELSI through its workshops and grantees. Were ELSI to routinely to serve as a conduit for getting information into the decision-making apparatuses of government, there would better information about the use of genetic technologies throughout the government so that those with the authority to govern could make more informed decisions. The statement on the ADA was one of the few instances where the Working Group rapidly took a strong stand on issues important to them. A lack of response from the EEOC reflects the strength of the legislative compromise that led to the enactment of the ADA. Amendments, no matter where they arise, will be difficult to achieve.

CONCLUSIONS

The ELSI program is a unique effort aimed at assessing the social consequences of the Human Genome Project. To date, it is the only extant national forum that can speak with authority about the ethical, legal, and social implications of genetic technologies. As such, it has both great potential and tremendous drawbacks. In many ways, the future policy-making power of the ELSI program lies within its Working Group and its willingness to change its direction, expand its mandate, assert itself, and produce results that are not only accessible but far reaching. Although ELSI, the grant-making body, has been conferred branch status in the NIH bureaucracy, ELSI, the policymaking body, seems very much a temporary organization. If it is to be deliberative, offering judgment and policy, then its base is far too narrow and its staff much too small.

ELSI has the potential to contribute in numerous ways to the policy debate about genetic technology. Given its place in the federal bureaucracy, it is in a unique position to advise the Public Health Service on issues related to genetic research and clinical genetics. Its ability to do this has been demonstrated through its work on CF pilot projects and pedigree studies. It can also serve a useful reconnaissance or watchdog function by alerting other federal agencies about genetics issues that fall within their domain, as it did with its statement to the EEOC regarding the Americans with Disabilities Act. But if it is to pursue these activities with due diligence then it must demand a research staff skilled in such policy tasks. Furthermore, it must find a mechanism for publishing its deliberations. In fact, one of ELSI's most tenable contributions is its potential to improve professional and public understanding of genetic issues.

The ELSI program has the power to do what a broad-based commission cannot, fund the development of educational materials regarding clinical genetics and the human genome. Among its education support activities, for example, is support of a two-year project by the Council of State Governments to educate state government officials and legislators about genetic issues. This type of direct communication of information to state policymakers is useful and fills a void. ELSI's support of educational activities will contribute to stimulating public interest and sophistication about the social issues of the Human Genome Project.

Commissions can be representative, build public support, add authority or legitimate activity, or reassure. Or, in the words of political scientist David Flitner, they can be "used as a tool for surmounting the pathologies of organizational complexity" (1986). It is not clear that the ELSI program, as currently configured, can do any of these things. Although it remains untested, its ability to surmount the pathologies of organizational complexity within the Department of Health and Human Services is dubious. It is worth mentioning that if the Ethics Advisory Board (EAB) of the NIH is reconstituted, some of the issues addressed in theory by ELSI grantees might be considered in practice by a body charged with the review of specific controversial research protocols. It is possible that the current uncertainty regarding the reestablishment of a national forum for bioethics contributes to the tentative nature of ELSI's policymaking powers.

If the ELSI Working Group is to confront issues in a timely manner, reliance on the extramural grants process is too elitist and far too slow. Were the ELSI Working Group to become a larger, more diverse group of individuals, it might rely on the courage of its convictions to forge ahead of the grantees is issuing policy recommendations. The narrow base of the current group precludes this confidence. As Tom Murray stated in the quote that introduced this manuscript, the Working Group as currently constituted "lack[s] the moral and political authority to decide what ought to be done." Members of the Working Group are keenly aware of these limitations, and themselves face the quandary of how to engage in policy.

The growth of the field of bioethics and growth in the number of individuals who are described as bioethicists has enhanced the analytical capacity of the nation to discuss bioethical issues. These developments also run the risk of breeding discussions that are ingrown and out of touch with the real world of the practitioner or the public. Thus, any new organization developed to address social and ethical issues must be representative of society, not just organized bioethics and science policy. The ELSI program, in its current configuration, runs the risk of being an overly academic, highly inbred mechanism for addressing issues of broad social impact. In order for it to be effective, it must diversify. And, ELSI must find a way to analyze, synthesize, and disseminate the results of its deliberations. Otherwise, it will be remembered as a missed opportunity to aggressively address the complex social issues raised by the Human Genome Project.

NOTE

1. The Biomedical Ethics Advisory Committee (BEAC) was a 14-member group whose multidisciplinary membership was appointed by the Biomedical Ethics Board (BEB), comprised of 12 members of Congress—three each from the majority and minority parties of the House and Senate. The BEAC ceased to exist before ever issuing a single report as a result of irresoluble moral conflicts over abortion rights on the part of the BEB.

REFERENCES

American Council of Life Insurance and Health Insurance Association of America. 1991. Report of the ACLI-HIAA Task Force on Genetic Testing. Washington, DC: American Council of Life Insurance.

Annas, G.J., and S. Elias. 1992. Social Policy Research Priorities for the Human Genome Project. In G.J. Annas and S. Elias (eds.) *Gene Mapping: Using Law and Ethics as Guides.* New York: Oxford University Press.

Chase, D. 1992. Genetic Testing: Emotionally Charged Issue Threatens Biggest Risk Classification Battle Yet. *Council Review* 17(4):2–6, July.

Cook-Deegan, R.M. 1991. "The Human Genome Project: The Formation of Federal Policies in the United States, 19861990," in K.E. Hanna (ed.) *Biomedical Politics.* Washington, D.C.: National Academy Press.

Cook-Deegan, R.M., ELSI Working Group member, personal communication, May 1993.

Cook-Deegan, R.M. 1994. *The Gene Wars: Science, Politics, and the Human Genome Project.* New York: W.W. Norton.

Fletcher, J.C. 1990. Evolution of the Ethical Debate about Human Gene Therapy. *Human Gene Therapy* 1(1):55–68.

Flitner, D. 1986. *The Politics of Presidential Commissions: A Public Policy Perspective.* Dobbs Ferry, N.Y.: Transnational Publications.

Fredrickson, D.S. 1991. Asilomar and Recombinant DNA: The End of the Beginning. In K.E. Hanna (ed.) *Biomedical Politics.* Washington, D.C.: National Academy Press.

Hall, S.S. 1990. James Watson and the Search for Biology's "Holy Grail" (Human Genome Initiative). *Smithsonian* 20(11):40–50.

Hanna, K.E., Cook-Deegan, R.M., and R. Nishimi. (1993). Finding a Forum for Bioethics in Public Policy. *Politics and the Life Sciences.* August. Vol. 12, No. 2, pp. 205–219.

Holtzman, N.A. 1989. *Proceed With Caution: Predicting Genetic Risks in the Recombinant DNA Era.* Baltimore, MD: The Johns Hopkins University Press.

Human Genome News. 1992. Healy Elevates NCHGR ELSI Program to Branch Status. Vol. 4(2):4, July.

Institute of Society, Ethics, and the Life Sciences, Research Group on Ethical, Social, and Legal Issues in Genetic Counseling and Genetic Engineering. 1972. Ethical and Social Issues in Screening for Genetic Disease. *New England Journal of Medicine* 286:1129–1132.

Joint Working Group on Ethical, Legal, and Social Issues. 1991. Genetic Discrimination and the Americans with Disabilities Act. Statement submitted to the Equal Employment Opportunity Commission. April 29.

Juengst, E., Director, Ethical, Legal, and Social Implications Program, National Center for Human Genome Research, personal communication, April 1993.

King, P., ELSI Working Group member, personal communication, May 1993.

Lewin, R. 1986a. Proposal to sequence the human genome stirs debate. *Science* 232:1598–1600.

Lewin, R. 1986b. Shifting sentiments over sequencing the human genome. *Science* 233:620–621.

Li, F.P., Garber, J.E., Friend, S.H., et al. 1992. "Recommendations on predictive testing for germ line p53 mutations among cancer-prone individuals," *Journal of the National Cancer Institute* 84(15):1156–1160.

Murray, T.H. 1990. Human Gene Therapy, the Public, and Public Policy. *Human Gene Therapy* 1(1):49-54.

Murray, T.H. 1992. Speaking Unsmooth Things about the Human Genome Project. In G.J. Annas and S. Elias (eds.) *Gene Mapping: Using Law and Ethics as Guides.* New York: Oxford University Press.

National Academy of Sciences. 1975. *Genetic Screening: Procedural Guidance and Recommendations.* Washington, D.C.: National Academy Press.

National Center for Human Genome Research. 1990. *Annual Report IFY 1990.* Bethesda, MD: National Institutes of Health, 1990.

National Center for Human Genome Research. 1993. *Funding Status Report, February 1993.* Bethesda, MD: National Institutes of Health.

National Center for Human Genome Research. 1993. *Draft Annual Report.* Bethesda, MD: National Institutes of Health.

National Institutes of Health-Department of Energy Joint Working Group on Ethical, Legal, and Social Implications in Human Genome Research. 1990. Workshop on the Introduction of New Genetic Tests. 10 September.

National Institutes of Health-Department of Energy Joint Working Group on Ethical, Legal and Social Implications of Human Genome Research. 1991. "Genetic Discrimination and the Americans With Disabilities Act," *Human Genome News* 3 (3):12–13.

National Institutes of Health-Department of Energy Working Group on Ethical, Legal, and Social Implications of Human Genome Research. 1993. Genetic Information and Health Insurance: Report of the Task Force on Genetic Information and Insurance, Department of Health and Human Services.

National Research Council. 1988. *Mapping and Sequencing the Human Genome.* Washington, D.C.: National Academy Press.

National Research Council, Committee on DNA Typing. 1992. *DNA Technology in Forensic Science.* Washington, D.C.: National Academy Press.

Powledge, T.M., and J.C. Fletcher. 1979. A Report from the Genetics Research Group of Hastings Center Institute of Society, Ethics, and Life Sciences. *New England Journal of Medicine* 300(4):168-172.

President's Commission for the Study of Ethical Problems in Medicine and Biomedical and Behavioral Research. 1982. *Splicing Life.* Washington, D.C.: U.S. Government Printing Office.

President's Commission for the Study of Ethical Problems in Medicine and Biomedical and Behavioral Research. 1983. *Screening and Counseling for Genetic Conditions.* Washington, D.C.: U.S. Government Printing Office.

Roberts, L. 1989. New game plan for genome mapping. *Science* 245:1438–1440.

Roberts, L. 1990. Cystic Fibrosis Pilot Projects Go Begging. *Science* 250:1076–1077.

Swazey, J. 1992. "Those Who Forget Their History: Lessons from the Human Genome Quest," in G.J. Annas and S. Elias (eds.) *Gene Mapping: Using Law and Ethics as Guides.* New York: Oxford University Press.

U.S. Congress, House of Representatives, Committee on Government Operations, Subcommittee on Government Information, Justice, and Agriculture. 1991. October 17, 1991 hearing on *Possible Uses and Misuses of Genetic Information.* Washington, D.C.: U.S. Government Printing Office.

U.S. Congress, House of Representatives, Committee on Government Operations. 1992. *Designing Genetic Information Policy: The Need for an Independent Policy Review of the Ethical, Legal, and Social Implications of the Human Genome Project.* Washington, D.C.: U.S. Government Printing Office, April 2.

U.S. Congress, Office of Technology Assessment. 1983. *The Role of Genetic Testing in the Prevention of Occupational Disease.* OTA-BA-194. Washington, D.C.: U.S. Government Printing Office.

U.S. Congress, Office of Technology Assessment. 1984. *Human Gene Therapy: A Background Paper.* OTA-BP-BA-32. Washington, D.C.: U.S. Government Printing Office.

U.S. Congress, Office of Technology Assessment. 1987. *New Developments in Biotechnology, 1: Ownership of Human Tissues and Cells. Special Report* OTA-BA-337. Washington, D.C.: U.S. Government Printing Office; also reprinted by J. B. Lippincott, Philadelphia, PA.

U.S. Congress, Office of Technology Assessment. 1988. *New Developments in Biotechnology, 4. U.S. Investment in Biotechnology.* OTA-BA-360. Washington, D.C.: U.S. Government Printing Office.

U.S. Congress, Office of Technology Assessment. 1988. *Mapping Our Genes—Genome Projects: How Big? How Fast?* OTA-BA-373. Washington, D.C.: U.S. Government Printing Office, also reprinted by Johns Hopkins University Press.

U.S. Congress, Office of Technology Assessment. 1989. *New Developments in Biotechnology. 5. Patenting Life*. OTA-BA-370. Washington, D.C.: U.S. Government Printing Office; reprinted by Marcel Dekker, New York, NY.

U.S. Congress, Office Technology Assessment. 1990. *Genetic Witness: Forensic Uses of DNA Tests*. Washington, D.C.: U.S. Government Printing Office.

U.S. Congress, Office of Technology Assessment. 1991. *Genetic Monitoring and Screening in the Workplace*. OTA-BA-455. Washington, D.C.: U.S. Government Printing Office

U.S. Congress, Office of Technology Assessment. 1992. *Cystic Fibrosis and DNA Tests: Implications of Carrier Screening*. OTA-BA-532. Washington, D.C.: U.S. Government Printing Office.

U.S. Congress, Office of Technology Assessment. 1993. *Biomedical Ethics in U.S. Public Policy*. OTA-BP-BBS-105. Washington, D.C.: U.S. Government Printing Office.

U.S. Department of Health and Human Services and U.S. Department of Energy. 1990. *Understanding Our Genetic Inheritance. The U.S Human Genome Project: The First Five Years, FY 1991–1995*, NIH Publication No. 90–1580. Bethesda, MD: National Institutes of Health.

Walsh, J., and J. Marks. 1990. Sequencing the Human Genome. *Nature* 322:590.

Walters, L. 1992. A National Advisory Committee on Genetic Testing and Screening. In G.J. Annas and S. Elias (eds.) *Gene Mapping: Using Law and Ethics as Guides*. New York: Oxford University Press.

Watson, J.D. 1988. NIH Press Conference: Appointment of James D. Watson to Head NIH Office of Human Genome Research. 26 September. Videotape, Bethesda, MD: National Center for Human Genome Research; also available at the National Reference Center for Bioethics Literature, Georgetown University.

Watson, J.D. 1990. The Human Genome Project: Past, Present, and Future. *Science* 248 (6 April): 44–49.

AIDS, Ethics, and Activism: Institutional Encounters in the Epidemic's First Decade

RONALD BAYER, Ph.D.

Professor, Columbia University School of Public Health

It is an extraordinary fact that no medical dimension of the epidemic of HIV infection has escaped ethical scrutiny. Among the issues that have drawn attention are: the duty of physicians to care for those who are in need,[1] the limits and significance of medical confidentiality,[2] the obligation to seek informed consent before testing and commencing treatment,[3] the functions of counseling infected individuals about their duties to partners[4] and of assisting women who are infected as they are compelled to make reproductive decisions,[5] the clash between the canons of research and the canons of care,[6] the limits of acceptable underwriting by insurance companies,[7] and, finally, the rights of individuals with costly medical conditions to emigrate.[8]

Despite the extraordinary context of the epidemic during the past decade, what is striking about the issues that have been pressed to the fore is that they are not new. They are subjects that have drawn the attention of ethicists and humanists over the past two decades as they have considered the role of medicine in society. What is new is the intensity of the discussion, the broad participatory nature of the debate, the political forces called into play, the demands their representatives have made, and the solutions they have sought to impose.

It is that political context that has given definition to the role ethicists have sought to assume in shaping policy on AIDS; it is that political context that has fostered an unusual series of institutional efforts to engage activists in the process of establishing guidelines for AIDS policy. What was unique about these efforts was not that those who spoke on behalf of the vulnerable were engaged at some level, but rather that representatives of vulnerable populations were sought out as collaborators. In the first years of the epidemic this process was facilitated by the existence of a politically organized, sophisticated gay community with the professional and intellectual resources that were crucial for the process of collaboration. It was the political strength and potential influence of the gay community and the widespread recognition that effective AIDS policy would require its involvement that necessitated an effort to engage it in a collaborative process.

In this paper I would like to examine the role of consultation between ethicists and those at risk for HIV infection in confronting a series of critical policy questions raised by the AIDS epidemic, each of which entailed a potential clash over the interests of privacy and individual rights on the one hand and communal well-being on the other. Five such instances will be examined: the development of guidelines for the protection of the subjects of epidemiological research, 1984; the development of guidelines for HIV screening, 1986; the development of policy options on testing of pregnant women and newborns, 1990; the development of a consensus policy on clinical research, 1991; policy recommendations for the control of tuberculosis, 1992.*

CREATING GUIDELINES FOR CONFIDENTIALITY IN RESEARCH ON AIDS

That the debate over bathhouse closure, with its implications for restrictions on gay sexual behavior, and the relevance of the public health power of quarantine to the control of AIDS would have directly engaged gay political leaders is not surprising. More unusual was their close and watchful involvement in the conduct of public and private research into the etiology, course, and epidemiology of AIDS even before HIV was identified. Fear of being labeled, of being incarcerated, and of being deprived of access to employment and insurance marked the tension between the representatives of the gay community concerned with privacy and researchers who asserted that the public health required the conduct of epidemiological studies based upon the most intimate details about AIDS patients' lives and identities. The conflict arose early as the Centers for Disease Control sought the names of AIDS patients reported to public health authorities throughout the country. Recognizing the critical importance of longitudinal studies to a broad research program, gay leaders were nevertheless fearful that providing federal health officials with such data would

---

*In all but the effort to draft recommendations on the testing of pregnant women and newborns, I was a direct project participant. In the projects on epidemiological research, HIV screening, and tuberculosis, I was a project co-director. Thus this paper relies on and has all the strengths and weaknesses of a study based on participant observation.

create the circumstances for the deprivation of the civil rights of gay men, intravenous drug users, and undocumented aliens. For them, the technical requirements of research had to be viewed within a broad political and ethical context.

How much did federal researchers need to know? Could codes be substituted for names? Were codes inviolable? Could the CDC's professional scientists be trusted to protect the confidentiality of their data? What were the links between public health researchers and public health enforcers? These were the questions that proved so troublesome. Doubts about the capacity or willingness of federal researchers to protect the privacy interests of AIDS patients came from many sources. The commissioner of health in the District of Columbia thus stated:

> I wouldn't trust the CDC one moment not to give up to the FBI, the CIA, or the Social Security Administration. The CDC is a federal agency. You and I both know that federal agencies do exchange information, and they will always do that on what they understand to be an appropriate need-to-know basis. And they will not consider that a breach of confidentiality.[9]

Virginia Apuzzo, executive director of the National Gay Task Force, underscored the social context of the confidentiality debate:

> In this country we [gays] are illegal in half of the states. We can't serve in the armed forces, we can't raise our own kids in many states, and we sure as hell can't teach other people's kids. When you tell us you're interested in our social security numbers, when we know we are not permitted to have security clearance, we would . . . be naive, at best, not to ask "What will you do with the information? Can we trust you enough?"[10]

The dilemma posed for gay leaders was pinpointed by Jeff Levi of the National Gay Task Force: "We could not be more interested in the gathering of accurate information about AIDS, but we also firmly believe that reporting mechanisms must guarantee confidentiality."[11]

While some believed that no tension existed between the imposition of ironclad protections and the conduct of epidemiological research, others felt it imperative to note that, while it was possible to strike a compromise position, all such efforts involved trade-offs in the speed and ease with which data could be gathered and subjected to analysis. The *New York Native,* a gay newspaper, soberly observed:

> Confidentiality and epidemiology may not be as mutually compatible as some gay leaders would have us think. Confidentiality and epidemiology are matters of tense negotiation, not marriage. We are in a gray area in which abuses on both sides could occur. On the one hand, someone could illegally obtain a list of people with AIDS and try to create havoc. On the other hand, some well-intentioned gay leaders who think that AIDS is primarily a civil liberties issue may be "endangering" research.[12]

In a remarkable and quite unusual process, all the more striking since it occurred during the conservative Reagan years, representatives of gay organizations entered into a complex set of negotiations over the nature of the confidentiality protections that were to be afforded to AIDS research subjects. Out of this process of negotiation and confrontation, compromises were fashioned for the protection of confidentiality. While some have asserted that the interests of public health were sacrificed, others acknowledged that the volatile setting of AIDS research required such adjustments. A refusal to yield would have produced inadequate or inaccurate reporting. James Allen of the CDC thus noted, "It clearly is a compromise position, which will make it more difficult to do our work. But if we are not getting reports, we can't do it either."[13]

It was within this context that the first institutional response to AIDS on the part of those professionally involved with bioethics occurred. In 1982, Daniel Callahan, the director of the Hastings Center, was called by Dr. Mathilde Krim (a member of the Center's board of directors and among the researchers first concerned about the emerging epidemic) to ask him to send a representative to a meeting at the New York City Department of Health that was to discuss the issue of confidentiality and epidemiological research. More specifically, the meeting was to discuss the question of the reporting of AIDS cases by name to the Centers for Disease Control. It was as a result of attendance at that session that Carol Levine, editor of the *Hastings Center Report* and managing editor of *IRB: A Review of Human Subjects Research,* became engaged in the complex set of questions being posed by the new disease.

Issues of confidentiality and the ethics of research were not new to the Hastings Center, and so it seemed only a natural extension of its institutional mission to confront these questions. Through the efforts of Dr. Krim, the Center was able to receive a small grant from the Charles A. Dana Foundation to undertake its work. This was the first private foundation grant to support work on AIDS in the United States.

From its very inception, the project on confidentiality, which lasted for approximately one year (1983–1984), was marked by the unique sensitivities that were to characterize work on ethical issues raised by the AIDS epidemic. In addition to experts on the ethics and law of human subjects research, public health representatives, and specialists on civil liberties, the group created to examine the question of confidentiality and research included representatives of the gay community. A physician who was among the first to seek a cure for those with AIDS, a patient of his who had early emerged as a spokesperson for people with AIDS, representatives from the Lambda Legal Defense and Education Fund, and the National Gay Task Force were all involved. Additionally, since Haitians were at that time thought to be at increased risk, efforts were made to engage representatives of that community.

Over the period of several months when the group met, discussions were often spirited, revealing the depths of suspicion on the part of those who were at risk for both the new disease and breaches of confidentiality, as well as the impatience that could sometimes characterize those committed to the efficient conduct of research. By design the discussions sought to underscore the points of consensus as well as to make manifest the points of disagreement. As a matter of principle, it appeared critical to the project's directors to avoid language that would mask the differences with well-meaning banalities.

The guidelines, broadly agreed to by the group and endorsed by much larger constituencies of experts on ethics as well as by representatives of the gay community, were published at the end of 1984.

Any investigation involving a possibly communicable disease poses a tension between an individual's desire to control personal information and the desire of others to have access to that information. Although this tension is not unique to AIDS, it is particularly sharply drawn in this case because those groups that have been identified as at high risk are also highly vulnerable socially, economically, and politically. Because in the early 1980s so much was unknown about AIDS, researchers believed they had to explore many intimate aspects of an individual's medical, social, and behavioral history and had to keep these data for an extended period. Investigators had to seek information that revealed, for example, that a subject had engaged in homosexual or other sexual practices that are illegal in many states and are subject to social stigma; had injected drugs obtained illegally; had engaged in criminal activities, such as prostitution; or had entered the country illegally. The guidelines thus argued:

> Furthermore, disclosure of a diagnosis of AIDS—or perhaps even involvement in AIDS research—carries a stigma that can adversely affect a person's interests socially, politically, and economically. Potential subjects, either individually or through organizations representing their interests, have sought recognition of these risks and assurances that appropriate measures will be taken to protect their privacy. For these reasons we believe that special guidelines are necessary for AIDS research.[14]

Clearly the guidelines embraced the concerns of the vulnerable. Despite a remarkable degree of consensus on the need to embrace confidentiality protections, to prevent the misuse of research data, and to employ personal identifiers only when critical to the task of linking research records in longitudinal studies, disagreement persisted on the topic of whether social security numbers should be used in AIDS research. For the advocates of such identifiers, they presented the greatest potential for matching data sets; for those who opposed their use, they posed the greatest threat to confidentiality.

Recognizing the prospect of an ever-expanding series of questions posed by research into AIDS, the guidelines proposed the creation of a national board that would consider such matters. Although never acted upon, this recommendation reflected the emerging commitment to a broad consultative model, which would include representatives of the communities most at risk for AIDS, for conducting work on the ethical issues posed by the AIDS epidemic.

It was this model of collaboration that was to inform the next major undertaking of the Hastings Center as it confronted the question of the tension between public health and civil liberties in the context of the AIDS epidemic. With support from the recently organized AIDS Medical Foundation (later to be called the American Foundation for AIDS Research) and a number of small liberal foundations, a much larger and more ambitious project commenced in 1985. It took as its agenda the exploration of the fundamentals of public health in light of contemporary ethical and constitutional standards for the limitation of the powers of the state. Reflecting of its broader scope, the project brought together leaders from the national gay community, health officials from the epidemic's epicenters (New York, San Francisco), and experts on ethics, law, and history.

For the project's organizers the involvement of representatives of the gay community was critical not only because they believed it necessary to hear their opinions. As important, it was necessary to learn from those who could uniquely convey the insights, fears, and needs of those most at risk for AIDS. Not long after it began its discussions the Hastings group elected to focus its work on the ethical challenges posed by the prospect of serological screening for HIV infection. Here, too, the Center was able to bring its long-time concern with the ethics of population screening to bear on the special problems posed by AIDS.

THE ETHICS OF SCREENING FOR HIV

From the outset the test developed to detect antibody to the AIDS virus—and first used on a broad scale in blood banking—was mired in controversy. Uncertainty about the significance of the test's findings and about its quality and accuracy provided the technical substrate of disputes that inevitably took on a political character, since issues of privacy, communal health, social and economic discrimination, coercion, and liberty were always involved. For those who feared that public anxiety about AIDS would turn individuals identified as infected with the AIDS virus into targets of irrational social policy and practice, the antibody test became emblematic of the most threatening prospect in the community's response to

AIDS. Vigorous encouragement of testing would ineluctably lead to mandatory approaches as the impatient appealed to the authoritarian history of public health. Since confidentiality would not be preserved, the consequences would be stigmatization and deprivation of the right to work, go to school, and obtain insurance. Most ominously, the identification of the infected could threaten freedom itself. No marginal advance of the public health, those who argued against wide-scale testing asserted, could warrant such a catastrophic array of personal burdens.

"Don't take the test" became the rallying cry of the leaders of the gay community. In an editorial, the *New York Native* wrote: "No gay or bisexual man should allow his blood to be tested. . . . The meaning of the test remains completely unknown. Scientists and physicians agree that a positive test result cannot be used to diagnose anything." What was far from uncertain, however, was the

> personal anxiety and socioeconomic oppression that [would] result from the existence of a record of a blood test result. . . . Will test results be used to identify the sexual orientation of millions of Americans? Will a list of names be made? How can such information be kept confidential? Who will be able to keep this list out of the hands of insurance companies, employers, landlords, and the government itself?

What was critical was for gay and bisexual men to modify their behaviors in order to protect their own health and that of their sexual partners. For those purposes, what role could such an ambiguous and potentially dangerous test play? "If you test positive, will you act with any more wisdom or concern than if you test negative? Will you be less or more conscious of following safe and health sexual guidelines?"[15]

Those who believed that the identification of the infected or potentially infected provided an opportunity for strategically targeted measures designed to modify risky behavior saw in the test a great opportunity. Some advocates of testing, opposed to the use of coercion and attentive to matters of privacy so forcefully articulated by gay groups, stressed the importance of preserving the right of each individual to determine whether to be tested, protecting the confidentiality of tests results, and guaranteeing the social and economic rights of those whose test results revealed infection with HIV. Theirs was a posture that sought to demonstrate the compatibility of an aggressive defense of the public health with a commitment to the privacy and social interests of the infected and those at risk of infection. The stress on voluntariness was reflected in the early policy statements of the national organization of state public health officials, the Association of State and Territorial Health Officials (ASTHO).

In August 1985, ASTHO convened a national consensus conference devoted to the antibody test. On this occasion, earlier doubts about the test, its use, and what recommendations should be made to those who tested positive had all but gone. ASTHO's published report declared: "With less than six months' experience, it is clear that [the tests] are more than simply measures to screen donated blood. Their high sensitivity, specificity, and in higher prevalence groups, their predictive powers for exposure to HTLV-III will substantially assist the disease prevention effort. When properly used, test information may also enhance the education efforts which remain for now the principal intervention to prevent HTLV-III transmission."[16] But an increased reliance on voluntary testing was predicated on the capacity to protect the confidentiality of test results. Acknowledging the skepticism of the gay community—indeed, at least one representative of the gay community was involved in the process of drafting the ASTHO report—the document stressed the importance of convincing those at risk that all measures would be taken to preclude the unwarranted disclosure of test findings."[17] The defense of confidentiality was not antithetical to the protection of public health; it provided the condition for the required interventions.

There were, of course, those who rejected the emphasis on voluntariness. Some argued for "routine screening." Others asserted that the defense of the public health required coercion and limitations on the liberty of the infected. For them screening on a compulsory basis was both necessary and inevitable. Assertions that the public health would not require such efforts merely masked, they argued, the willingness to sacrifice the communal welfare to private interests. The specter of such coercion haunted the discussion of all public health efforts, even the apparently voluntary attempts to facilitate identification of the infected.

Ultimately, the debate over testing and other public health measures designed to identify the infected would force a confrontation over which proposed interventions could most effectively contribute to the transformation of the private behaviors linked to the spread of HIV infection and the development of a public culture that would encourage and reinforce such changes. Bold moves might advance the cause of public health in the face of the AIDS epidemic, or they might subvert that very cause. Caution might represent wisdom or a failure to grasp the opportunity to affect the pattern of HIV transmission. Appeals to the history of public health would inform the perspectives of those who encountered each other as antagonists; so too would profound differences over the weight to be given to communal well-being and personal liberty. Empirical considerations, historical perspectives, and philosophical commitments each thus helped to shape the fractious struggles that characterized the politics of identification.

Given the profound gulf that separated those who believed that HIV testing was crucial to the strategy of preventing the spread of a lethal infection and those who saw in such testing not only a misdirection of public efforts but a potentially dangerous approach to the epidemic, it would have been futile in 1986 to seek a common ground on the question of the place of testing in the campaign against AIDS. What was possible, however, was to provide the ethical foundations for an approach that rejected mandatory screening. Relying on the principles first enunciated in *The Belmont Report,* as well as on constitutional principles, limiting the exercise of state power in the name of the public health and welfare, it was possible for the directors of the Hastings project to provide a clear enunciation of the case for voluntary HIV testing. More specifically the guidelines, published in the *Journal of the American Medical Association,* provided a response to the concerns voiced by gay leaders. Arguments for the protection of confidentiality and against discrimination were clearly asserted. So too was the necessity of informed consent with pretest counseling—requirements that were to become the platform of those committed to liberal AIDS policies.

The Hastings Center authors were unencumbered by a commitment to produce a consensus report. Nevertheless, they worked to elicit broad support for the guidelines from their working group. Drafts were repeatedly circulated. Comments and criticisms were considered carefully. It was, however, the relative independence of the guidelines' authors that made it possible for them to take a rather striking position in favor of wide-scale voluntary testing and against the moral right of those who had been tested not to know their status. "We conclude," stated the guidelines, "that given the disastrous consequences of HIV infection and the imperative of the harm principle, those who are infected have an obligation to know their antibody status, to inform their sexual partners, and to modify their behavior."[18] As a consequence those who had elected to undergo testing had no moral claim to shield themselves from those results. But that posture, in defense of what was perceived to be a public health imperative, was for the Hastings group intimately linked to the defense of the liberal values that inspired the voluntarist strategy for dealing with AIDS. Thus the guidelines concluded:

> We believe that the greatest hope for stopping the spread of HIV infection lies in the voluntary cooperation of those at higher risk—their willingness to undergo testing and to alter their personal behavior and goals in the interests of the community. But we can expect this voluntary cooperation—in some cases, sacrifice—only if the legitimate interests of these groups and individuals in being protected from discrimination are heeded by legislators, professionals, and the public. Yet voluntary testing is not enough. We must proceed with vigorous research and educational efforts to eliminate both the scourge of AIDS and the social havoc that has accompanied it.

TESTING PREGNANT WOMEN AND NEWBORNS

The approach to consultation with those at risk adopted by the Working Group on HIV Testing of Pregnant Women and Newborns, organized under the aegis of the Johns Hopkins University School of Public Health, was more conventional than that which had been adopted by the Hastings Center. Described by its chair, Dr. Ruth Faden, as a "self-appointed group," it included a range of experts in public health, law, ethics, and policy drawn from the Hopkins community, the Georgetown Law Center, and the Kennedy Institute of Ethics.[19] Funded by the American Foundation for AIDS Research, the group undertook, through a series of meetings in the late 1980s, an examination of a range of complex screening issues involving women and newborns.

Given the epidemiology of HIV infection in women, this was a project that had to confront a set of questions with enormous implications for women of color. Like the Hastings Center group, the Working Group on HIV Testing of Pregnant Women and Newborns demonstrated a singular commitment to the privacy rights of those who might be the target of screening and efforts at prevention. Most critically, the group sought to underscore its commitment to the reproductive rights of those with HIV: ". . . we reject the implementation of counseling and screening, policies that interfere with women's reproductive freedom or that result in the unfair stigmatization of vulnerable social groups."[20]

Incorporating the well-established ethical principles that inform genetic counseling, the Working Group explicitly rejected efforts to discourage pregnancy on the part of HIV-infected women. In so doing the Working Group had adopted a position long advocated by feminists but one that stood in sharp contrast to the formal policy of the Centers for Disease Control and many state health departments which urged HIV-infected women to consider the postponement of pregnancy. Even more striking was the position adopted by the Working Group on the question of whether information and screening resources should be targeted to those communities at greatest risk for HIV infection—poor inner-city communities of color. Here the Working Group was initially divided, with some favoring such targeting as the rational application of public health principles and others believing that programs that targeted poor black and Latina women would be stigmatizing. On this topic the group was ultimately strongly influenced by its one-time consultation with representatives of a number of organizations representing the interests of African American and Latina women. It was this encounter, which occurred as part of a daylong session with representatives of communities at risk as well as public health officials, that led the Working Group to define as "unjust" any program that either implicitly or explicitly targeted women of color and to state that, "to add the stigma of AIDS contagion to poor women of color is to further harm a group of persons who are already unfairly disadvantaged."[21]

In considering the unique impact that the one-time consultation had played, the Working Group chair, Dr. Faden, has lamented the fact that limited resources had not permitted a more systematic and ongoing involvement of those at risk—the poor women themselves as well as the advocacy groups that spoke on their behalf. Nevertheless, even the modest consultation that did occur represented more than had been undertaken in the past. Was it AIDS itself that had pressed Faden and her group in a new direction? "Probably," she has said. But as important was the commitment to developing a consensus, one that was "in tune" with the communities of color affected by the threat of AIDS.

Going beyond the consultative efforts of both the Hastings and the Hopkins groups were there those which were undertaken in response to the challenge posed by AIDS to the process of new drug development in the United States. Here the search for a new consensus necessitated a level of collaboration that was unprecedented.

THE ETHICS OF DRUG TRIALS

In the mid-1970s, the National Commission for the Protection of Human Subjects of Biomedical and Behavioral Research issued *The Belmont Report,* which codified a set of ethical principles that sought to inform the work of researchers. Those norms provided the foundations for regulations subsequently enacted by the Department of Health and Human Services and the Food and Drug Administration. At the core of those guidelines was the radical distinction between research designed to produce socially necessary, generalizable knowledge and therapy designed to benefit individuals. Against the former, *The Belmont Report* held, individuals—especially those who are socially vulnerable—need protection against conscription.

AIDS has forced a reconsideration of this formulation. There had been challenges to federal protections in the past, for example, when prisoners at Jackson State Prison in Michigan demanded that they be permitted to serve as research subjects because participation provided them with *social* advantages. But the HIV epidemic has provided the circumstances for the emergence of a broad and potent political movement that has sought to reshape radically the conditions under which research is undertaken. The role of the randomized clinical trial, the importance of placebo controls, the centrality of academic research institutions, the dominance of scientists over subjects, the sharp distinction between research and therapy, and the protectionist ethos of *The Belmont Report* have all been brought into question.

Although scholars concerned with the methodological demands of sound research and ethicists committed to the protection of research subjects have played a crucial role in the ensuing discussions, both as defenders of the received wisdom and as critics, the debate has been driven by the articulate demands of those most threatened by AIDS. Most prominent have been groups such as the People with AIDS Coalition and ACT-UP, organizations made up primarily of white, gay men. But advocates of women's, children's, and prisoners' rights have also made their voices heard. What has been so stunning, disconcerting to some, and exciting to others has been the rhythm of challenge and response. Rather than the careful exchange of academic arguments, there has been the mobilization of disruptive and effective political protest.

The threat of death has hovered over the process. As Carol Levine has noted, "the shortage of proven therapeutic alternatives for AIDS and the belief that trials are, in and of themselves, beneficial have led to the claim that people have a right to be research subjects. This is the exact opposite of the tradition started with Nuremberg—that people have a right *not* to be research subjects."[22] That striking reversal has resulted in a rejection of the model of research conducted at remote academic centers, with restrictive (protective) standards of access, and strict adherence to the "gold standard" of the randomized clinical trial. Blurring the distinction between research and treatment—"A Drug Trial Is Health Care Too"—those insistent on radical reform have sought to open wide the points of entry to new "therapeutic" agents both within and outside of clinical trials; they have demanded that the paternalistic ethical warrant for the protection of the vulnerable from research be replaced by an ethical regime informed by respect for the autonomous choice of potential subjects who could weigh, for themselves, the potential risks and benefits of new treatments for HIV infection. Moreover, the revisionists have demanded a basic reconceptualization of the relationship between researchers and subjects. In place of protocols imposed from above, they have proposed a more egalitarian and democratic model in which negotiation would replace a scientific authority.

The reformulation of the ethics of research that has begun under the brutal impact of AIDS has implications that go far beyond the epidemic of HIV disease because the emerging new conceptions and standards could govern the conduct of the entire research enterprise. Furthermore, the role of the carefully controlled clinical trial as providing protection against the wide-scale use of drugs whose safety and efficacy have not yet been proven no longer commands unquestioned respect.

Protagonists who have been locked in often acrimonious debate foretell very different consequences of the changing social standards of research. Proponents of a revised ethos hold out the prospect of a new regime that is both respectful of individual rights and the requirements of good science. Martin Delaney of Project Inform in San Francisco, for example, has stated:

> Regulatory practices contribute to the failure of science, demean the public good, and tread heavily on our civil liberties. . . . Scientist and patient alike would be better served by a system that permits life-threatened patients some form of access to the most promising experimental therapies, peacefully coexisting alongside a program of unencumbered clinical research.[23]

Those who are less sanguine have spoken in a different voice. George Annas has warned that the blurring of the distirction between research and treatment can only harm the desperate: "It is not compassionate to hold out false hope to terminally ill patients so that they spend their last dollars on unproven remedies that they might live longer."[24] Jerome Groopman of New England Deaconess Hospital n Boston has gone further, viewing liberalization as a threat to the research enterprise itself: "If the philosophy is that anyone can decide at any point what drugs he or she wants to take, then you will not be able to do a clinical."[25]

Here was an issue that raised questions somewhat different from those involved in the confrontation between public health and privacy. Nevertheless, it was an issue that entailed a clash between differing conceptions of the demands of the common good and of the priority that ought to be accorded to those demands. For the American Foundation for AIDS Research (AmFAR), which had been instrumental in funding virtually every effort on AIDS and ethics, the debate over drug trials was of central importance. That Mathilde Krim, AmFAR's founding co-chair, was an early and persistent critic of the research orthodoxies was, of course, a critical contributing factor. But most important, the challenge to the research establishment by AIDS activists made the question of the conduct of research trials a topic that no one concerned about AIDS could ignore. It was the existence of such activism that would fundamentally shape the design of the project funded by AmFAR to examine the issues at hand.

The project directors, Carol Levine, Robert Levine, and Nancy Dubler, had long and distinguished records for examining issues involving human experimentation. But for a project that was charged with the responsibility of forging a new consensus on research ethics, one that would "entail a reappraisal of the ethical balance between protecting the rights and welfare of subjects and expanding their options for possibly beneficial but still unproven drugs,"[26] it would have been unthinkable to approach the questions without fully involving those who had forced the issue onto the national agenda. And indeed the task force constituted represented the most serious effort to date to develop a fully collaborative relationship between activists and ethicists. Community-based researchers, members of ACT-UP, representatives of minority communities, as well as lawyers, ethicists, and policymakers, were recruited. That collaboration was especially crucial since the project goal was to develop a consensus document that would serve as a platform for reforming drug trials in the United States.

The degree to which the task force was successful in achieving its goal of consensus was in no small part a function of the care and skill of its directors in selecting the participants. "We could have had a total standoff on any issue if there had been noncompromisers in the group," said Carol Levine. "We [sought out] people who could hear other points of view and who could accept something less than the full incorporation of their own views and values in a final document."[27] In the process of seeking a "negotiated settlement," it was crucial to lay the foundations for the broad points of agreement, thus moving those questions upon which consensus could not be reached to the margins, no matter how important they were.

When finally published in *IRB: A Review of Human Subjects Research* in 1991, the report, "Building a New Consensus: Ethical Principles and Policies for Clinical Research on HIV/AIDS," reflected agreement on the need to replace the overly protective and paternalistic ethos that had informed the regulation of research and to open wide access to therapeutic trials to those who had previously been excluded or who had faced severe restrictions—women, prisoners, drug users, members of minority groups. Reflecting the political demands of AIDS activists, the consensus not only stressed the critical importance of community consultation but argued that such consultation should not be viewed as a way to obtain acceptance of an already agreed-upon protocol; the task of shaping the protocol itself "must be a partnership." Thus did the process of arriving at a consensus on research through the joint efforts of ethicists and activists produce a recommendation for partnership in the enterprise of investigating new drugs.

Despite the spirit of cooperation that animated the process of consensus building, there was one issue that remained intractable: the question of whether research participants were morally obligated to be truthful with investigators on matters of compliance and criteria for inclusion in trials. At stake, in a fundamental way, was the extent to which participants in research trials had obligations to others that could constrain their behavior. Failure to reach consensus thus represented in an acute way the profound tension between a perspective driven by a commitment to the survival interests of individuals with HIV and that which while sympathetic to those interests did not view them as trumping all other concerns. Rather than disguise the clash of perspectives, the consensus statements openly acknowledge them. Those who held that participants had a duty to candor believed that a failure to adhere to such a norm represented a violation of the trust of the researchers that could "harm the interests of current and future patients because the trial may result in scientifically invalid data and have a negative effect on their care." To others the legacy of injustice in research and the health care system made it difficult to demand compliance from those who viewed access to a drug trial as providing the only access to a potentially lifesaving drug. In the face of this irresolvable conflict the consensus document retreated from the task of making normative statements and instead underscored the prospect for improving candor and compliance if a number of meliorative measures were taken.

The experience of preparing the report on drug trials thus revealed both the strengths and limitations of efforts at consensus building between ethicists and activists. Those who believed that consensus was always possible simply did not understand the extent to which unbridgeable ideological differences might surface in the course of joint effort. It was these limitations that would be revealed in 1992 when a task force was constituted to examine the ethical challenges posed by the resurgence of tuberculosis in the face of the AIDS epidemic.

PUBLIC HEALTH AND TUBERCULOSIS CONTROL

From the mid-1980s on, the century-long decline in the incidence of tuberculosis came to an end. Fueled by a rise in poverty, homelessness, untreated drug addiction, and the crowding of prisons, this stark shift was fundamentally linked to the HIV epidemic. Those who are dually infected with HIV and microbacterium tuberculosis are at sharply increased risk for developing tuberculosis disease. Complicating the epidemiological picture was the dramatic increase in multiple-drug-resistant tuberculosis, the treatment of which involves toxic drugs and is costly, long and often ineffective. The rise in drug-resistant tuberculosis has been attributed to the failure of those who commence treatment to complete the course of therapy. In New York City, only slightly more than half of those who are diagnosed with tuberculosis complete treatment. In that city 20 percent of diagnosed cases are resistant to two or more drugs.

Tuberculosis is, of course, not AIDS. It is airborne and can be transmitted through casual contact. It is these factors that provide the biological foundations for the strategy of TB control which is compulsory at its core, standing in marked contrast to the voluntaristic strategy for dealing with HIV. To those whose first extended engagement with the public health challenges posed by a communicable disease was the AIDS epidemic, the resurgence of tuberculosis provoked profound concerns.

Given the epidemiology of the tuberculosis epidemic, its relationship to HIV infection, and the fact that it is the most socially marginalized individuals who are typically sick or at risk, there was a danger that the demands by the public for increased health protections would create a climate within which the rights and interests of those with tuberculosis *and* HIV would be disregarded. Additionally, there was the potential that the policies created during the first decade of the AIDS epidemic that promoted and protected individual choice and confidentiality and that sought to prevent unwarranted acts of discrimination could be subverted in the name of tuberculosis control.[28] Finally, the resurgence of tuberculosis necessitated an examination of the compatibility of the voluntaristic strategy for dealing with HIV and the compulsory tradition of dealing with tuberculosis.

These concerns inspired two ethicists (Ronald Bayer and Nancy Dubler) and a physician (Sheldon Landesman) long associated with work on the AIDS epidemic to constitute a working group under the auspices of the United Hospital Fund in New York City, with additional funding by AmFAR. Emboldened by the experience of past working groups that had successfully achieved broad consensus on critical policy issues posed by the HIV epidemic, the three project directors constituted a panel that was built on the model of the first Hastings Center working group on AIDS. It included clinicians, lawyers, philosophers, public health officials and representatives of the gay community. Although an explicit decision was made not to develop a consensus report, every effort was to be made to achieve consensus on all critical issues.

When the report *Tuberculosis in the 1990s: Ethical, Legal and Policy Issues in Screening, Treatment and the Protection of Those in Congregate Facilities* was issued at the end of 1992, it did, in fact, reflect the successful attainment of agreement on a number of issues that the working group had struggled with over time: there was no need to initiate mandatory HIV testing in order to effectively conduct compulsory or routine TB screening; resources should be made available to provide the social and support services necessary to enhance the capacity of the poor, the homeless, the mentally ill, and the drug addicted to comply with their TB treatment; those with HIV infection should not be excluded from work settings where they might be exposed to tuberculosis.

Where consensus eluded the group was when it confronted the question of a mandatory system of directly observed therapy for all tuberculosis patients in the postacute phase of treatment. Here the chasm between those whose perspective was informed by a primary commitment to the preventive values became clear. Despite repeated efforts the gap was unbridgeable. In the end two working group members—representatives of the Gay Men's Health Crisis and the Lesbian and Gay Rights Project of the American Civil Liberties Union—refused to sign the report. In summarizing this controversy the authors of the report wrote:

Some have argued that requiring all patients to submit to directly observed therapy is an unacceptable intrusion on privacy and liberty.[29] Why should those who have no prior record of failure to adhere to treatment be subjected to a regime that is appropriate only for those who cannot be trusted to take their medication? Wouldn't such a requirement be overbroad? Wouldn't it represent a violation of the constitutional principle that for each individual the least restrictive alternative should be relied on in pursuing the goals of public health? Opponents of such a requirement also argue that the cost of directly observed therapy in all instances represents a misallocation of scarce public health resources. We recognize that a requirement that all patients undergo directly observed therapy will entail impossible supervision on some patients who might otherwise complete the course of treatment without such oversight. Nevertheless, we believe that the marginal intrusions on privacy and restrictions on autonomy represented by supervised therapy are justified, on balance, by the public health benefits that could be achieved. Given the social costs of noncompliance, the expenditure of resources on mandated directly observed therapy, at least during the initial phase of treatment, clearly would represent a cost-effective approach to tuberculosis control.[30]

CONCLUSIONS

As ethicists have sought to make an impact on the shaping of public health policy in the context of the AIDS epidemic—an undertaking that has perforce required an extension of the principles first developed in the context of the challenges posed by the clinical encounter—they have tended to develop positions most compatible with the political perspectives of those most at risk. In part the ideological content of the work of ethicists during the first decade of the AIDS epidemic reflected their own political identification as American liberals; in part it reflected the extension of the concern for the subordinate party in the clinical encounter that so shaped the development of medical ethics since the late 1960s. Finally, the preeminent place of the values of liberal individualism in contemporary bioethics was critical in forging an identification between those whose professional work centered on bioethics and those most at risk for HIV infection who for historical reasons harbored deep suspicions about the role of the state and its agencies. But the challenges of public health were not completely analogous to those of the clinical setting. After all, the public health authority could be deployed to protect vulnerable communities in a way that was fundamentally different from the paternalistic exercise of physician authority over a nonconsenting competent adult.

It was the concern over the protection of the community—whether involving the advocacy of voluntary HIV testing at a time when gay organizations saw in the test a terrible threat, the protection of the research enterprise from subversion by those who failed to comply with protocols, or the recommendation for universal directly observed therapy for tuberculosis—that the gap between the ideological perspective of bioethicists drawn to the issue of AIDS and the most articulate proponents of the rights of those groups most at risk was manifest.

Nevertheless, the lessons of the past decade have made clear that to the extent that bioethics seeks to enter the policy arena there are considerable advantages to open collaborative relationships with activists. In some instances it is only through such collaboration that bioethicists can learn about the complexity of the issues to which they will bring their analytical tools, and can fully appreciate the contextual forces that shape the lives of the individuals who will be affected by particular policy choices. Most important, such collaboration will be enhanced if those selected for various working parties are committed to the possibility and value of compromise. But on some matters it may not be possible to identify such individuals. There are occasions when compromise will be viewed as an unacceptable capitulation to expedience rather than as a virtue. (Needless to say, the unyielding adherence to principle or position may characterize ethicists or activists.) Under such circumstances fruitful collaboration may not be possible. At best it may be possible only to agree to disagree.

Fortunately, that was not, for the most part, the case during the first decade of the AIDS epidemic. At a time when national administrations were indifferent, even hostile, to the concerns of those with HIV it was vital for ethicists and activists to find common ground in shaping perspectives that were both humane and effective. That they did so was a singular achievement.

NOTES

1. Zuger, A., and S.H. Miles. 1987. Physicians, AIDS and occupational risk: Historic traditions and ethical obligations. *JAMA* 258:1924–1928.

2. Dickens, B. 1989. Confidentiality and the duty to warn. In L. Gostin, ed., *AIDS and the Health Care System*. New Haven: Yale University Press.

3. Bayer, R., C. Levine, and S. Wolf. 1986. HIV antibody screening: An ethical framework for evaluating proposed programs. *JAMA* 256:1768–1774.

4. Shoeman, F. 1991. AIDS and privacy. In F. Reamer, ed., *AIDS and Ethics*. New York: Columbia University Press.

5. Bayer, R. 1991. AIDS and the future of reproductive freedom. In D. Wilkin, D. Nelkin, and S. Paris, eds., *A Disease of Society: Cultural and Institutional Responses to AIDS*. New York: Cambridge University Press.

6. Levine, C., N.N. Dubler, and R.J. Levine. 1991. Building a new consensus: Ethical principles and policies for clinical research on HIV/AIDS. *IRB: A Review of Human Subjects Research* 13:1–17.

7. Oppenheimer, G.M., and R.A. Padgug. 1991. AIDS and the crisis of health insurance. In F. Reamer, ed., *AIDS and Ethics*. New York: Columbia University Press.

8. Gostin, L., P. Cleary, K. Mayer, et al. 1990. Screening immigrants and international travelers for the human immunodeficiency virus. *New England Journal of Medicine* 322:1743–1746.

9. *The Washington Post,* July 18, 1983, p. 4.

10. *The Washington Post,* July 18, 1983.

11. "'Confidentiality' Issue May Cloud Epidemiologic Studies of AIDS," *JAMA,* Oct. 21, 1983, p. 1945.

12. *New York Native,* Nov. 7–20, 1983.

13. *The Washington Post,* July 18, 1983.

14. *IRB: A Review of Human Subjects Research,* 1984, 6(6).

15. *New York Native,* October 8–21, 1984, 5.

16. Association of State and Territorial Health Officials, *ASTHO Guide to Public Health Practice: HTLVIII Antibody Testing and Community Approaches.* Washington, D.C.: Public Health Foundation, 1985, 16.

17. *Ibid.*

18. Bayer, R., C. Levine, and S.M. Wolf. 1986. HIV antibody screening: an ethical framework for evaluating proposed programs. *JAMA* 256:1768–1774.

19. Interview with Ruth Faden.

20. Working Group in HIV Testing of Pregnant Women and Newborns. 1990. "HIV Infection, Pregnant Women, and Newborns: A Policy Proposal for Information and Testing." *JAMA* 264(18).

21. Working Group on HIV Testing of Pregnant Women and Newborns. 1990. HIV infection, pregnant women, and newborns: a policy proposal for information and testing. *JAMA* 264:2416–2420.

22. Levine, C. 1988. Has AIDS changed the ethics of human subjects research. *Law, Medicine and Health Care* 16:167–173.

23. Parallel track system defended. 1989. *CDC AIDS Weekly.* December 11, 3.

24. Annas, G.J. 1989. Faith, healing, hope and charity at the FDA: The politics of AIDS drug trials. *Villanova Law Review* 34:771–797.

25. Parallel track system defended. 1989. *CDC AIDS Weekly* December 11, 3.

26. *IRB: A Review of Human Subjects Research,* 1991, 13(1–2).

27. Interview with Carol Levine.

28. Bayer, R. 1991. *Private Acts, Social Consequences: AIDS and the Politics of Public Health.* New Brunswick, NJ: Rutgers University Press.

29. Gostin, L. 1993. Controlling the re-emergent tuberculosis epidemic: A fifty-state survey of TB statutes and proposals for reform. *JAMA* 269:255–261.

30. Bayer, R., N.N. Dubler and S. Landesman. 1993. The dual epidemics of tuberculosis and AIDS: Ethical and policy issues in screening and treatment. *American Journal of Public Health* 83:649–654.

"La Pénible Valse Hésitation"[1]:
Fetal Tissue Research Review and the Use of Bioethics Commissions in France and the United States

R. ALTA CHARO, J.D.

Assistant Professor, Program in Medical Ethics, School of Law, University of Wisconsin, Madison

[Unlike the naive rationality of the French Revolution, in which ignorance was always bad for mankind,] it is understood today that ignorance is not the only enemy of man, and that science must submit to a superior morality if it is to continue to be his ally. Oppenheimer had already faced this conflict when he stood before the atom bomb. The advances in genetics that bring benefits but also exceptional risks to humanity lead us to the same dilemma. . . . Our society has as much need of philosophers as it does of scientists.[2]

The unyielding antiabortion stance of the Bush and Reagan administrations, combined with the continuing mutual distrust between abortion rights advocates and antiabortion forces in Congress, has created a growing paralysis on vital bioethical matters. For example:

• The congressional Biomedical Ethics Advisory Committee and the board that appointed it collapsed in a political squabble centered on abortion. The committee was supposed to report to Congress on such issues as human genetic research, fetal research, and the withholding of food and water from dying patients.

• Experiments deemed scientifically worthwhile by National Institutes of Health reviewers have gone unfunded because a federal ethics board that must review them doesn't exist.

• Candidates for scientific posts in the Department of Health and Human Services under the Reagan and Bush administrations were asked their positions on abortion and fetal tissue transplants, leading some to withdraw from consideration.

• Potentially valuable drugs, such as RU-483, are left relatively un-investigated in the United States because the private sector perceives the likelihood of a biased federal review and hostile public reaction.

Both the United States and France have attempted to use bioethics commissions to overcome these tensions, and to smooth the way toward coordinated public policy, whether in the form of executive action or legislation. The French experience, however, may prove somewhat more successful. In part this is due to the differing political traditions of the two nations. In part, it reflects a simpler conflict to be addressed by the French commissions.

The long history of central government, whether by monarchy or Paris-based national legislatures, has made the French public more apt to accept the pronouncements of national commissions. And a comparative review of national bioethics commissions by Sonia Le Bris of the University of Montreal found that centralized nations tended, not surprisingly, to have centralized (though still purely advisory) bioethics commissions.[3]

The correlate to this phenomenon is that French commissions appear to take far longer to develop their positions, as there is no federalist system by which local commissions can experiment with different legal approaches to the same problem. Further, in the absence of the laboratory of state governments, the French commissions appear to make a genuine effort to ground their pronouncements in an appeal to universal values, often characterized as philosophical precepts.[4] "If it's not scientific, it's not ethics,"[5] declared Jean Bernard, former chairman of the French national bioethics commission (the "Comité Consultatif National d'Éthique pour la Santé et les Sciences de la Vie" or CCNE)[6]. And from a political viewpoint, the French parliament viewed much of the CCNE's work as consistent with the very definition of a "liberal" (in the European sense of the word) democracy:

> We wanted to set the least restrictive rules of a tolerant society, each person being free to impose upon himself or herself the strictest possible code consonant with his or her convictions and free to forgo possibilities offered under the law. To want to impose upon all a religious morality that, by definition applies only to the individual, would not only be a grave error vis-à-vis our fellow citizens, but also would seriously overstep the authority of Parliament. We must, at any price avoid a moral order which, imposed by some, would tell others what is good and bad.[7]

This attitude helped to maintain the impression that the conclusions of this commission were somehow inevitable, rather than merely reactions to the political and legal temperament of the times. For example, the French view the experience of German commissions, which have been extraordinarily strict with regard to biotechnology, as a continuing response to the Nazi era. Spain's unusually liberal rules on assisted reproduction are viewed as a reaction to Franco's years of conservative rule. And, of course, American deliberations are seen as reflecting, more than anything else, the political divide created by legal abortion. In France, politicians and philosophers like to think that their reflections are less driven by political history and more by ethical analysis.[8]

This paper will briefly compare the CCNE with the U.S. commission appointed to examine the use of fetal tissue in federally funded research.[9] As the French have had little to say on the issue of fetal tissue,[10] the examination of the French commission will review its history and its reception by French politicians, researchers, the medical community, and leading commentators.[11]

Overall, the most remarkable difference between the French and U.S. experiences lies in the nature of the central conflict to be resolved by the ethics commission. In France, the fundamental debate still appears to be one over the control of science. Specifically, does government have the right and the duty to limit scientific inquiry or practice in the name of inchoate political or cultural values? In the United States this same question is asked. But in general the research community in the United States has long grown accustomed to political control, at least by virtue of funding priorities. Thus, U.S. debates tend more to be about whether a particular application of political control—for example, the ban on the use of fetal tissue—is wise or effective. This in turn relates closely to the political popularity of the goal of the research or moratorium, and thus makes the American commission discussions more responsive to grass-roots political movements.

The significance of this observation lies in its implications for the structure and membership of future commissions. In France, where the ongoing struggle is between the technical and political communities, the credibility of a commission's conclusions lies in their persuasiveness within the research community. French physicians, who (unlike their American counterparts) have little financial stake in proffering novel technologies, tend to have interests aligned with the research community, i.e., the "producers" of new biotechnologies. It is no accident, therefore, that the new director of the French commission is a leading French scientist, or that the commission's "public hearings" consisted of prepared statements by 17 luminaries and prepared questions by a number of leading theologians and intellectuals.[12]

In the United States, where the debate is somewhat less about limiting the freedom of researchers and somewhat more about limiting the freedom of potential patients (service consumers) or physicians (service retailers), the credibility of commissions lies in their persuasiveness within the lay and medical communities. This in turn would seem to argue for commission leadership that is political rather than technical, and for hearings

that are open to the general public. It also means that a commission's work
will be far more subject to the vagaries of the general public's political
sensibilities on issues such as abortion or the role of religious teachings in
public policy.

FETAL TISSUE RESEARCH: THE U.S. EXPERIENCE

Fetal research has led to a vaccine for polio, to improved treatments
for diseases of both fetus and expectant mother, and now, through transplantation, to prospects for curing Parkinson's disease and juvenile diabetes. Perhaps most important, it has helped develop basic understanding of
cell biology, particularly of cancer cells. In the words of R. J. Levine, "Even
this incomplete list should serve to demonstrate the enormous value of
fetal research."[13] And sensitivity to the potential ethical problems raised by
the use of fetal tissue prompted the creation of a national panel of medical,
ethical, and legal experts as early as December 1986, meeting at Case
Western Reserve University in Cleveland to quietly endorse such research
as "ethically acceptable."[14]

But the American experience with reviewing the use of fetal tissue in
research and transplantation, while seemingly raising lofty questions of
morality, has in fact been mired in far more sticky political problems.
Indeed, the effort to ground the process in serious epidemiology discussing cause-and-effect (would permitting research increase the number of
abortions?) or philosophical concepts of responsibility (does a good use of
data derived from arguably evil procedures make the researcher and ben-
eficiary complicit in the evil act?) was drowned out by the admittedly symbolic issue at hand: whether allowing anything of any value[15] to emerge
from the abortion decision would destigmatize the procedure to the point
of weakening political opposition to it.[16]

The Uniform Anatomical Gift Act, passed by all 50 states and the District of Columbia between 1969 and 1973, authorizes donation of "all or
part of the body" of an aborted fetus for research or therapeutic purposes.
But individual states also can regulate or restrict fetal tissue donation, and
the 25 state laws on the subject contain vague and sometimes conflicting
provisions. Some of the state laws do not even define what a fetus is or what
constitutes fetal research. For example, Arizona bans the use of "any human fetus or embryo" in nontherapeutic research. California bans nontherapeutic research upon the "product of conception," Illinois upon a
"fetus," Oklahoma and Pennsylvania upon the "unborn child."[17] The all-
inclusive Missouri law, by contrast, covers "the offspring of human beings
from the moment of conception until birth at every state of its biological
development, including the human conceptus, zygote, morula, blastocyst,
embryo and fetus." Many of the laws regulating research on aborted fe-

tuses "seem designed to preclude any medical or social benefits of elective abortion," according to reproductive rights specialist Lori Andrews.[18]

The first major flap at the federal level over fetal research occurred in the 1970s, when reports surfaced of experiments on live aborted fetuses. The image was so distasteful that it helped Congress to pass the National Research Act in 1974,[19] creating the National Commission for the Protection of Human Subjects of Biomedical and Behavioral Research (National Commission). Meanwhile, a moratorium was imposed halting all research "on a living human fetus, before or after the induced abortion of such fetus, unless such research is done for the purposes of assuring the survival of such fetus." The act also set up a national commission charged with recommending the circumstances, if any, under which the moratorium should be lifted.

In 1975, the National Commission issued its report *Research on the Fetus*,[20] in which it outlined proposed limitations on research with dead fetuses and fetal tissue. These proposals, eventually adopted and codified[21] by the Department of Health, Education, and Welfare, followed the National Commission's unanimous proposal that "use of the dead fetus, fetal tissue, and fetal material for research purposes be permitted, consistent with local law, the Uniform Anatomical Gift Act and commonly held convictions about respect for the dead."[22]

By the mid-1980s, promising research in Sweden and Mexico on the use of fetal tissue transplantation for the treatment of Parkinson's disease made this form of research far more visible than it had been. By the same time, anti-abortion forces had expanded the scope of their efforts to include a number of collateral issues, including the development of new abortifacients; use of alcohol and other drugs among pregnant women; regulation of in vitro fertilization; and mandatory contraception for female child abusers.[23] In late 1987, consistent with its promise to reward the anti-abortion movement for its help in two successive elections, President Reagan, through the auspices of his White House staffer Gary Bauer, made it clear that fetal tissue research would no longer be financed without some further review.

On March 22, 1988, the Reagan administration rejected a request from the National Institutes of Health for permission to transplant fetal tissue into the brain of a patient with severe Parkinson's disease, and imposed a moratorium on all research using tissue from aborted fetuses.[24] The protocol, which had already been passed for scientific value by NIH, was held up while NIH director Jim Wyngaarden sought guidance from assistant secretary of health Robert Windom. The guidance he received consisted of a letter from Windom, directing Wyngaarden to convene an outside advisory panel to look at the ethics of fetal tissue transplantation, and listing specific questions to be answered.[25]

That panel was appointed in 1988, and was known as the Human Fetal Tissue Transplantation Research Panel (HFTTR). An ad hoc selection committee deliberately chose a politically acceptable chair, Arlin Adams. Known as a conservative opponent of abortion, Adams nonetheless took seriously the appearance of impartiality flowing from his position as a federal judge. A prominent physician (Kenneth Ryan), ethicist (Leroy Walters), and abortion opponent (James Bopp) were added to the roster to round out appearances and leadership, and an additional 17 panel members were selected by NIH's internal ad hoc committee.[26]

On September 9, 1988, during the week before the NIH panel opened its hearing, a draft executive order from President Reagan banning all fetal tissue research was disclosed. The order appeared to have been drafted and circulated by White House domestic policy adviser Gary Bauer. According to a published news account, "Some committee members expressed dismay that the White House would draft such an order before the NIH advisory panel had a chance to hear a word of testimony, but spokesman Marlin Fitzwater said the draft did not represent the official White House position."[27] From the beginning, then, the efforts of this national panel to provide dispassionate advice leading to a consensus on research regulations had a bit of a farcical quality; political considerations seemed clearly to dominate ethical concerns.

Nonethless, on September 14–16, 1988, the NIH special advisory panel held three days of hearings on fetal tissue research. While most speakers urged the panel to consider the scientific value and ethical acceptability of fetal tissue research apart from controversy over abortion, the abortion issue quickly dominated the debate. At the conclusion of the hearings, the panel voted 19 to 0, with two abstentions, that use of tissue from legally aborted fetuses for medical research and treatment is "acceptable." Chairman Adams called that vote "tentative," but said it meant that "we are willing to go ahead with the use of fetal tissue in medical research if we could take a series of steps to insure that the abortion procedure is sufficiently insulated from the medical research that comes afterward."[28] The vote was preliminary and unbinding, however, and the panel carefully took no stand on the morality of abortion. Indeed, Kenneth Ryan, the NIH panel's scientific chairman, said the committee would try to "steer a conciliatory, practical approach to policy" on fetal tissue research, despite the volatility of the abortion issue.[29]

A month later the NIH advisory committee met again to continue its work on its advisory report to NIH officials. The panel attempted, within severe time constraints and the subject matter limitations of Windom's charge to the committee, to arrive at a consensus concerning the principles and values that ought to guide fetal research. Those included (1) the moral status of the fetus and of abortion; (2) the possibility that deriving good from abortion is an example of complicity in evil; (3) the possibility that deriving good from abortion would increase the number of abortions (i.e., the level of evil in the world); and (4) the possibility that the decision to abort deprived a woman of the usual moral authority a parent has over the disposition of a child's remains.

The attack on fetal research was grounded partly on the idea of complicity: "Investigators, who do not themselves perform the abortions, were portrayed as accomplices whose work creates the impression that the 'abortion industry' is legitimate."[30] It also relied on the incorrect belief that, contrary to evidence from countries where such research is permitted, a woman who for moral reasons is ambivalent about having an abortion might decide to proceed if she is reassured that some good might come of it—for example, that a Parkinson's-disease patient might receive therapy. Worse, a woman might choose to get pregnant merely to produce research material; perhaps she could sell her fetus or give it to a relative who has diabetes. Fetal research was also denounced as being unethical because the subject cannot give informed consent and no one appears to have the standing to give proxy consent—surely a mother who has chosen to end the life of her "unborn child" cannot be relied on to guard its interests."[31]

Underlying all these discussions, but particularly those concerning the moral status of the fetus, was a tension between the value of fetal life and the value of adult life that might be helped by the use of the tissue. In other words, the conflict was not one between science for the sake of science versus the potentially immoral effects of yielding to the technological imperative. Rather, it was a more pragmatic balancing of the benefits of applied science for one group of people (Parkinson's patients) against the disadvantages to another group (fetuses and their defenders). And as neither group of persons could claim moral primacy based on biology alone,[32] the fetuses won moral primacy based upon their symbolic value and the political efforts of the well-organized anti-abortion movement.

In the end, therefore, despite efforts to reach a consensus by accepting for the sake of argument the evil nature of abortion and then working forward to whether this prohibits some good from emerging from its practice, the panel failed. Dissenting opinions were written, and the 18–3 vote of the panel to lift the moratorium was ignored. During the subsequent Bush administration, secretary of health and human services Louis Sullivan rejected the panel's report on the dubious excuse that he was not convinced by the epidemiological evidence that abortion frequency would remain unchanged should fetal tissue donation be permitted.

But the fundamental dynamic at play concerned appearances, not fine analytical reasoning. As suggested by panel member Rabbi David Bleich, "federal funding conveys an unintended message of moral approval for every aspect of the research program."[33] In the end the issue here was not primarily one of whether fetal tissue transplantation was a potentially valuable therapy for living adults, or whether restrictions on this research via federal funding moratoria constituted an untoward invasion into the pursuit of scientific reason. Rather, the issue was one of pure politics and appearances. To the extent that fetal tissue research offended the sensibilities of abortion opponents, it could legitimately be discouraged. Efforts by panel members such as John Robertson or Leroy Walters to analyze *why* social legitimation of abortion does not follow from use of fetal tissue (just as social legitimation of homicide or drunk driving does not follow from use of cadaveric tissue) were futile because they were directed at the merits rather than the emotional content of the social legitimation argument.

By November 1989, newspapers were reporting that the scientific community had reached an impasse with the administration and its willingness to let political concerns over the abortion issue block promising research and promising therapies. A sample:

> Frustration has been building among medical researchers for the last year, according to several interviewed this week. They said the seemingly irreconcilable split over abortion has created a climate in which one bioethical issue after another has become politically too hot to handle—or even discuss.
>
> Concern rose to a new pitch last week when the secretary of health and human services, Louis W. Sullivan, extended a ban on research using transplants of tissue from aborted fetuses. Sullivan ignored the advice of a special federal panel that had concluded that the research could help millions of afflicted people and would not increase the number of abortions.
>
> "In effect, this is a suppression of legitimate science at the federal level," said John Fletcher, a bioethicist at the University of Virginia. "When political considerations dominate science, it concerns me very, very deeply."[34]

The failure of the federal commission to reach an *effective* consensus led to a series of private efforts by medical societies, whose members specialized in therapies hampered by the absence of good fetal research, to rally public support through self-regulation of fetal tissue research. For example, a report titled "Medical Applications of Fetal Tissue Transplants" was issued by the American Medical Association in June 1989, calling for the use of fetal tissue grafts. Under guidelines approved by the AMA panel, the use of fetal tissue for transplantation was considered ethically permissible when it is not provided for profit and when the recipient is not designated by the donor. A woman's decision to have an abortion should be made before any discussion of the transplantation use of the fetal tissue is initiated, according to the report, and doctors who participate in the abortion should not receive any benefit from the transplantation of the tissue.[35]

Another effort was led by ACOG and AFS, who created a privately funded organization called the National Advisory Board on Ethics in Reproduction (NABER). Kenneth Ryan, a member of the NABER board and an advocate of developing guidelines said: "Research on fetal tissue and reproductive technologies is going on in this country and will continue with or without Government regulation," said Ryan. "The time is ripe for a private group to shoulder the task of setting standards to insure that such research is ethically and scientifically sound." But Douglas Johnson, legislative director of the National Right to Life Committee, which opposes legalized abortion, objected to the new, private board, saying: "I see this in part as an attempt to undermine the policies that the Federal Government has established. I also oppose it to the extent that it will be a tiny elite clique deciding fundamental ethical issues, such as when we can treat human beings like laboratory animals." Arthur Caplan, director of the Center for Biomedical Ethics at the University of Minnesota, supported the privatization of ethical review of fetal tissue transplantation, noting: "There is a vacuum on public policy in these areas. We are moving by conscious inaction. There is abortion gridlock, and in the Government there is also just plain fear of any issue pertaining to reproduction."[36]

The federal government, faced with this revolt by patient-consumers and their provider-advocates, stepped in again in the form of congressional action, when legislation was introduced in 1992 to overturn the fetal tissue ban as part of an overall NIH funding bill. The bill passed with substantial majorities in both houses of Congress, prompting a wave of public advertisements[37] and public statements[38] on both sides of the issue, directed at President Bush and his veto power.

In June 1992, however, as expected, President Bush vetoed legislation that would have overturned a federal ban on fetal tissue research, saying that such work is "inconsistent with our nation's deeply held beliefs" and that many Americans find it "morally repugnant."[39] Bush, who made it clear early in the bill's history that he would never support research that involved using tissue obtained from elective abortions, said he found the legislation "unacceptable to me on almost every ground: ethical, fiscal, administrative, philosophical and legal."[40] The House immediately scheduled an override vote, but supporters of the legislation could not muster the two-thirds vote needed.[41] Thus the ban remained in place until its removal by exective order upon Bill Clinton's ascension to the White House in January 1993.

Interestingly enough, the U.S. experience is not generally representative of North American experience. Canadian concerns about fetal tissue research centered not on its effect on the frequency or morality of abortion, but rather on commercialization of this and other forms of organ donation.

The Royal Commission on New Reproductive Technologies was established by the Canadian federal government in October 1989. Its mandate directs it to examine medical and scientific developments around new reproductive technologies, in particular their social, ethical, health, research, legal, and economic implications, and their impact on women, children, and society as a whole. The Commission has established a multifaceted Consultations program to enable it to hear the views and opinions of people from all sectors of Canadian society. It has also set in motion a comprehensive and multidisciplinary program of research and evaluation to provide rigorous, credible, and timely information about, and critical analysis of, the issues surrounding new reproductive technologies.

In response to requests from academics and policymakers for raw data and underlying analysis, the Royal Commission began releasing copies of its working papers to the public. The paper on fetal research, entitled "The Use of Human Embryos and Fetal Tissues: A Research Architecture,"[42] examines the decades—long use of human fetal tissue by pharmaceutical and biotechnology companies to develop vaccines and to test the efficacy of new pharmaceutical products. It notes that it has more recently been a critical tool in viral research on infections such as human influenza, hepatitis B, measles, and human immunodeficiency virus (HIV). The paper concludes that, while the scope of application for human embryo and fetal tissue research is increasing, there is a lack of public policy to address the social, ethical, legal, and regulatory issues their use raises.

The French Experience: The Comité Consultatif National d'Éthique

The CCNE, the first national bioethics commission in Europe, was created by executive decree in February of 1983. At the request of Jacques Chirac, prime minister, the CCNE's reflections were developed into a voluminous report by Guy Braibant. This study, entitled "Sciences de la vie: de l'éthique au droit" ("Life Sciences: From Ethics to Law"), was submitted to the government and to the public in early 1988, and listed more than 150 specific measures that could be taken by executive or parliamentary action to bring French law into conformity with the advisory opinions of the CCNE.[43]

The Braibant report is notable for its attempt to propose an enormous number of legal changes consistent with a few thematic conclusions of the CCNE. These included the indivisibility of body and soul, and the resulting importance of bodily integrity and the noncommercialization of body parts,[44] principles endorsed by the Ministry of Justice:

> It's the inalienability of the body that makes it wrong both to touch my body without my consent or to make my body the object of patrimony or commercialization: the body is not an element that can be regarded as the object of property rights, either of others or of one's self.[45]

A later prime minister, Michel Rocard, extended this work by requesting that the Braibant report be transformed into discrete pieces of draft legislation. Thus, beginning in early 1989, a drafting effort was led by Claude Evin, health minister, and Pierre Arpaillage, minister of justice. Rocard hoped to present amendments to the civil code and the public health code by the spring of that year, in time to coincide with the bicentennial celebrations. But that was not to be:

> Michel Rocard's preferred schedule was ignored from the beginning, and thus began the hesitation waltz that would last for three long years. Voices quickly were raised to protest the Braibant proposals, in more or less radical fashion and to denounce all precipitous action. . . . The need for a bioethics law fed an intense cacophony in the government at this time. By the end of 1989, . . . the minster of research was saying that a legislative initiative was no longer at all desirable. Claude Evin . . . was taking the position that the draft law project should be reduced in scope, while Pierre Arpaillage . . . was calling for a rapid parliamentary review of the entire text. [46]

All eyes looked to Mitterrand to unblock the legislative path toward a bioethics law. After some two years of delay he appointed the "maitre des requêtes" Noelle Lenoir to the Council of State,[47] to oversee a report by the parliamentary office of technology and science assessment (the Serusclat report) and a parliamentary advisory report (the Bioulac report).

Further movement would await the efforts of deputy minister of justice Michel Sapin, who called in September 1991 for a declaration of the "rights of the biological being" and an embodiment in the civil code of a legally defined status for the human body. By March 1992, Sapin had persuaded the Council of Ministers to adopt three draft law projects, which then were sent to the National Assembly, with health minister Kouchner as their proponent.[48]

Thus, by March 1992, the French cabinet had adopted a biomedical code of ethics to prevent the alteration of genes, a trade in organs, surrogate motherhood, or the use of artificial insemination except for women who are sterile or whose husbands have genetic diseases.[49] Based upon the decade-long efforts of the CCNE, the code would ban manipulation of genes except for specific therapeutic purposes, and limit the use of genetic identification techniques to establish a child's parentage. It would also outlaw payment for donated blood or organs, and keep all donors anonymous. It would ban the use of any part of a person's body without prior consent.

The French code proposal followed years of heated debate over whether to limit innovative scientific techniques. Critics feared such innovations could lead to nightmarish experiments; others argued that scientific progress must not be impeded. It took eight months for the cabinet's adoption of the code to be accepted by the National Assembly.[50] Despite the series of commissions since the mid-1980s, each created to review the recommendations of the purely advisory CCNE, and despite the call for action by French president Mitterrand,[51] further legislative action stalled again in May 1993, and Senate review and action was not expected until late 1993.[52] This occurred despite Mitterrand's enthusiastic vision of a bioethics law that transcends political party or even national boundaries and which would, incidentally, position France as the leader in the European bioethics movement: As Mitterrand stated in April 1993:

> The Parliamentary debates . . . have shown that political divisions did not affect this kind of discussion. . . . Besides, the principle of respect for persons has universal appeal, so despite some differences in ideas or sensitivities . . . it is desirable that all European countries find their way toward a common set of values. [53]

As in the United States, some of the resistance to implementing Mitterrand's vision lay in the politics of the abortion movement. For example, there was the pressure of researchers fighting anti-abortionists over the issue of sanctity of research versus embryonic life, and general fear that unforeseeable consequences of the new technologies would outstrip legislative, religious, and philosophical efforts.[54] The American anti-abortion movement exported some of its most violent forms of debate to France in the form of Operation Rescue. In its local incarnation, the movement focused mostly on clinic services, but it did register opposition to the bioethics law project as well, using the public hearings as an occasion on which to attack the underlying law concerning abortion.[55]

And the National Assembly debates did feature some very forceful anti-abortion rhetoric. For example, the appointment of member Yvette Roudy as the chair of the assembly's ad hoc committee to examine the law proposals (Bioulac was its rapporteur) drew a blistering response by conservative member Christine Boutin, who charged that the appointment was an "open provocation," as Roudy was known to be a woman "leading the struggle against the defense of the embryo, and therefore against life."[56]

On the other hand, another commentator characterized the procedure by which the CCNE opinions became legislative proposals as one that "does honor to French democracy." He noted that, in the beginning of the process ten years ago, the project was universally embattled "by three contradictory forces: the conservatives, for whom any law would be too liberal; the liberals, for whom any debate risked a return to debate over abortion law; and some researchers, for whom any law would be a potential obstacle to pursuing biological and medical research."[57] But the sincere desire of French politicians to sink their teeth into a significant and sexy subject seems to have countered those forces inherently inclined toward the status quo:

"Since becoming a member of the Parliament," explained one politician, "I have rarely had, other than today, the simultaneously exhilarating and anguishing feeling of exercising a decisive responsibility with regard to the French people, and, at the same time, to express my values in accomplishing the central calling of politics, by knowing how to reconcile my ethics of personal conviction with my ethics of public responsibility."[58]

And indeed the politicians did take advantage of their opportunity to reflect upon the subject. The Roudy-Bioulac parliamentary report did not slavishly follow CCNE recommendations. Instead, a number of amendments were made to the proposed law project, including: protection of financial interests in cell lines and other products derived from tissues and cells (although the original donation of unimproved tissue would remain uncompensated); special procedures for the conservation of embryos for future implantation; and creation of a national registry to ensure accurate transcription of each person's wishes concerning potential organ donation upon death. But most interesting, perhaps, are the amendments that sought to reinforce the CCNE's original position that reproductive technologies are to be used for "medical" purposes only.[59] These amendments concerned prenatal diagnosis:

> These would be strictly limited to the prevention or treatment of "an affliction of particular gravity, and in the interest of the child to be born" . . . [subject to] confirmation by two physicians, at least one of whom is affiliated with an authorized center; and the creation of registries permitting identification of the causes for therapeutic abortions and verification of the accuracy of the prenatal diagnosis. . . .[60]

In an article reflecting upon the ten years of the CCNE's work, one commentator suggested that the fundamental dilemma posed by new reproductive technologies, and indeed, most new medical technologies, was one of competing claims to power by the medical and political communities:

> Ten years after the creation of the national bioethics commission, the following question still remains: are physicians morally obligated to satisfy every request for services made to them for the simple reason that the technology exists? If they do so, they become mere retailers of services; if they do not, they become sole judges. Therefore, it is urgent that we create social regulations that do not depend only upon physicians' own conceptions, but also upon the fact that society is made of humanity. Medicine is a human affair, treated on a case-by-case basis, but within a framework that spells out which things are legal and which are not (e.g., setting a maximum limit of twelve weeks for the performance of abortions).[61]

With the prenatal diagnosis amendments, the National Assembly reinforced the notion that these technologies ought to be developed within the boundaries of a "superior morality" that governs the potential consumer class. Physicians are appointed to enforce that morality by virtue of their role as interpreters of the law. This sort of power sharing among elite classes—the political elite and the technical elite—is one reason for the effectiveness of the consensus development on bioethics issues that has taken place in France since 1983. It creates a unified front against which religious leaders, feminists, leftist and rightist radicals, or any other marginalized group must struggle.

One of France's leading researchers, Jacques Testart, has written about the various possible formulations for a commission reviewing genetic planning. Interestingly, he concludes that no commission will be able to resist the power of researchers and physicians, because it is they who will give meaning to the terms "infertility" or "grave genetic malformation." To the extent that any commission uses such terms in an effort to define legal and illegal uses of genetic planning or in vitro fertilization, the law will ultimately return power wholly to the hands of practitioners.[62] He notes that this is exactly what has stymied the national commission on biology and reproductive medicine, created in 1988 to implement the CCNE advisory opinions, and thus he is critical of almost all "regulatory" proposals to date.

But the most recent political dam was created more by the vagaries of the legislative session than by any substantive concern over the proposed laws themselves. Despite anti-abortion action during the National Assembly debates, for example, the legislation was passed with a large majority reflecting a broad coalition encompassing all but the extreme right and left ends of the political spectrum.[63] But the Senate debates were delayed by overlapping committee jurisdictions and the failure to appoint in their stead an ad hoc committee, the decline of Mitterrand's socialist party in the most recent elections, and the loss of Prime Minister Pierre Beregevoy.[64]

One commentator feared that any further delay in Senate action to translate policy into law would subject France to another series of "media coups" that awaken patient demands based on outlandish examples of reproductive technology, such as "insemination of young virgins, pregnancy after menopause, or gender selection, which stir up people's fancies for three or four days—the time for which the media hopes to temporarily increase its sales or audience share—and leave physicians to face the resulting requests for services."[65] These controversial uses of reproductive technologies, in turn, could scuttle the effort of years to put into place basic law governing the donation of tissues and cells in a manner that reduces risk of viral transmission.[66] And further delay could mean that the legislative proposals would need to be reviewed yet again:

> The role of the legislator is so sensitive that the rapidity of scientific progress and the evolution of social mores can render obsolete a piece of legislation that has just been passed."[67]

The Senate adopted the CCNE proposal in January 1994 to have its recommendations definitively made into law, the CCNE itself is hoping to enlarge its scope of activities beyond consideration of medical research to all aspects of medical practice. This is largely in reaction to Mitterrand's call for its greater involvement in the question of AIDS policy and the CCNE's own three efforts to shape public screening proposals.[68] This expansion of its role is not favored, however, by the Council of the Order of Physicians,[69] as it would theoretically enlarge the CCNE's role to encompass nearly every aspect of medical practice. But the CCNE has already been expanding its activities even within its current advisory, executive branch, research-oriented structure, and the pace at which it issues its opinions has quickened since 1988. Senate passage of the legislation discussed above would authorize the CCNE by statute and its opinions legal force subject to review each five years for their conformity with technical, political, and philosophical developments.[70]

As of May 1993, the future of the CCNE was a bit uncertain. While its continued existence was not in doubt, its membership and mission were subject to change. Some commentators continued to deplore the presence of researchers on the commission, asserting that they are unable to act in a disinterested manner, and called instead for a commission made up entirely of philosophers and theologians. "The researchers propose, and society disposes," one commentator suggested. "Briefly, there must be ethics for the sake of ethics."[71]

Others confronted the divide between research and law even more directly, and worried openly that the appointment of scientist Pierre Changeux to replace philosopher Jean Bernard as head of the body was inconsistent with the very premise of a bioethics commission:

> First of all, science is not beyond the reach of the law. . . . The desire to see research placed literally outside the law has been expressed by some scientists, first by opposing the very idea of a bioethics law, and then, this first battle lost, by wanting to write into the preamble of the law the principle of the development of science under the same heading and level as the principle of respect for the person. This sentiment was particularly expressed by Pierre Changeux . . . [who says]

> "Man was conceived as a moral being whose free will must distinguish between good and evil, particularly in the face of the new scientific horizons that open before him. Science, however well circumscribed by law, must remain in second place. . . . It is man who creates science, and chooses only its beneficial fruits; it is not science that creates man."[72]

Indeed, Pierre Changeux may prove to be the beginning of a profoundly different path for the CCNE. Although he, like his predecessor Jean Bernard, hopes to enlarge the scope of CCNE's charge, Changeux is

much more modest in his vision of social control over science. As mentioned above, his is one of the voices that called for a preamble to the
bioethics law that would express the importance of scientific progress as a
fundamental principle of French society.

Further, and perhaps more subtly, Changeux does not share a rhetoric
of man as a "social" and "natural" being, or as an animal with a spirit and a
body. Instead, Changeux's lengthy career in neurobiology has made him a
leading exponent of biological reductionism, in which all behavior and
thought can ultimately be explained in terms of molecular biology and
gross neural structure. This in turn has led to speculation that his views on
the "status" of the human body will be profoundly shaped by the presence
or absence of consciousness, laying the groundwork for liberal law on
abortion, euthanasia, and embryo or fetal research. Under the leadership
of Jean Bernard, the CCNE approached these questions with an underlying assumption that the spirit is indivisible from, and in some fashion
sanctifies, the body.[73] Changeux, on the other hand, rejects the metaphysi-
cal out of hand:

> Any scientist who refuses to succumb to the comfortable mental split of
> the believer and who wants to remain internally consistent and to endeav-
> or to reject all reference to the metaphysical must search for the natural
> bases of ethics. [This is nothing more than a rediscovery of the underly-
> ing premises of the French Revolution] with the considerable benefits we
> can procure from recent advances in neuroscience, cognitive science,
> and social anthropology. The most important function of science is to
> permanently chase away all irrationality in order to obtain objective knowl-
> edge.[74]

Overall, then, the French experience with its bioethics commission has
been one of abstract argumentation and a political accommodation among
elite segments of society. Although the subject of innumerable newspaper
articles, bioethics regulation remains a topic largely divorced from the
general population.

Conclusion

The United States is a fundamentally more decentralized, egalitarian,
and religiously observant country than France. Its conflicts are different.
Therefore, the structure and mission of a successful bioethics commission
in the United States must be different.

The French commission has a subtle but rather well-contained mission: to balance in a rather thematic way the competing principles of free
scientific investigation and protection of the public order and morale.
This is a classic debate in France, dating back most notably to the French
Revolution. And the events of 1789 have for 200 years stood for the victory

of reason over superstition, secularism over clericalism, and knowledge over ignorance. Thus, the main task left to the government today is to work out an accommodation between necessary public health regulation and the chafed sensibilities of the research and medical communities. The discussion between the two groups, although heavily covered in the daily newspapers, are rather abstract and largely distant from the day-to-day concerns of the general population.

By contrast, bioethics in the United States has devolved largely into a debate on the autonomy of service consumers and providers. Thus it pits government against the individual, and opens classic debates about the degree to which moral teachings ought to be imposed upon the population in the name of good order and morale. This in turn generates a rights-based discussion, in which competing interests of competing groups of persons are pragmatically weighed against one another, subject to occasional limits based on principles embedded in the Constitution and the Bill of Rights. Such a discussion, which is inherently political, is an invitation to grass-roots politicking. Any bioethics commission created for the U.S. government will have to be responsive to this political reality.

NOTES

1. "The Wearisome Hesitation Waltz." The title "La Pénible Valse Hésitation" is taken from an article by Jean-Yves Nau in the French daily, *Le Monde*.

2. "Évoquons aussi la fameuse formule attribuée au professeur Jean Bernard, 'Tout ce qui n'est pas scientifique n'est pas éthique.'" Cette formule faussement rationnelle et vraiment idéologique renverse la charge de la prévue en exigeant d'une position éthique qu'elle se soumette d'abord aux refles de la logique scientifique. La loi bioéthique retrouve le chemin interrompu de l'humanisme. L'homme y est conçu comme un être moral dont le libre jugement doit séparer le bien du mal, en particulier face aux nouveaux horizons scientifiques qui s'ouvrent devant lui. La science, désormais encadrée par la loi, retrograde à la second place, derrière le primat moral. C'est l'homme qui produit la science et en choisit les seuls fruits positifs; ce n'est pas la science qui produit l'homme. On comprend aujourd'hui que l'ignorance n'est pas la seule ennemie de l'homme et que la science doit se soumettre à une morale supérieure pour demeurer son alliée. Oppenheimer devant l'atome avait déja rencontré ce débat. Les découvertes de la biologie génétique porteuses de bénéfices mais aussi de risques exceptionnels pour l'humanité conduisent aux mêmes dilemmes. . . . Notre société a autant besoin de philosophes que de scientifiques." Stasse, F-X, "Santé, éthique, et argent," *Le Monde*, 5 February 1993.

3. Nau, J-Y, "L'éclosion internationale de la bioéthique," *Le Monde*, 20 May 1992.

4. The four principles are "le bénévolat, la gratuité, l'anonymat et le volontariat" (benevolence, non-commercialization, anonymity, and autonomy), and are equally applicable to reproductive technologies, AIDS screening, or organ donation. See Nau, J-Y, "La Pénible Valse Hésitation," *Le Monde*, 19 March 1993.

5. "Tout ce qui n'est pas scientifique n'est pas éthique." Stasse, F-X, "Santé, éthique, et argent" *Le Monde*, 5 February 1993.

6. The CCNE consists of members appointed from a variety of disciplines. They include: five members representing a "family of philosophical and theological thought," appointed by

the President; fifteen others appointed by virtue of their "interest and competency" in bio-ethics, nominated in varying numbers by several minstries (health, social affairs, education family, industry, justice, research, labor); and one member each appointed by the Prime Minister (who may be of a different party than the President), the President of the National Assembly, the President of the Senate, the President of the Cours de Cassation, and the Vice-President of the Council of State. An additional fifteen members are appointed by various organizations within the medical and research communities. Members are to serve two year terms, with half the membership changing every second year. Nau, J-Y, "Dans l'attente du renouvellement de ses effectifs et de son président: Le Comité national d'éthique est au bord de l'asphyxie," Le Monde, 13 May 1992.

7. "Nous avons voulu fixer les règles minimales d'une société tolérante, chacun étant libre de s'imposer des règles plus strictes en fonction de ses convictions et de ne pas recourir aux possibilités offertes par la loi. Vouloir imposer à la collectivité une morale religieuse qui, par définition, ne s'applique qu'à l'individu, non seulement serait une erreur vis-à-vis de nos concitoyens, mais outrepasserait gravement le rôle du Parlement . . . Il faut éviter à tout prix l'ordre moral, qui, impose par les uns, dirait aux autres ce qui est bien et ce qui est mal. . . ." Paris, G., "A l'Assemblée nationale: Les députés souhaitent que les textes sur la bio-éthique soient adoptés avant la fin de la législature," Le Monde, 23 November 1992.

8. Paris, G., "A l'Assemblée nationale: Les députés souhaitent que les textes sur la bio-éthique soient adoptés avant la fin de la législature," Le Monde, 23 November 1992.

9. The IOM requested an international comparative study on fetal tissue panels. This paper will be more an international comparison than a study of fetal tissue panels, because no other country seems to have devoted as much time to the subject as the United States.

10. The CCNE originally endorsed a moratorium on embryo research and the use of fetal tissue, but lifted the moratorium within a year.

11. As per request by the committee, this paper will be very brief, and will be based upon publicly available sources only. Thus, the CCNE review will be based upon its own documents and upon a review of over 137 articles in the French newspaper Le Monde.

12. Nau, J-Y, "L'audition publique de dix-sept 'grands témoins': Une loi-cadre pourrait être proposée pour la bioéthique," Le Monde, 27 March 1991.

13. Levine, R.J., "Fetal research: the underlying issue; Human fetal research," Scientific American 261(2):112 (August 1989).

14. Timothy J. McNulty, "Murky Moral Issues Surround Fetal Research," Chicago Tribune, July 27, 1987, at Pg. 1.

15. Other than a woman's own satisfaction at ending her pregnancy.

16. For a more complete review of the internal squabbles of the Fetal Tissue Panel, see Childress, J.F., "Deliberations of the Human Fetal Tissue Transplantation Research Panel," in Institute of Medicine (K. Hanna, ed.), Biomedical Politics (National Academy Press, 1991). For a review of congressional efforts to overturn the ban, see Vawter, D.E., "Fetal Tissue Transplantation Policy in the United States," 12(1) Politics and the Life Sciences 79:85 (February 1993). President Clinton lifted the moratorium shortly after taking office.

17. U.S. Congress, Office of Technology Assessment, Infertility: Medical and Social Choices (OTA-BA-358) (U.S. G.P.O.; Washington, D.C.: 1988). As of 1988, restrictions on fetal research existed in 25 states. Id.

18. Don Colburn, "The Fetus, Medicine, Law, and Morality," Washington Post, October 18, 1988, at Health Section, Pg. 16.

19. P.L. 93-348; 88 stat. 348.

20. National Commission for the Protection of Human Subjects of Biomedical and Behavioral Research, "Research on the Fetus: Report and Recommendations" (DHEW-OS-76-128) (U.S. G.P.O., Washington, D.C.: 1975).

21. See 45 CFR Part 46, Subpart B.

22. On the other hand, the proposed regulations also provided stringent safeguards for research on living fetuses, such as requiring that such research be done only when therapeutic for the fetus or when it posed minimal risk to the fetus and the information to be gained was compellingly important and impossible to otherwise obtain. These proposals were subsequently adopted as regulations. *See generally* 45 C.F.R. Part 46. The regulations provided for a federal Ethics Advisory Board (EAB) that could issue waivers from that restrictive policy on a case-by-case basis, but the EAB granted only one waiver before it was dissolved and has never been reappointed.

23. Charo, R.A., "Mandatory Contraception in the U.S.," The Lancet 1992; 339:1104–1105 (5/2/92); Charo, R.A., "A Political History of RU-486," in Institute of Medicine (K. Hanna, ed.) *Biomedical Politics* (National Academy Press, 1991).

24. "Note that this moratorium deals only with the use of tissues and cells of dead fetuses. The 1974 commission had considered such use to be relatively unproblematic; its central concerns were, rather, over the possibility that a living fetus might be harmed or wronged to serve research interests. Although the morality of abortion has always figured in the debate over the ethical permissibility of fetal research, it is notable that those who oppose the transplantation of fetal tissues seem to consider it the only issue." Levine, R.J., "Fetal research: the underlying issue; human fetal research," *Scientific American* 261(2):112 (August 1989).

25. Letter from Robert Windom to James Wyngaarden, 22 March 1988.

26. 1988 HFTTR Panel: Arlin Adams (Chair), Schnader, Harrison, Segal & Lewis, Philadelphia; Kenneth Ryan (Chair, Scientific Issues), Brigham and Women's Hospital, Boston; LeRoy Walters (Chair, Ethical and legal issues), Kennedy Institute of Ethics, Washington D.C.; David Bleich, Cardozo Law School, New York City; James Bopp, Brames, McCormick, Bopp & Abel, Terre Haute, IN; James Burtchaell, University of Notre Dame, Notre Dame, IN; Robert Cefalo, University of North Carolina School of Medicine, Chapel Hill; James Childress, University of Virginia, Charlottesville; K. Danner Clauser, Pennsylvania State University, Hershey; Dale Cowan, Marymount Hospital, Garfield Heights, OH; Jane Delgado, National Coalition of Hispanic and Human Services Organizations, Washington, DC; Bernadine Healy, Cleveland Clinic Foundation, Cleveland; Dorothy Height, National Council of Negro Women, Alexandria, VA; Barry Hoffer, University of Colorado Department of Pharmacy, Denver; Patricia King, Georgetown University Law Center, Washington, DC; Paul Lacy, Washington University School of Medicine, St. Louis; Joseph Martin, Massachusetts General Hospital, Boston; Aron Moscona, University of Chicago Department of Molecular Biology, Chicago; John Robertson, University of Texas Law School, Austin; Daniel Robinson, Georgetown University Department of Psychology, Washington, DC; Charles Sweezey, Union Theological Seminary, Richmond, VA.

27. Don Colburn, "The Fetus, Medicine, Law, and Morality," *Washington Post*, October 18, 1988, at Health Section, Pg. 16.

28. Don Colburn, "The Fetus, Medicine, Law, and Morality," *Washington Post*, October 18, 1988, at Health Section, Pg. 16.

29. Don Colburn, "The Fetus, Medicine, Law, and Morality," *Washington Post*, October 18, 1988, at Health Section, Pg. 16. The article notes that: "The issue of fetal research has generated a range of opinions that sometimes cut across traditional political lines. A group called The Value of Life Committee last week called on President Reagan to ban federally funded research using tissue from aborted fetus. Signers of the letter to Reagan included not only anti-abortion activist Bernard Nathanson but also libertarian *Village Voice* columnist Nat Hentoff and Pulitzer Prize-winning novelist Walker Percy, a physician. On the other hand, syndicated columnist James J. Kilpatrick, whose credentials as a conservative are unimpeachable, endorsed fetal tissue research in a recent column because 'I believe the living may benefit from the dead' and because it 'might permit at least the rationalization that a fetus has not died in vain.'"

30. Levine, R.J., "Fetal research: the underlying issue; Human fetal research," *Scientific American* 261(2):112 (August 1989).

31. "Note that this moratorium deals only with the use of tissues and cells of dead fetuses. The 1974 commission had considered such use to be relatively unproblematic; its central concerns were, rather, over the possibility that a living fetus might be harmed or wronged to serve research interests. Although the morality of abortion has always figured in the debate over the ethical permissibility of fetal research, it is notable that those who oppose the transplantation of fetal tissues seem to consider it the only issue."

32. That argument, i.e., that live-born persons matter more than fetuses, circled directly back to the underlying conflict on abortion. Those wishing to overturn the ban tried very hard to make arguments that were not based on rehashing the abortion debate directly.

33. Bleich, D.J., "Dissenting Statement, Fetal Tissue Research and Public Policy," pp. 39–43, in vol. 1 of the Report of the Fetal Tissue Transplantation Research Panel (Bethesda, MD; DHHS 1988).

34. Richard Saltus, "Research, ethical issues stalled by abortion debate," *The Boston Globe*, November 10, 1989, Friday, City Edition, Pg. 1.

35. G. Croucher, "AMA issues fetal tissue, life support guidelines," U.P.I. June 21, 1989, Wednesday, BC cycle.

36. Phillip Hilts, "Groups Set Up Panel On Use of Fetal Tissue," *New York Times*, January 8, 1991, Tuesday, Section C; Pg. 3; Col. 1.

37. For example, the following is the text of an advertisement that ran in the May 12, 1992 edition of the congressional newspaper "Roll Call":

Does fetal tissue research have anything to do with abortion?

Ask NARAL: The National Abortion Rights Action League (NARAL) intends to score H.R. 2507, a bill to provide taxpayer funding of abortion-dependent fetal research, in their annual congressional roll call scorecard.

Ask Ted Kennedy: On April 5, 1992, Ted Kennedy told a cheering pro-abortion rally on Capitol Hill that Senate passage of H.R. 2507 proved "your message is getting through, in a very important and significant way. Make no doubt about it."

Ask Laurence Tribe: Harvard Law Professor Laurence Tribe testified that medical demand for fetal tissue gives Congress constitutional authority to pass the so-called "Freedom of Choice Act" to ensure a nationwide policy of abortion on demand.

Abortion advocates agree: H.R. 2507 has everything to do with abortion.

— A congressional vote to fund abortion-dependent fetal tissue research would give the abortion industry something it's never been able to achieve on its own: respectability.

— Such a vote will make the abortion industry look good, but make Congress look awfully bad. Especially when Congress can use these funds for other, equally promising, research methods that do not require an unprecedented alliance with the abortion industry.

— 63 percent of Americans oppose spending tax dollars for transplant research that uses tissue from induced abortions (January 1992 Wirthlin poll).

— Americans want limits to abortion on demand. So why does Congress think now is the time to begin collaborating with the very industry that performs and profits from it?

Why should Congress give the abortion industry a good name and taxpayer dollars? Vote No on H.R. 2507!

The Committee on Research Ethics; National Right to Life Committee; Southern Baptist Christian Life Commission; Christian Coalition; Doctors for Life; American Association of Pro-Life OB/Gyns; National Association of Pro-Life Nurses; United States Catholic Conference; American Association of Pro-Life Pediatricians; American Academy of Medical Ethics;

Black Americans for Life; Pharmacists for Life; Catholic Women's Institute; Christian Action Council; Knights of Columbus; American Life League; National Conference of Catholic Women; Ad Hoc Committee in Defense of Life; University Faculty for Life; Value of Life Committee; Life Issues Institute; Concerned Women for America; National Association of Evangelicals; Capitol Hill Women for Life; Women Exploited by Abortion; Jewish Anti-Abortion League; Women for Faith and Family; Women for Women; Fortress International; Family Research Council; Professional Women's Network; Traditional Values Coalition; American Victims of Abortion; Presbyterians for Life; Scientists for Life; Feminists for Life; Eagle Forum; Jews for Morality.

38. For example, here is the text of statement by American Jewish Congress, May 19, 1988, in support of H.R. 2507.

"It is truly unfortunate that fetal tissue transplantation research, which holds great promise for treating a number of devastating diseases, has become a battlefield in the ongoing national debate over abortion. After extensive study by a distinguished Task Force on Bio-Ethics, AJCongress has reached the conclusion that women should be permitted to donate fetal remains so that they may be used for research and treatment that could preserve and extend human life.

"Opponents of such research argue that elective abortions will increase if transplantation of fetal tissue becomes successful, either because of financial incentives or because some women will choose to abort in order to save the lives of others. The National Institutes of Health Reauthorization, however, contains stringent safeguards that would both eliminate any financial incentive to encourage abortions and which would insulate a woman's decision to abort from her consent to the use of fetal remains. And it is highly unlikely that even ambivalent women would be influenced in such a difficult decision by a desire to donate the fetal remains to an anonymous recipient.

"The current moratorium on fetal tissue transplant research wholly ignores the suffering of millions of Americans who endure the diseases which such research could ameliorate. We therefore urge that the current ban on federal funding of fetal tissue transplantation research be rescinded."

39. Marlene Cimons, "Bush vetoes repeal of fetal tissue research ban," *Los Angeles Times*, June 24, 1992, Part A; Pg. 6; Col. 2.

40. Marlene Cimons, "Bush vetoes repeal of fetal tissue research ban," *Los Angeles Times*, June 24, 1992, Part A; Pg. 6; Col. 2.

41. When the chamber approved the bill, the vote was 260 to 148. In the Senate, 85 members voted for the legislation.

42. Copies of this publication, as well as information about the Royal Commission on New Reproductive Technologies, are available by calling the Commission at 1-800-668-7060.

43. Nau, J-Y, "L'Assemblée nationale examine trois projets de loi sur la bioéthique: Les garde-fous de la science," *Le Monde*, 20 November 1992.

44. Nau, J-Y, "L'Assemblée nationale examine trois projets de loi sur la bioéthique: Les garde-fous de la science," *Le Monde*, 20 November 1992.

45. "C'est à la fois l'indisponibilité du corps Bianco, ministre des affaires sociales et de l'intégration, Hubert Curien, ministre de la recherche et de la technologie, et Michel Sapin, ministre délégué à la justice. Dans un entretien au Monde, ce dernier précise les orientations choisies par le gouvernement.

. . . statut du corps humain. Il devra correspondre à un certain nombre de grands principes.

Lesquels? C'est à la fois l'indisponibilité du corps on ne peut pas toucher à mon corps sans mon consentement et là on ne peut pas toucher à mon corps sans mon consentement et là non-patrimonialité ou non-commercialité: le corps n'est pas un élément qui peut faire l'objet d'une propriété, ni des autres ni de soi-même." Statement by Michel Sapin, Deputy

Minister of Justice, in Nau, J-Y, Nouchi, F., and Michel Sapin. "Un entretien avec M. Michel Sapin" *Le Monde*, 19 December 1991.

46. "Le calendrier souhaité par M. Rocard ne put être respecté et on assista au début d'une valse-hésitation qui devait au total durer trois longues années. Rapidement, des voix s'élevèrent pour contester, de manière plus ou moins radicale, le travail réalisé sous l'autorité de M. Braibant et dénoncer toute précipitation. La necessité d'une loi sur la bioéthique alimenta à cette époque une intense cacophonie gouvernementale. Fin 1989, M. Hubert Curien, ministre de la recherche, déclarait qu'une initiative législative n'était nullement souhaitable. M. Claude Evin, ministre de la santé et de la protection sociale, prenait position en faveur d'un "tronçonnage" de l'avant-projet de loi alors que M. Pierre Arpaillange, (ministre de la justice), souhaitait une discussion rapide au Parlement du texte dans sa globalité." Nau, J-Y, "L'Assemblée nationale examine trois projets de loi sur la bioéthique: Les garde-fous de la science," *Le Monde*, 20 November 1992.

47. Director of appeals?

48. Nau, J-Y, "L'Assemblée nationale examine trois projets ce loi sur la bioéthique: Les garde-fous de la science," *Le Monde*, 20 November 1992.

49. Reuters Library Report, "French Cabinet Adopts Bio-Ethics Code," 25 March 1992.

50. Nau, J-Y, "Le dixième anniversaire du Comité national d'éthique; M. Beregovoy souhaite que la future Assemblée adopte au plus vite les projets de loi sur la bioéthique," *Le Monde*, 10 February 1993.

51. "Dans un entretien au journal *La Vie* François Mitterrand souhaite l'adoption définitive des projets de loi sur la bioéthique" (unauthored column), *Le Monde*, 15 April 1993.

52. "Malgré le colloque "De l'éthique au droit," suivi du rapport Braibant, puis du rapport Lenoir, du travail de la commission parlementaire, du travail de la commission senatoriale, de l'adoption en première lecture à l'Assemblée nationale au mois de novembre 1992 (ce, à une très large majorité), le vote définitif des projets de loi relatifs à l'éthique biomédicale, faute de la convocation d'une session extraordinaire du Parlement, n'est pas intervenu." Frydman, R., "Procréation médicalement assistée: De l'éthique au droit: le piège de la politique," *Le Monde*, 10 February 1993.

53. "Les débats parlementaires (. . .) ont démontré que les clivages politiques n'affectaient pas ce type de discussion," affirme-t-il. En outre, puisque "les principes de respect de la personne humaine" ont "vocation universelle," et malgre "des differences de conception ou de sensibilité," M. Mitterrand estime "souhaitable que tous les pays d'Europe se retrouvent autour de valeurs communes." "Dans un entretien au journal *La Vie*, François Mitterrand souhaite l'adoption définitive des projets de loi sur la bioéthique" (unauthored column), *Le Monde*, 15 April 1993.

54. "Pourquoi une telle frilosité? Les explications sont nombreuses: poids d'un lobby qui voit certains milieux de la recherche soutenus en l'espèce par des courants confessionnels violemment opposés à ce que la loi traité du statut de l'embryon humain; craintes du pouvoir devant les conséquences imprévisibles que pourrait avoir une démarche législative dans un domaine où les conceptions philosophiques, morales et religieuses l'emportent presque toujours sur la logique des partis. . . ." Nau, J-Y, "Regards sur la Législature Bioéthique: Une penible valse-hésitation," *Le Monde*, 19 March 1993.

55. Chombeau, C., "Le retour des "croises" de l'avortement: La multiplication des actions anti-IVG, a l'image d'un mouvement qui se développe aux États-Unis, conduit le gouvernement à réagir," *Le Monde*, 9 January 1991.

56. "Mme Roudy présidera la commission spéciale sur les projets de bioéthique" (unsigned column), *Le Monde*, 30 April 1992.

57. "La procédure par laquelle la loi bioéthique s'est construite fait honneur à la démocratie française. Il faut, en effet, rappeler qu'à l'origine le projet de loi fut combattu par trois forces contradictoires: les conservateurs, pour qui toute loi serait trop libérale; les libéraux pour qui tout débat risquerait de voir remise en cause la loi Veil sur l'interruption volontaire

de grossesse; certains scientifiques, pour qui toute loi constituerait un obstacle potentiel à la poursuite de la recherche biologique et médicale." Stasse, F-X, "Santé, éthique et argent," *Le Monde*, 5 February 1993.

58. "Depuis que je suis parlementaire, a expliqué M. Toubon, j'ai rarement eu, autant qu'aujourd'hui, le sentiment à la fois exaltant et angoissant d'exercer une responsabilité déterminante à l'égard des Français et, en même temps, d'exprimer mes valeurs en accomplissant ce que la vocation du politique a d'essentiel, à savoir concilier mon éthique de conviction avec mon éthique de responsabilité." Paris, G., "Le débat sur la bioéthique: Les députés affirment l'inviolabilité et l'indisponibilité du corps humain," *Le Monde*, 23 November 1993.

59. To that end, for example, the law projects specified that artificial insemination by donor was to be used only when husbands carried genes for genetic disorders resulting in early childhood death or when husbands were sterile. Other uses, for "convenience" or by a single woman, would be subject to legal punishment.

On the other hand, the government proceeded to declare itself in favor of private sperm banks, despite CCNE's opinion to the contrary. CCNE had said that private sperm banks would not only put the non-commercialization of gamete donation at risk, but would be harder to control in the effort to restrict use of the sperm to those with "medical" needs. Nau, J-Y, "En contradiction avec l'avis du Comité national d'éthique: Le ministère de la santé pourrait autoriser les laboratoires privés à créer des banques de sperme," *Le Monde*, 10 August 1992.

60. "Celui-ci serait limité à la prévention ou au traitement d'une affection d' 'une particulière gravité dans l'intérêt de l'enfant à naître.' L'encadrement passerait par les dispositions suivantes: confirmation du diagnostic prénatal par deux praticiens agréés dont l'un au moins doit exercer son activité dans un centre autorisé; création de régistres permettant d'établir les causes des interruptions thérapeutiques de grossesse et de vérifier l'authenticité de l'anomalie décelée par diagnostic prénatal." Nau, J-Y, "La protection du corps humain et de l'identité génétique," *Le Monde*, 20 November 1992.

61. "Dix ans après la création du Comité national d'éthique, la question suivante demeure: le médecin a-t-il l'obligation morale de satisfaire toutes les demandes qui lui sont faites sous prétexte qu'il possède la technique? S'il répond oui, il devient prestataire de services; s'il répond non, il devient le seul juge. Il y a donc besoin urgent de créer des règles sociales qui ne dépendent pas que de la conception des médecins et correspondent à l'idée que la société se fait de l'homme. La médecine est une affaire humaine traitée au cas par cas mais dans un certain cadre qui autorise ce qui est licite et ce qui ne l'est pas (par exemple douze semaines pour le terme maximum de l'IVG)." Frydman, R., "Procréation médicalement assistée: De l'éthique au droit: le piège de la politique," *Le Monde*, 10 February 1993.

62. Testart, J., "Sélectionne humaine," *Le Monde*, 26 November 1992.

63. Paris, G., "A l'Assemblée nationale: Les députés ont adopté les trois projets de loi sur la bioéthique," *Le Monde*, 26 November 1993.

64. Nau, J-Y, "Le dixième anniversaire du Comité national d'éthique: M. Beregovoy souhaite que la future Assemblée adopte au plus vite les projets de loi sur la bioéthique," *Le Monde*, 10 February 1993.

65. "La période qui s'ouvre sera interrompue comme à l'accoutumée par decoups médiatiques" du genre insemination de jeunes filles vierges, grossesse après la menopause, choix du sexe, qui agiteront les esprits trois ou quatre jours, le temps pour les médias d'espérer augmenter transitoirement leur chiffre de vente ou leur taux d'écoute et de laisser les médecins face à des demandes réactivées." Frydman, R., "Procréation médicalement assistée: De l'éthique au droit: le piège de la politique," *Le Monde*, 10 February 1993.

66. The fear is not misplaced. By 20 May 1993, the next two controversies had broken—a regional court denial of a widow's request for the frozen embryos created with the gametes

from her late husband, and the revelation of the destruction of over thirty frozen embryos by an IVF center. "Une législation sur la bioéthique est devenue d'une urgente necessité" (unauthored column), *Le Monde*, 20 May 1993.

67. "Le rôle du législateur est d'autant plus délicat que la rapidité du progrès scientifique et l'évolution des moeurs peuvent rendre obsolète une norme législative qui vient d'être adoptée." Paris, G., "Le débat sur la bioéthique: à l'Assemblée nationale M. Kouchner: la loi doit tracer une frontière entre ce qui est possible et ce qui est souhaitable." *Le Monde*, 21 November 1993.

68. Nau, J-Y, "Après les déclarations du président de la République sur la bioéthique. Le Comité national d'éthique souhaite élargir son champ d'activité." *Le Monde*, 17 April 1993.

69. This organization is roughly equivalent to the A.M.A. in the United States.

70. Nay, J-Y, "Le Pénible Valse Hésitation," *Le Monde*, 19 March 1993.

71. "Au tribunal, les experts ne font pas partie du jury. On peut imaginer un comité d'éthique formé uniquement de représentants de la société civile et religieuse, faisant appel aux avis parfois contradictoires d'experts médicaux. Les chercheurs proposent, la société dispose. . . . En bref, il faut une éthique pour l'éthique." Dumaz, Y, "Bioéthique: Entre la dérive et le progrès," *Le Monde*, 26 November 1993.

72. "Deux principes majeurs en émergent: Tout d'abord, la science n'est pas au-dessus de la loi. Je me place ici sur le plan philosophique, et non sur le plan juridique. La volonté de mettre la science littéralement hors la loi a été exprimée par certains scientifiques, d'abord en s'opposant à l'idée même d'une loi bioéthique, puis, cette première bataille perdue, en voulant faire inscrire dans le préambule de la loi le principe de la protection du développement de la science au même titre et au même rang que le principe du respect de la personne. Cette prétention a été exprimée en particulier par M. Jean-Pierre Changeux, ce qui laisse perplexe de la part du nouveau président du Comité national d'éthique.

. . .

L'homme y est conçu comme un être moral dont le libre jugement doit séparer le bien du mal, en particulier face aux nouveaux horizons scientifiques qui s'ouvrent devant lui. La science, désormais encadrée par la loi, retrograde à la seconde place, derrière le primat moral. C'est l'homme qui produit la science et en choisit les seuls fruits positifs; ce n'est pas la science qui produit l'homme." Stasse, F-X, "Santé, éthique, et argent," *Le Monde*, 5 February 1993.

73. Nouchi, F., "Succédant au professeur Jean Bernard: Le professeur Jean-Pierre Changeux va présider le Comité national d'éthique," *Le Monde*, 3 June 1992.

74. "Tout scientifique qui refuse de succomber [au clivage mental confortable] du croyant, qui souhaite rester cohérent avec lui-même [et s'efforce de rejeter toute référence à la métaphysique], devra tenter, dans sa réflexion, de rechercher les bases naturelles de l'éthique. Ce n'est, somme toute, que réactualiser la démarche des Lumières et de la Révolution française, avec le bénéfice considérable que peuvent nous procurer les résultats récents des neurosciences, des sciences cognitives et de l'anthropologie sociale." [En résumé:] "La science a pour vocation première de pourchasser, en permanence, l'irrationnel pour atteindre la connaissance objective." Nouchi, F., "Succédant au professeur Jean Bernard: Le professeur Jean-Pierre Changeux va présider le Comité national d'éthique," *Le Monde*, 3 June 1992

APPENDIX

Past Commissions and
Advisory Boards

This Appendix is an expansion of the background information on some of the past commissions and advisory boards that have served to consider social, ethical, or legal issues related to advances in biomedicine. These are the:

- Ethics Advisory Board of the Department of Health, Education, and Welfare (DHEW);
- National Commission for the Protection of Human Subjects of Biomedical and Behavioral Research (National Commission);
- President's Commission for the Study of Ethical Problems in Medicine and Biomedical and Behavioral Research (President's Commission);
- NIH Recombinant DNA Advisory Committee;
- Working Group on Ethical, Legal, and Social Implications of the Human Genome Project (ELSI Working Group);
- Biomedical Ethics Advisory Committee;
- New York State Task Force on Life and the Law; and
- New Jersey Bioethics Commission.

ETHICS ADVISORY BOARD OF THE DEPARTMENT OF HEALTH, EDUCATION, AND WELFARE (DHEW)

Dates of operation: 1978–1980

Sponsorship/appointing authority: DHEW Secretary

Function: to consult on all DHEW programs and policies, review of waiver submissions for proposals of fetal research potentially exceeding existing standards of risk, and advise the DHEW Secretary regarding such projects' approval or disapproval

Scope: DHEW only

Membership characteristics: rotating; included attorneys, theologians, and physicians

Members:

Chairman
James C. Gaither, J.D.
Cooley, Godward, Castro, Huddleson
　and Tatum
San Francisco, California

Vice Chairman
David A. Hamburg, M.D.
President, Carnegie Corporation of
　New York
Member, Institute of Medicine

Members
Sissela Bok, Ph.D.
Lecturer in Medical Ethics
Harvard University

Jack T. Conway
Senior Vice President
United Way of America
Washington, D.C.

Henry W. Foster, M.D.
Professor and Chairman
Department of Obstetrics and
　Gynecology
Meharry Medical College

Donald A. Henderson, M.D.
Dean, School of Hygiene and Public
　Health
Johns Hopkins University

Maurice Lazarus
Chairman, Finance Committee
Federated Department Stores, Inc.
Boston, Massachusetts

Richard A. McCormick, S.T.D.
Professor of Christian Ethics
Kennedy Institute for the Study of
　Reproduction and Bioethics
Georgetown University
Washington, D.C.

Robert F. Murray, M.D.
Chief, Division of Medical Genetics
College of Medicine
Howard University

Mitchell W. Spellman, M.D.
Dean for Medical Services and
　Professor of Surgery
Harvard Medical School

Daniel C. Tosteson, M.D.
Dean, Harvard Medical School

Agnes N. Williams, LL.B.
Potomac, Maryland

Eugene M. Zwieback, M.D.
Surgeon in Private Practice
Omaha, Nebraska

Report:
Report and Conclusions: Support of Research Involving Human In Vitro Fertilization and Embryo Transfer, 1979

THE NATIONAL COMMISSION FOR THE PROTECTION OF HUMAN SUBJECTS OF BIOMEDICAL AND BEHAVIORAL RESEARCH (NATIONAL COMMISSION)

Dates of operation: 1974–1978

Sponsorship/appointing authority: U.S. Congress (under National Research Act of 1974, P.L. 93-348); appointments made by the Secretary of the Department of Health, Education, and Welfare (DHEW)

Function: to identify basic ethical principles that should underlie the conduct of biomedical and behavioral research involving human subjects, develop guidelines that should be followed in such research to assure that it is conducted in accordance with such principles, and make recommendations to the DHEW Secretary regarding the development of regulations

Scope: limited to research conducted or funded by the DHEW, study topics were congressionally mandated

Membership characteristics: 5 scientists, 3 lawyers, 2 ethicists, and 1 social worker

Members:

Chairperson
Kenneth J. Ryan, M.D.
Chief of Staff
Boston Hospital for Women

Members
Joseph V. Brady, Ph.D.
Professor of Behavioral Biology
Johns Hopkins University

Robert E. Cooke, M.D.
President
Medical College of Pennsylvania

Dorothy I. Height
President
National Council of Negro Women,
  Inc.

Albert R. Jonsen, Ph.D.
Associate Professor of Bioethics
University of California, San Francisco

Patricia King, J.D.
Associate Professor of Law
Georgetown University Law Center

Karen Lebacqz, Ph.D.
Associate Professor of Christian Ethics
Pacific School of Religion

David W. Louisell, J.D.
Professor of Law
University of California, Berkeley

Donald W. Seldin, M.D.
Professor and Chairman
Department of Internal Medicine
University of Texas at Dallas

Eliot Stellar, Ph.D.
Provost of the University
Professor of Physiological Psychology
University of Pennsylvania

Robert H. Turtle, LL.B.
Attorney
VomBaur, Coburn, Simmons & Turtle
Washington, D.C.

Reports:

Report and Recommendations: Research on the Fetus, 1975
Appendix to Report and Recommendations: Research on the Fetus, 1975
Proceedings of the March 14–15, 1975 Meeting
*The Belmont Report: Ethical Principles and Guidelines for the Protection of
  Human Subjects of Research,* 1978
*Appendix (Volumes I and II) to The Belmont Report: Ethical Principles and
  Guidelines for the Protection of Human Subjects of Research,* 1978
Report and Recommendations: Research Involving Prisoners, 1976
Appendix to Report and Recommendations: Research Involving Prisoners, 1976
Report and Recommendations: Research Involving Children, 1977
Appendix to Report and Recommendations: Research Involving Children, 1977
Report and Recommendations: Psychosurgery, 1977
Appendix to Report and Recommendations: Psychosurgery, 1977
Disclosure of Research Information Under the Freedom of Information Act, 1977
*Report and Recommendations: Special Study: Implications of Advances in
  Biomedical and Behavioral Research, 1978*
*Report and Recommendations: Research Involving Those Institutionalized as
  Mentally Infirm,* 1978
*Appendix to Report and Recommendations: Research Involving Those
  Institutionalized as Mentally Infirm,* 1978
Report and Recommendations: Institutional Review Boards, 1978
Appendix to Report and Recommendations: Institutional Review Boards, 1978
*Report and Recommendations: Ethical Guidelines for Delivery of Health Services
  by DHEW,* 1978
*Appendix to Report and Recommendations: Ethical Guidelines for Delivery of
  Health Services by DHEW,* 1978

PRESIDENT'S COMMISSION FOR THE STUDY OF ETHICAL PROBLEMS IN MEDICINE AND BIOMEDICAL AND BEHAVIORAL RESEARCH (PRESIDENT'S COMMISSION)

Dates of Operation: January 1980–March 1983

Sponsorship/appointing authority: U.S. Congress (under: Biomedical Research and Training Amendments of 1978, P.L. 95-622); appointments made by the President

Function: to advise the President and Congress on bioethical issues

Scope: report topics mandated by Congress, but commission also had authority to undertake studies upon its own initiative

Membership characteristics: rotating; as specified by law, there were 11 active commissioners at a time, 3 of whom were active in the practice of medicine, 3 biomedical or behavioral researchers, and 5 members from other fields

Members:

Chairman
Morris B. Abram, J.D., L.L.D.
New York, New York
(July 1979–March 1983)

Members
H. Thomas Ballantine, Jr., M.D., M.S., D.Sc.
Harvard Medical School
(Aug. 1982–March 1983)

George R. Dunlop, M.D.
University of Massachusetts
(Feb. 1982–March 1983)

Renee C. Fox, Ph.D., D.H.L.
University of Pennsylvania
(July 1979–Feb. 1982)

Mario Garcia-Palmieri, M.D.
University of Puerto Rico
(July 1979–Aug. 1982)

Franes K. Graham, Ph.D.
University of Wisconsin
(May 1980–Jan. 1982)

Bruce Kelton Jacobson, M.D.
Southwestern Medical School
Fort Worth, Texas
(Aug. 1982–March 1983)

Albert R. Jonsen, S.T.M., Ph.D.
University of California, San Francisco
(July 1979–Aug. 1982)

Patricia A. King, J.D.
Georgetown University
(July 1979–May 1980)

Mathilde Krim, Ph.D.
Sloan-Kettering Institute for Cancer Research
(July 1979–Oct. 1981)

Donald N. Medearis, M.D.
Harvard University
(July 1979–Feb. 1982)

John J. Moran, B.S.
Houston, Texas
(Aug. 1982–March 1983)

Arno G. Motulsky, M.D.
University of Washington
(July 1979–March 1983)

Daher B. Rahi, D.O.
St. Clair Shores, Michigan
(Feb. 1982–March 1983)

Fritz C. Redlich, M.D.
University of California, Los Angeles
(July 1979–Feb. 1980)

Anne A. Scitovsky, M.A.
Palo Alto Medical Research
  Foundation
(July 1979–Aug. 1982)

Seymour Siegel, D.H.L.
Jewish Theological Seminary
New York, New York
(Feb. 1982–March 1983)

Lynda Hare Smith, B.S.
Colorado Springs, Colorado
(March 1982–March 1983)

Kay Toma, M.D.
Bell, California
(Aug. 1982–March 1983)

Charles J. Walker, M.D.
Nashville, Tennessee
(July 1979–March 1983)

Carolyn A. Williams, Ph.D.
University of North Carolina, Chapel
  Hill
(Sept. 1980–Aug. 1982)

Executive Director
Alexander Morgan Capron, LL.B.
(Dec. 1979–March 1983)

Deputy Director
Barbara Mishkin, M.A., J.D.
(Jan. 1980–Jan. 1983)

Assistant Directors
MEDICINE
Joanne Lynn, M.D., M.A.
(Jan. 1981–March 1983)

LAW
Alan Meisel, J.D.
(Aug, 1982–Dec. 1982)

Alan J. Weisbard, J.D.
(Jan. 1980–Aug. 1982)

Professional Staff
ECONOMICS
Mary Ann Baily, Ph.D.
(March 1980–Feb. 1983)

ETHICS
Dan Brock, Ph.D.
(July 1981–July 1982)

Allen Buchanan, Ph.D.
(Jan. 1982–Dec. 1982)

HEALTH POLICY
Kathryn Kelly, M.S., M.S.W.
(Oct. 1981–Dec. 1982)

Susan Morgan
(Feb. 1981–Feb. 1983)

SOCIOLOGY
Marian Osterweiss, Ph.D.
(Jan. 1981–Jan. 1983)

PUBLIC HEALTH
Renie Schapiro, M.P.H.
(March 1980–Feb. 1983)

ETHICS
Daniel Wikler, Ph.D.
(Sept. 1980–Aug. 1981)

Continuing Consultants
SOCIOLOGY
Bradford E. Gray, Ph.D.
(Aug. 1981–Dec. 1982)

ETHICS
Dorothy E. Vawter
(March 1980–Feb. 1983)

Reports:

Defining Death: A Report on the Medical, Legal, and Ethical Issues in the Determination of Death, 1981

Protecting Human Subjects: The Adequacy and Uniformity of Federal Rules and their Implementation, 1981

Whistleblowing in Biomedical Research: Policies and Procedures for Responding to Reports of Misconduct, 1981

Making Health Care Decisions: A Report on the Ethical and Legal Implications of Informed Consent in the Patient–Practitioner Relationship. Volume 1: Report, 1982

Making Health Care Decisions: A Report on the Ethical and Legal Implications of Informed Consent in the Patient–Practitioner Relationship. Volume 2: Appendices, Empirical Studies of Informed Consent, 1982

Making Health Care Decisions: A Report on the Ethical and Legal Implications of Informed Consent in the Patient–Practitioner Relationship. Volume 3: Appendices, Studies of the Foundations of Informed Consent, 1982

Splicing Life: A Report on the Social and Ethical Issues of Genetic Engineering with Human Beings, 1982

Compensating for Research Injuries: The Ethical and Legal Implications for Programs to Redress Injured Subjects, 1982

Deciding to Forego Life-Sustaining Treatment: A Report on the Ethical, Medical, and Legal Issues in Treatment Decisions, 1983

Implementing Human Research Regulations: Second Biennial Report of the Adequacy and Uniformity of Federal Rules and Policies, and of their Implementation, for the Protection of Human Subjects, 1983

Screening and Counseling for Genetic Conditions: The Ethical, Social, and Legal Implications of Genetic Screening, Counseling, and Education Programs, 1983

Securing Access to Health Care: The Ethical Implications of Differences in the Availability of Health Services. Volume 1: Report, 1983

Securing Access to Health Care: The Ethical Implications of Differences in the Availability of Health Services. Volume 2: Appendices, Sociocultural and Philosophical Studies, 1983

Securing Access to Health Care: The Ethical Implications of Differences in the Availability of Health Services. Volume 3: Appendices, Empirical, Legal, and Conceptual Studies, 1983

Summing Up: Final Report on Studies of the Ethical and Legal Problems in Medicine and Biomedical and Behavioral Research, 1983

NIH RECOMBINANT DNA ADVISORY PANEL

Dates of operation: authorized in February 1975, ongoing

Sponsorship/appointing authority: Department of Health, Education, and Welfare, National Institutes of Health, Office of Recombinant DNA Activities

Function: to provide guidance to the NIH on issues in the field of recombinant DNA research, review protocols for federally funded recombinant DNA research, and develop guidelines for the conduct of this research

Scope: research conducted or supported by the NIH

Membership characteristics: size has ranged from 15 to 40 members; today RDAC has 24 members, including lawyers, ethicists, political scientists, researchers, and clinicians

Members:

Chairman
LeRoy B. Walters, Ph.D.
Kennedy Institute of Ethics
Georgetown University
Washington, D.C.

Members
Constance E. Brinckerhoff, Ph.D.
Dartmouth Medical School
Hanover, New Hampshire

Nancy L. Buc, L.L.B.
Well, Gotshal, and Manges
Washington, D.C.

Alexander M. Capron, L.L.B.
The Law Center
University of Southern California
Los Angeles, California

Ira H. Carmen, Ph.D.
University of Illinois
Urbana, Illinois

Gary A. Chase, Ph.D.
The Johns Hopkins University
Baltimore, Maryland

Patricia A. DeLon, Ph.D.
University of Delaware
Newark, Delaware

Roy H. Doi, Ph.D.
University of California
Davis, California

Krishna R. Dronamraju, Ph.D.
Foundation for Genetic Research
Houston, Texas

E. Peter Geiduschek, Ph.D.
University of California, San Diego
La Jolla, California

Mariann Grossman
Institute of Human Gene Therapy
Philadelphia, Pennsylvania

Robert Haselkorn, Ph.D.
University of Chicago
Chicago, Illinois

Susan S. Hirano, Ph.D.
University of Wisconsin
Madison, Wisconsin

Donald J. Krogstad, M.D.
Tulane University School of Medicine
New Orleans, Louisiana

Abbey S. Meyers
National Organization for Rare
   Disorders
New Fairfield, Connecticut

Dusty A. Miller, Ph.D.
Fred Hutchinson Cancer Research
  Center
Seattle, Washington

Arno G. Motulsky, M.D.
University of Washington Medical
  School
Seattle, Washington

Robertson Parkman, M.D.
Childrens Hospital of Los Angeles
Los Angeles, California

Leonard E. Post, Ph.D.
Parke-Davis Pharmaceutical Division
Ann Arbor, Michigan

Marian G. Secundy, Ph.D.
Howard University College of
  Medicine
Washington, D.C.

Brian R. Smith, M.D.
Yale University School of Medicine
New Haven, Connecticut

Stephen E. Straus, M.D.
National Institutes of Health
Bethesda, Maryland

Doris T. Zallen, Ph.D.
Virginia Polytechnic Institute and State
  University
Blacksburg, Virginia

Executive Secretary
Nelson A.Wivel, M.D.
Office of Recombinant DNA Activities
National Institutes of Health
Bethesda, Maryland

Reports:

Points to Consider in the Design and Submission of Human Somatic-Cell Gene Therapy Protocols, 1985 (Human Gene Therapy Subcommittee)

WORKING GROUP ON ETHICAL, LEGAL, AND SOCIAL IMPLICATIONS OF THE HUMAN GENOME PROJECT (ELSI WORKING GROUP)

Dates of operation: 1988, ongoing

Sponsorship/appointing authority: NIH Center for Human Genome Research and the Department of Energy

Function: to stimulate research on issues through grantmaking; to refine the research agenda through workshops, commissioned papers, and invited lectures; to solicit public input through town meetings and public testimony; to support the development of educational materials; to encourage international collaboration in this area. In terms of policy-making, the goals of the ELSI Working Group are to clarify the ethical, legal, and social consequences of mapping and sequencing the human genome through a program of targeted research; to develop policy options at professional, institutional, governmental, and societal levels to ensure that genetic information is used to maximize the benefit to individuals and society; to improve understanding of the issues and policy options through educational initiatives at public, professional, and policy-making levels; and, to stimulate public discussion of the issues and policy options.

Scope: all social, legal, and ethical issues relating to the Human Genome Project

Membership characteristics: with the exception of the chairperson, members are ad hoc technical consultants representing basic and clinical genetics, law, and ethics

Members:

Chairperson
Nancy Wexler, Ph.D.
Hereditary Disease Foundation, and
Department of Neurology and
  Psychiatry
College of Physicians and Surgeons
Columbia University
New York

Members
Jonathan Beckwith, Ph.D.
Department of Microbiology and
  Molecular Genetics
Harvard Medical School
Boston, Massachusetts

Robert Cook-Deegan, M.D.
Institute of Medicine
National Academy of Sciences
Washington, D.C.

Patricia King, J.D.
Professor of Law
Georgetown University Law Center
Washington, D.C.

Victor McKusick, M.D.
Division of Medical Genetics
Johns Hopkins Hospital
Baltimore, Maryland

Robert F. Murray, Jr., M.D.
Department of Pediatrics
Howard University College of Medicine
Washington, D C.

Thomas H. Murray, Ph.D.
Center for Biomedical Ethics
School of Medicine
Case Western Reserve University
Cleveland, Ohio

Reports:
Workshop on the Introduction of New Genetic Tests, 1990
Genetic Discrimination and the Americans with Disabilities Act, 1991

THE BIOMEDICAL ETHICS ADVISORY COMMITTEE (BEAC)

Dates of operation: September 1988–September 1989

Sponsorship/appointing authority: Congressional Biomedical Ethics Board (BEB); (under Health Research Extension Act, May 1985)

Function: to study and report to Congress on a continuing basis on ethical issues arising from health care delivery and biomedical and behavioral research

Scope: mandated by BEB; first three reports mandated were on (1) implications of human genetic engineering, (2) fetal research, and (3) nutrition and hydration in dying patients

Membership characteristics: 14 members appointed from the fields of law, ethics, biomedical research, and clinical care, including two lay members; appointment process took almost two and a half years

Members:

Julianne Beckett
Associate Director for Consumer
    Affairs
National Maternal and Child Health
    Resource Center
University of Iowa

James Bopp, Jr. Esq.
Brames, McCormick, Bopp & Abel
Terre Haute, Indiana

Watson Allen Bowes, Jr., M.D.
Professor, Department of Obstetrics
    and Gynecology
University of North Carolina
    School of Medicine

Alexander Morgan Capron
University Professor of Law, Medicine
    and Public Policy
The Law Center
University of Southern California

Christine K. Cassel, M.D., F.A.C.P.
Chief, Section of Internal Medicine
Pritzker School of Medicine
University of Chicago

James Franklin Childress, Ph.D.
Professor, Department of Religious
    Studies
University of Virginia

Theodore Friedmann. M.D.
Center for Genetics
Department of Pediatrics
University of California School of
    Medicine
San Diego

Ms. Sylvia Drew Ivie
Executive Director
T.H.E. Clinic for Women, Inc.
Los Angeles, California

Reverend Donald G. McCarthy, Ph.D.
Church of Saint Antoninus
Cincinnati, Ohio

Edmund D. Pellegrino, M.D.
Director, Kennedy Institute of Ethics
Georgetown University
Washington, D.C.

Kenneth N. Rosenbaum, M.D.
Childrens' Hospital National Medical
    Center
Washington, D.C.

Kenneth John Ryan, M.D.
Brigham and Women's Hospital
Boston, Massachusetts

Stanley Burton Troup, M.D.
Professor of Medicine, Health Care,
   and Human Values
Department of Internal Medicine
University of Cincinnati College of
   Medicine

Members of Congressional Bioethics Board
SENATE MEMBERS
Albert Gore (D-TN), Vice Chair
Dale Bumpers (D-AK)
David Durenberger (R-MN)
Gordon Humphrey (R-NH)
Edward Kennedy (D-MA)
Lowell Weiker (R-CT)*

HOUSE MEMBERS
Willis Gradison (R-OH), Chair
Thomas Bliley (R-VA)
Thomas Luken (D-OH)
J. Roy Rowland (D-GA)
Thomas Tauke (R-IA)
Henry Waxman (D-CA)

---

* Replaced in 1988 by Don Nickles (R-OK)

NEW YORK STATE TASK FORCE ON LIFE AND THE LAW

Dates of operation: March, 1985 to present

Sponsorship/appointing authority: New York Governor Mario Cuomo

Function: to develop recommendations for New York State public policy (in the form of proposed legislation, regulation, public education, and other measures) on a wide range of issues arising from recent advances in medical technology; reports seek to inform and focus public debate

Scope: such issues as the determination of death, the withdrawal and withholding of life-sustaining treatment, new reproductive technologies (artificial insemination and in vitro fertilization), surrogate parenting, the treatment of disabled newborns, organ transplantation, and, in a more limited context, abortion

Membership characteristics: 25 members; includes prominent physicians, nurses, lawyers, academics, and representatives of numerous religious communities

Members:

Karl Adler, M.D.
Dean, New York Medical College

Rev. Msgr. John A. Alesandro
Chancellor, Roman Catholic Diocese
   of Rockville Centre

John Arras, Ph.D.
Clinical Associate Professor of
   Bioethics
Albert Einstein College of Medicine
Montefiore Medical Center

Mario L. Baeza, Esq.
Debevoise & Plimpton

The Right Rev. David Ball
Bishop, Episcopal Diocese of Albany

Rabbi J. David Bleich
Professor of Talmud, Yeshiva
   University
Professor of Jewish Law and Ethics
Benjamin Cardozo School of Law

Evan Calkins, M.D.
Professor of Medicine, Emeritus
SUNY Buffalo

Richard J. Concannon, Esq.
Kelley, Drye & Warren

Myron W. Concvitz, M.D.
Attending Physician, North Shore
   University Hospital
Clinical Associate Professor of
   Medicine
Cornell University Medical College

Saul J. Farber, M.D.
Dean and Provost
Chairman, Department of Medicine
New York University School of
   Medicine

Alan R. Fleishman, M.D.
Director, Division of Neonatology
Albert Einstein College of Medicine
Montefiore Medical Center

Samuel Gorovitz, Ph.D.
Dean, College of Arts and Sciences
Professor of Philosophy
Syracuse University

Jane Greenlaw, J.D., R.N.
Director, Division of Medical
 Humanities
University of Rochester School of
 Medicine and Dentistry

Beatrix A. Hamburg, M.D.
Chairman, Division of Child and
 Adolescent Psychiatry
Mount Sinai School of Medicine

Denise Hanlon, R.N., M.S.
Clinical Specialist
Rehabilitation and Gerontology
SUNY Buffalo, School of Nursing

Rev. Donald W. McKinney
First Unitarian Church of Brooklyn
Chairman Emeritus, Choice in Dying

Maria I. New, M.D.
Chief, Department of Pediatrics
New York Hospital
Cornell Medical Center

John J. Regan, J.S.D.
Professor of Law
Hofstra University School of Law

Rabbi A. James Rudin
National Director of Interreligious
 Affairs
The American Jewish Committee

Rev. Betty Bone Schiess
Episcopal Diocese of Central New York

Barbara Shack
The New York Civil Liberties Union

Rev. Robert S. Smith
Director, Institute for Medicine in
 Contemporary Society
SUNY Health Science Center at Stony
 Brook

Elizabeth W. Stack
Commissioner, New York State
 Commission on Quality of Care for
 the Mentally Retarded

Reports:

The Required Request Law, March 1986
Do Not Resuscitate Orders, April 1986
The Determination of Death, July 1986
*Life-Sustaining Treatments: Making Decisions and Appointing a Health Care
 Agent,* July 1987
*Transplantation in New York State: The Procurement and Distribution of Organs
 and Tissues,* January 1988
Fetal Extrauterine Survivability, January 1988
Surrogate Parenting: Analysis and Recommendations for Public Policy, May 1988
When Others Must Choose: Deciding for Patients Without Capacity, March 1992

NEW JERSEY COMMISSION ON LEGAL AND ETHICAL PROBLEMS IN THE DELIVERY OF HEALTH CARE

Dates of operation: 1985 to 1991

Sponsorship/appointing authority: Governor of New Jersey, New Jersey Senate President, and Speaker of the General Assembly

Function: to provide a comprehensive and scholarly examination of the impact of advancing technology on health care decisions and to recommend policies to the governor, legislature, and citizens of New Jersey

Scope: focused on three areas: surrogate motherhood, decision making about medical treatment (especially advance directives), and determination of death

Membership characteristics: 26 members, including 4 legislators, 9 representatives of executive agencies and major statewide professional and health care organizations, as well as representatives from the fields of law, medicine, nursing, science, humanities, theology, and health care administration

Members:

Chairman
Paul W. Armstrong, M.A., J.D., LL.M.
Councellor at Law

Members
Sr. Jane Frances Brady
President, St. Joseph's Medical Center

Thomas P. Brown, M.A.
Acting Ombudsman for the
   Institutionalized Elderly

The Hon. Gerald Cardinale, D.D.S.
Senator—District 39

Diana Czarepuszko, R.N., L.N.H.A.
Executive Director, Cheshire Home

Robert W. Deaton
Director of Long Term Care
Diocese of Camden

Joseph Fennelly, M.D.
Vice Chairman, Bioethics Committee
Medical Society of New Jersey

J. Richard Goldstein, M.D.
President, Stopwatch, Inc.

Noreen Haveron, R.N., B.S.N.
Assistant Nursing Supervisor
Nutley Nursing Service

Lois Hull
Director, Division of Aging

The Hon. C. Richard Kamin
Assemblyman—District 23

Rabbi Charles A. Kroloff
Rabbi, Temple Emanu-El

The Hon. David C. Kronick
Assemblyman—District 32

Paul Langevin, M.A.
Assistant Commissioner for Health
   Facilities Evaluation

Mary K. Lindner, R.N., M.A.
Senior Vice President, Patient Services
   and Executive Director of Nursing
Overlook Hospital

Rita Martin
Legislative Director
N.J. Citizens Concerned for Life

Russell L. Mcintyre, Ph.D.
Associate Professor (Medical Ethics)
University of Medicine and Dentistry of
    New Jersey
Robert Wood Johnson Medical School

Patricia Ann Murphy, R.N., Ph.D.
Clinical Specialist (Bereavement)
Newark Beth Israel Medical Center

Michael Nevina, M.D.
Internist, Chairman, Bioethics
    Committee
Pascack Valley Hospital

Sally Nunn, R.N.
Chair, Bioethics Committee
Shore Memorial Hospital

Robert L. Pickens, M.D.
Chairman, Bioethics Committee
Medical Society of New Jersey

David Rogoff, M.S.
Director, Haven Hospice
John F. Kennedy Medical Center

RitaMarie G. Rondum
Member, State Legislative Committee
American Association of Retired
    Persons

Mary S. Strong
Chair, Citizens' Committee on
    Biomedical Ethics

Joseph F. Suozzo, Esq.
Assistant Director of Litigation

Edward Tetalman, Esq.
Assistant Commissioner for
    Intergovernmental Affairs

Robert S. Olick, M.A., J.D., Executive
    Director
Michael Vollen, M.A., Associate
    Director
Adrienne Asch, M.D., Ph.D., Associate
    in Social Science and Policy
Anne Reichman Schiff, LL.M.,
    Associate in Law
Ellen B. Friedland, Esq. Consultant
Sally Sulphen, B.A., Admnistrative
    Assistant

Reports:

*Problems and Approaches in Health Care Decision Making: The New Jersey
    Experience,* 1990
*Advance Directives for Health Care: Planning Ahead for Important Health Care
    Decisions,* 1991
*The New Jersey Advance Directives for Health Care and Death Acts: Statutes,
    Commentaries, and Analyses,* 1991
After Baby M: The Legal, Ethical, and Social Dimensions of Surrogacy, 1992
Death and the Brain-Damaged Patient, 1992
*The New Jersey Advance Directives for Health Care Act (and the Patient Self-
    Determination Act): A Guidebook for Health Care Professionals,* 1992

Index

Spring, In re, 314, 316
State governments
    abortion regulation, 106, 342
    bioethics advisory bodies, 6, 99-100
    bioethics commissions, 99-100
    constitutional authority, 346
    death and dying legislation, 105,
        313-316
    executive branch in policymaking,
        351-353
    fetal tissue research regulation, 480-
        481
    genetic testing regulation, 175
    in health care policymaking, 335-336
    national commission findings and,
        103, 185
    political process, 45
    President's Commission influence,
        272, 286
    recommendations for, 18-19, 176-
        177, 183-185
    See also specific states
Sterilization, 118
Stevenson-Wydler Act, 59
Storar, In re, 314, 316, 317
*Superintendent of Belchertown Hospital v.
    Saikewicz*, 314, 315-316
Supra-agency ethics commission
    action-forcing powers, 21-22, 191
    advantages of, 20, 187
    advisory role, 21-22, 190-191
    appointment process, 21, 189-190
    dissemination of findings, 190-191
    duration, 20, 22, 192
    educational role, 21
    external advisory committee for,
        23
    funding and staff, 22, 191
    government sponsorship, 189
    interim operations, 23, 192-193
    mandate, 20-21, 186-188
    membership structure, 21, 22, 189
    models for, 15
    in multitiered system, 15-16, 174-
        175
    public participation, 190
    recommendations for, 19-23, 186-
        193
    resources for, 22

Surrogate decision making
    in absence of patient guidance, 326-
        327
    best interest standard, 315, 324,
        326, 327
    documentation for, 329
    health care agent for, 325-326
    in home care, 329
    for incompetent patients, 313, 318-
        319
    legal environment, 342
    legal instruments in, 326
    New York State Task Force, 99,
        324
    parents in, 315
    state statutes, 313, 314, 316
    substituted judgment standard, 309,
        315, 316, 324, 326, 327
Surrogate parenting, 99, 100, 106, 118,
    162, 342
    practitioner guidelines, 120
Swine flu vaccine, 306 n.8

T

Tay-Sachs disease, 140-141
Technology transfer
    genetic science, 40-41
    legislation, 59
    university-industry collaborations
        and, 61
Teel, Karen, 409-410
Terminally ill patients, 94, 99, 119, 266
    artificial nutrition and hydration
        guidelines, 121-122, 309, 314
    do not resuscitate orders, 163-164,
        323-325, 328-330
    legal guidelines for treatment
        decisions, 342-343
    as research subjects, 124, 469-470
    See also Life-sustaining procedures/
        technologies
Testart, Jacques, 490
Texas, 313, 314
Theological thought
    basic questions in, 385 n.3
    in bioethics, 73-74, 134, 383-385
    concept of human loyalties in, 377-
        379